Medicinal Chemistry of Neglected and Tropical Diseases

Advances in the Design and Synthesis of Antimicrobial Agents

T0186234

Editors

Venkatesan Jayaprakash
Associate Professor
Department of Pharmaceutical Sciences & Technology
Birla Institute of Technology, Mesra
Ranchi, India

Daniele Castagnolo
Institute of Pharmaceutical Science
King's College London
London, UK

Yusuf Özkay
Faculty of Pharmacy
Department of Pharmaceutical Chemistry
Anadolu University
Eskisehir, Turkey

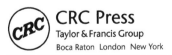

CRC Press
Taylor & Francis Group
Boca Raton London New York

CRC Press is an imprint of the
Taylor & Francis Group, an **informa** business

A SCIENCE PUBLISHERS BOOK

Cover credit
- Top right figure: Figure 6a from Chapter 4 – Reproduced by permission of the authors, Drs. J. Jonathan Harburn and G. Stuart Cockerill.
- Middle left figure: Figure 1 of Chapter 14 – Curcuma Plant photograph taken from article 'On the identity of turmeric: the typification of Curcuma longa L. (Zingiberaceae)' published in Botanical Journal of the Linnean Society, Wiley, 2008.
- Middle right figure: Figure 4c from Chapter 11. Reproduced by permission of the authors, Drs. Andrea Ilari and Gianni Colotti.
- Bottom right figure: Figure 1 from Chapter 6. Reproduced by permission of the authors, Drs. D. Velmurugan, K. Manish and D. Gayathri.
- Bottom left figure: Figure created by Dr. Daniele Castagnolo.

CRC Press
Taylor & Francis Group
6000 Broken Sound Parkway NW, Suite 300
Boca Raton, FL 33487-2742

First issued in paperback 2021

© 2019 by Taylor & Francis Group, LLC
CRC Press is an imprint of Taylor & Francis Group, an Informa business

No claim to original U.S. Government works

Version Date: 20190516

ISBN 13: 978-0-367-77925-2 (pbk)
ISBN 13: 978-1-138-54124-5 (hbk)

Library of Congress Cataloging-in-Publication Data
Names: Jayaprakash, Venkatesan, editor.
Title: Medicinal chemistry of neglected and tropical diseases : advances in the design and synthesis of antimicrobial agents / editors, Venkatesan Jayaprakash, Associate Professor, Department of Pharmaceutical Sciences & Technology, Birla Institute of Technology, Mesra, Ranchi, India, Daniele Castagnolo, Institute of Pharmaceutical Science, King's College London, London, UK, Yusuf èOzkay, Faculty of Pharmacy, Department of Pharmaceutical Chemistry, Anadolu University, Eskisehir, Turkey.
Description: Boca Raton, FL : CRC Press, Taylor & Francis Group, [2018]	Includes bibliographical references and index.
Identifiers: LCCN 2019013026	ISBN 9781138541245 (hardback)
Subjects: LCSH: Tropical medicine.	Drug development.
Classification: LCC RC961 .M467 2018	DDC 616.9/883--dc23
LC record available at https://lccn.loc.gov/2019013026

Visit the Taylor & Francis Web site at
http://www.taylorandfrancis.com

and the CRC Press Web site at
http://www.crcpress.com

Preface

The book "Medicinal Chemistry of Neglected and Tropical Diseases: Advances in the Design and Synthesis of Antimicrobial Agents" comes as an attempt to consolidate the modern drug discovery approaches employed to date to develop effective chemotherapeutic agents for the treatment of Neglected Tropical Diseases (NTDs). According to the definition of WHO, NTDs are "*a diverse group of communicable diseases that prevail in tropical and subtropical conditions in 149 countries, affect more than one billion people and cost developing economies billions of dollars every year.*" NTDs are caused by a variety of pathogens including viruses, bacteria, protozoa and helminths and are mainly common in low-income populations in developing regions of Africa, Asia, and the Americas. Currently, twenty diseases such as dengue and chikungunya infections, African and American trypanosomiasis (Sleeping sickness and Chagas disease), leishmaniasis as well as several worm infestations are listed in the WHO portfolio. Other diseases, widely spread in tropical regions, such as tuberculosis and malaria have been removed from the WHO NTDs list due to the greater treatment and research funding that they received in the last decades. However, despite the increasing investments, tuberculosis and malaria still affect millions of people worldwide and, due to the emergence of drug-resistance strains, the eradication of these diseases is still far from succeeding. Today, the majority of neglected tropical diseases are widely spread in the poorest regions of the world, where substandard housing, lack of access to safe water and sanitation, chronic hunger, filthy environments, and abundant insects and other vectors contribute to their efficient transmission. Diseases like dengue or chikungunya, and more recently zika, have been confined mainly in tropical regions since they are transmitted by mosquitoes living at these latitudes. However, due to climate changes, an increasing number of mosquitoes are adapting to live in subtropical regions, thus contributing to spread of viral infections outside their usual areas, as demonstrated by the presence of cases of chikungunya infections in southern Europe (France and Italy) in 2017–2018. Other neglected diseases, such as worm infestations (helminthiasis), are widely spread in almost any part of the world, regardless of the latitude, and currently affect more than 1 billion of people. However, despite the high number of cases, only a few drugs are available in the market to efficiently treat helminthiasis, making this a class of truly neglected diseases.

The aim of this book is to highlight the progresses made to date in the field of drug design, discovery and development of novel treatments active against neglected diseases such as vector borne viral infections, trypanosomiasis, worm infections as well as those tropical diseases such as tuberculosis and malaria which, even if they are no longer considered neglected by funding investment and research, still represent a major health threat worldwide.

The first three chapters of the book describe some general approaches currently used in the identification and design of novel drugs active against neglected and tropical diseases, such as fragment-based drug design and molecular hybridization of established lead molecules.

Chapters 4, 5 and 6 are focused on three vector borne viral diseases, namely dengue, zika and chikungunya. Although no drugs are currently available in the market to treat these diseases, a few promising lead candidates, described in these chapters, are currently under development. In addition, the development of effective vaccine strategies as well as approaches aimed at preventing and controlling the spread of these diseases are reported.

The Chapters 7, 8 and 9 will be focused on the two main non-neglected tropical diseases, tuberculosis and malaria. The most recent repositioning strategies for the treatment of tuberculosis by using non-antibiotic drugs are reviewed in Chapter 7 while Chapter 8 describes the recent progresses made in the synthesis of nitrogen heterocycles as antitubercular agents. Finally, Chapter 9 is focused on the recent developments made in the field of antimalarial drugs with a focus on their mechanism of action and screening of novel hit molecules.

Chapters 10, 11, 12 and 13 will describe in depth all the drugs currently available for the treatment of kinetoplastid diseases, such as leishmaniasis and African and American trypanosomiasis. The Chapter 10 describes a general and comprehensive overview of the design and synthesis of currently available anti-kinetoplastid drugs, while the Chapters 11 and 12 are more focused on drugs targeting the trypanothione metabolism and on nitroaromatic drugs, respectively. Finally, Chapter 13 is specifically dedicated to anti-leishmanial drugs.

The book is completed by Chapter 14 where the use of a natural product, namely curcumin, in the treatment of NTDs is presented, and by Chapter 15, which is entirely focused on the synthesis and pharmaceutical properties of currently available drugs in the treatment of worm infections.

Each chapter has been designed in such a way that it caters to the need of the medicinal chemists who work in the field of the chemotherapeutics development for NTDs, as well as a guide to budding those scientists, not only chemists, who wish to work in this area of research. We believe that this book will be of interest and use for all those scientists working in the big field of NTDs and whose expertise ranges widely from chemistry to biology, pharmacology and drug development. Moreover, we hope that the book would be of inspiration for the next generation of young scientists at the beginning of their studies and careers, with the wish that they could discover novel treatments to efficiently fight neglected and tropical diseases.

Finally, we want to give a special and warm thanks to all the authors who devoted themselves to this book and contributed to make it a reality.

Contents

Chapter **1**

Key Concepts in Assay Development, Screening and the Properties of Lead and Candidate Compounds

Sheraz Gul

Introduction

The drug discovery process lies at the interface of biology and chemistry and can be divided into two main phases, namely the pre-clinical and the clinical phase (Blass 2015, Ng 2015, Li and Corey 2013, Marshall et al. 2018). The former begins with the identification of a biological target that is implicated in a particular disease and ends with a candidate compound which is suitable for entering First Time in Human (FTIH) studies (Bergstrom 2017). For most drug discovery projects, it is commonplace that the duration of the pre-clinical phase is in the region of five years and costs 5–10 million Euros. The pre-clinical phase can itself be sub-divided into three stages, namely Target-to-Hit, Hit-to-Lead and Lead-to-Candidate (Mignani et al. 2018, Parker et al. 2015, Vaswani 2016). Associated with these stages are compound centric milestones such as identification of a hit compound series which will have modest potency against the biological target which it has been screened against, limited selectivity and toxicity information (Tobinaga et al. 2018, Uliassi et al. 2018, Xia et al. 2018, Yang et al. 2018, Zhang et al. 2018). Significant optimisation of a Hit compound series with respect to a number of properties is necessary, often in an iterative manner, which will yield a Lead compound series that has defined properties relating to its bio-activity, physico-chemical properties and various toxicity determinations (Chiarelli et al. 2018, Thompson et al. 2018, Xie et al. 2018). Due to the costs involved in further optimisation, the most promising Lead compound is further optimised resulting in the generation of a Candidate which has extensive data relating to its *in vitro* and *in vivo* efficacy and safety profile such that it is suitable for progression to clinical trials (Dias Viegas et al. 2018, Forkuo et al. 2018, Gao et al. 2018a, Huang et al. 2018, Wu et al. 2018).

Head of Drug Discovery, Fraunhofer Institute for Molecular Biology & Applied Ecology - ScreeningPort, Schnackenburgallee 114, D-22525 Hamburg, Germany.
Email: Sheraz.Gul@ime.fraunhofer.de

The main processes in pre-clinical drug discovery are reviewed herein and these cover target identification, assay development, compound screening, Hit identification and properties of a Lead series and Candidate compound. A summary of the key compound centric activities in the pre-clinical drug discovery value chain are shown in Figure 1.

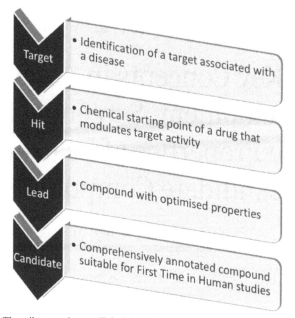

Figure 1. The milestones in pre-clinical drug discovery relating to compound progression.

Target Identification

Prior to initiating a drug discovery project, a biological target that is implicated in a disease needs to be selected. The success of the entire drug discovery process is dependent on choosing the right target for a particular disease, therefore, a strong biological rationale for target selection is necessary (Cowell et al. 2018, Kurata et al. 2018, Neggers et al. 2018, Storer et al. 2017). Despite all efforts and due diligence that can be taken to ensure selection of a suitable target, proof that its modulation will treat a disease will only be known during a suitably powered clinical trial (Lok et al. 2017, Shapiro et al. 2018).

The sequencing of the human genome has been a major technological achievement and has led to the identification of thousands of proteins that function in concert leading to a healthy human (Venter et al. 2001). These proteins can be classified into various biological target classes; for example, there are approximately 400 GPCR, 50 nuclear receptor, 500 kinase and 400 protease targets, all of which are now well established to be tractable classes of proteins from a drug discovery perspective (Ferguson and Gray 2018, Fernandez 2018, Hauser et al. 2017, Turk 2006). A significant proportion of the human genome has therefore not been explored and it is likely that only a small fraction of these genes are actually tractable with respect to a small molecule or biologics therapeutic approach. This may be due to potential target redundancy and the existence of alternative biological pathways and it may explain the lack of efficacy that has been observed for many Candidate compounds in clinical trials (Hwang et al. 2016, Jones et al. 2017). Thus, a major challenge in drug discovery is to focus the efforts on valid targets (Floris et al. 2018, Rouillard et al. 2018, Xu et al. 2018).

In light of the above challenges, target validation involves demonstrating that the target itself is directly involved in a disease process and modulation of its activity would control disease progression. For this, a comprehensive understanding of the biological pathways the target protein is involved in is necessary. However, this is usually not possible when evaluating the target in isolation or in a non-physiological environment which often occurs in the early stages of drug discovery programs. The best validated targets are generally identified as the result of extensive studies in disease biology that may have taken many years to accomplish by researchers in academia and industry.

The ranking of the confidence in target validation can conveniently be classified using a score ranging from 1 (least confidence) through to 4 (most confidence), as shown in Figure 2. The ranking is also consistent with the progression of most drug discovery projects as the initial steps are biology focused and upon understanding target mechanism of action. The attention then shifts to a chemistry focus where compounds are designed, synthesised and evaluated *in vitro* and *in vivo* to confirm that they are able to modulate the activity of the biological target in a manner that could be therapeutically relevant (Bhullar et al. 2018, García-Aranda and Redondo 2017, Mohs and Greig 2017). The best assessment for validating a particular target from a drug discovery perspective would come from the existence of a therapeutic agent that has successfully been shown to yield clinical benefit. However, this scenario is not optimal when searching for novel first-in-class drugs as the existence of a competitor molecule would impact the revenue generating potential of an additional drug.

The latest trends in pre-clinical drug discovery appear to emphasise the importance of developing lower-throughput but more physiologically relevant assay systems such as those that make use of patient derived cells (O'Duibhir et al. 2017), stem cells (Di Baldassarre et al. 2018, Robbins and Price 2017, Watmuff et al. 2017), complex 3D models (Miranda et al. 2018, Weeber et al. 2017), fluorescence-activated cell sorting (Fu et al. 2014), cellular thermal shift (Martinez et al. 2018, McNulty et al. 2018), high fidelity toxicity (Lin et al. 2014) and technologies such as label-free electrical impedance (Atienzar et al. 2013, Doornbos et al. 2018, Peters et al. 2015) and gene editing (Ahmad and Amiji 2018, Lino et al. 2018).

A confounding aspect of target validation is when a single target is implicated in different disease processes. For example, 3-hydroxy-3-methylglutaryl-CoA reductase (HMG-CoA reductase) is a drug target for statins (Istvan and Deisendorfer 2001) and is therefore involved in lowering blood cholesterol concentrations, but it has also been implicated in other diseases including neurodegeneration (Saravi et al. 2017), periodontal disease (Muniz et al. 2018), cancer (Zaleska et al. 2018) and Alzheimer's disease (Daneschvar et al. 2015), albeit to varying degrees of confidence. Therefore, robust target validation relating to disease association is often lacking, especially for novel drug targets.

A powerful technique that can be used to identify novel targets is Genome Wide Association Studies (GWAS) which can provide evidence for disease associated gene loci even if it often lacks detailed characterisation (Breen et al. 2016, Schunkert et al. 2001, Shu et al. 2018, Sud et al. 2017, Wijmenga and Zhernakova 2018). Although this offers the opportunity to discover first-in-class drugs, progressing small

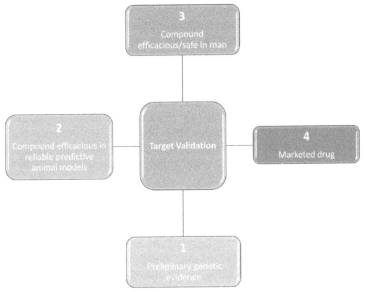

Figure 2. The criteria for ranking target validation in pre-clinical drug discovery.

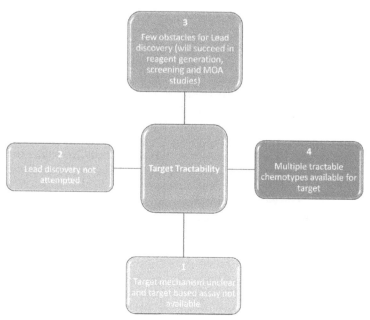

Figure 3. The criteria for ranking target tractability in pre-clinical drug discovery.

molecule drug discovery projects for such targets is often extremely challenging as the function of many of such genes is unknown (Gaspar and Breen 2017).

Another important aspect to consider in the early stages of drug discovery is whether the activity of the target can be modulated by a drug (often referred to as target tractability). A scoring system that captures the key facets of target tractability are summarised in Figure 3. This ranking is also conveniently classified using a score ranging from 1 (least confidence) through to 4 (most confidence). This scoring system has been devised taking into account the past successes and failures in drug discovery. For example, approximately 25% of all small molecule drugs target the GPCR family and these therefore have the highest score for target validation and target tractability (Hauser et al. 2017). Although only a relatively few kinase drugs have been approved for clinical use, the kinase target class of proteins also score high for both target validation and target tractability (Markham 2018). This target tractability concept is based upon factors such as the understanding of the mechanism of action of the protein, and the ability to obtain sufficient amounts of biological reagents that can lead to *in vitro* assays that are compatible with screening against compounds, ultimately leading to chemical starting points for drug discovery.

Understanding whether a protein can be targeted by a small molecule often relies upon the protein possessing a pocket that can accommodate a small molecule that subsequently has the ability to modulate protein activity. Many protein target classes are known to be druggable such as GPCRs, nuclear receptor and kinase proteins as they have been extensively characterised and are known to possess druggable binding sites (Fuller et al. 2009, Ma and Nussinov 2014, Pérot et al. 2010, Wenthur et al. 2014). Although many of such sites described in the literature are typically located in the active centre of protein, unique allosteric binding sites offer significant advantages as they may allow for selectivity to be achieved for proteins that otherwise have similar structures.

Assay Development

Having identified a biological target to investigate, in the case of small molecule drug discovery, it is necessary to develop an assay that has sufficient throughput so that it can be screened against libraries of compounds. These assays should be compatible for automated screening against small molecule libraries in High Throughput Screening (HTS) campaigns to identify compounds that are capable of modulating the activity of the target in a potentially therapeutically meaningful manner (Baggio et al. 2018, Cook et al. 2018, Roy 2018, Taylor et al. 2018).

The enzyme target class are well validated in drug discovery, with many drugs having been approved for clinical use that modulate their activities. There are many different types of enzymes and these are generally classified depending upon the nature of the catalytic machinery that is responsible for catalysis. For example, in the case of protease enzymes, the most common members are the serine, cysteine, aspartyl and metallo-proteases (Rawling and Salvesen 2013). As the protease enzymes are found ubiquitously in living organisms, in particular in significant amounts in plants, enzymes from these sources have historically been studied with a view to translate the findings to human enzymes. Although the plant proteases are not directly of therapeutic value, studies making use of them have provided extremely valuable insights into protease mechanism of action, specificity characteristics, structural information and the design and development of substrates and inhibitors (Gul et al. 1997, 2006, 2008, Hussain et al. 2011, Noble et al. 2000, Pinitglang et al. 1997). A number of strategies can be explored when developing enzyme assays which are subsequently employed in screening. In the case of an enzyme target, it is desirable to make use of full-length protein that has been expressed in a suitable system so as to generate it in a form that is as physiologically relevant as possible. A tag is also often expressed at the terminus of the protein to facilitate its purification and this should be removed by the inclusion of a suitable cleavage site between protein and tag. With regards to the substrate of an enzyme target, a number of options are available and a careful thought needs to be given as to which of the possible substrates should be utilised for assay development and subsequent screening. The importance of choosing the most appropriate substrate stems from the fact that protease enzymes contain an active centre which is composed of a catalytic site, where the residues directly involved in the cleavage of the substrate are located, and a binding site where the substrate can interact with the enzyme and confer substrate specificity characteristics upon it. Early studies on proteases made use of simple chromogenic substrates such as 4-nitrophenyl acetate (Figure 4a) with the reaction monitored by measuring the accumulation of 4-nitrophenol at 410 nm (Kezdy and Bender 1962). Although this substrate allows the detection of protease activity, it contains no specificity features for any particular protease. Therefore, compounds which are substrate competitive are unlikely to be identified using this approach. As the measured activity may be due to other contaminant proteases within the preparation, significant care is required when utilising such non-specific substrates as these need to be fully validated. This includes appropriate benchmarking against reference compounds of known potencies if available. The consequences of utilising artificial substrates are that they may lead to the identification of inhibitors of protease activity whose properties may not translate to more physiologically relevant assays. The use of peptide based substrates for protease enzymes that have more of a resemblance to physiological substrates offers significant advantages over 4-nitrophenyl-acetate as they will incorporate some of the specificity requirements of the enzyme (Lottenberg et al. 1982). Early peptide substrate based protease assays made use of unlabelled substrates which, after undergoing cleavage to generate lower molecular mass products, would be separated by methods such as thin layer chromatography (Zhang et al. 2015) or HPLC (Chen et al. 2018), only after which the activity of the protease could be determined. However, such assays are very low throughput and not compatible with screening large libraries of compounds. Thus the use of appropriately labelled peptide substrates (chromogenic or fluorogenic) allows them to be used without any separation steps and in most cases can be used to monitor protease activity kinetically in real time. Chromogenic substrates release a chromophore following protease mediated cleavage with a concomitant colour change which can be followed spectrophotometrically. These types of substrates are not ideally suited for compound screening activities due to their lack of sensitivity and their susceptibility towards optical interference. In the case of 4-nitroanilide derived peptide substrates (Figure 4b), the chromophore that is produced (4-nitroaniline) can be monitored by measuring the absorbance at 410 nm.

The commonly used fluorogenic protease substrates (which are significantly more sensitive than chromogenic substrates) contain the 7-amino-4-methyl coumarin (AMC) group (Figure 4c). Upon catalytic cleavage of the substrate, the AMC product is detected by excitation of the system at 380 nm and detects the emission at 460 nm. Alternative fluorogenic substrates make use of quenched peptides that contain a donor and quencher chemically coupled to residues within the peptide substrate which are in close spatial proximity. An example of such a substrate is one that contains the fluorescent AMC group that is

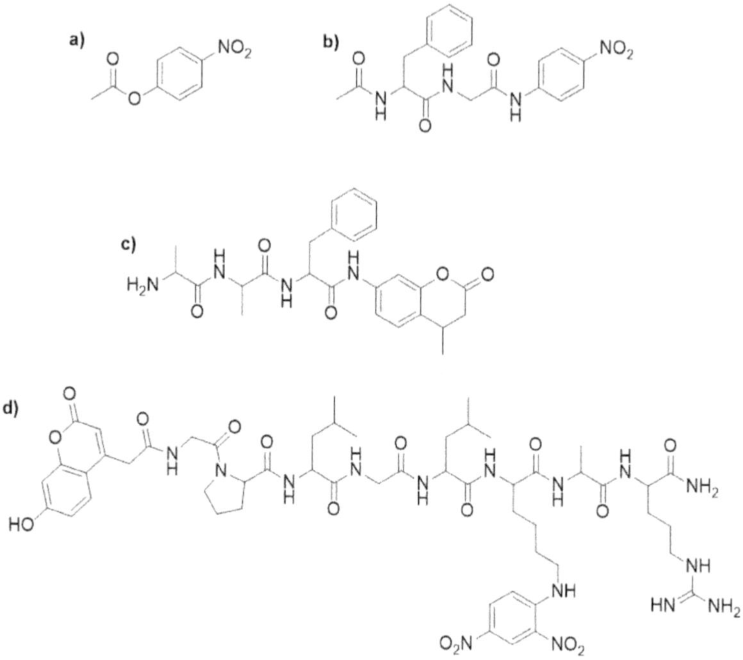

Figure 4. Structures of (a) 4-nitrophenyl acetate substrate, (b) Ac-Phe-Gly-4-nitroanilide peptide substrate, (c) Ala-Ala-Phe-7-amido-4-methylcoumarin peptide substrate, (d) MCA-Gly-Pro-Leu-Gly-Leu-Lys(DNP)-Ala-Lys quenched peptide substrate.

quenched by resonance energy transfer to the 2,4-dinitrophenyl (DNP) group (Figure 4d) (McCartney et al. 2018). Upon catalytic cleavage of the peptide, these two groups are spatially separated, quenching is overcome and the extent of product that is produced can be determined by excitation of the system at 320 nm and detecting the emission at 405 nm. Although the fluorogenic substrates are an improvement from chromogenic substrates, they still have the unnatural fluorophore moiety within the substrate molecule that could compromise the binding modes with the enzyme.

As the catalytic action of proteases upon their substrates produces products that have a newly generated epitope that is absent in the initial substrate molecule, this feature can be exploited in the development of a protease assay. If the substrate is a protein, the cleavage site within it is known and if antibodies that specifically recognise the newly generated epitope are available, its use in conjunction with another antibody that recognises the total protein (e.g., N- or C- terminus antibody) will enable the development of proximity based assays such as Time Resolved-Fluorescence Resonance Energy Transfer (TR-FRET) (Engels et al. 2009) or Amplified Luminescence Proximity Homogeneous Assay (AlphaScreen™) technologies (Ren et al. 2013). However, a prerequisite to developing these types of assays are the appropriate labelling of the antibodies.

One method of overcoming the issues associated with the development of artificial substrates in assay systems is to use label free methods that obviate the requirement for the alteration of molecules in assays that could interfere with binding modes with the protein target and substrate of interest. Many of these label free techniques (e.g., biacore and isothermal titration calorimetry (Shoji et al. 2017)) are very powerful in that they allow the quantitative characterisation of interactions. The main disadvantage with these techniques is that they usually are not amenable to screening large numbers of compounds and can also consume large amounts of protein. However, strides are being made to increase their throughput and reduce reagent consumption.

Microfluidics based assays have a role in screening and significant advances have been made with respect to the design, development and manufacture of such devices. Of particular note is their ability to contain multiple fine channels that offer the possibility of mixing small volumes of various reagents and monitoring their effects on the activity of the protein target (Gupta et al. 2016, Regnault et al. 2018). For biochemical assays, it is possible to create "plugs" of various reagents (enzyme, substrate and compound) which can be allowed to come into contact at specific times and concentrations. It is also possible to design chambers within these devices that can mimic individual organs in the body and cellular changes can be measured upon their exposure to compound. For cell-based assays, microfluidic based assays offer the potential to measure the activity of individual cells whilst applying a concentration gradient of compound.

Compound Screening Activities

A key requirement for executing HTS campaigns is access to a suitable compound library. These can vary in size from a few hundred compounds in a focussed library up to many millions in a diverse library (Butler et al. 2014, Gong et al. 2017, Peng 2013, Spear and Brown 2017, Zimmermann and Neri 2016). Purchasing a library can be an expensive endeavour and requires reliable hardware and IT infrastructure to manage the libraries. These extra functionalities require significant financial investment which usually can only be found in industry. As a result of the variation in the sizes of compound libraries, researchers require varying degrees of automated solutions. In those cases where a few relatively simple manual tasks are carried out, off the shelf solutions are usually sufficient. At the other extreme, there may be a need to cater for throughputs in excess of 100,000 tests per day (Hassig et al. 2014).

Compound screening activities (CSA) of drug targets against compound libraries is now a mature and validated approach to identifying the chemical starting points of drugs. There are broadly two main screening types, namely phenotypic (often termed systems-based and target-agnostic) and target-based (using hypothesis-driven) approaches (Gul 2017). These approaches have been comprehensively analysed in relation to the Food and Drug Administration (FDA) approval of 113 first-in-class drugs in the US between 1999 and 2013 and suggested that the majority of the first-in-class drugs were discovered through target-based approaches with a minority originating from phenotypic screening (Eder et al. 2014). This analysis contrasts with another study in which the FDA approval of 259 agents between 1999 and 2008 showed that the contribution of phenotypic screening to the discovery of first-in-class small-molecule drugs exceeded that of target-based approaches (Swinney and Anthony 2011). It is also important to acknowledge that the definitions of the various screening methods have changed over time and as we move forward, the contributions of both phenotypic and target-based methodologies will be important in discovering new medicines and they should be seen as complementing rather than competing against each other.

The most widely utilised method for the screening of biological targets considered to be suitable for therapeutic intervention in drug discovery efforts uses microtiter plate based assays that conform to the Society of Biomolecular Screening (SBS) plate standard (96, 384 and 1536 wells per plate), all of which allow for a significant throughput and reduction in reagent consumption (Brostromer et al. 2007). These microtiter plate based assays have also had a positive impact on manufacturers of equipment such as liquid handlers, microtiter plate readers, compound storage facilities and data analysis software.

It is now commonplace to perform entire HTS campaigns using primary cells. These cell-based assays offer the potential to overcome some of the undesirables associated with biochemical assays (Auld et al. 2008, Hall et al. 2016, Hsieh 2016, Jadhav et al. 2010, Thorne et al. 2012). Cell-based assays can also be configured to allow the identification of compounds that are activators or inhibitors of the target of interest. When searching for inhibitors in a cell-based assay, a cytotoxic compound would yield an "apparent inhibition" profile (a false positive). When searching for activators, a genuine activator of the target may not be identified if the compound is also cytotoxic (a false negative). In light of these complications, there is a need to put into place appropriate control assays that are suitable for identifying such assay artefacts that can manifest themselves in cell-based assays, especially when compounds are cytotoxic (Mervin et al. 2016). If a compound also appears inactive in an appropriate and well validated target-based secondary assay, then the observation in the HTS assay may not be mediated via the target of interest. However, if the activity of compounds is confirmed in the target-based secondary assay, then such compounds can be progressed with more confidence.

High Content Screening (HCS) has become a firmly established technology that can aid the reduction in the high attrition rates in drug discovery (Mandavilli et al. 2018, Smith et al. 2018, Xia and Wong 2012). Too often, the identification of compounds that exhibit the ability to modulate the activity of a therapeutically relevant target in isolation fails to translate their behaviour when evaluated in a cellular context. Compounds identified from screening activities against libraries carried out in a HCS setting may be better starting points for drug discovery efforts. This has been possible as a result of the fusion of the outcomes of the advances in microscopy, image acquisition and analysis software, computer processing power, integration into automated platforms, and molecular biological techniques to construct tagged target proteins with suitable labels, e.g., Green Fluorescent Protein (GFP). HCS also offers the possibility of evaluating the effect of compounds on both phenotypic end-points as well as on individual cellular events (Kain 1999).

Automated compound handling has usually been treated separately from the liquid handling of bulk reagents for assays. Compounds are usually stored in 100% v/v DMSO as the solvent for their dissolution in microtiter plates (Chen et al. 2013, Liu et al. 2012, Popa-Burke and Russel 2014, Zaragoza-Sundqvist et al. 2009). Usually, assays will contain DMSO at concentrations in the region of 1% v/v; therefore, a 100-fold dilution of compound will need to be carried out. Thus, for an assay with a volume of 10 μl, the volume of the compound solution required will be 0.1 μl which is usually added to assay plates first. This is then followed by the addition of bulk biological reagents, e.g., in the case of a simple *in vitro* assay, one addition of substrate (5 μl) and a second addition of enzyme (5 μl) to initiate the reaction and a third addition (10 μl) to stop the reaction prior to reading the microtiter plate. The types of liquid handling equipment employed to dispense compounds and bulk reagents are usually kept separate as the volumes required are substantially different. Numerous technologies have been developed that are capable of reliable dispensing of sub-microlitre volumes of compounds in DMSO whilst maintaining sufficient throughput for the production of plates containing compounds for screening activities. One such example is based on capillary action using specially designed tips for fixed volume dispensing (Genomic Solutions® Hummingbird). In this case, as the same tips are re-used, they need to be washed sufficiently after each dispenses to prevent cross contamination. This washing is usually done with DMSO (the same solvent that is used to dissolve the compounds) to prevent their precipitation within the tips and blocking them. A more recent development for dispensing low volumes of solutions of DMSO is based on a contactless method using acoustic droplet ejection and is exploited by the Labcyte Echo®. As a result of the contactless dispense method, there is no need for the use of disposable tips, the need for washing is overcome, no waste DMSO is generated and compound adsorption is obviated.

Hit-to-Lead

A Hit molecule identified from a biological screen may not always be a suitable basis for a medicinal chemistry optimisation programme. The purpose of the Hit-to-Lead phase is to identify one or more molecules upon which such an optimisation could be successful (Bruno et al. 2017, Dinges et al. 2016, Gao et al. 2018b). Thus, the first part of this phase involves the validation of the Hit compounds in terms of confirming chemical structure and purity. This will usually involve a re-synthesis of the most interesting Hit compounds. Once Hit validation has been completed, analogues of the most promising Hit molecules are investigated, in terms of biological activity, selectivity and drugability in order to identify one or more high quality molecules that meet agreed pre-defined criteria. The typical information required for a Lead compound is summarised in Table 1.

Ultimately, a Lead compound will typically be associated with sub-micromolar potency against the biological target it was designed to modulate the activity of and limited selectivity, physicochemical and ADMET properties (Barberis et al. 2017, Shirai et al. 2018). As in the case of the choice of assay for CSA against any drug target, numerous assays are available to characterise the *in vitro* properties in the Hit-to-Lead phase and this is illustrated here by cell viability assays. Cell viability is often based on the integrity of the cell membrane, key cellular biochemical reactions and specific cellular markers (Méry et al. 2017). Knowledge of the extent of cytotoxicity that is induced by compounds is a parameter that needs to be determined prior to progressing them in the drug discovery value chain.

A variety of microtiter plate-based cytotoxicity assays in colorimetric, fluorometric and luminescence detection technologies are available. The colorimetric based methods have historically been the most widely

Table 1. Summary of the attributes of a typical Lead compound.

Property	Attribute	Annotation
Chemical properties	Hit validation to confirm activity in screening assay	Confirmed activity (usually μM range)
	Resynthesis and screening of Hit compounds	Confirmed activity
	Structure identity and purity	Purity level (> 95%)
	Synthesis of analogue compounds	Confirmed
	Synthetically accessible and tractable chemistry	Confirmed
	Measurement of physicochemical properties of library compounds	Confirmed properties
	Potential for patent protection	Assessment undertaken
	Confirmed structure supported by X-ray crystal structure	Confirmed
Pharmacological properties	SAR information suggestive that optimisation is possible	Confirmed activity
	Suitable selective profile against biological targets	Positive results (usually > 10-fold selective)
Pharmacokinetics	Bioavailability for route of administration	Positive results
	Half-life and bio-distribution for route of administration	Positive results
Safety and toxicity	*In vitro* ADMET studies on compounds to include CYP450 inhibition and induction and *h*ERG inhibition	Positive results (usually > 10-fold selective)
	Absence of cytotoxicity in human cell-lines	Positive results (usually > 10-fold selective)

utilised and are well validated. These include quantification of (1) mitochondrial succinate dehydrogenase activity of cells using the tetrazoles XTT and MTT (Berridge et al. 2005), (2) extracellular lactate dehydrogenase activity by measuring NADH consumption (Decker and Lohmann-Matthes 1998), (3) acid phosphatase activity as a marker of lysosomal activity (Ivanov et al. 2017), (4) remaining glucose in cell culture medium using a glucose oxidase-peroxidase assay (Wong and Huang 2014), (5) cell proliferation using crystal violet dye accumulation in the nucleus (Feoktistova et al. 2016), (6) lysosomal accumulation of a cationic dye neutral red (Ates et al. 2017) and (7) protein synthesis using sulforhodamine B binding to proteins (Shaik et al. 2013).

Fluorometric based cytotoxicity assays are also available and include those that quantify (1) lactate dehydrogenase activity assay using a coupled reaction that results in the conversion of resazurin into resorufin (CytoTox-ONE™ Assay) (Shaife et al. 2017), (2) protease activity that is released from cells with a compromised cell membrane and a non-cell permeable fluorogenic peptide substrate (CytoTox-Fluor™ Cytotoxicity Assay) (Shaik et al. 2013) and (3) the activity of two proteases using cell permeable (giving the live cell measurement) and non-cell permeable (giving the dead cell measurement) substrates (MultiTox-Fluor Multiplex Cytotoxicity Assay) (Niles et al. 2009).

Luminescence based assays are also available and include those that quantify (1) the activity of a protease that is released from cells that no longer retain an intact cell membrane using a luminogenic peptide substrate (CytoTox-Glo® Cytotoxicity Assay) (Schorpp et al. 2016), (2) glutathione-5-transferase activity using a luciferin derived substrate, the product of the reaction being a substrate of firefly luciferase (Slim et al. 2000) and (3) intracellular ATP using a luciferase reaction (CellTiter-Glo® Luminescent Cell Viability Assay) (Lhuissier et al. 2017). There is also a multiplex assay that uses a fluoresence and luminescence readout essentially the same as the MultiTox-Fluor Multiplex cytotoxicity assay mentioned above but the substrate for dead cells is luminogenic instead of being fluorogenic (Trumpi et al. 2015).

Thus, a suitable cytotoxicity assay is essential to quantify the potential liabilities associated with a Lead compound. As there are many such assays, a thorough approach to evaluating the effects of compound induced cytotoxicity should be carried out in order to identify the best compounds with the aim of reducing attrition in the later stages of drug discovery.

Lead-to-Candidate

The optimisation of a Lead molecule into a Candidate is a very challenging multiparameter process (Forkuo et al. 2018, Mikami et al. 2017, Landis et al. 2018, Zhang et al. 2016). It should lead to the identification of a molecule that satisfies pre-defined criteria with regard to *in vitro* and *in vivo* activity, pharmacokinetics, toxicological and pharmaceutical properties, and complexity of chemical synthesis (Table 2). It will typically have nano-molar potency against its primary biological target and will have undergone significant medicinal chemistry optimisation, comprehensive *in vitro* selectivity screening, determination of physicochemical and pharmaceutical properties and initial formulation studies, detailed *in vitro* ADMET studies, mutagenicity testing, detailed secondary pharmacology studies, detailed *in vivo* pharmacodynamics and pharmacokinetic studies, and comprehensive toxicological profiling.

Table 2. Summary of the attributes of a typical Candidate.

Property	Attribute	Annotation
Chemical properties	• Physicochemical properties • Chemistry and Patents	• MW • CLogP and cLogD • tPSA • H-bond donors and H-bond acceptors • Physiochemical properties determined and no major issues identified • Aqueous solubility pH 7.4 • Synthetic route appropriate for progression to development stage • Scalable (50 g batch prepared) • Purity level > 95% • Acceptable stability and formulation • Appropriate crystalline (salt) form identified and single enantiomer • Back-ups identified • Clinical development plan • Patent life target 15 years or greater
Mechanism of action and pharmacology	• Biological activity and Mode of Action Studies • Cytotoxicity (against mammalian cells) • *In vivo* efficacy studies	• Mode of Action understood • Selective potent *in vitro* activity • Dose response relationship defined • Activity in a relevant animal model • Pharmacodynamics determined • Oral bioavailability in rat, dog or marmoset • No major effects on human CYP450 metabolism • Metabolism in human liver S9 fractions determined
Absorption, distribution, metabolism and excretion (ADME)	• *In vitro* and *in vivo* DMPK • Bioanalytical methodology • *In vitro* metabolism • Plasma Protein Binding • Pharmacokinetic Studies	• Intrinsic clearance in hepatic microsomes • Intrinsic clearance in hepatocytes • Preferred human plasma protein binding < 95% • Preferred bioavailability: F > 20% • Appropriate permeability (PAMPA) • Appropriate pK_a • Appropriate drug efflux pump profile • Stability in Simulated Gastric Fluid Stability, plasma and blood stability (mouse/human), Media, Milli-Q water, FeSSIF and FaSSIF
Toxicology	• *In vitro* cell toxicity • Selectivity Index and Safety Profile • Cardiac Safety • Gene toxicity • CYP450 inhibition • *In vivo* rat safety studies	• No issues identified in secondary pharmacology assays • No *h*ERG inhibition • No effect in zebrafish and Ames test • Minimum lethal dose (rat) suggestive of an acceptable therapeutic ratio • No deaths or major organ damage following 7-day dosing at 100 mg/kg in rat

An additional component of this phase is preparation of a dossier in order to obtain regulatory approval for FTIH studies following Investigational New Drug (IND) filing. This will include determination of compound formulation and packaging information including:

- Synthesis of Active Pharmaceutical Ingredient (API) to Good Manufacturing Practice (GMP)
- Analytical method development and its validation
- Selection of optimal formulation
- Manufacture of formulated drug product
- Two (or more if necessary) species toxicological evaluation
- Further *in vivo* evaluation
- Stability studies of API and formulated drug product.

Pre-clinical Drug Discovery Cycle Time and Costs

It is important to set clear target cycle times and progression criteria for each project and terminate projects that fail to meet the prescribed criteria in a timely manner. However, it is difficult to precisely quantify what resources are required over what time period to provide success for each of the drug discovery phases since each particular biological target will provide its own set of challenges. This is because certain targets are more tractable than others in terms of finding Hit molecules from screening and the ease with which such Hits can be optimised to give Candidates with good pharmaceutical properties. Nevertheless, ranges can be estimated based on bench-marking analysis and previous experience. Table 3 summaries the duration and resources for each stage of a Target-to-IND programme. The shortest total cycle time for a project would be around 3 years whilst the longest cycle time would be 5.5 years.

Table 3. Summary of the typical timeline and costs associated with a Target to Candidate project.

Stage	Duration (months)	Cost range (EUR)
Target to Hit	12–24	100,000–1,000,000
Hit-to-Lead	12–24	100,000–1,000,000
Lead-to-Candidate	12–18	2,000,000–5,000,000

Conclusions

It is important to ensure that a common set of definitions is used in the drug discovery value chain so that all stakeholders have a common basis for expectations when evaluating compounds. Commonly accepted definitions in the pre-clinical stages are:

Biological Target: A macromolecule with known function, disease association and involvement, and ideally 3-dimensional structure.

Validated Hit: A molecule with robust dose-response activity in an assay that utilises the target protein with confirmed structure and preliminary SAR information.

Lead Compound: A representative compound series which satisfies predefined criteria (see Table 1) for progression to Lead-to-Candidate optimisation.

Candidate: A representative compound that satisfies predefined criteria (see Table 2) for progression to subsequent IND submission.

When initiating a drug discovery process, the end goal has to be clearly defined and this can take the shape of a Target Product Profile (TPP) which describes how the product will be utilised by the end-user (https://www.fda.gov/downloads/drugs/guidancecomplianceregulatoryinformation/guidances/ucm080593. pdf [Last accessed 03-04-2019]). A variety of formats for a TPP exists and the FDA have provided draft guidelines to assist with its preparation. A total of 17 specific aspects of the drug were considered to be necessary to be included in a TPP and these are (1) Indications and use, (2) Dosage and administration, (3)

Dosage forms and strengths, (4) Contraindications, (5) Warnings and precautions, (6) Adverse reactions, (7) Drug interactions, (8) Use in specific populations, (9) Drug abuse and dependence, (10) Over-dosage, (11) Description, (12) Clinical pharmacology, (13) Nonclinical toxicology, (14) Clinical studies, (15) References, (16) How supplied/storage and handling and (17) Patient counselling information. A well-defined TPP will ensure the entire drug discovery team are aligned in terms of understanding the attributes that are required to ensure the overall success of the project. Any TPP that is devised needs careful consideration as they will be bespoke for a given disease (Lambert 2010) and these have been exemplified for a number of diseases including malarial (Burrows et al. 2017) and parasitic diseases (Wyatt et al. 2011).

Although drug discovery is fraught with challenges, the prospect of discovering a new drug is highly rewarding as it offers the potential for mankind to live healthier and longer lives. This is particularly relevant as life expectancy has increased significantly in the past century, but drugs are still lacking to treat diseases that afflict the elderly such as Alzheimer's and Parkinson's disease. With the plethora of research taking place in industry and academia, it is anticipated that in the coming decades many novel drug treatments will be available to treat diseases which currently curtail the quality of life.

Acknowledgment

The author acknowledges the European Union's Seventh Framework Programme for research, technological development and demonstration under grant agreement no. 603240 (NMTrypI—New Medicines for Trypanosomatidic Infections).

References

Ahmad, G. and M. Amiji. 2018. Use of CRISPR/Cas9 gene-editing tools for developing models in drug discovery. Drug Discov. Today. 23: 519–533.

Ates, G., T. Vanhaecke, V. Rogiers and R.M. Rodrigues. 2017. Assaying cellular viability using the neutral red uptake assay. Methods Mol. Biol. 1601: 19–26.

Atienzar, F.A., H. Gerets, K. Tilmant, G. Toussaint and S. Dhalluin. 2013. Evaluation of impedance-based label-free technology as a tool for pharmacology and toxicology investigations. Biosensors (Basel). 3: 132–156.

Auld, D.S., N. Thorne, D.T. Nguyen and J. Inglese. 2008. A specific mechanism for nonspecific activation in reporter-gene assays. ACS Chem. Biol. 3: 463–470.

Baggio, C., L. Cerofolini, M. Fragai, C. Luchinat and M. Pellecchia. 2018. HTS by NMR for the identification of potent and selective inhibitors of metalloenzymes. ACS Med. Chem. Lett. 9: 137–142.

Barberis, C., N. Moorcroft, J. Pribish, E. Tserlin, A. Gross, M. Czekaj et al. 2017. Discovery of N-substituted 7-azaindoles as Pan-PIM kinase inhibitors-Lead series identification—Part II. Bioorg. Med. Chem. Lett. 27: 4735–4740.

Bergstrom, M. 2017. The use of microdosing in the development of small organic and protein therapeutics. J. Nucl. Med. 58: 1188–1195.

Berridge, M.V., P.M. Herst and A.S. Tan. 2005. Tetrazolium dyes as tools in cell biology: new insights into their cellular reduction. Biotechnol. Annu. Rev. 11: 127–152.

Bhullar, K.S., N.O. Lagarón, E.M. McGowan, I. Parmar, A. Jha, B.P. Hubbard et al. 2018. Kinase-targeted cancer therapies: progress, challenges and future directions. Mol. Cancer. 17: 48.

Blass, B.E. 2015. Basic Principles of Drug Discovery and Development. Academic Press, USA, pp. 580.

Breen, G., Q. Li, B.L. Roth, P. O'Donnell, M. Didriksen, R. Dolmetsch et al. 2016. Translating genome-wide association findings into new therapeutics for psychiatry. Nat. Neurosci. 19: 1392–1396.

Brostromer, E., J. Nan and X.D. Su. 2007. An automated image-collection system for crystallization experiments using SBS standard microplates. Acta Crystallogr. D Biol. Crystallogr. 63: 119–125.

Bruno, A., G. Costantino, L. Sartori and M. Radi. 2017. The in silico drug discovery toolbox: applications in lead discovery and optimization. Curr. Med. Chem. In press.

Burrows, J.N., S. Duparc, W.E. Gutteridge, R. Hooft van Huijsduijnen, W. Kaszubska, F. Macintyre et al. 2017. New developments in anti-malarial target candidate and product profiles. Malar. J. 16: 26.

Butler, M.S., F. Fontaine and M.A. Cooper. 2014. Natural product libraries: assembly, maintenance, and screening. Planta Med. 80: 1161–1170.

Chen, A., X. Zhao, L. Mercer, C. Su, L. Zalameda, Y. Liu et al. 2013. Assessment of the integrity of compounds stored in assay-ready plates using a kinase sentinel assay. Comb. Chem. High Throughput Screen. 16: 644–651.

Chen, H., P. Shi, F. Fan, M. Tu, Z. Xu, X. Xu et al. 2018. Complementation of UPLC-Q-TOF-MS and CESI-Q-TOF-MS on identification and determination of peptides from bovine lactoferrin. J. Chromatogr. B. 1084: 150–157.

Chiarelli, L.R., G. Mori, B.S. Orena, M. Esposito, T. Lane, A.L. de Jesus Lopes Ribeiro et al. 2018. A multitarget approach to drug discovery inhibiting Mycobacterium tuberculosis PyrG and PanK. Sci. Rep. 8: 3187.

Cook, E., J. Hermes, J. Li and M. Tudor. 2018. High-content reporter assays. Methods Mol. Biol. 1755: 179–195.

Cowell, A.N., E.S. Istvan, A.K. Lukens, M.G. Gomez-Lorenzo, M. Vanaerschot, T. Sakata-Kato et al. 2018. Mapping the malaria parasite druggable genome by using *in vitro* evolution and chemogenomics. Science. 359: 191–199.

Daneschvar, H.L., M.D. Aronson and G.W. Smetana. 2015. Do statins prevent Alzheimer's disease? A narrative review. Eur. J. Intern. Med. 26: 666–669.

Decker, T. and M.L. Lohmann-Matthes. 1988. A quick and simple method for the quantification of lactate dehydrogenase release in measurements of cellular cytotoxicity and tumor necrosis factor (TNF) activity. J. Immunol. Methods. 115: 61–69.

Di Baldassarre, A., E. Cimetta, S. Bollini, G. Gaggi and B. Ghinassi. 2018. Human-induced pluripotent stem cell technology and cardiomyocyte generation: Progress and clinical applications. Cells. 7: 48.

Dias Viegas, F.P., M. de Freitas Silva, M. Divino da Rocha, M.R. Castelli, M.M. Riquiel, R.P. Machado et al. 2018. Design, synthesis and pharmacological evaluation of N-benzyl-piperidinyl-aryl-acylhydrazone derivatives as donepezil hybrids: Discovery of novel multi-target anti-alzheimer prototype drug candidates. Eur. J. Med. Chem. 147: 48–65.

Dinges, J., C.M. Harris, G.A. Wallace, M.A. Argiriadi, K.L. Queeney, D.C. Perron et al. 2016. Hit-to-lead evaluation of a novel class of sphingosine 1-phosphate lyase inhibitors. Bioorg. Med. Chem. Lett. 26: 2297–2302.

Doornbos, M.L.J., I. Van der Linden, L. Vereyken, G. Tresadern, A.P. IJzerman, H. Lavreysen et al. 2018. Constitutive activity of the metabotropic glutamate receptor 2 explored with a whole-cell label-free biosensor. Biochem. Pharmacol. 152: 201–210.

Eder, J., R. Sedrani and C. Wiesmann. 2014. The discovery of first-in-class drugs: origins and evolution. Nat. Rev. Drug Discov. 13: 577–587.

Engels, I.H., C. Daguia, T. Huynh, H. Urbina, J. Buddenkotte, A. Schumacher et al. 2009. A time-resolved fluorescence resonance energy transfer-based assay for DEN1 peptidase activity. Anal. Biochem. 390: 85–87.

Feoktistova, M., P. Geserick and M. Leverkus. 2016. Crystal violet assay for determining viability of cultured cells. Cold Spring Harb Protoc. 2016: 4.

Ferguson, F.M. and N.S. Gray. 2018. Kinase inhibitors: the road ahead. Nat. Rev. Drug Discov. 17: 353–377.

Fernandez, E.J. 2018. Allosteric pathways in nuclear receptors—Potential targets for drug design. Pharmacol. Ther. 183: 152–159.

Floris, M., S. Olla, D. Schlessinger and F. Cucca. 2018. Genetic-driven druggable target identification and validation. Trends Genet. 34: 558–570.

Forkuo, G.S., A.N. Nieman, R. Kodali, N.M. Zahn, G. Li, M.S. Rashid Roni et al. 2018. A novel orally available asthma drug candidate that reduces smooth muscle constriction and inflammation by targeting GABAA receptors in the lung. Mol. Pharm. 15: 1766–1777.

Fu, Y., Y.L. Chen, M. Herve, F. Gu, P.Y. Shi and F. Blasco. 2014. Development of a FACS-based assay for evaluating antiviral potency of compound in dengue infected peripheral blood mononuclear cells. J. Virol. Methods. 196: 18–24.

Fuller, J.C., N.J. Burgoyne and R.M. Jackson. 2009. Predicting druggable binding sites at the protein-protein interface. Drug Discov. Today. 14: 155–161.

Gao, X., J. Li, M. Wang, S. Xu, W. Liu, L. Zang et al. 2018a. Novel enmein-type diterpenoid hybrids coupled with nitrogen mustards: Synthesis of promising candidates for anticancer therapeutics. Eur. J. Med. Chem. 146: 588–598.

Gao, D.D., H.X. Dou, H.X. Su, M.M. Zhang, T. Wang, Q.F. Liu et al. 2018b. From hit to lead: Structure-based discovery of naphthalene-1-sulfonamide derivatives as potent and selective inhibitors of fatty acid binding protein 4. Eur. J. Med. Chem. 154: 44–59.

García-Aranda, M. and M. Redondo. 2017. Protein kinase targets in breast cancer. Int. J. Mol. Sci. 18: 2543.

Gaspar, H.A. and G. Breen. 2017. Drug enrichment and discovery from schizophrenia genome-wide association results: an analysis and visualisation approach. Sci. Rep. 7: 12460.

Gong, Z., G. Hu, Q. Li, Z. Liu, F. Wang, X. Zhang et al. 2017. Compound libraries: Recent advances and their applications in drug discovery. Curr. Drug Discov. Technol. 14: 216–228.

Gul, S., A. Clarke, B. Field, M.P. Thomas, F. Willenbrock, S. Pinitglang et al. 1997. Investigation of the electrostatic field of the papain active centre by using monoprotonated and diprotonated pyridyl (Py) disulphides as reactivity probes. Biochem. Soc. Trans. 25: 91S.

Gul, S., G.W. Mellor, E.W. Thomas and K. Brocklehurst. 2006. Temperature-dependences of the kinetics of reactions of papain and actinidin with a series of reactivity probes differing in key molecular recognition features. Biochem. J. 396: 17–21.

Gul, S., S. Hussain, M.P. Thomas, M. Resmini, C.S. Verma, E.W. Thomas et al. 2008. Generation of nucleophilic character in the Cys25/His159 ion pair of papain involves Trp177 but not Asp158. Biochemistry. 47: 2025–2035.

Gul, S. 2017. Epigenetic assays for chemical biology and drug discovery. Clin. Epigenetics. 9: 41.

Gupta, N., J.R. Liu, B. Patel, D.E. Solomon, B. Vaidya and V. Gupta. 2016. Microfluidics-based 3D cell culture models: Utility in novel drug discovery and delivery research. Bioeng. Transl. Med. 1: 63–81.

Hall, M.D., A. Simeonov and M.I. Davis. 2016. Avoiding fluorescence assay interference-the case for diaphorase. Assay Drug Dev. Technol. 14: 175–179.

Hassig, C.A., F.Y. Zeng, P. Kung, M. Kiankarimi, S. Kim, P.W. Diaz et al. 2014. Ultra-high-throughput screening of natural product extracts to identify proapoptotic inhibitors of Bcl-2 family proteins. J. Biomol. Screen. 19: 1201–1211.

Hauser, A.S., M.M. Attwood, M. Rask-Andersen, H.B. Schiöth and D.E. Gloriam. 2017. Trends in GPCR drug discovery: New agents, targets and indications. Nat. Rev. Drug Discov. 16: 829–842.

Hsieh, J.H. 2016. Accounting artifacts in high-throughput toxicity assays. Methods Mol. Biol. 1473: 143–152.

https://www.fda.gov/downloads/drugs/guidancecomplianceregulatoryinformation/guidances/ucm080593.pdf [Last accessed 03-04-2019].

Huang, B., X. Liu, Y. Tian, D. Kang, Z. Zhou, D. Daelemans et al. 2018. First discovery of a potential carbonate prodrug of NNRTI drug candidate RDEA427 with submicromolar inhibitory activity against HIV-1 K103N/Y181C double mutant strain. Bioorg. Med. Chem. Lett. 28: 1348–1351.

Hussain, S., A. Khan, S. Gul, M. Resmini, C.S. Verma, E.W. Thomas et al. 2011. Identification of interactions involved in the generation of nucleophilic reactivity and of catalytic competence in the catalytic site Cys/His ion pair of papain. Biochemistry. 50: 10732–10742.

Hwang, T.J., D. Carpenter, J.C. Lauffenburger, B. Wang, J.M. Franklin and A.S. Kesselheim. 2016. Failure of investigational drugs in late-stage clinical development and publication of trial results. JAMA Intern. Med. 176: 1826–1833.

Istvan, E.S. and J. Deisenhofer. 2001. Structural mechanism for statin inhibition of HMG-CoA reductase. Science. 292: 1160–1164.

Ivanov, D.P., A.M. Grabowska and M.C. Garnett. 2017. High-throughput spheroid screens using volume, resazurin reduction, and acid phosphatase activity. Methods Mol. Biol. 1601: 43–59.

Jadhav, A., R.S. Ferreira, C. Klumpp, B.T. Mott, C.P. Austin, J. Inglese et al. 2010. Quantitative analyses of aggregation, autofluorescence, and reactivity artifacts in a screen for inhibitors of a thiol protease. J. Med. Chem. 53: 37–51.

Jones, M.R., H. Lim, Y. Shen, E. Pleasance, C. Ch'ng, C. Reisle et al. 2017. Successful targeting of the NRG1 pathway indicates novel treatment strategy for metastatic cancer. Ann. Oncol. 28: 3092–3097.

Kain, S.R. 1999. Green fluorescent protein (GFP): applications in cell-based assays for drug discovery. Drug Discov. Today. 4: 304–312.

Kezdy, F.J. and M.L. Bender. 1962. The kinetics of the alpha-chymotrypsin-catalyzed hydrolysis of p-nitrophenyl acetate. Biochemistry. 1: 1097–1106.

Kurata, M., K. Yamamoto, B.S. Moriarity, M. Kitagawa and D.A. Largaespada. 2018. CRISPR/Cas9 library screening for drug target discovery. J. Hum. Genet. 63: 179–186.

Lambert, W.J. 2010. Considerations in developing a target product profile for parenteral pharmaceutical products. AAPS PharmSciTech. 11: 1476–1481.

Landis, M.S., S. Bhattachar, M. Yazdanian and J. Morrison. 2018. Commentary: Why pharmaceutical scientists in early drug discovery are critical for influencing the design and selection of optimal drug candidates. AAPS PharmSciTech. 19: 1–10.

Lhuissier, E., C. Bazille, J. Aury-Landas, N. Girard, J. Pontin, M. Boittin et al. 2017. Identification of an easy to use 3D culture model to investigate invasion and anticancer drug response in chondrosarcomas. BMC Cancer. 17: 490.

Li, J.J. and E.J. Corey (eds.). 2013. Drug Discovery: Practices, Processes, and Perspectives. Wiley, USA, pp. 570.

Lin, D., A.W. Wyatt, H. Xue, Y. Wang, X. Dong, A. Haegert et al. 2014. High fidelity patient-derived xenografts for accelerating prostate cancer discovery and drug development. Cancer Res. 74: 1272–1283.

Lino, C.A., J.C. Harper, J.P. Carney and J.A. Timlin. 2018. Delivering CRISPR: a review of the challenges and approaches. Drug Deliv. 25: 1234–1257.

Liu, X., M.X. Kolpak, J. Wu and G.C. Leo. 2012. Automatic analysis of quantitative NMR data of pharmaceutical compound libraries. Anal. Chem. 84: 6914–6918.

Lok, A.S., F. Zoulim, G. Dusheiko and M.G. Ghany. 2017. Hepatitis B cure: From discovery to regulatory approval. J. Hepatol. 67: 847–861.

Lottenberg, R., J.A. Hall, J.W. 2nd Fenton and C.M. Jackson. 1982. The action of thrombin on peptide p-nitroanilide substrates: hydrolysis of Tos-Gly-Pro-Arg-pNA and D-Phe-Pip-Arg-pNA by human alpha and gamma and bovine alpha and beta-thrombins. Thromb. Res. 28: 313–332.

Ma, B. and R. Nussinov. 2014. Druggable orthosteric and allosteric hot spots to target protein-protein interactions. Curr. Pharm. Des. 20: 1293–1301.

Mandavilli, B.S., R.J. Aggeler and K.M. Chambers. 2018. Tools to measure cell health and cytotoxicity using high content imaging and analysis. Methods Mol. Biol. 1683: 33–46.

Markham, A. 2018. Fostamatinib: First global approval. Drugs. 78: 959–963.

Marshall, L.J., C.P. Austin, W. Casey, S.C. Fitzpatrick and C. Willett. 2018. Recommendations toward a human pathway-based approach to disease research. Drug Discov. Today. In press.

Martinez, N.J., R.R. Asawa, M.G. Cyr, A. Zakharov, D.J. Urban, J.S. Roth et al. 2018. A widely-applicable high-throughput cellular thermal shift assay (CETSA) using split Nano Luciferase. Sci. Rep. 8: 9472.

McCartney, C.E., J.A. MacLeod, P.A. Greer and P.L. Davies. 2018. An easy-to-use FRET protein substrate to detect calpain cleavage *in vitro* and *in vivo*. Biochim. Biophys. Acta. 1865: 221–230.

McNulty, D.E., W.G. Bonnette, H. Qi, L. Wang, T.F. Ho, A. Waszkiewicz et al. 2018. A high-throughput dose-response cellular thermal shift assay for rapid screening of drug target engagement in living cells, exemplified using SMYD3 and IDO1. SLAS Discov. 23: 34–46.

Mervin, L.H., Q. Cao, I.P. Barrett, M.A. Firth, D. Murray, L. McWilliams et al. 2016. Understanding cytotoxicity and cytostaticity in a high-throughput screening collection. ACS Chem. Biol. 11: 3007–3023.

Méry, B., J.B. Guy, A. Vallard, S. Espenel, D. Ardail, C. Rodriguez-Lafrasse et al. 2017. *In vitro* cell death determination for drug discovery: A landscape review of real issues. J. Cell Death. 10: 1.

Mignani, S., J. Rodrigues, H. Tomas, R. Jalal, P.P. Singh, J.P. Majoral et al. 2018. Present drug-likeness filters in medicinal chemistry during the hit and lead optimization process: how far can they be simplified? Drug Discov. Today. 23: 605–615.

Mikami, S., S. Nakamura, T. Ashizawa, I. Nomura, M. Kawasaki, S. Sasaki et al. 2017. Discovery of clinical candidate N-((1S)-1-(3-Fluoro-4-(trifluoromethoxy)phenyl)-2-methoxyethyl)-7-methoxy-2-oxo-2,3-dihydropyrido[2,3-b]pyrazine-4(1H)-carboxamide (TAK-915): A highly potent, selective, and brain-penetrating phosphodiesterase 2A inhibitor for the treatment of cognitive disorders. J. Med. Chem. 60: 7677–7702.

Miranda, C.C., T.G. Fernandes, M.M. Diogo and J.M.S. Cabral. 2018. Towards multi-organoid systems for drug screening applications. Bioengineering (Basel). 5. pii: E49.

Mohs, R.C. and N.H. Greig. 2017. Drug discovery and development: Role of basic biological research. Alzheimers Dement (N Y). 3: 651–657.

Muniz, F.W.M.G., K. Taminski, J. Cavagni, R.K. Celeste, P. Weidlich and C.K. Rösing. 2018. The effect of statins on periodontal treatment-a systematic review with meta-analyses and meta-regression. Clin. Oral. Investig. 22: 671–687.

Neggers, J.E., B. Kwanten, T. Dierckx, H. Noguchi, A. Voet, L. Bral et al. 2018. Target identification of small molecules using large-scale CRISPR-Cas mutagenesis scanning of essential genes. Nat. Commun. 9: 502.

Ng, R. 2015. Drugs: From Discovery to Approval. Wiley-Blackwell, USA, pp. 552.

Niles, A.L., R.A. Moravec and T.L. Riss. 2009. *In vitro* viability and cytotoxicity testing and same-well multi-parametric combinations for high throughput screening. Curr. Chem. Genomics. 3: 33–41.

Noble, M.A., S. Gul, C.S. Verma and K. Brocklehurst. 2000. Ionization characteristics and chemical influences of aspartic acid residue 158 of papain and caricain determined by structure-related kinetic and computational techniques: multiple electrostatic modulators of active-centre chemistry. Biochem. J. 1: 723–733.

O'Duibhir, E., N.O. Carragher and S.M. Pollard. 2017. Accelerating glioblastoma drug discovery: Convergence of patient-derived models, genome editing and phenotypic screening. Mol. Cell Neurosci. 80: 198–207.

Parker, D.L. Jr, S. Walsh, B. Li, E. Kim, A. Sharipour, C. Smith et al. 2015. Rapid development of two factor IXa inhibitors from hit to lead. Bioorg. Med. Chem. Lett. 25: 2321–2325.

Peng, Z. 2013. Very large virtual compound spaces: construction, storage and utility in drug discovery. Drug Discov. Today Technol. 10: e387–e394.

Pérot, S., O. Sperandio, M.A. Miteva, A.C. Camproux and B.O. Villoutreix. 2010. Druggable pockets and binding site centric chemical space: a paradigm shift in drug discovery. Drug Discov. Today. 15: 656–667.

Peters, M.F., S.D. Lamore, L. Guo, C.W. Scott and K.L. Kolaja. 2015. Human stem cell-derived cardiomyocytes in cellular impedance assays: bringing cardiotoxicity screening to the front line. Cardiovasc. Toxicol. 15: 127–139.

Pinitglang, S., A.B. Watts, M. Patel, J.D. Reid, M.A. Noble, S. Gul et al. 1997. A classical enzyme active center motif lacks catalytic competence until modulated electrostatically. Biochemistry. 36: 9968–9982.

Popa-Burke, I. and J. Russell. 2014. Compound precipitation in high-concentration DMSO solutions. J. Biomol. Screen. 19: 1302–1308.

Rawlings, N.D. and G. Salvesen (eds.). 2013. Handbook of Proteolytic Enzymes. Academic Press, USA, pp. 4094.

Regnault, C., D.S. Dheeman and A. Hochstetter. 2018. Microfluidic devices for drug assays. High Throughput. 7: 18.

Ren, Z., D. Tam, Y.Z. Xu, D. Wone, S. Yuan, H.L. Sham et al. 2013. Development of a novel β-secretase binding assay using the AlphaScreen platform. J. Biomol. Screen. 18: 695–704.

Robbins, J.P. and J. Price. 2017. Human induced pluripotent stem cells as a research tool in Alzheimer's disease. Psychol. Med. 47: 2587–2592.

Rouillard, A.D., M.R. Hurle and P. Agarwal. 2018. Systematic interrogation of diverse Omic data reveals interpretable, robust, and generalizable transcriptomic features of clinically successful therapeutic targets. PLoS Comput. Biol. 14: e1006142.

Roy, A. 2018. Early probe and drug discovery in academia: A minireview. High Throughput. 7: 4.

Saravi, S.S.S., S.S.S. Savari, A. Arefidoust and A.R. Dehpour. 2017. The beneficial effects of HMG-CoA reductase inhibitors in the processes of neurodegeneration. Metab. Brain Dis. 32: 949–965.

Schorpp, K., I. Rothenaigner, J. Maier, B. Traenkle, U. Rothbauer and K. Hadian. 2016. A multiplexed high-content screening approach using the chromobody technology to identify cell cycle modulators in living cells. J. Biomol. Screen. 21: 965–977.

Schunkert, H., I.R. König, S. Kathiresan, M.P. Reilly, T.L. Assimes, H. Holm et al. 2011. Large-scale association analysis identifies 13 new susceptibility loci for coronary artery disease. Nat. Genet. 43: 333–338.

Shafaie, S., V. Hutter, M.B. Brown, M.T. Cook and D.Y.S. Chau. 2017. Influence of surface geometry on the culture of human cell lines: A comparative study using flat, round-bottom and v-shaped 96 well plates. PLoS One. 12: e0186799.

Shaik, J.S., M. Ahmad, W. Li, M.E. Rose, L.M. Foley, T.K. Hitchens et al. 2013. Soluble epoxide hydrolase inhibitor trans-4-[4-(3-adamantan-1-yl-ureido)-cyclohexyloxy]-benzoic acid is neuroprotective in rat model of ischemic stroke. Am. J. Physiol. Heart Circ. Physiol. 305: H1605–H1613.

Shapiro, M.D., H. Tavori and S. Fazio. 2018. PCSK9: From basic science discoveries to clinical trials. Circ. Res. 122: 1420.

Shirai, J., Y. Tomata, M. Kono, A. Ochida, Y. Fukase, A. Sato et al. 2018. Discovery of orally efficacious RORγt inverse agonists, part 1: Identification of novel phenylglycinamides as lead scaffolds. Bioorg. Med. Chem. 26: 483–500.

Shoji, A., Y. Suenaga, A. Hosaka, Y. Ishida, A. Yanagida and M. Sugawara. 2017. Inhibitory assay for degradation of collagen IV by cathepsin B with a surface plasmon resonance sensor. J. Pharm. Biomed. Anal. 145: 79–83.

Shu, L., M. Blencowe and X. Yang. 2018. Translating GWAS findings to novel therapeutic targets for coronary artery disease. Front Cardiovasc. Med. 5: 56.

Slim, R., M. Toborek, L.W. Robertson, H.J. Lehmler and B. Hennig. 2000. Cellular glutathione status modulates polychlorinated biphenyl-induced stress response and apoptosis in vascular endothelial cells. Toxicol. Appl. Pharmacol. 166: 36–42.

Smith, K., F. Piccinini, T. Balassa, K. Koos, T. Danka, H. Azizpour et al. 2018. Phenotypic image analysis software tools for exploring and understanding big image data from cell-based assays. Cell Syst. 6: 636–653.

Spear, K.L. and S.P. Brown. 2017. The evolution of library design: crafting smart compound collections for phenotypic screens. Drug Discov. Today Technol. 23: 61–67.

Storer, R.I., A. Pike, N.A. Swain, A.J. Alexandrou, B.M. Bechle, D.C. Blakemore et al. 2017. Highly potent and selective NaV1.7 inhibitors for use as intravenous agents and chemical probes. Bioorg. Med. Chem. Lett. 27: 4805–4811.

Sud, A., B. Kinnersley and R.S. Houlston. 2017. Genome-wide association studies of cancer: current insights and future perspectives. Nat. Rev. Cancer. 17: 692–704.

Swinney, D.C. and J. Anthony. 2011. How were new medicines discovered? Nat. Rev. Drug Discov. 10: 507–519.

Taylor, I.R., B.M. Dunyak, T. Komiyama, H. Shao, X. Ran, V.A. Assimon et al. 2018. High-throughput screen for inhibitors of protein-protein interactions in a reconstituted heat shock protein 70 (Hsp70) complex. J. Biol. Chem. 293: 4014–4025.

Thompson, A.M., P.D. O'Connor, A.J. Marshall, A. Blaser, V. Yardley, L. Maes et al. 2018. Development of (6 R)-2-Nitro-6-[4-(trifluoromethoxy)phenoxy]-6,7-dihydro-5 H-imidazo[2,1- b][1,3]oxazine (DNDI-8219): A new lead for visceral leishmaniasis. J. Med. Chem. 61: 2329–2352.

Thong, B., J. Pilling, E. Ainscow, R. Beri and J. Unitt. 2011. Development and validation of a simple cell-based fluorescence assay for dipeptidyl peptidase 1 (DPP1) activity. J. Biomol. Screen. 16: 36–43.

Thorne, N., M. Shen, W.A. Lea, A. Simeonov, S. Lovell, D.S. Auld et al. 2012. Firefly luciferase in chemical biology: a compendium of inhibitors, mechanistic evaluation of chemotypes, and suggested use as a reporter. Chem. Biol. 19: 1060–1072.

Tobinaga, H., T. Kameyama, M. Oohara, N. Kobayashi, M. Ohdan, N. Ishizuka et al. 2018. Pyrrolinone derivatives as a new class of P2X3 receptor antagonists. Part 1: Initial structure-activity relationship studies of a hit from a high throughput screening. Bioorg. Med. Chem. Lett. 28: 2338–2342.

Trumpi, K., D.A. Egan, T.T. Vellinga, I.H. Borel Rinkes and O. Kranenburg. 2015. Paired image- and FACS-based toxicity assays for high content screening of spheroid-type tumor cell cultures. FEBS Open Bio. 5: 85–90.

Turk, B. 2006. Targeting proteases: successes, failures and future prospects. Nat. Rev. Drug Discov. 5: 785.

Uliassi, E., L. Piazzi, F. Belluti, A. Mazzanti, M. Kaiser, R. Brun et al. 2018. Development of a focused library of triazole-linked privileged-structure-based conjugates leading to the discovery of novel phenotypic hits against protozoan parasitic infections. ChemMedChem. 13: 678–683.

Vaswani, R.G., V.S. Gehling, L.A. Dakin, A.S. Cook, C.G. Nasveschuk, M. Duplessis et al. 2016. Identification of (R)-N-((4-Methoxy-6-methyl-2-oxo-1,2-dihydropyridin-3-yl)methyl)-2-methyl-1-(1-(1-(2,2,2-trifluoroethyl)piperidin-4-yl)ethyl)-1H-indole-3-carboxamide (CPI-1205), a potent and selective inhibitor of histone methyltransferase EZH2, Suitable for phase I clinical trials for B-Cell lymphomas. J. Med. Chem. 59: 9928–9941.

Venter, J.C., M.D. Adams, E.W. Myers, P.W. Li, R.J. Mural, G.G. Sutton et al. 2001. The sequence of the human genome. Science. 291: 1304–1351.

Vichai, V. and K. Kirtikara. 2006. Sulforhodamine B colorimetric assay for cytotoxicity screening. Nat. Protoc. 1: 1112–1116.

Watmuff, B., B. Liu and R. Karmacharya. 2017. Stem cell-derived neurons in the development of targeted treatment for schizophrenia and bipolar disorder. Pharmacogenomics. 18: 471–479.

Weeber, F., S.N. Ooft, K.K. Dijkstra and E.E. Voest. 2017. Tumor organoids as a pre-clinical cancer model for drug discovery. Cell Chem. Biol. 24: 1092–1100.

Wenthur, C.J., P.R. Gentry, T.P. Mathews and C.W. Lindsley. 2014. Drugs for allosteric sites on receptors. Annu. Rev. Pharmacol. Toxicol. 54: 165–184.

Wijmenga, C. and A. Zhernakova. 2018. The importance of cohort studies in the post-GWAS era. Nat. Genet. 50: 322–328.

Wong, A.I. and D. Huang. 2014. Assessment of the degree of interference of polyphenolic compounds on glucose oxidation/peroxidase assay. J. Agric. Food Chem. 62: 4571–4576.

Wu, Y., Z. Jiang, Z. Li, J. Gu, Q. You and X. Zhang. 2018. Click chemistry-based discovery of [3-Hydroxy-5-(1H-1,2,3-triazol-4-yl)picolinoyl]glycines as orally active hypoxia-inducing factor prolyl hydroxylase inhibitors with favorable safety profiles for the treatment of anemia. J. Med. Chem. 61: 5332–5349.

Wyatt, P.G., I.H. Gilbert, K.D. Read and A.H. Fairlamb. 2011. Target validation: linking target and chemical properties to desired product profile. Curr. Top. Med. Chem. 11: 1275–1283.

Xia, J., H. Hu, W. Xue, X.S. Wang and S. Wu. 2018. The discovery of novel HDAC3 inhibitors via virtual screening and *in vitro* bioassay. J. Enzyme. Inhib. Med. Chem. 33: 525–535.

Xia, X. and S.T. Wong. 2012. Concise review: a high-content screening approach to stem cell research and drug discovery. Stem Cells. 30: 1800–1807.

Xie, Z., D. Cheng, L. Luo, G. Shen, S. Pan, Y. Pan et al. 2018. Design, synthesis and biological evaluation of 4-bromo-N-(3,5-dimethoxyphenyl)benzamide derivatives as novel FGFR1 inhibitors for treatment of non-small cell lung cancer. J. Enzyme. Inhib. Med. Chem. 33: 905–919.

Xu, C., O. Nikolova, R.S. Basom, R.M. Mitchell, R. Shaw, R.D. Moser et al. 2018. Functional precision medicine identifies novel druggable targets and therapeutic options in head and neck cancer. Clin. Cancer Res. 24: 2828–2843.

Yang, K., K. Nong, Q. Gu, J. Dong and J. Wang. 2018. Discovery of N-hydroxy-3-alkoxybenzamides as direct acid sphingomyelinase inhibitors using a ligand-based pharmacophore model. Eur. J. Med. Chem. 151: 389–400.

Zaleska, M., O. Mozenska and J. Bil. 2018. Statins use and cancer: an update. Future Oncol. 14: 1497–1509.

Zaragoza-Sundqvist, M., H. Eriksson, M. Rohman and P.J. Greasley. 2009. High-quality cost-effective compound management support for HTS. J. Biomol. Screen. 14: 509–514.

Zhang, C.H., K. Chen, Y. Jiao, L.L. Li, Y.P. Li, R.J. Zhang et al. 2016. From lead to drug candidate: Optimization of 3-(Phenylethynyl)-1H-pyrazolo[3,4-d]pyrimidin-4-amine derivatives as agents for the treatment of triple negative breast cancer. J. Med. Chem. 59: 9788–9805.

Zhang, G., J. Xing, Y. Wang, L. Wang, Y. Ye, D. Lu et al. 2018. Discovery of novel inhibitors of Indoleamine 2,3-Dioxygenase 1 through structure-based virtual screening. Front Pharmacol. 29: 9–277.

Zhang, Y., R. Chen, H. Ma and S. Chen. 2015. Isolation and identification of dipeptidyl peptidase IV-Inhibitory peptides from trypsin/chymotrypsin-treated goat milk casein hydrolysates by 2D-TLC and LC-MS/MS. J. Agric. Food Chem. 63: 8819–8828.

Zimmermann, G. and D. Neri. 2016. DNA-encoded chemical libraries: foundations and applications in lead discovery. Drug Discov. Today. 21: 1828–1834.

Chapter **2**

The Application of Fragment-based Approaches to the Discovery of Drugs for Neglected Tropical Diseases

Christina Spry[1],* and *Anthony G. Coyne*[2]

Introduction

The term *neglected tropical disease* (NTD) is used to describe a diverse collection of communicable diseases prevalent in tropical and subtropical regions, which predominantly affect the poor. The World Health Organization (WHO) currently identifies a set of twenty diseases,[†] chiefly caused by parasites, bacteria and viruses, as priority NTDs (WHO 2018a). Although these diseases have not attained the notoriety of the "big three" infectious diseases—malaria, tuberculosis and HIV—most are highly debilitating, several cause chronic diseases, and some are lethal. They currently affect more than a billion people in 149 countries (WHO 2018a) and impart a substantial economic and social burden, thereby perpetuating the cycle of poverty and disease. Through implementation of five main strategies (preventative chemotherapy, innovative and intensified disease management, vector ecology and management, veterinary public health services and the provision of safe water, sanitation and hygiene), great strides have been made toward the goals of controlling, eliminating and eradicating NTDs set forth by the WHO in 2012 (WHO 2017). However, in order to meet targets set for 2020 and beyond, it has become evident that new control tools, including drugs, are needed. For some NTDs no safe, affordable and orally active drugs are available, and where they are, alternatives are required for combination therapies and as backups for when efficacy is lost and/or resistance emerges. Despite the high NTD burden, in the period between 2000 and 2011, just 0.6% of new therapeutics were for neglected diseases and none of these were new chemical entities (Pedrique et al. 2013), highlighting the unmet medical need.

---

[1] Research School of Biology, The Australian National University, ACT, 2601, Australia.
[2] Department of Chemistry, University of Cambridge, Cambridge, CB2 1EW, United Kingdom.
* Corresponding author: christina.spry@anu.edu.au
[†] At of the time of publication, the WHO NTD portfolio includes: (1) Buruli ulcer, (2) Chagas disease, (3) Dengue and Chikungunya, (4) Dracunculiasis, (5) Echinococcosis, (6) Foodborne trematodiases, (7) Human African trypanosomiasis, (8) Leishmaniasis, (9) Leprosy, (10) Lymphatic filariasis, (11) Mycetoma, chromoblastomycosis and other deep mycoses, (12) Onchocerciasis, (13) Rabies, (14) Scabies and other ectoparasites, (15) Schistosomiasis, (16) Soil-transmitted helminthiases, (17) Snakebite envenoming, (18) Taeniasis, (19) Trachoma, and (20) Yaws.

Phenotypic (or whole-cell) screening has dominated over target-based approaches in drug discovery for NTDs (Gilbert 2013, Martin-Plaza and Chatelain 2015, Behnam et al. 2016). There are two main reasons:

(i) The success of any target-based approach is underpinned by the careful choice of a well-validated drug target. In the case of NTDs, few validated drug targets have been identified. This, at least in part, is because the genetic tools for target validation in the pathogens causing NTDs (except perhaps *Trypanosoma brucei*) are lacking, and the modes of action of existing drugs are poorly understood (Gilbert 2013).

(ii) In phenotypic screens, molecules with access to a given molecular target, which possess activity in the context of the cell (where permeability barriers and efflux mechanisms exist and mechanisms of metabolic plasticity and regulation operate), are identified from the onset. This is particularly advantageous for pathogens with intracellular stages such as *Leishmania* (the cause of leishmaniasis).

Despite the above advantages of phenotypic screening for hit identification, subsequent hit-to-lead and lead optimization can be a significant challenge. Elucidation of the molecular target(s) of a hit greatly facilitates hit-to-lead optimization, however, this is no trivial task. Metabolomic analysis is one approach that has been used successfully to provide clues to the mode of action of antitrypanosomal and antileishmanial compounds (Vincent and Barrett 2015). Nonetheless, even when the molecular target of a phenotypic screening hit can be confidently identified, improving target affinity while also achieving the required drug-like properties is challenging and requires intensive medicinal chemistry efforts.

Over the past two decades, fragment-based approaches have gained traction as alternative and complementary hit finding mechanisms to target-based and phenotypic high-throughput screening (HTS) (Erlanson et al. 2016). By contrast with HTS, which involves screening of a large library (typically tens to hundreds of thousands) of drug-like compounds in a high-throughput assay, a classical fragment-based approach begins with the screening of a small library (typically 1000–5000) of fragments (chemicals of low molecular weight and complexity), primarily using biophysical techniques. The goal of a fragment screen is to identify chemicals that bind a target efficiently. As a consequence of their low molecular weight and size, fragments invariably bind with low affinity, and therefore metrics are used that attempt to normalize affinity for properties such as molecular weight. The most popular metric is ligand efficiency (LE), in which the free energy of binding of a compound is divided by the number of non-hydrogen atoms (NHA) that compound has (reported in units of $kcal.mol^{-1}.NHA^{-1}$) (Hopkins et al. 2004). Provided sufficient structural information is available, weakly, but efficiently binding fragment hits can be elaborated iteratively into higher affinity binders with drug-like properties. Fragments are commonly elaborated by *growing* (the iterative addition of moieties designed to pick up interactions in neighboring regions of a binding site), *merging* (the amalgamation of fragments binding in overlapping binding sites into a single molecule), or *linking* (the fusion of two fragments binding in adjacent regions of a binding site through a chemical linker). For a review of fragment screening approaches and discussion of fragment elaboration strategies, the reader is referred to Scott et al. (2012).

Although typically only compatible with target-based approaches, fragment-based approaches have a number of advantages over HTS approaches, the first of which is that fragments form high quality interactions with a target. This stems from their low complexity and, as a consequence, the greater probability they will complement a binding pocket as compared with more complex drug-like molecules where the optimal binding modes of key moieties may be hindered by unfavorable interactions with other moieties (Hann et al. 2001). The second reason is that fragments are efficient probes of chemical space; the chemical space associated with molecules of drug-like size is estimated to be 13 orders of magnitude greater than that associated with fragment-sized chemicals (Ruddigkeit et al. 2012, Erlanson et al. 2016). Hence a small fragment library more efficiently samples the fragment chemical space than a large library of drug-like compounds samples drug-like chemical space. For this reason, fragment-based approaches offer a means by which to overcome the chemical diversity limitations of HTS libraries. Higher hit rates are encountered in fragment-based approaches, providing more choice for chemical starting points, and smaller and more easily maintained libraries are used, facilitating implementation of fragment-based approaches also in an academic setting. Fragment-based approaches are now used widely in academia and industry and have produced more than 45 clinical candidates and at least four drugs approved by the US Food and Drug Administration (Erlanson et al. 2016, Peplow 2017, Erlanson 2019).

In this chapter, we describe how fragment-based approaches are being applied in projects aimed at the discovery of new drugs for NTDs, either alone or in conjunction with HTS. The examples discussed, which have been classified according to pathogen, highlight the power of fragment-based approaches to reveal binding hot-spots and novel allosteric binding sites, and to identify efficient starting points for drug discovery. They also show how fragment-based approaches can facilitate optimization of hits identified by other means and enable careful control of drug-like properties during the optimization of a chemical series.

Fragment-based Approaches in Antitrypanosomal Drug Discovery

Chagas disease and Sleeping Sickness are two NTDs caused by protozoan parasites of the genus *Trypanosoma*. Chagas disease, which is also known as American trypanosomiasis, affects approximately 6–7 million people, predominantly in Latin America (although increasing numbers of cases are being detected elsewhere around the world (Schmunis and Yadon 2010)), and results in over 10,000 deaths annually (WHO 2017, 2018b). The disease is caused by *Trypanosoma cruzi*, which is primarily transmitted by the triatomine bug, but can also be transmitted through blood transfusion from infected donors, or from mother to child during pregnancy or childbirth. There is no vaccine for Chagas disease, but the disease can be cured with the antiparasitic drugs benznidazole or nifurtimox if treatment is initiated during onset of the acute phase of the disease. Unfortunately, however, drug efficacy diminishes with time since infection and 40% of patients suffer from adverse effects due to treatment (WHO 2017). Hence, new drugs with improved safety and efficacy are needed.

Sleeping Sickness, which is also known as Human African trypanosomiasis or HAT, is caused by two subspecies of *T. brucei* (*T. b. gambiense* and *T. b. rhodesiense*) that are transmitted predominantly through the bite of an infected tsetse fly. In the first stage of the disease, parasites multiply in subcutaneous tissues, blood and lymph, before crossing the blood-brain barrier and infecting the central nervous system in the second stage of the disease. Without treatment, sleeping sickness is invariably fatal (WHO 2017). Currently, five drugs, each with undesirable side effects, are available for the treatment of sleeping sickness, and the stage of the disease dictates which should be administered. As for Chagas disease, early treatment provides better prospects for a cure. Unfortunately, the drugs required to treat the second stage of the disease are challenging to administer and/or toxic (and, in some cases, lethal) (WHO 2018c). Hence, although the incidence of sleeping sickness has been declining due to sustained control efforts, and in 2017 there were just 1447 new cases (WHO 2018d), there is a need for safe and effective new drugs.

As illustrated in the examples highlighted below, fragment-based approaches have been utilized in several antitrypanosomal drug discovery projects spanning more than two decades. They have revealed binding hot spots and previously unidentified binding pockets, provided chemical starting points for novel inhibitors (only some of which have been pursued), and facilitated optimization of antitrypanosomal HTS hits.

Targeting the peroxin 5-peroxin 14 interaction using a fragment-guided approach

Trypanosomes and other kinetoplastids uniquely possess a membrane-bound, peroxisomal-like organelle known as a glycosome, in which glucose metabolism and other metabolic reactions occur (Haanstra et al. 2016). Biogenesis of this organelle depends on proteins called peroxins or PEX. For example, the import receptor PEX5 mediates import of glycosomal enzymes from the cytoplasm into the organelle through a process dependent on an interaction with the N-terminus of PEX14, a glycosomal-membrane associated protein (Haanstra et al. 2016). After determining the solution NMR structure of the N-terminal domain of *T. brucei* PEX14 (*Tb*PEX14) that interacts with the intrinsically-disordered N-terminus of PEX5, Dawidowski et al. (2017) embarked on an *in silico* screen of a subset of the ZINC library. In doing so, they identified a pyrazolo[4,3-*c*]pyridine derivative (**1**, Figure 1) that binds the N-terminus of PEX14 with modest affinity, disrupts its interaction with PEX5 ($K_i = 61.6 \mu M$, LE = 0.19), and kills blood-stage *T. brucei* ($EC_{50} = 21 \mu M$) more effectively than mammalian cells. The authors thereafter used a fragment-based approach to facilitate optimization of this inhibitor. To guide the design of inhibitors with improved affinity, they screened an in-house library of 1500 fragments (initially in cocktails of five, each at a concentration of 1 mM) for binding to ^{15}N-labeled PEX14 using ^{1}H-^{15}N-Heteronuclear Multiple-Quantum Correlation (HMQC) NMR. This screen yielded twelve fragments binding with K_D values below 2 mM and revealed a tendency of the protein to bind fused bicyclic aromatic ring systems (Table 1). This in turn led the researchers

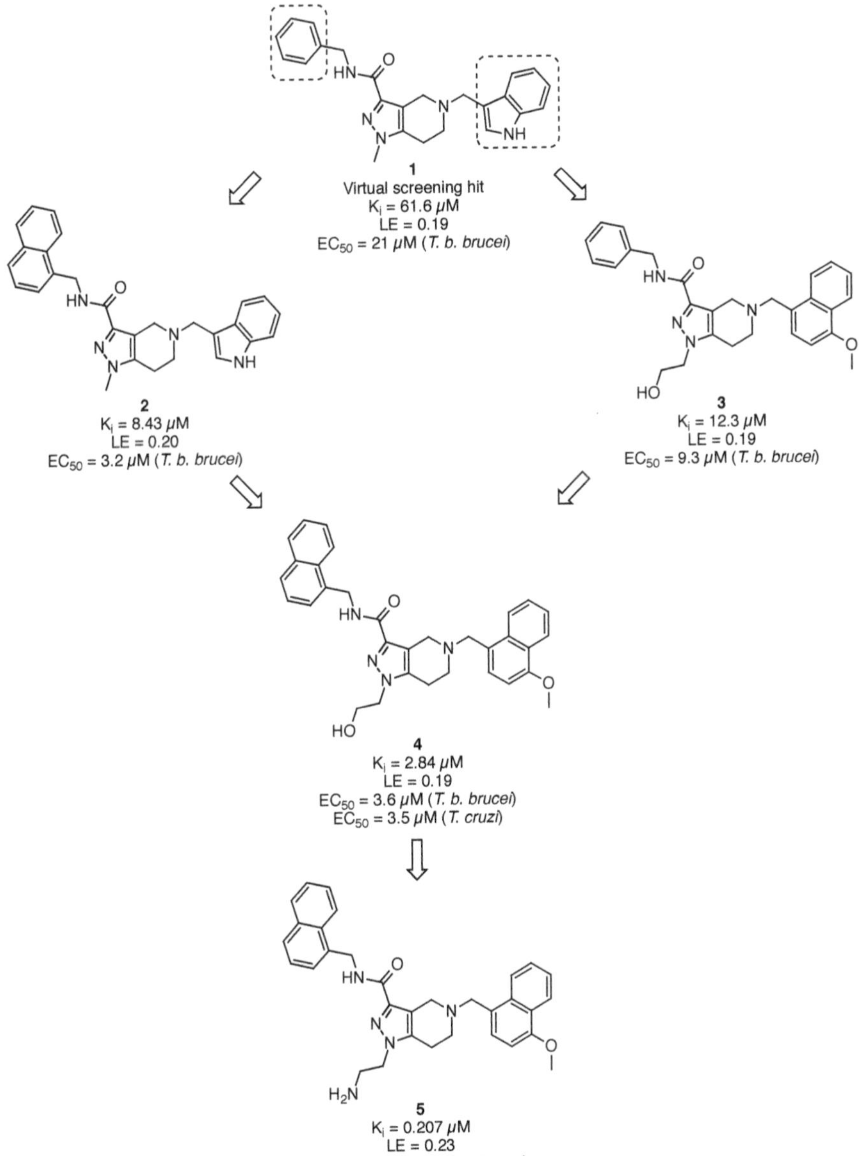

Figure 1. Fragment-guided optimization of an inhibitor of the interaction between *T. brucei* PEX14 and PEX5 identified in a virtual screen. Terminal aromatic moieties of virtual screening hit **1** (dashed rectangles) were replaced with naphthyl moieties, a common scaffold among the fragment hits (Table 1). K_i, inhibition constant; LE, ligand efficiency = $(-RT\ln(K_i))$/NHA, in kcal.mol^{-1}.NHA^{-1}; EC_{50}, half maximal effective concentration as measured in whole-cell assays.

Table 1. Examples of fragment-based approaches applied to antitrypanosomal drug discovery.

Target	Approach	Selected fragment hit(s)	Elaborated compound(s)	Reference
*Tb*PEX14-PEX5	Fragment-guided optimization. ^{1}H-^{15}N-HMQC-based screen of 1500 fragments performed		**5** ^{a}K$_i$ = 0.207 μM ^{b}LE = 0.23 ^{c}EC$_{50}$ (*T. b. brucei*) = 0.186 μM EC$_{50}$ (*T. cruzi*) = 0.57 μM	Figure 1 Dawidowski et al. (2017)
*Tc*SpdSyn	DSF and SPR-based fragment screen, followed by enzyme assay and X-ray crystallography	^{d}IC$_{50}$ = 180 μM LE = 0.46 IC$_{50}$ = 460 μM LE = 0.41 IC$_{50}$ = 9.1 μM LE = 0.33 IC$_{50}$ = 0.051 μM LE = 0.83	N/A	Amano et al. (2015)

Table 1 contd. ...

...Table 1 contd.

Target	Approach	Selected fragment hit(s)	Elaborated compound(s)	Reference
*Tb*PDEB1	Enzyme assay (luminescence-based) screen of 1040 fragments followed by whole-cell tests	IC$_{50}$ = 50 µM LE = 0.34 IC$_{50}$ = 12.5 µM LE = 0.32 IC$_{50}$ = 63 µM LE = 0.22 IC$_{50}$ = 100 µM LE = 0.45	*a*IC$_{50}$ (parasite) = 2.0–7.9 µM IC$_{50}$ (parasite) = 0.2–63 µM	Blaazer et al. (2015)
	Fragment growing guided by scintillation proximity assay data	**6** IC$_{50}$ = 12 µM LE = 0.30	**14** IC$_{50}$ (*Tb*PDEB1)= 49 nM IC$_{50}$ (*T. brucei*) = 520 nM LE = 0.25	Figure 2 Orrling et al. (2012)

Table 1 contd. ...

...Table 1 contd.

Target	Approach	Selected fragment hit(s)	Elaborated compound(s)	Reference
*Tc*HisRS	X-ray crystallography-based screen of 680 fragments, followed by DSF and aminoacylation assay. Fragment growing and tethering	**15** $IC_{50} > 2$ mM LE < 0.33	**18** $IC_{50} = 0.85$ mM LE = 0.28 **19** $IC_{50} = 1.65$ mM LE = 0.24	Figure 3 Koh et al. (2015)
Rhodesain	Fragment tethering. Enzyme assay-based screen of 200 cysteine-reactive fragments	$k_{inact}/K_i = 18.3$ M^{-1}.s^{-1} IC_{50} (*T. brucei*) = 30 μM $K_{inact}/K_i = 13.2$ M^{-1}.s^{-1} IC_{50} (*T. brucei*) = 43 μM	N/A	McShan et al. (2015)
*Tb*RFK	Ultrafiltration-based screen of 134 fragments		N/A	Shibata et al. (2011)
*gTb*REL1	*In silico* (CrystalDock) fragment hit identification and fragment-assisted optimization			Durrant et al. (2011)

Table 1 contd. ...

...Table 1 contd.

Target	Approach	Selected fragment hit(s)	Elaborated compound(s)	Reference
*Tb*PTR1	Virtual screen of 26,084 fragments. Prioritized fragments tested in enzyme assay	 **20** $^hK_i^{app} = 10.6$ μM LE = 0.62	 **23** $K_i^{app} = 0.007$ μM LE = 0.44 $EC_{50} = 10$ μM	Figure 4 Mpamhanga et al. (2009), Spinks et al. (2011)
*Tb*6PGDH	Virtual screen of 64,000 fragments. Prioritized fragments tested in enzyme assay	 $IC_{50} = 45$ μM LE = 0.40 $IC_{50} = 43$ μM LE = 0.66 $IC_{50} = 28$ μM LE = 0.52	N/A	Ruda et al. (2010)
*Tb*NDRT	X-ray crystallographic fragment screen of 304 fragments	 EC_{50} (*T. brucei*) = 0.12 mM EC_{50} (*T. brucei*) = 0.25 mM EC_{50} (*T. brucei*) = 0.41 mM EC_{50} (*T. brucei*) = 1.3 mM	N/A	Verlinde et al. (2009), Bosch et al. (2006)

[a]K_i, inhibition constant; [b]LE, ligand efficiency = (−RTln(K_D/K_i/IC_{50}))/NHA, in kcal.mol[−1].NHA[−1]; [c]EC_{50}, half maximal effective concentration as measured in whole-cell assays; [d]IC_{50}, concentration causing 50% inhibition as measured in enzyme assays, unless otherwise specified; [e]Range of IC_{50} values measured in whole-cell assays against *T. brucei, T. cruzi, L. infantum, P. falciparum*; [f]k_{inact}, rate of inactivation; [g]Compounds shown in the *Tb*REL1 row are *in silico* predicted binders. Binding has not been experimentally confirmed; [h]K_i^{app}, the apparent value of K_i.

to introduce naphthyl substituents in place of two terminal aromatic moieties that were predicted by docking to bind in adjacent hydrophobic cavities that accommodate two aromatic residues of PEX5. Introduction of one or two naphthyl moieties improved inhibitory activity in an AlphaScreen-based competition assay (K_i = 8.4 or 12.3 μM for compounds **2** and **3**, respectively, each with a single naphthyl substituent, or 2.8 μM for compound **4**, which has two naphthyl moieties) and also enhanced trypanocidal activity (EC_{50} = 3.2 and 9.3 μM for compounds **2** and **3**, respectively, or 3.6 μM for compound **4**) (Figure 1). X-ray crystal structures of the optimized inhibitors showed that the naphthyl rings filled the hydrophobic pockets as intended. Replacement of a hydroxyl moiety of compound **4** with an amine, produced compound **5**, which inhibits the PEX14-PEX5 interaction with a K_i of 207 nM (LE = 0.23) and demonstrates antitrypanocidal activity against *T. b. brucei*, *T. b. rhodesiense* and the intracellular amastigote form of *T. cruzi* with EC_{50} values of 0.186, 0.021 and 0.57 μM, respectively. Key differences between the N-termini of PEX14 from trypanosomes and humans were considered during inhibitor design and, favorably, compound **5** shows selectivity for trypanosomal PEX14 over the human variant (IC_{50} (*T. brucei* PEX14) = 1.34 μM vs IC_{50} (human PEX14) = 37.8 μM), and lower toxicity against mammalian cell lines tested.

Dawidowski et al. (2017) went on to show that in the presence of compound **5**, glycosomal enzymes mislocalize to the cytosol and trypanosomal ATP levels are reduced as was predicted if hexokinase and phosphofructokinase mislocalize, and glucose phosphorylation is, as a consequence, unregulated. These data, and the observed correlation between affinity for PEX14 and antitrypanosomal activity for the pyrazolo[4,3-*c*]pyridine derivatives tested, are consistent with the antitrypansomal activity of the PEX14-PEX5 inhibitors being on target, and hence validate PEX5-PEX14 as a trypanosomal drug target. Following modification of the lead PEX5-PEX14 inhibitor to reduce plasma protein binding, antitrypanosomal activity could be observed also in a murine model of HAT. A reduction in parasitemia, with no adverse effects on the mice, was observed when the compound was administered at 100 mg/kg twice a day for five days. Further optimization of absorption, distribution, metabolism and excretion (ADME) properties is expected to yield a clinical candidate.

Targeting spermidine synthase

Trypanothione is a bis(gluthionyl)-spermidine conjugate essential for, and unique to, kinetoplastids such as trypanosomes and leishmania (Fairlamb et al. 1985). It functions to protect the cells from oxidative stress (Krauth-Siegel and Comini 2008). In light of the parasites' requirement for trypanothione, the enzymes involved in its biosynthesis—including spermidine synthase, which catalyses the conversion of putrescine to spermidine—have attracted attention as potential antiparasitic drug targets (Birkholtz et al. 2011). Using a fragment-based approach, Amano et al. (2015) set out to identify novel inhibitors of *T. cruzi* spermidine synthase (*Tc*SpdSyn). In order to target the putrescine binding site of *Tc*SpdSyn, rather than the pocket that tightly binds the decarboxylated *S*-adenosyl-L-methionine (dcSAM) also required for the reaction, fragment screening was performed in the presence of dcSAM. In their approach, fragments were screened both by differential scanning fluorimetry (DSF; at a concentration of 2 mM) and surface plasmon resonance (SPR; at a concentration of 250 μM). Fragments observed to stabilize the protein to thermal-denaturation in the DSF assay and/or bind the protein in the SPR assay were selected for *Tc*SpdSyn crystal soaking experiments and evaluation of inhibitory activity in an enzyme assay. Amano et al. (2015) describe co-crystal structures of six fragments identified in the screen. Two of the fragment hits were observed to bind the putrescine-binding pocket, interacting with both the protein and bound dcSAM. These fragments inhibit the enzyme with IC_{50} values of 180 and 460 μM, corresponding to LE values of 0.46 and 0.41, respectively (Table 1). Interestingly, the remaining four fragment hits were observed to bind at the interface of the two monomers in the *Tc*SpdSyn dimer, with one fragment binding covalently. All four of the interface-binding fragments inhibit the enzyme allosterically. The most potent of the non-covalently bound fragments binding at the interface inhibits the enzyme with an IC_{50} value of 9.1 μM (LE = 0.33), and the covalently bound fragment, which was observed to bind twice (forming disulfide bonds with Cys239 of each monomer) inhibits *Tc*SpdSyn with an IC_{50} value of 0.051 μM (LE = 0.83) (Table 1). This study not only identified ligand efficient fragments that could serve as starting points for novel *Tc*SpdSyn inhibitors, but also revealed two binding sites, including an allosteric site composed of residues not conserved between *Tc*SpdSyn and its human orthologue, that could be exploited for further structure-based design of selective *Tc*SpdSyn inhibitors.

Targeting 3',5'-cyclic nucleotide phosphodiesterase

Cyclic nucleotide phosphodiesterases (PDEs) play a key role in regulating levels of cyclic nucleotides in cells through hydrolysis of the phosphodiester bond of cAMP and/or cGMP. Two 3',5'-cyclic nucleotide phosphodiesterases (PDEB1 and B2, which are 76.2% similar to each other) have been shown using RNAi (Oberholzer et al. 2007), as well as with a small molecule inhibitor (de Koning et al. 2012), to be essential for proliferation of *T. brucei in vitro* and *in vivo* when knocked down together. Two distinct fragment-based approaches targeting these enzymes have been published.

Blaazer et al. (2015) screened a commercially available library of 1040 fragments (with slightly higher molecular weight and complexity than a rule-of-three compliant fragment library) against *T. brucei* PDEB1 (*Tb*PDEB1) using a luminescence-based biochemical assay. In parallel, fragments were tested against a human PDE (PDE4D) in order to facilitate prioritization of fragment hits selective for the parasite enzyme. A set of twelve fragments that inhibit *Tb*PDEB1 by more than 90% at a concentration of 200 μM was identified in the screen, as was a set of seven fragments that show selectivity for *Tb*PDEB1 over human PDE4D. Blaazer et al. (2015) focused on a set of four fragment hits (Table 1) that shared similarity with the scaffolds of known drugs. These fragments, along with analogues of each chosen from in-house libraries of drug-like compounds, were then tested for whole-cell activity against a panel of parasites (*T. brucei, T. cruzi, Leishmania infantum* and *Plasmodium falciparum*) as well as human cells. The two fragment hits with the highest molecular weight (which share a biphenyl core) showed antiparasitic activity against multiple parasites, as did a number of analogues. Two analogues (Table 1) with improved antiparasitic activity (meeting or surpassing that of benznidazole and miltefosine against *T. cruzi* and *L. infantum*, respectively) and selectivity are under further investigation (Blaazer et al. 2015). Whether the antiparasitic effect of these compounds is a consequence of PDE inhibition remains to be reported.

Orrling et al. (2012) identified a catechol pyrazolinone fragment (compound **6**, Figure 2a) that inhibits *Tb*PDEB1 with an IC_{50} value of 12 μM (LE = 0.30) in a follow up of chemotypes related to a HTS hit (compound **7**, Figure 2b; IC_{50} (*Tb*PDEB1) = 4 nM, LE = 0.27, IC_{50} (*T. brucei*) = 80 nM) (Orrling et al. 2012). The fragment carries multiple structural features present in known inhibitors of *T. brucei* (compound **8**, Figure 2b) or human PDEs (compounds **9** and **10**, Figure 2b), enzymes that have been extensively studied as drug targets for human diseases. Orrling et al. (2012) performed docking experiments with a homology model of *Tb*PDEB1 based on the structure of *Leishmania major* PDEB1 (which shares 66% sequence identity), to predict how the fragment and related human PDE inhibitors bind the enzyme. Based on docking poses, the researchers identified two opportunities for growth of the fragment—from the pyrazolinone nitrogen, and through replacement of the cyclopentyl ring, which was positioned at the entrance to a parasite-specific pocket named the P-pocket. Growth of the fragment from the pyrazolinone nitrogen through introduction of an aliphatic substituent (namely a cycloheptyl moiety) increased potency against *Tb*PDEB1 in a scintillation proximity assay (IC_{50} = 0.41 μM, LE = 0.30); however, this molecule (compound **11**, Figure 2c), like the parent fragment, lacked whole-cell activity. Replacement of the cyclopentyl moiety with a benzyl moiety increased the potency against the enzyme just twofold (compound **12**, IC_{50} = 6.3 μM, LE = 0.30) but, encouragingly, conferred activity against the parasite (IC_{50} = 8.6 μM). Furthermore, introduced together, as in compound **13**, these two modifications yielded an inhibitor with IC_{50} values of 0.5 μM (LE = 0.28) and 6.3 μM against the enzyme and parasite, respectively. Encouragingly, compound **13** was without effect on a human fibroblast cell line at the concentrations tested. Further chemical synthesis was focused on growing the molecule to pick up interactions in the P-pocket. Inspired by the structure of HTS hit **7**, a butyloxy linker was introduced between the phenyl moieties and a tetrazole substituent was introduced (compound **14**). This increased the potency against both *Tb*PDEB1 and *T. brucei* (IC_{50} = 0.049 μM (LE = 0.25) and 0.52 μM, respectively). Although the compound was also a potent inhibitor of a panel of human PDEs it showed selectivity at the whole-cell level (IC_{50} (human fetal lung fibroblasts) > 64 μM). Orrling et al. (2012) additionally presented evidence that the antitrypanosomal activity of the final compound was indeed a consequence of PDE inhibition; the compound was shown

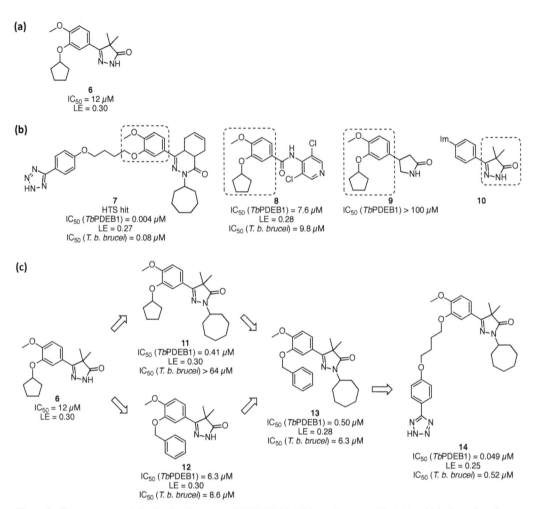

Figure 2. Fragment growth in the development of *Tb*PDEB1 inhibitors. Fragment hit **6 (a)**, which shares key features of HTS hit **7** and other known *Tb*PDEB1 (compound **8**) or human PDE (**9** and **10**) inhibitors **(b)**, was shown to inhibit *Tb*PDEB1. Dashed rectangles highlight common structural features. Fragment **6** was elaborated using a fragment growing strategy **(c)**. IC_{50} values for inhibition of *Tb*PDEB1 activity or *T. b brucei* proliferation are shown. LE, ligand efficiency = $(-RT\ln(IC_{50}(TbPDEB1)))/NHA$, in $kcal.mol^{-1}.NHA^{-1}$.

to (i) increase cAMP levels in an engineered trypanosome strain with a FRET-based cAMP sensor, and (ii) cause phenotypic changes (formation of duplicate/multiple nuclei and kinetoplasts) consistent with changes observed following genetic or chemical knock-down of *Tb*PDEs (Oberholzer et al. 2007, de Koning et al. 2012).

Targeting histidyl-tRNA synthetase using a fragment-tethering approach

Aminoacyl-tRNA synthetases are well-validated parasite drug targets (Kalidas et al. 2014, Pham et al. 2014). Having previously solved X-ray crystal structures of *T. cruzi* histidyl-tRNA synthetase (*Tc*HisRS), *T. brucei* HisRS, and human cytosolic HisRS (Merritt et al. 2010, Koh et al. 2014), and identified trypanosomal-specific pockets (Koh et al. 2014), Koh et al. (2015) sought to identify chemical starting points for parasite-selective HisRS inhibitors by performing an X-ray crystallographic fragment screen of the Medical Structural Genomics of Pathogenic Protozoa (MSGPP) fragment library. Histidine-complexed

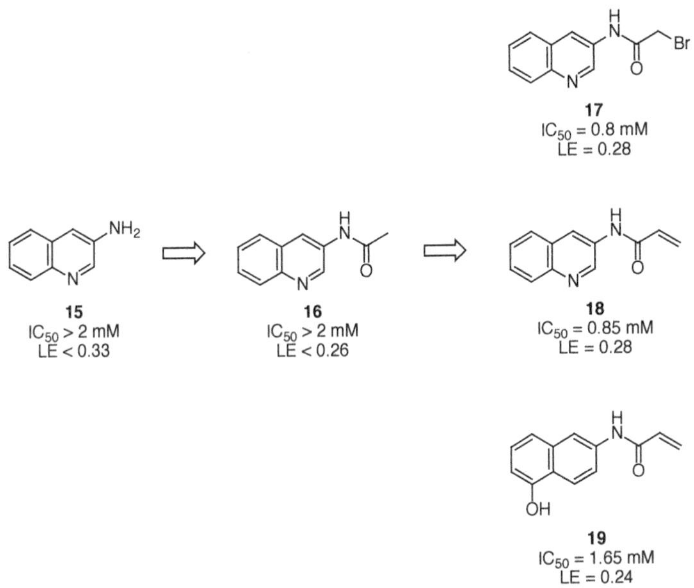

Figure 3. Application of a fragment tethering approach in the elaboration of a *Tc*HisRS-binding fragment hit. IC_{50} values measured in an aminoacylation assay are shown. LE = $(-RTln(IC_{50}))/NHA$, in $kcal.mol^{-1}.NHA^{-1}$.

*Tc*HisRS crystals were soaked with 68 different fragment cocktails of ten fragments each. Co-crystal structures were solved for fifteen fragments (2.2% hit rate), and all fifteen fragments were observed to bind to the same site—a narrow groove adjacent to the histidine binding site that is not present in the crystal structure without the fragments bound. The site is in very close proximity to the binding site of the adenine ring of the histidyl-AMP reaction intermediate and it is likely that fragment binding will interfere with ATP/histidyl-AMP binding. Although fragment binding was observed by X-ray crystallography, binding of only one of the fifteen fragments could be detected by DSF, when fragments were tested at 1 mM. Additionally, the fragments showed little inhibitory activity in an aminoacylation assay; at a concentration of 2 mM, the most active fragments (including the fragment that gave rise to a thermal shift in the DSF assay) inhibited aminoacylation by 20–39%.

With detailed knowledge of the fragment binding mode, Koh et al. (2015) attempted to grow fragment hit **15** (Table 1, Figure 3). Three analogues with substituents on the 3-amino group, intended to extend the fragment toward the histidine binding site, were synthesized (e.g., compound **16**, Figure 3). A co-crystal structure of *Tc*HisRS with compound **16** (which showed similar inhibitory activity to the parent fragment) was obtained, but interestingly it revealed that the substituent caused the fragment to flip in the binding site. The researchers took advantage of the finding that the substituent (an acetamide moiety) was now in close proximity to a cysteine residue (Cys365) not present in the human enzyme, and in a fragment tethering approach, synthesized reactive fragments with an electrophile introduced (compounds **17–19**, Figure 3). Co-crystal structures were obtained for two of the three reactive fragments (compounds **18** and **19**, both with acrylamide moieties replacing the acetonide group) and these showed the fragments to bind as intended, with the electron density around the acrylamide group consistent with covalent bond formation. Although these compounds did not increase the melting temperature of the protein by DSF, they did show improved and selective activity in the aminoacylation assay (IC_{50} = 0.85 and 1.65 mM against *Tc*HisRS vs IC_{50} > 2 mM against human cytosolic and mitochondrial HisRS; Table 1, Figure 3).

Targeting rhodesain with reactive fragments

Rhodesain, a major cathepsin L-like cysteine protease, is required for survival of *T. b. rhodesiense* (Steverding et al. 2012, Ettari et al. 2013). Furthermore, the *T. cruzi* homologue of rhodesain (cruzain) is the target of a drug candidate that has progressed to late-stage preclinical development (K777; McKerrow et al. 2009). McShan et al. (2015) recently screened a library of 200 cysteine-reactive electrophilic fragments against rhodesain using a biochemical assay. Two fragments that reproducibly inhibit the protease by ≥ 85% at a concentration of 10 μM were identified (Table 1). Encouragingly, the fragments also possess antitrypanosomal activity (IC$_{50}$ (*T. brucei*) = 30 and 43 μM) and demonstrate selectivity (IC$_{50}$ (Hep G2) > 150 μM).

Targeting riboflavin kinase using an ultrafiltration-based fragment screen

To validate an ultrafiltration-based fragment screening approach, Shibata et al. (2011) screened a library of 134 fragments against *T. brucei* riboflavin kinase (*Tb*RFK). From 134 fragments screened in 23 cocktails, each containing five to nine fragments, three fragment hits were identified (Table 1). Subsequent competitive binding assays revealed that flavin mononucleotide (FMN) decreased binding of each of the fragments, while ADP-Mg increased binding. These observations are consistent with the fragments binding in the FMN binding site, which is reported to be stabilized upon ADP-Mg binding (Bauer et al. 2003, Karthikeyan et al. 2003).

In silico *fragment-assisted optimization of an inhibitor of RNA editing ligase 1*

To demonstrate the utility of CrystalDock, an algorithm designed to identify fragments likely to bind a protein pocket, Durrant et al. (2011) used the algorithm to identify fragments likely to bind to the adenylation domain of *T. brucei* RNA editing ligase 1 (*Tb*REL1). The algorithm identified three clusters of fragments likely to bind in the *Tb*REL1 active site. One cluster of hydrophobic fragments was interestingly predicted to bind in close proximity to the predicted binding site of a low-μM naphthalene-based inhibitor (Durrant et al. 2010), in a small pocket not previously exploited for drug discovery. This presented the opportunity to improve the affinity of the naphthalene-based inhibitor through fragment linking. One of the hydrophobic fragments—a toluene fragment (Table 1)—was positioned such that it could be linked via a methylene linker to the inhibitor. Subsequent binding energy calculations are consistent with the elaborated inhibitor (Table 1) binding with higher affinity; however, this needs to be experimentally validated.

Targeting PTR1

Tryanosomes require pterin for growth, yet lack enzymes for its *de novo* synthesis, rendering the parasites dependent on the salvage of oxidized pteridines, such as biopterin, and their subsequent reduction by pteridine reductase (PTR1). Following the demonstration that *T. brucei* PTR1 (*Tb*PTR1) is required for survival of blood stage *T. brucei* parasites *in vitro* (Sienkiewicz et al. 2010), Mpamhanga et al. (2009) set out to validate *Tb*PTR1 chemically and identify leads for novel HAT drugs. The need to identify novel *Tb*PTR1 inhibitors was a primary factor that motivated the use of a fragment-based approach; many existing PTR1 inhibitors were derived from dihydrofolate reductase (DHFR) inhibitors, and also inhibit human and *T. brucei* DHFR. Such activity would render any *Tb*PTR1 inhibitor unsuitable for use as a chemical probe or drug lead. Furthermore, existing inhibitors, which primarily have a 2,4-diaminopteridine, 2,4-diaminoquinazoline, or 2,4-diaminopyrimidine core (Figure 4a), have relatively high polar surface areas (PSAs; 77–100 Å^2), which is an undesirable property of a lead required to permeate the blood-brain barrier. A second key factor in choosing a fragment-based approach was the availability of multiple *Tb*PTR1 (and *L. major* PTR1) X-ray crystal structures, which showed a well-defined binding cleft.

The fragment-based approach used to target *Tb*PTR1 began with an *in silico* screen of 26,084 fragment-like compounds against a representative *Tb*PTR1 crystal structure. The fragment library, which was derived from a database of lead-like compounds filtered to retain only compounds with < 20 heavy atoms, ≤ 2 ring systems, at least one hydrogen-bond donor, < 4 rotatable bonds and a clogP or clogD < 3.5, was docked into the active site of *Tb*PTR1. A set of 2725 compounds predicted to interact with the

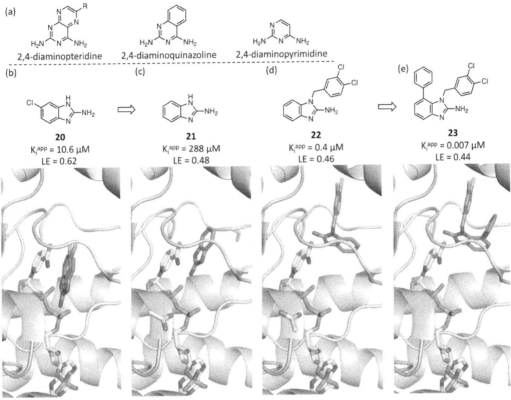

Figure 4. Fragment-based approach to identifying novel inhibitors targeting *Tb*PTR1. (a) Common scaffolds of known PTR1 and DHFR inhibitors. **(b)** Crystal structure showing binding of an aminobenzimidazole fragment hit (carbons in magenta) identified in a virtual fragment screen, to *Tb*PTR1 (with bound NADP$^+$ cofactor, carbons in yellow) [PDB ID: 2WD7]. The fragment was observed to bind in two overlapping poses. **(c–e)** Crystal structures of analogues of fragment **20** in complex with *Tb*PTR1-NADP$^+$ [PDB IDs: 3GN1, 3GN2, 2WD8]. An acetate molecule (carbons in grey) can be seen in the crystal structures shown in (c) and (d). LE = (−RTln(K_i^{app}))/NHA, in kcal.mol^{-1}.NHA^{-1}.

> **Color version at the end of the book**

β-phosphate of the enzyme's NADP$^+$ cofactor and participate in additional hydrogen bonding interactions observed in previously obtained inhibitor-complexed *Tb*PTR1 crystal structures, were prioritized for further analysis. Following removal of compounds containing scaffolds of known PTR1 inhibitors and consideration of (i) scaffold diversity, (ii) PSA of the scaffolds (ideally to be < 70 A^2), (iii) results of minimization, and (iv) shape complementarity with the binding site, the researchers arrived at a list of 59 compounds, 45 of which were commercially available. These compounds were purchased and three fragments were shown to inhibit *Tb*PTR1 by more than 50%, and a further seven between 30 and 50%, in a biochemical assay.

Although Mpamhanga et al. (2009) were unable to co-crystallize the aminobenzothiazole fragment with the second highest activity (K_i^{app} = 21 μM, LE = 0.46), they did obtain a co-crystal structure of the aminobenzimidazole fragment with the highest activity (compound **20**, Figure 4b and Table 1; K_i^{app} = 10.6 μM, LE = 0.62) bound to *Tb*PTR1 (Figure 4b). Interestingly, the ligand was found to adopt two distinct binding poses, both of which involved hydrogen bonding with the phosphate moiety of NADP$^+$, and the predominant pose was in close agreement with the highest scoring docking pose. Co-crystal structures of two closely related aminobenzimidazole fragments (compounds **21** and **22**) were also obtained but interestingly, despite sharing an aminobenzimidazole core, the fragments adopted distinct binding poses (Figures 4c and d). Compound **22**, the more potent of the two analogues (with a K_i^{app} an order of magnitude lower than the original fragment hit; $K_i^{app} = 0.4$ μM), was observed to bind 3.7 Å away from the nicotinamide moiety of NADP$^+$ and to not form any hydrogen bonds with the cofactor. The co-crystal structure revealed hydrophobic pockets adjacent to the aminobenzimidazole core and in an attempt to improve the affinity of compound **22**, derivatives with substituents introduced to fill the largest pocket were tested. This ultimately produced aminobenzimidazole derivative **23**, which inhibits *Tb*PTR1 with a K_i^{app} of 7 nM (Table 1, Figure 4e). This time a co-crystal structure showed that the binding mode of the aminobenzimidazole was maintained. Favorably, none of the *Tb*PTR1 inhibitors identified showed appreciable activity against human or *T. brucei* DHFR as hoped, and the lead aminobenzimidazole has physicochemical properties suitable for cell and CNS penetration (molecular weight of 368 Da, PSA of 55 Å, and logD of 3.7). However, disappointingly, the EC_{50} measured against *T. brucei* in cell culture was 10 μM, over a thousand fold higher than the K_i^{app} measured against the enzyme. Based on the results of knock-down and additional kinetic studies, it seems likely that to see the level of antitrypanosomal activity required in a drug candidate, potency against PTR1 will need to be increased by at least two orders of magnitude (Spinks et al. 2011).

Targeting 6-phosphogluconate dehydrogenase

Ruda et al. (2010) used a similar *in silico* fragment screening approach to that used against PTR1, to target 6-phosphogluconate dehydrogenase of *T. brucei* (*Tb*6PGDH). This essential pentose phosphate pathway enzyme (Hanau et al. 2004) catalyzes the oxidative decarboxylation of 6-phosphogluconate (a molecule with phosphate, carboxylate and hydroxyl groups) and, as a consequence, has an active site composed of several polar residues. Potent and selective substrate-like inhibitors of the enzyme have been reported, but they lack trypanocidal activity (e.g., Dardonville et al. (2004)), presumably due to poor cellular permeability resulting from their charge and polarity.

In this study, a library of 64,000 fragments was compiled from the available chemicals and screening compounds directories (ACD-SCD). Compounds were required to be < 320 Da in size and possess a phosphonate, sulfonate, sulfonic acid, sulfonamide, carboxylic acid or tetrazole to mimic the phosphate group of known inhibitors. The inclusion of such functional groups was anticipated to facilitate binding to the positively charged site that accommodates the phosphate of 6-phosphogluconate but produce less polar starting points for drug discovery compared with the known phosphate-containing inhibitors. Although the crystal structure of *Tb*6PGDH had been solved, the structure of *Lactococcus lactis* 6PGDH was used as the template for docking because of the availability of cofactor, substrate and inhibitor co-crystal structures. Substrate-binding residues are fully conserved between the two proteins. The docking approach involved placement of the phosphate isosteres in the phosphate binding site, and was first validated by docking of known inhibitors. Binding modes were predicted for 5836 of the 64,000 fragments, and following clustering and visual inspection of the predicted binding poses of high-scoring compounds, a set of 71 fragments was purchased and tested against *Tb*6PGDH in a biochemical assay. Ten compounds showed > 80% inhibition when tested at a concentration of 200 μM, and IC_{50} values below 50 μM were determined for three 5-membered carboxylic acid-containing heterocycles among these (corresponding to LEs of 0.40–0.66; Table 1). Fifty-three analogues of the initial ten hits were purchased, leading to the identification of a further three compounds with IC_{50} values below 50 μM and LEs between 0.48 and 0.60, albeit with two showing hill slopes ≥ 2, possibly indicative of non-specific inhibition. Pending structural validation of the proposed binding modes, the inhibitory fragments—invariably 5-membered heterocycles containing a carboxylic acid as a phosphate replacement—provide ligand efficient chemical starting points for the development of novel *Tb*6PGDH inhibitors. With higher partition coefficients, lower total PSAs and predicted improved human intestinal absorption, the fragments have the potential to yield more drug-like inhibitors than those identified previously.

Targeting nucleoside 2-deoxyribosyltransferase

Nucleoside 2-deoxyribosyltransferase functions in the nucleoside salvage pathway, catalyzing the transfer of deoxyribose between nucleobases. As *T. brucei* lacks the enzymes required for *de novo* purine synthesis and is dependent on purine nucleoside scavenging, the enzyme was proposed as a potential drug target (Bosch et al. 2006). This enzyme is particularly attractive as a target because humans are devoid of nucleoside 2-deoxyribosyltransferases (and instead rely on purine and pyrimidine phosphorylases), and as such it should be possible to design inhibitors that selectively target the pathogen. After solving the X-ray crystal structure of *T. brucei* nucleoside 2-deoxyribosyltransferase (*Tb*NDRT) in the *apo* form (to 1.8 Å), Bosch et al. (2006) performed an X-ray crystallographic fragment screen against the enzyme.

In the screen, *Tb*NDRT crystals were soaked with 304 fragments (an earlier version of the fragment library screened against *Tc*HisRS) in 31 different cocktails of approximately 10 fragments each. Four fragments (Table 1), as well as glycerol (originating from the protein buffer), were observed to bind in the active site of *Tb*NDRT. The fragments bind with their ring systems essentially all binding to the same region of the pocket, in close proximity to the glycerol, which binds deep in the hydrophilic "tip" of the active site. By comparison with the X-ray structure of the ribosylated ester intermediate of *Lactobacillus helveticus* NDRT (with a ribose moiety bound covalently and adenine bound non-covalently), it could be seen that the aromatic fragments bind in a similar position to the adenine ring, whereas the glycerol mimics part of the bound ribose. The ligand binding sites observed shed new light on opportunities for the design of higher affinity inhibitors, and all four fragments showed some inhibition of *T. brucei brucei* growth *in vitro* (Table 1). Whether this effect was on target was not, however, investigated, and the fragments will require elaboration to improve affinity.

Targeting triosephosphate isomerase

In an early form of an X-ray crystallographic fragment screen against a putative NTD target, Verlinde et al. (1997) screened three cocktails of 128 fragments each against *T. brucei* triose-phosphate isomerase (*Tb*TIM). For one of the three cocktails, additional electron density was identified; however, the poor resolution (2.8 Å) prevented identification of the fragment, and subsequent soaks with subsets of the 128 fragments failed to reveal the ligand. This was possibly due to production of a binder from the chemical reaction of two ligands. Significant improvements to the method of X-ray crystallographic fragment screening along with several important technological advances has led to this approach now being used with great success both in the NTD drug discovery field as illustrated by examples discussed here, and in other areas (Murray and Blundell 2010).

Fragment-based Approaches in Antileishmanial Drug Discovery

Leishmaniases are a group of diseases caused by protozoan parasites of the genus *Leishmania* that are transmitted by *Phlebotomus* sandflies during a blood meal. It is estimated that there are between 700,000 to one million new cases each year, resulting in 20–30,000 deaths (WHO 2018e). There are three main forms of leishmaniasis:

(i) Visceral leishmaniasis—a disease characterized by bouts of fever, weight loss, anemia, and an enlarged spleen and liver. If untreated, it is fatal in > 95% of cases. There are estimated to be 50–90,000 new cases each year, predominantly in Brazil, East Africa and South-East Asia.

(ii) Cutaneous leishmaniasis—a disease characterized by skin lesions on exposed parts of the body that can cause permanent scarring. With an estimated 600,000–1 million new cases each year, it is the most common form of leishmaniasis, with most cases occurring in the Americas, the Mediterranean basin, the Middle East and Central Asia.

(iii) Mucocutaneous leishmaniasis—a disease in which the mucous membranes of the nose, mouth and throat are destroyed. The disease is predominantly found in Bolivia, Brazil, Ethiopia and Peru.

Currently, there is no vaccine to prevent leishmaniases, and disease prevention relies primarily on reducing contact with sandflies. Leishmaniases are currently treated with pentavalent antimonial compounds that have been in use for several decades, as well as the newer drugs amphotericin B, paromomycin and miltefosine. However, as yet, drugs are not available to those in need, and only miltefosine can be administered orally. Furthermore, as current therapies do not clear parasites from the body, treatment failure, relapse and mortality are high among HIV co-infected patients unless antiretroviral therapy is given (WHO 2018e).

Although there is a need for new therapies, the development of antileishmanials is challenging as drugs must not only be able to traverse multiple membranes to gain access to the amastigote-stage parasite that resides within macrophages and other mononuclear phagocytic cells, but must also be stable to the acidic pH of macrophages. Fewer published examples of fragment-based approaches being applied primarily to the discovery of antileishmanials can be found, as compared with the number of published fragment-based approaches applied to antitrypanosomal drug discovery. Some examples are discussed below and summarized in Table 2.

Table 2. Examples of fragment-based approaches applied to antileishmanial drug discovery.

Target	Approach	Selected fragment hit(s)	Elaborated compound	Reference
L. major coproporphyrinogen III oxidase	X-ray crystallographic fragment screen		N/A	Verlinde et al. (2009)
L. major adenylate kinase	X-ray crystallographic fragment screen		N/A	Verlinde et al. (2009)
L. naiffi uracil-DNA glycosylase	X-ray crystallographic fragment screen followed by enzyme assay	[a]IC_{50} = 15 mM [b]LE = 0.21	IC_{50} = 15 μM LE = 0.44	Verlinde et al. (2009)
L. amazonensis and *L. donovani*	Whole-cell screen of 1604 fragments	[c]EC_{50} = 4 μM EC_{50} = 31 μM	N/A	Ayotte et al. (2018)

[a]IC_{50}, concentration causing 50% inhibition as measured in enzyme assays; [b]LE, ligand efficiency = $(-RT\ln(IC_{50}))/NHA$ in kcal.mol^{-1}.NHA; [c]EC_{50}, half maximal effective concentration as measured in whole-cell assays.

Screening fragments by X-ray crystallography to identify novel chemical starting points for antileishmanial drug design

The MSGPP Consortium performed a number of X-ray crystallographic fragment screens to identify chemical starting points for inhibitors of leishmanial proteins crystallized by the consortium (Verlinde et al. 2009). A collection of fragment cocktails created in-house (the Biomolecular Structure Center (BMSC) collection), which was also used in the X-ray crystallographic fragment screens performed against *Tb*NDRT and *Tc*HisRS described in the previous section, was utilized for the screens.

Crystals of *L. major* coproporphyrinogen III oxidase, an enzyme involved in porphyrin biosynthesis, were soaked with 66 different fragment cocktails. Co-crystal structures were obtained for two fragments each from different cocktails (Table 2). Interestingly, one of the two fragment hits, cyclopentyl acetate, was observed to bind at three positions within the active site. In the same structure, one molecule of acetate (co-purified with the enzyme) was also bound. The four carboxylates contributed by the three fragment molecules and the acetate molecule were predicted to occupy the binding sites of the four carboxylates of the natural substrate coproporphyinogen-III.

Crystals of a putative *L. major* adenylate kinase were also soaked with fragment cocktails, and a single fragment hit—4-amino-2-methyl-quinoline—binding to the protein was identified (Table 2).

Uracil-DNA glycosylase (UDG) catalyses excision of misincorporated uracil from DNA and initiates "base-excision repair" (Pena-Diaz et al. 2004). Having solved the structure of a putative uracil-DNA glycosylase from *Leishmania naiffi*, crystals of the enzyme were soaked with 68 cocktails each containing ten fragments. Four fragments were observed to bind to the enzyme (Table 2), as was DMSO. A derivative of one fragment hit (5-chloro-2-methoxybenzoic acid) was designed and found to inhibit the activity of the enzyme 1000-fold more potently than the parent fragment (IC_{50} = 15 µM (LE = 0.44) vs 15 mM (LE = 0.21); Table 2). Recently, and since this fragment screen, Mishra et al. (2018) have shown that expression of the gene coding for UDG is upregulated in *Leishmania donovani* in response to treatment with commonly used antileishmanial drugs, and that drug-resistant clinical isolates of *L. donovani* show higher levels of the transcript encoding UDG. For these reasons, the enzyme has been proposed as a potential target for new combination therapies. The hits identified here may therefore serve as good starting points for development of tool compounds/new drugs targeting this enzyme.

Fragment-based phenotypic screening to identify leishmanicidal agents

Ayotte et al. (2018) used a hybrid strategy incorporating aspects of a fragment-based approach and a phenotypic screen, to identify fragments with leishmanicidal activity. From an initial set of 8000 fragments, a library of 1604 fragments was compiled. The starting set was refined using cheminformatic filters (to enrich for desirable substructures and maximize chemical diversity), as well as ^{1}H NMR analysis (to ensure all compounds included in the library were sufficiently soluble, and showed no signs of degradation or aggregation). The library was tested in 169 pools of 7–12 compounds against axenic cultures of promastigote-stage *Leishmania amazonensis* and *L. donovani* parasites, each at a concentration of 166 µM. Fifty fragment pools were found to show high leishmanicidal activity against both parasites at this concentration, as determined by microscopic examination, and 16 of these showed selectivity (having little/no cytotoxic effect on macrophages). Subsequently, fragments in the five pools showing the greatest leishmanicidal activity but no cytotoxic effect on macrophages, were tested individually at the same concentration. In this process, two fragments with selective leishmanicidal activity were identified (Table 2). These compounds—an indazole and an indole—were subsequently also shown to inhibit intracellular amastigote-stage *L. amazonesis* parasites within murine bone-marrow derived macrophages (EC_{50} values of 4 and 31 µM, determined respectively, Table 2), and have no effect on the macrophages even at a concentration of 500 µM (corresponding to a selectivity index > 125 for the most active compound). Interestingly, indoles and indazoles are scaffolds of a number of published leishmanicidal lead compounds. Close analogues of the two hits were also tested to establish structure-activity relationships, and in the process two compounds with modest increases

(2.8–3.7-fold) in potency were identified, as were modifications that were detrimental to the activity. The activity and selectivity of the lead indole and indazoles identified warrant further investigations into their potential as lead leishmanicidal compounds and/or tool compounds to reveal novel targets.

Fragment-based Approaches in Dengue Drug Discovery

Dengue is a viral infection that is transmitted by female *Aedes* mosquitoes, primarily of the species *Aedes aegypti*. The disease is widespread in tropical and subtropical regions, and has an increasing global incidence due to a growing number of outbreaks and spread to previously unaffected regions (WHO 2017). Although it is difficult to quantify the disease burden, it has been estimated that there are 390 million infections per year, and 96 million people presenting with clinical manifestations (Bhatt et al. 2013). The dengue virus (DENV) gives rise to flu-like symptoms, from which a patient typically recovers within 2–7 days (WHO 2018f). However, in a small proportion of patients, the disease develops into potentially lethal Dengue Haemorrhagic Fever (also known as severe dengue) or Dengue Shock Syndrome (Rajapakse 2011). Four DENV serotypes (DENV-1, DENV-2, DENV-3 and DENV-4) cause dengue in humans, and although infection with one serotype provides lifelong immunity to that serotype, it increases the risk of developing severe dengue upon subsequent infection with another serotype (WHO 2018f). Currently, there are no specific drugs for prevention or treatment of dengue, and disease control relies primarily on reducing contact with mosquitoes (WHO 2018a). Dengvaxia®, the first Dengue vaccine, was licensed in 2015 and approved for use in 9–45 year olds in endemic areas of 20 countries. However, retrospective analysis has revealed that the vaccine confers an increased risk of severe dengue to those not previously infected and as such is only recommended in persons with evidence of a previous infection (WHO 2018f). Currently, disease treatment is limited to supportive care and fluid resuscitation (WHO 2009), and as such small molecule drugs that could be used for chemoprophylaxis/treatment could be transformative.

The DENV has an approximately 11 kb, positive-sense, single-strand RNA genome, encoding three structural proteins and seven non-structural proteins (NS) (Noble et al. 2010). These virus-encoded proteins, along with host proteins required for viral replication, have been explored as potential antiviral drug targets (Behnam et al. 2016). The examples discussed below and summarized in Table 3, illustrate how fragment-based approaches have been used to target four DENV-encoded proteins.

Targeting DENV protease using principles of a fragment-based approach

The NS2B-NS3 protease complex is one of the best-studied targets for the development of drugs against the DENV (Behnam et al. 2016). This complex catalyzes the post-translational cleavage of the DENV polyprotein and is essential for viral replication; the proteolytic activity is localized to the N-terminus of NS3, while NS2B contributes to substrate recognition (Nitsche et al. 2014). A number of inhibitors of the DENV protease have been identified and these can be broadly classified into (i) peptidic and peptidomimetic inhibitors and (ii) non-peptidic small molecule inhibitors (reviewed by Nitsche et al. (2014)).

Behnam et al. (2014) utilized a fragment merging strategy to improve the potency of the tripeptide Bz-Arg-Lys-Nle-NH$_2$ found in a previous study (Nitsche et al. 2012) to inhibit DENV-2 protease (compound **24**, Figure 5, IC$_{50}$ = 13.3 µM, K$_i$ = 11.2 µM). Guided by docking studies performed using the DENV-3 protease crystal structure, they synthesized and tested a series of peptides with different C-terminal moieties. Replacement of the C-terminal residue with a phenylglycine moiety improved activity fourfold (peptide **25**, Figure 5, IC$_{50}$ = 3.3 µM, K$_i$ = 2.1 µM). Furthermore, they were able to improve the activity a further fivefold by merging the peptide with previously identified peptide **26** (Figure 5, IC$_{50}$ = 2.5 µM, K$_i$ = 1.8 µM) with a variant N-terminal cap associated with improved membrane permeability, protease inhibitor activity, and antiviral activity (Nitsche et al. 2013) (peptide **27**, Figure 5, IC$_{50}$ = 0.6 µM, K$_i$ = 0.4 µM).

In a follow up study, Behnam et al. (2015) applied a fragment growing strategy to improve activity against the DENV protease, as well as the related West Nile virus (WNV). Initially, a benzyloxyether was added at the *para* position of the C-terminal phenylglycine moiety of peptide **25** (peptide **28**, Figure 5), which improved potency against the DENV-2 protease ninefold (IC$_{50}$ = 0.367 µM) and WNV protease by 80-fold

Table 3. Examples of fragment-based approaches applied to anti-DENV drug discovery.

Target	Approach	Selected fragment hit(s)	Elaborated compound	Reference
NS2B-NS3	Fragment merging and growing	N/A	**32** ^aK_i (DENV-2 protease) = 176 nM $^bEC_{50}$ (DENV-2) = 3.4 µM	Figure 5 Behnam et al. (2014), Behnam et al. (2015)
RdRp	X-ray crystallographic screen of 1408 fragments. Elaboration by growing	**35** $^cIC_{50}$ (DENV-4 RdRp) = 730 µM ^dK_D (DENV-3 & 4 RdRp) = 210 and 610 µM $^eLE = 0.24–0.28$	**40** IC_{50} (DENV-4 RdRp) = 0.17 µM K_D (DENV-4 RdRp) = 0.07 µM LE = 0.30 EC_{50} (DENV-1-4) = 1.8–2.3 µM	Figure 6 Noble et al. (2016), Yokokawa et al. (2016)
MTase	DSF screen of 500 fragments, followed by X-ray crystallography and enzyme assays. Elaboration by fragment linking	**41** $^fIC_{50}$ (2'O) = 9.3 mM LE = 0.28 $^gIC_{50}$ (N7) ≥ 10 mM **42** IC_{50} (2'O) = 2.8 mM LE = 0.32 IC_{50} (N7) ≥ 10 mM	**45** IC_{50} (2'O) = 91 µM LE = 0.16 IC_{50} (N7) = 1.1 mM **46** IC_{50} (2'O) = 110 µM LE = 0.16 IC_{50} (N7) = 742 µM **47** IC_{50} (2'O) = 24 µM LE = 0.15	Coutard et al. (2014), Benmansour et al. (2017), Hernandez et al. (2019)

^aK_i, inhibition constant; $^bEC_{50}$, half maximal effective concentration as measured in whole-cell assays; $^cIC_{50}$, concentration causing 50% inhibition as measured in enzyme assays; ^dK_D, dissociation constant; ^eLE, ligand efficiency = $(-RTln(K_D/IC_{50}))/NHA$, in kcal.mol^{-1}.NHA^{-1}; $^fIC_{50}$ (2'O), IC_{50} determined in a 2'-*O*-MTase assay using DENV-3 MTase; $^gIC_{50}$ (N7), IC_{50} determined in a N7-MTase assay using DENV-3 MTase.

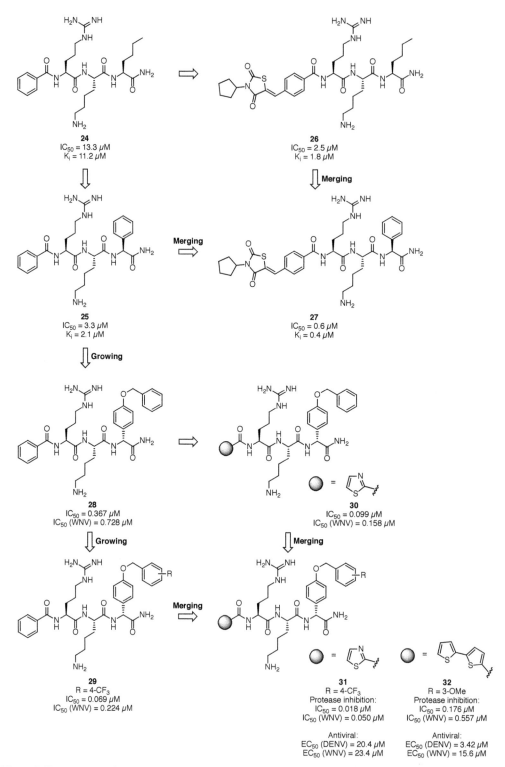

Figure 5. Fragment merging and growing strategies applied to the optimization of a peptidic inhibitor of DENV-2 protease. Unless otherwise specified, IC_{50} and K_i values shown were determined from DENV-2 protease activity assays. As indicated, IC_{50} values for inhibition of the WNV protease and for antiviral activity against DENV-2 and WNV are also shown in some cases.

(IC$_{50}$ = 0.728 μM). Subsequent addition of a trifluoromethyl group (peptide **29**, Figure 5) led to a further fivefold improvement in activity against the DENV-2 protease (IC$_{50}$ = 0.069 μM) and threefold improvement against the WNV protease (IC$_{50}$ = 0.224 μM). In parallel, they searched for the optimal N-terminal cap; a range of peptide **28** derivatives in which the benzoyl moiety was replaced with various small chemical groups was tested. Substitution of the benzoyl moiety with a thiazole ring (peptide **30**) produced the most potent inhibitor of DENV-2 and WNV protease (IC$_{50}$ = 0.099 and 0.158 μM, respectively). The most productive N and C terminal modifications were then combined into a single molecule through merging of peptides **29** and **30**. The resultant peptide (**31**) was observed to inhibit DENV-2 and WNV protease with IC$_{50}$ values of 18 and 50 nM, respectively, corresponding to a 180-fold increase in activity against the DENV-2 protease and a > 1000-fold increase in activity against WNV protease relative to peptide **25**. Furthermore, peptide **31** also possesses antiviral activity against both DENV-2 and WNV (EC$_{50}$ = 20.4 and 23.4 μM, respectively). However, a less potent inhibitor of DENV-2 protease showed the highest antiviral activity (peptide **32**, Figure 5, EC$_{50}$(DENV) = 3.42 μM and EC$_{50}$(WNV) = 15.6 μM), presumably due to improved permeability.

Targeting RNA polymerase

DENV RNA-dependent RNA polymerase (RdRp) forms the C-terminal part of NS5, the largest DENV protein and the most highly conserved protein across the DENV serotypes (Yap et al. 2007). The N-terminus of NS5 functions as a methyltransferase (discussed in the next section). DENV RdRp is an attractive drug target because it is required for viral replication, has no mammalian counterpart, and because its conservation across DENV serotypes should facilitate identification of inhibitors effective against all serotypes (Lim et al. 2015). Furthermore, viral polymerases have been clinically-validated as drug targets (Tsai et al. 2006), and X-ray crystal structures of DENV RdRp have been determined (Yap et al. 2007, Zhao et al. 2015), enabling structure-based drug design. Nucleoside and non-nucleoside inhibitors of RdRp have been identified to date, with some nucleoside inhibitors having entered clinic trials, albeit with limited success (reviewed by Lim et al. 2015, Behnam et al. 2016).

Researchers at Novartis previously performed a HTS campaign against RdRp (Yin et al. 2009, Niyomrattanakit et al. 2010). *N*-Sulfonyl anthranilic acid **33** (Figure 6a), which inhibits DENV-2 RdRp with an IC$_{50}$ value of 7.2 μM, was identified as a hit in this screen. Subsequent SAR investigations and optimization led to a highly lipophilic molecule (compound **34**, Figure 6a) with improved activity against the enzyme (IC$_{50}$ = 0.26 μM), but without antiviral activity in cell cultures (Yin et al. 2009). As the HTS campaign failed to produce specific DENV RdRp inhibitors with suitable physicochemical properties, a fragment-based approach was explored as an alternative method to identify lead compounds targeting RdRp.

Noble et al. (2016) screened the Novartis library of 1408 fragments in pools of eight against RdRp using X-ray crystallography. DENV-3 RdRp crystals were soaked with a total of 176 fragment pools, with each fragment tested at a concentration of 625 μM. This led to the identification of a single fragment hit (compound **35**) that was subsequently shown by SPR to bind DENV-3 and DENV-4 RdRp with K$_D$ values of 210 and 610 μM, respectively (LE = 0.28 and 0.24, respectively). The structure of DENV-3 RdRp, like that of other polymerases, resembles a right hand with subdomains that mimic the fingers, palm and thumb. The fragment hit was observed to bind in a novel allosteric pocket of *apo* DENV-3 RdRp, between the thumb and palm subdomains and the priming loop that regulates binding of the RNA template and polymerization. Importantly, binding at this site was also shown to translate into an inhibitory effect on enzyme activity, with an IC$_{50}$ value of 730 μM determined against DENV-4 RdRp in a *de novo* initiation/elongation assay. Replacement of the terminal phenyl moiety of fragment **35** with a thiophene produced a fragment (**36**, Figure 6b) with two-to-seven-fold improved affinity and the same binding mode. Guided by X-ray crystallography, this thiophene fragment was subsequently elaborated using a fragment growing strategy (Yokokawa et al. 2016).

As shown in Figure 6b, initially a propargyl alcohol moiety was added to fill a narrow cavity in the protein and displace a water molecule. This modification increased the affinity by > 100-fold. The subsequent removal of a methylene group and addition of a methyl group improved affinity by a further

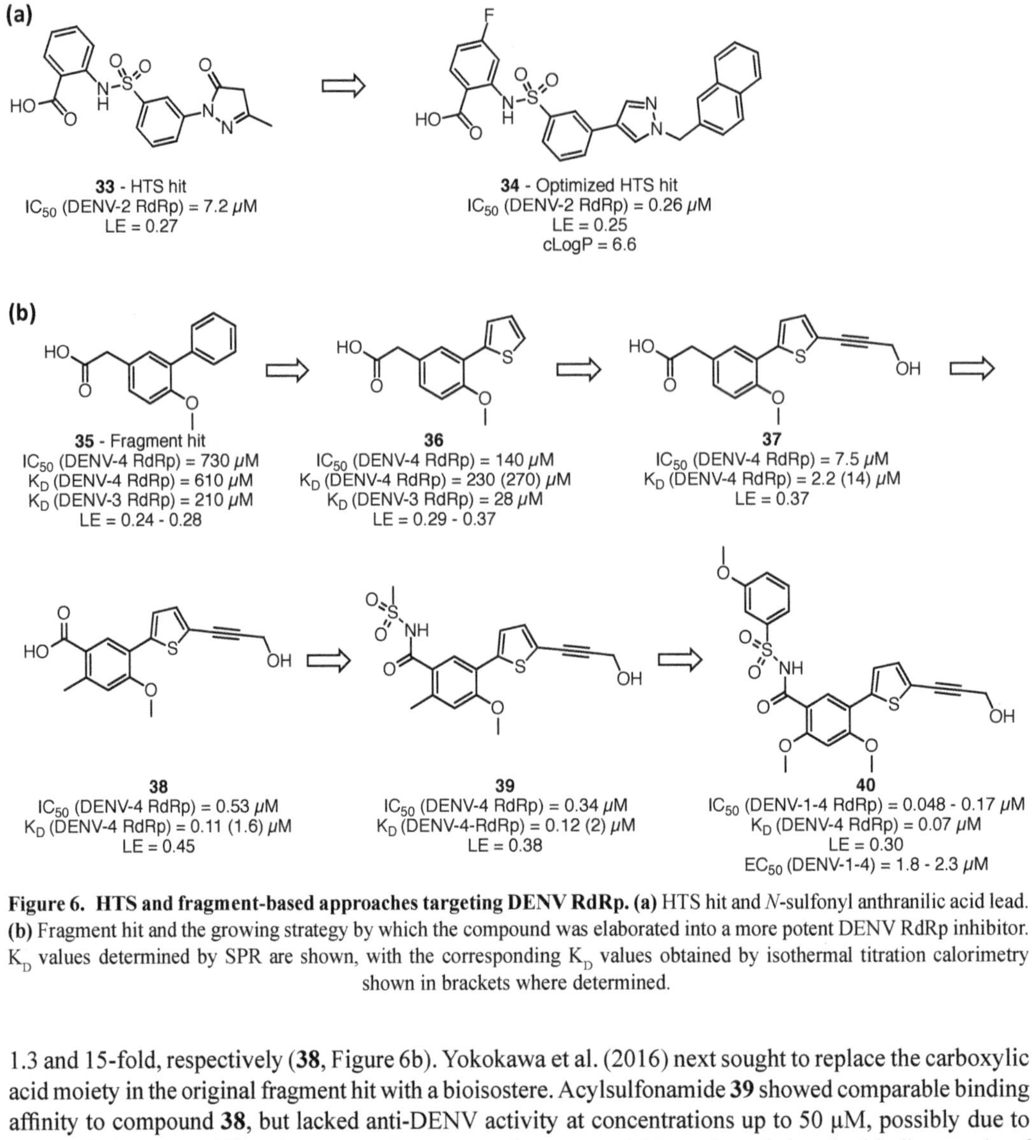

Figure 6. HTS and fragment-based approaches targeting DENV RdRp. (a) HTS hit and *N*-sulfonyl anthranilic acid lead. **(b)** Fragment hit and the growing strategy by which the compound was elaborated into a more potent DENV RdRp inhibitor. K_D values determined by SPR are shown, with the corresponding K_D values obtained by isothermal titration calorimetry shown in brackets where determined.

1.3 and 15-fold, respectively (**38**, Figure 6b). Yokokawa et al. (2016) next sought to replace the carboxylic acid moiety in the original fragment hit with a bioisostere. Acylsulfonamide **39** showed comparable binding affinity to compound **38**, but lacked anti-DENV activity at concentrations up to 50 μM, possibly due to poor cellular permeability. A co-crystal structure of compound **39** confirmed that the binding mode of the parent fragment was retained, and that the propargyl alcohol and acylsulfonamide moieties formed two and three hydrogen-bonds with the protein, respectively. They additionally showed that the methyl group of the acylsulfonamide was solvent exposed. With the aim of improving the physicochemical properties without reducing affinity for the enzyme, various replacements for this methyl group were investigated. Ultimately, replacement of the methyl substituent with a 3-methoxyphenyl substituent produced compound **40**, which binds RdRp with a K_D of 0.07 μM (DENV-4) and inhibits DENV-1-4 RdRp with IC_{50} values of 0.05–0.17 μM (Figure 6b), corresponding to a > 4000-fold improvement in activity relative to the parent fragment, and a slight overall improvement in ligand efficiency (0.30). Importantly, this compound demonstrated anti-DENV activity against all four DENV serotypes, with EC_{50} values between 1.8 and 2.3 μM measured, and the antiviral activity was demonstrated to be on target (Lim et al. 2016). The study by Yokokawa et al. (2016) is the first to describe RdRp inhibitors with pan-serotype antiviral activity in cell cultures.

Targeting DENV helicase and methyltransferase

Coutard et al. (2014) utilized a fragment-based approach to target two key components of the DENV replication complex, the NS3 Helicase (Hel) and the NS5 methyltransferase (MTase). Hel forms the C-terminus of the NS3 protein, and catalyzes activities involved in RNA capping and replication of the DENV genome—nucleotide and RNA triphosphate hydrolysis and RNA unwinding (Benarroch et al. 2004, Yon et al. 2005). MTase forms the N-terminus of the NS5 protein, and catalyzes two sequential methylation reactions involved in formation of the cap structure at the 5'-end of the RNA genome: (i) methylation of the cap guanine at the N7-position, and (ii) methylation at the 2'-*O*-position of the first nucleotide that is transcribed (Dong et al. 2010). The Hel and N7-MTase activities are essential for viral replication, and while moderate replication is possible when 2'-*O*-MTase activity is defective, 2'-*O*-MTase activity is required for virulence *in vivo* (Matusan et al. 2001, Dong et al. 2010, Zust et al. 2013). These findings highlight the potential of Hel and MTase as novel targets for antiviral therapies for the prevention or treatment of dengue. As crystal forms of DENV NS3 Hel and NS5 MTase yielding high-resolution X-ray structures had previously been obtained (Luo et al. 2008, Lim et al. 2011), Coutard et al. (2014) anticipated that the proteins would be suitable for targeting using a fragment-based approach.

In an attempt to identify novel binding sites and/or starting points for inhibitor development, a library of 500 rule-of-three compliant fragments was screened against each of the target proteins using DSF. In this primary screen, in which fragments were tested at a concentration of 2 mM, 36 and 32 fragments increased the melting temperature of Hel (from DENV-4) and MTase (from DENV-3) by > 0.5°C, respectively, consistent with binding. These fragments were therefore progressed to X-ray crystallography experiments for hit confirmation and binding mode determination. Unfortunately, in the case of Hel, crystal-soaking experiments did not produce a single fragment co-crystal structure and as such none of the fragment hits were confirmed by X-ray crystallography. By contrast, a total of seven fragments were observed by X-ray crystallography to bind *S*-adenosyl-L-methionine (SAM)-bound DENV-3 MTase. Furthermore, the seven fragments were found to bind at four distinct sites—one fragment was observed to bind in a site overlapping with the GTP binding site, while the remaining six fragments bind at one of three novel binding sites. The inhibitory effect of the MTase fragment hits on DENV-3 MTase activity was also determined and five of the seven X-ray crystallography-confirmed hits were found to inhibit 2'-*O*-MTase activity with IC_{50} values between 180 µM and 9 mM, with the most active 2'-*O*-MTase inhibitor also inhibiting N7-MTase activity (IC_{50} = 2 mM). Notably, the fragment binding at the GTP-binding site showed little-to-no inhibition of MTase activity. Hel and MTase inhibitors were also found among Hel and MTase fragment hits that did not yield crystal structures in soaking experiments (or, where attempted, co-crystallization experiments); however, because detailed knowledge of a fragment's binding mode is important for fragment elaboration, these fragments were not progressed. The failure to obtain any Hel-fragment co-crystal structures despite some of the DSF fragment hits possessing weak inhibitory activity against the enzyme in an ATPase assay, was hypothesized to be a consequence of the fragment hits inducing a conformational change in the protein that cannot occur in the crystal; previous studies had shown the protein to be highly dynamic (Luo et al. 2008).

In a subsequent study, two of the MTase fragment hits (fragments **41** and **42**, Table 3, Figure 7) were used as the basis for a fragment-linking strategy aimed at developing higher affinity and selective DENV MTase inhibitors (Benmansour et al. 2017). The two fragments selected were observed to bind in adjacent positions in a novel binding site in close proximity to the binding site of the natural substrate SAM (Figure 7). Informed by docking experiments, different linking strategies were considered. Compounds in which the fragments were linked by a 3-unit urea or amide linker were predicted to allow the fragments to adopt their desired binding poses and form linker-mediated hydrogen bonding interactions, and were therefore synthesized. A few close analogues were also synthesized, the design of which was inspired by a third fragment hit observed to bind in a site overlapping with fragment **41**. Crystal soaking experiments yielded co-crystal structures for two urea-linked compounds, demonstrating that they are able to bind MTase; however, the binding site of the two analogues is shifted relative to the parent fragments (e.g.,

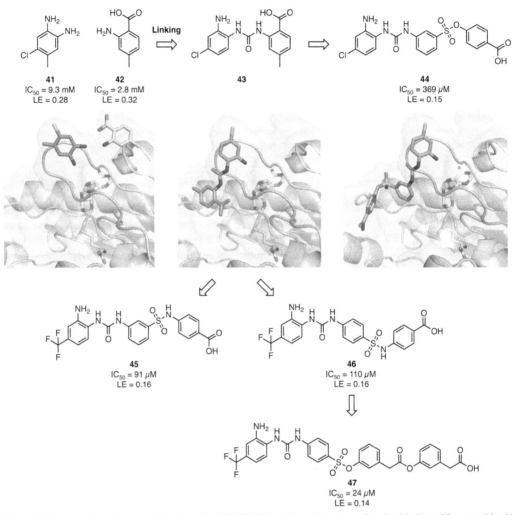

Figure 7. Fragment-based approach to targeting DENV MTase. Crystal structures showing binding of fragment hits **41** and **42** (carbons in magenta or cyan, respectively) and elaborated compounds **43** and **44** (carbons in orange) to DENV-3 MTase (with bound SAM, carbons in yellow) [PDB IDs: 5EKX, 5EIF, 5EC8 and 5EHG]. IC_{50} values measured in a 2'-*O*-MTase activity assay, and the corresponding LE values in kcal.mol^{-1}.NHA, are shown.

Color version at the end of the book

compound **43**, Figure 7). Sulfonamide and sulfone ester derivatives of the new urea-linked compounds designed to pick up additional interactions in adjacent areas of the MTase binding site were synthesized, soaked into DENV-3 MTase crystals and tested for inhibition of DENV-3 MTase activity. Co-crystal structures were obtained for two of the derivatives and showed that the binding mode of the original urea-linked compounds was maintained (e.g., compound **44**, Figure 7). The most active compounds (compounds **45** and **46**, Figure 7), which did not give rise to co-crystal structures, inhibit 2'-*O*-MTase activity with IC_{50} values of 91 and 110 µM. Although this represents a 25–100-fold improvement in the IC_{50} values relative to the parent fragments, this corresponds to a substantial drop in ligand efficiency relative to the parent fragments (Table 3, Figure 7). However, favorably, by contrast with the parent fragments, the elaborated compounds also inhibit N7-MTase activity (IC_{50} values of 1.1 and 0.7 mM for compound **45** and **46**, respectively). Unfortunately, however, when tested for antiviral activity against strains of DENV-1–3 in Vero E6 cells, no antiviral activity was detected at concentrations up to 20 µM. An elaborated sulfone ester analogue of **46** with approximately four-fold improved inhibitory activity in a DENV 2'-*O*-MTase assay was subsequently identified (**47**, Figure 7) (Hernandez et al. 2019). However, the analogue, which was without cytotoxicity at concentrations ≤ 100 μM, was also without effect on DENV-2 replication *in vitro* at concentrations ≤ 20 μM. Nevertheless, these studies have now produced a number of fragment and inhibitor co-crystal structures that could inform the future development of compounds with improved MTase inhibitory activity that also possess antiviral activity and have improved selectivity compared to known inhibitors, which primarily bind in the SAM binding site (Behnam et al. 2016).

Conclusions

Drug discovery in a NTD landscape is associated with a number of challenges. New drugs should be cheap and ideally orally administered to ensure they are accessible to those in need. Furthermore, NTDs are complex and diverse, and low investment, disproportionate to the disease burden, means there are fewer validated targets and often a lack of *in vivo* relevant assays compatible with HTS platforms (Martin-Plaza and Chatelain 2015). However, with new public-private partnerships entering the area, this is changing. Phenotypic screening is the favored hit finding mechanism in NTD drug discovery and has produced clinical candidates, e.g., fexinidazole and the oxaborole SCYX-7158 for the treatment of HAT (Hotez et al. 2016). Nonetheless, phenotypic screening is not without its shortcomings. For example, the approach requires access to screening libraries difficult to handle and maintain outside of an industry setting, and libraries invariably represent limited chemical space. Furthermore, it can be challenging to optimize HTS hits while achieving appropriate physicochemical properties. In this regard, fragment-based approaches, although target-based, have the key advantages that libraries are smaller and more efficiently explore chemical space, and more careful control of physicochemical properties is possible during optimization. Fragments are also valuable tools for identifying novel allosteric sites in a target (which can facilitate selective targeting), as seen in the fragment-based approaches targeting *Tc*SpdSyn and DENV RdRP, as well as binding hotspots. For these reasons, fragment-based approaches certainly hold value in NTD drug discovery either alone (provided they are paired with careful target validation) or in conjunction with phenotypic screening approaches.

In addition to the requirement for a well-validated target, a successful fragment-based approach generally also demands a target that can be expressed in a pure and soluble form and is suitable for binding mode studies by X-ray crystallography/protein NMR, as iterative structure determination is important for informing fragment elaboration. Fragment screens make use of a range of predominantly biophysical techniques from DSF, which is fast and inexpensive and employs a RT-PCR machine likely present in most academic institutions, to more specialized approaches like NMR and X-ray crystallography. As illustrated by the DENV Hel example discussed, the ability to obtain structural information on fragment binding remains a bottleneck. A number of the fragment-based approaches discussed involved an X-ray crystallography-based primary or secondary fragment screen, which is advantageous in that the binding mode is known early on. This, however, requires access to specialist equipment and expertise. Notably, the MSGPP Consortium has made significant contributions to the field, both in the form of structures and fragment cocktails for X-ray crystallography-based fragment screens. *In silico* approaches are also widely used, both in fragment screening and to guide fragment elaboration. However, it is important to be aware that experimental binding modes can deviate from those predicted, and *in silico* approaches will invariably identify only fragments binding to pre-formed pockets. Variations on a classical fragment-based approach are also being employed, for example, whole-cell screening of fragments, two examples of which were presented, and although innovation is welcomed, whether such approaches can produce optimizable hits remains to be seen.

The challenge, as with other target-based approaches, remains translating potency against an isolated target to on-target activity in cell cultures under *in vivo*-relevant conditions. Many of the published fragment-based approaches discussed here report only on fragment hit identification and as yet have not reached this hurdle, and at least in one case—the study targeting *Tb*PTR1—translation of potent enzyme inhibition to whole-cell activity proved difficult. Nonetheless, several other examples of fragment-based approaches producing on-target cell-active compounds—and in the case of compounds targeting *Tb*PEX14-PEX5, also with activity in an animal model—are presented, and we eagerly watch this space.

References

Amano, Y., I. Namatame, Y. Tateishi, K. Honboh, E. Tanabe, T. Niimi et al. 2015. Structural insights into the novel inhibition mechanism of *Trypanosoma cruzi* spermidine synthase. Acta Crystallogr. D Biol. Crystallogr. 71: 1879–1889.

Ayotte, Y., F. Bilodeau, A. Descoteaux and S.R. LaPlante. 2018. Fragment-based phenotypic lead discovery: cell-based assay to target leishmaniasis. ChemMedChem. 13: 1377–1386.

Bauer, S., K. Kemter, A. Bacher, R. Huber, M. Fischer and S. Steinbacher. 2003. Crystal structure of *Schizosaccharomyces pombe* riboflavin kinase reveals a novel ATP and riboflavin-binding fold. J. Mol. Biol. 326: 1463–1473.

Behnam, M.A., C. Nitsche, S.M. Vechi and C.D. Klein. 2014. C-Terminal residue optimization and fragment merging: discovery of a potent peptide-hybrid inhibitor of dengue protease. ACS Med. Chem. Lett. 5: 1037–1042.

Behnam, M.A., D. Graf, R. Bartenschlager, D.P. Zlotos and C.D. Klein. 2015. Discovery of nanomolar dengue and West Nile virus protease inhibitors containing a 4-benzyloxyphenylglycine residue. J. Med. Chem. 58: 9354–9370.

Behnam, M.A., C. Nitsche, V. Boldescu and C.D. Klein. 2016. The medicinal chemistry of dengue virus. J. Med. Chem. 59: 5622–5649.

Benarroch, D., B. Selisko, G.A. Locatelli, G. Maga, J.L. Romette and B. Canard. 2004. The RNA helicase, nucleotide 5'-triphosphatase, and RNA 5'-triphosphatase activities of Dengue virus protein NS3 are Mg^{2+}-dependent and require a functional Walker B motif in the helicase catalytic core. Virology. 328: 208–218.

Benmansour, F., I. Trist, B. Coutard, E. Decroly, G. Querat, A. Brancale et al. 2017. Discovery of novel dengue virus NS5 methyltransferase non-nucleoside inhibitors by fragment-based drug design. Eur. J. Med. Chem. 125: 865–880.

Bhatt, S., P.W. Gething, O.J. Brady, J.P. Messina, A.W. Farlow, C.L. Moyes et al. 2013. The global distribution and burden of dengue. Nature. 496: 504–507.

Birkholtz, L.M., M. Williams, J. Niemand, A.I. Louw, L. Persson and O. Heby. 2011. Polyamine homoeostasis as a drug target in pathogenic protozoa: peculiarities and possibilities. Biochem. J. 438: 229–244.

Blaazer, A.R., K.M. Orrling, A. Shanmugham, C. Jansen, L. Maes, E. Edink et al. 2015. Fragment-based screening in tandem with phenotypic screening provides novel antiparasitic hits. J. Biomol. Screen. 20: 131–140.

Bosch, J., M.A. Robien, C. Mehlin, E. Boni, A. Riechers, F.S. Buckner et al. 2006. Using fragment cocktail crystallography to assist inhibitor design of *Trypanosoma brucei* nucleoside 2-deoxyribosyltransferase. J. Med. Chem. 49: 5939–5946.

Coutard, B., E. Decroly, C. Li, A. Sharff, J. Lescar, G. Bricogne et al. 2014. Assessment of Dengue virus helicase and methyltransferase as targets for fragment-based drug discovery. Antiviral. Res. 106: 61–70.

Dardonville, C., E. Rinaldi, M.P. Barrett, R. Brun, I.H. Gilbert and S. Hanau. 2004. Selective inhibition of *Trypanosoma brucei* 6-phosphogluconate dehydrogenase by high-energy intermediate and transition-state analogues. J. Med. Chem. 47: 3427–3437.

Dawidowski, M., L. Emmanouilidis, V.C. Kalel, K. Tripsianes, K. Schorpp, K. Hadian et al. 2017. Inhibitors of PEX14 disrupt protein import into glycosomes and kill Trypanosoma parasites. Science. 355: 1416–1420.

de Koning, H.P., M.K. Gould, G.J. Sterk, H. Tenor, S. Kunz, E. Luginbuehl et al. 2012. Pharmacological validation of *Trypanosoma brucei* phosphodiesterases as novel drug targets. J. Infect. Dis. 206: 229–237.

Dong, H., D.C. Chang, X. Xie, Y.X. Toh, K.Y. Chung, G. Zou et al. 2010. Biochemical and genetic characterization of dengue virus methyltransferase. Virology. 405: 568–578.

Durrant, J.D., L. Hall, R.V. Swift, M. Landon, A. Schnaufer and R.E. Amaro. 2010. Novel naphthalene-based inhibitors of *Trypanosoma brucei* RNA editing ligase 1. PLoS Negl. Trop. Dis. 4: e803.

Durrant, J.D., A.J. Friedman and J.A. McCammon. 2011. CrystalDock: a novel approach to fragment-based drug design. J. Chem. Inf. Model. 51: 2573–2580.

Erlanson, D.A., S.W. Fesik, R.E. Hubbard, W. Jahnke and H. Jhoti. 2016. Twenty years on: the impact of fragments on drug discovery. Nat. Rev. Drug Discov. 15: 605–619.

Erlanson, D.A. 2019. April 16. Third fragment-based drug approved! [Blog post]. http://practicalfragments.blogspot.com/2019/04/third-fragment-based-drug-approved.html.

Ettari, R., L. Tamborini, I.C. Angelo, N. Micale, A. Pinto, C. De Micheli et al. 2013. Inhibition of rhodesain as a novel therapeutic modality for human African trypanosomiasis. J. Med. Chem. 56: 5637–5658.

Fairlamb, A.H., P. Blackburn, P. Ulrich, B.T. Chait and A. Cerami. 1985. Trypanothione: a novel bis(glutathionyl) spermidine cofactor for glutathione reductase in trypanosomatids. Science. 227: 1485–1487.

Gilbert, I.H. 2013. Drug discovery for neglected diseases: molecular target-based and phenotypic approaches. J. Med. Chem. 56: 7719–7726.

Haanstra, J.R., E.B. Gonzalez-Marcano, M. Gualdron-Lopez and P.A. Michels. 2016. Biogenesis, maintenance and dynamics of glycosomes in trypanosomatid parasites. Biochim. Biophys. Acta. 1863: 1038–1048.

Hanau, S., E. Rinaldi, F. Dallocchio, I.H. Gilbert, C. Dardonville, M.J. Adams et al. 2004. 6-Phosphogluconate dehydrogenase: a target for drugs in African trypanosomes. Curr. Med. Chem. 11: 2639–2650.

Hann, M.M., A.R. Leach and G. Harper. 2001. Molecular complexity and its impact on the probability of finding leads for drug discovery. J. Chem. Inf. Comput. Sci. 41: 856–864.

Hernandez, J., L. Hoffer, B. Coutard, G. Querat, P. Roche, X. Morelli et al. 2019. Optimization of a fragment linking hit toward Dengue and Zika virus NS5 methyltransferases inhibitors. Eur. J. Med. Chem. 161: 323–333.

Hopkins, A.L., C.R. Groom and A. Alex. 2004. Ligand efficiency: a useful metric for lead selection. Drug Discov. Today. 9: 430–431.

Hotez, P.J., B. Pecoul, S. Rijal, C. Boehme, S. Aksoy, M. Malecela et al. 2016. Eliminating the neglected tropical diseases: translational science and new technologies. PLoS Negl. Trop. Dis. 10: e0003895.

Kalidas, S., I. Cestari, S. Monnerat, Q. Li, S. Regmi, N. Hasle et al. 2014. Genetic validation of aminoacyl-tRNA synthetases as drug targets in *Trypanosoma brucei*. Eukaryot. Cell. 13: 504–516.

Karthikeyan, S., Q. Zhou, A.L. Osterman and H. Zhang. 2003. Ligand binding-induced conformational changes in riboflavin kinase: structural basis for the ordered mechanism. Biochemistry. 42: 12532–12538.

Koh, C.Y., A.B. Wetzel, W.J. de van der Schueren and W.G. Hol. 2014. Comparison of histidine recognition in human and trypanosomatid histidyl-tRNA synthetases. Biochimie. 106: 111–120.

Koh, C.Y., L.K. Siddaramaiah, R.M. Ranade, J. Nguyen, T. Jian, Z. Zhang et al. 2015. A binding hotspot in *Trypanosoma cruzi* histidyl-tRNA synthetase revealed by fragment-based crystallographic cocktail screens. Acta Crystallogr. D Biol. Crystallogr. 71: 1684–1698.

Krauth-Siegel, R.L. and M.A. Comini. 2008. Redox control in trypanosomatids, parasitic protozoa with trypanothione-based thiol metabolism. Biochim. Biophys. Acta. 1780: 1236–1248.

Lim, S.P., L.S. Sonntag, C. Noble, S.H. Nilar, R.H. Ng, G. Zou et al. 2011. Small molecule inhibitors that selectively block dengue virus methyltransferase. J. Biol. Chem. 286: 6233–6240.

Lim, S.P., C.G. Noble and P.Y. Shi. 2015. The dengue virus NS5 protein as a target for drug discovery. Antiviral. Res. 119: 57–67.

Lim, S.P., C.G. Noble, C.C. Seh, T.S. Soh, A. El Sahili, G.K. Chan et al. 2016. Potent allosteric dengue virus NS5 polymerase inhibitors: mechanism of action and resistance profiling. PLoS Pathog. 12: e1005737.

Luo, D., T. Xu, R.P. Watson, D. Scherer-Becker, A. Sampath, W. Jahnke et al. 2008. Insights into RNA unwinding and ATP hydrolysis by the flavivirus NS3 protein. EMBO J. 27: 3209–3219.

Martin-Plaza, J. and E. Chatelain. 2015. Novel therapeutic approaches for neglected infectious diseases. J. Biomol. Screen. 20: 3–5.

Matusan, A.E., M.J. Pryor, A.D. Davidson and P.J. Wright. 2001. Mutagenesis of the dengue virus type 2 NS3 protein within and outside helicase motifs: effects on enzyme activity and virus replication. J. Virol. 75: 9633–9643.

McKerrow, J.H., P.S. Doyle, J.C. Engel, L.M. Podust, S.A. Robertson, R. Ferreira et al. 2009. Two approaches to discovering and developing new drugs for Chagas disease. Mem. Inst. Oswaldo Cruz. 104 Suppl. 1: 263–269.

McShan, D., S. Kathman, B. Lowe, Z. Xu, J. Zhan, A. Statsyuk et al. 2015. Identification of non-peptidic cysteine reactive fragments as inhibitors of cysteine protease rhodesain. Bioorg. Med. Chem. Lett. 25: 4509–4512.

Merritt, E.A., T.L. Arakaki, J.R. Gillespie, E.T. Larson, A. Kelley, N. Mueller et al. 2010. Crystal structures of trypanosomal histidyl-tRNA synthetase illuminate differences between eukaryotic and prokaryotic homologs. J. Mol. Biol. 397: 481–494.

Mishra, A., M.I. Khan, P.K. Jha, A. Kumar, S. Das, P. Das et al. 2018. Oxidative stress-mediated overexpression of uracil DNA glycosylase in *Leishmania donovani* confers tolerance against antileishmanial drugs. Oxid. Med. Cell Longev. 2018: 4074357.

Mpamhanga, C.P., D. Spinks, L.B. Tulloch, E.J. Shanks, D.A. Robinson, I.T. Collie et al. 2009. One scaffold, three binding modes: novel and selective pteridine reductase 1 inhibitors derived from fragment hits discovered by virtual screening. J. Med. Chem. 52: 4454–4465.

Murray, C.W. and T.L. Blundell. 2010. Structural biology in fragment-based drug design. Curr. Opin. Struct. Biol. 20: 497–507.

Nitsche, C., M.A. Behnam, C. Steuer and C.D. Klein. 2012. Retro peptide-hybrids as selective inhibitors of the Dengue virus NS2B-NS3 protease. Antiviral. Res. 94: 72–79.

Nitsche, C., V.N. Schreier, M.A. Behnam, A. Kumar, R. Bartenschlager and C.D. Klein. 2013. Thiazolidinone-peptide hybrids as dengue virus protease inhibitors with antiviral activity in cell culture. J. Med. Chem. 56: 8389–8403.

Nitsche, C., S. Holloway, T. Schirmeister and C.D. Klein. 2014. Biochemistry and medicinal chemistry of the dengue virus protease. Chem. Rev. 114: 11348–11381.

Niyomrattanakit, P., Y.L. Chen, H. Dong, Z. Yin, M. Qing, J.F. Glickman et al. 2010. Inhibition of dengue virus polymerase by blocking of the RNA tunnel. J. Virol. 84: 5678–5686.

Noble, C.G., Y.L. Chen, H. Dong, F. Gu, S.P. Lim, W. Schul et al. 2010. Strategies for development of Dengue virus inhibitors. Antiviral. Res. 85: 450–462.

Noble, C.G., S.P. Lim, R. Arora, F. Yokokawa, S. Nilar, C.C. Seh et al. 2016. A conserved pocket in the dengue virus polymerase identified through fragment-based screening. J. Biol. Chem. 291: 8541–8548.

Oberholzer, M., G. Marti, M. Baresic, S. Kunz, A. Hemphill and T. Seebeck. 2007. The *Trypanosoma brucei* cAMP phosphodiesterases TbrPDEB1 and TbrPDEB2: flagellar enzymes that are essential for parasite virulence. FASEB J. 21: 720–731.

Orrling, K.M., C. Jansen, X.L. Vu, V. Balmer, P. Bregy, A. Shanmugham et al. 2012. Catechol pyrazolinones as trypanocidals: fragment-based design, synthesis, and pharmacological evaluation of nanomolar inhibitors of trypanosomal phosphodiesterase B1. J. Med. Chem. 55: 8745–8756.

Pedrique, B., N. Strub-Wourgaft, C. Some, P. Olliaro, P. Trouiller, N. Ford et al. 2013. The drug and vaccine landscape for neglected diseases (2000–11): a systematic assessment. Lancet Glob. Health. 1: e371–379.

Pena-Diaz, J., M. Akbari, O. Sundheim, M.E. Farez-Vidal, S. Andersen, R. Sneve et al. 2004. *Trypanosoma cruzi* contains a single detectable uracil-DNA glycosylase and repairs uracil exclusively via short patch base excision repair. J. Mol. Biol. 342: 787–799.

Peplow, M. 2017. Astex shapes CDK4/6 inhibitor for approval. Nat. Biotechnol. 35: 395–396.

Pham, J.S., K.L. Dawson, K.E. Jackson, E.E. Lim, C.F. Pasaje, K.E. Turner et al. 2014. Aminoacyl-tRNA synthetases as drug targets in eukaryotic parasites. Int. J. Parasitol. Drugs Drug Resist. 4: 1–13.

Rajapakse, S. 2011. Dengue shock. J. Emerg. Trauma Shock. 4: 120–127.

Ruda, G.F., G. Campbell, V.P. Alibu, M.P., Barrett, R. Brenk and I.H. Gilbert. 2010. Virtual fragment screening for novel inhibitors of 6-phosphogluconate dehydrogenase. Bioorg. Med. Chem. 18: 5056–5062.

Ruddigkeit, L., R. van Deursen, L.C. Blum and J.L. Reymond. 2012. Enumeration of 166 billion organic small molecules in the chemical universe database GDB-17. J. Chem. Inf. Model. 52: 2864–2875.

Schmunis, G.A. and Z.E. Yadon. 2010. Chagas disease: a Latin American health problem becoming a world health problem. Acta Trop. 115: 14–21.

Scott, D.E., A.G. Coyne, S.A. Hudson and C. Abell. 2012. Fragment-based approaches in drug discovery and chemical biology. Biochemistry. 51: 4990–5003.

Shibata, S., Z. Zhang, K.V. Korotkov, J. Delarosa, A. Napuli, A.M. Kelley et al. 2011. Screening a fragment cocktail library using ultrafiltration. Anal. Bioanal. Chem. 401: 1585–1591.

Sienkiewicz, N., H.B. Ong and A.H. Fairlamb. 2010. *Trypanosoma brucei* pteridine reductase 1 is essential for survival *in vitro* and for virulence in mice. Mol. Microbiol. 77: 658–671.

Spinks, D., H.B. Ong, C.P. Mpamhanga, E.J. Shanks, D.A. Robinson, I.T. Collie et al. 2011. Design, synthesis and biological evaluation of novel inhibitors of *Trypanosoma brucei* pteridine reductase 1. ChemMedChem. 6: 302–308.

Steverding, D., D.W. Sexton, X. Wang, S.S. Gehrke, G.K. Wagner and C.R. Caffrey. 2012. *Trypanosoma brucei:* chemical evidence that cathepsin L is essential for survival and a relevant drug target. Int. J. Parasitol. 42: 481–488.

Tsai, C.H., P.Y. Lee, V. Stollar and M.L. Li. 2006. Antiviral therapy targeting viral polymerase. Curr. Pharm. Des. 12: 1339–1355.

Verlinde, C.L., H. Kim, B.E. Bernstein, S.C. Mande and W.G. Hol. 1997. Anti-trypanosomiasis drug development based on structures of glycolytic enzymes. pp. 365–394. *In*: P. Veerapandian [ed.]. Structure-based Drug Design. Marcel Dekker Inc, New York.

Verlinde, C.L., E. Fan, S. Shibata, Z. Zhang, Z. Sun, W. Deng et al. 2009. Fragment-based cocktail crystallography by the Medical Structural Genomics of Pathogenic Protozoa Consortium. Curr. Top. Med. Chem. 9: 1678–1687.

Vincent, I.M. and M.P. Barrett. 2015. Metabolomic-based strategies for anti-parasite drug discovery. J. Biomol. Screen. 20: 44–55.

WHO. 2009. Dengue: guidelines for diagnosis, treatment, prevention and control—New edition. World Health Organization.

WHO. 2017. Integrating neglected tropical diseases into global health and development: fourth WHO report on neglected tropical diseases. World Health Organization.

WHO. 2018a. Neglected tropical diseases. World Health Organization. https://www.who.int/neglected_diseases/diseases/en/ (accessed December 12, 2018).

WHO. 2018b. Chagas disease (American Trypanosomiasis)—Epidemiology. World Health Organization. https://www.who.int/chagas/epidemiology/en/ (accessed December 12, 2018).

WHO. 2018c. Trypanosomiasis, human African (sleeping sickness). World Health Organization. https://www.who.int/news-room/fact-sheets/detail/trypanosomiasis-human-african-(sleeping-sickness) (accessed December 12, 2018).

WHO. 2018d. WHO outlines criteria to assess elimination of sleeping sickness. World Health Organization. https://www.who.int/neglected_diseases/news/criteria-eliminate-sleeping-sickness/en/ (accessed December 12, 2018).

WHO. 2018e. Leishmaniasis. World Health Organization. https://www.who.int/leishmaniasis/en/ (accessed December 12, 2018).

WHO. 2018f. Dengue and severe dengue. World Health Organization. https://www.who.int/news-room/fact-sheets/detail/dengue-and-severe-dengue (accessed December 12, 2018).

Yap, T.L., T. Xu, Y.L. Chen, H. Malet, M.P. Egloff, B. Canard et al. 2007. Crystal structure of the dengue virus RNA-dependent RNA polymerase catalytic domain at 1.85-angstrom resolution. J. Virol. 81: 4753–4765.

Yin, Z., Y.L. Chen, R.R. Kondreddi, W.L. Chan, G. Wang, R.H. Ng et al. 2009. *N*-Sulfonylanthranilic acid derivatives as allosteric inhibitors of dengue viral RNA-dependent RNA polymerase. J. Med. Chem. 52: 7934–7937.

Yokokawa, F., S. Nilar, C.G. Noble, S.P. Lim, R. Rao, S. Tania et al. 2016. Discovery of potent non-nucleoside inhibitors of dengue viral RNA-dependent RNA polymerase from a fragment hit using structure-based drug design. J. Med. Chem. 59: 3935–3952.

Yon, C., T. Teramoto, N. Mueller, J. Phelan, V.K. Ganesh, K.H. Murthy et al. 2005. Modulation of the nucleoside triphosphatase/RNA helicase and 5'-RNA triphosphatase activities of Dengue virus type 2 nonstructural protein 3 (NS3) by interaction with NS5, the RNA-dependent RNA polymerase. J. Biol. Chem. 280: 27412–27419.

Zhao, Y., T.S. Soh, J. Zheng, K.W. Chan, W.W. Phoo, C.C. Lee et al. 2015. A crystal structure of the Dengue virus NS5 protein reveals a novel inter-domain interface essential for protein flexibility and virus replication. PLoS Pathog. 11: e1004682.

Zust, R., H. Dong, X.F. Li, D.C. Chang, B. Zhang, T. Balakrishnan et al. 2013. Rational design of a live attenuated dengue vaccine: 2'-*O*-methyltransferase mutants are highly attenuated and immunogenic in mice and macaques. PLoS Pathog. 9: e1003521.

Chapter **3**

Chemical Hybridization Approaches Applied to Natural and Synthetic Compounds for the Discovery of Drugs Active Against Neglected Tropical Diseases

Elena Petricci,* Paolo Governa and *Fabrizio Manetti*

Introduction

Within the drug discovery process, serendipity is often counterposed to the rational design approach, in terms of both logic and chronology. There is in fact a significant number of literature reports published in scientific journals that describes approaches going from "serendipity to rational" drug design or discovery. In the popular imagination, serendipity means that there was something lucky during the experiments and the corresponding results came from fortunate events. Serendipity is a term coined by Walpole to describe accidental discoveries made by "the three princes of Serendip" who reached smart deductions and outstanding conclusions that were based on their powers of observation. Examples of serendipity can be found everywhere: Cristoforo Colombo who discovered America instead of reaching the Indies, Dante Alighieri who "goes looking for silver and apart from his intention finds gold" (Alighieri 1304) and many scientists who made the most spectacular discovery of their career. After all, we very well know that "*le hasard ne favorise l'invention que pour des esprits préparés aux découvertes par de patientes études et de persévérants efforts*" (Pasteur Vallery-Radot 1939). However, in disagreement with this latter statement, high-throughput screening approaches and phenotypic screening recently culminated the serendipity.

On the contrary, the tremendous and continuous advancements in both theoretical and experimental research fields led to the collection of a huge amount of information of the biological systems under study. Fruitfully, the knowledge of the molecular basis of the target-ligand interactions allowed flowering of many drug design strategies, such as structure-based and ligand-based drug design approaches.

Dipartimento di Biotecnologie, Chimica e Farmacia, Dipartimento di Eccellenza 2018-2022, Università di Siena, via A. Moro 2, 53100 Siena, Italy.
* Corresponding author: elena.petricci@unisi.it

One of the pioneering review that described the transition from serendipity to a rational approach in drug discovery was published about twenty years ago (Kubinyi 1999). In this context, the molecular hybridization approach to drug design could be part of the rational conception of new active compounds on the basis of ligand-based considerations. Given the availability of structurally different classes of biologically active compounds and the relationships between their structure and activity, molecular hybridization combines the pharmacophoric portions of these active molecules to design new hybrid chemical entities with an improved biological profile in terms of pharmacokinetics or pharmacodynamics, or both of them.

In the past, however, the term hybrid ligand or hybrid drug has been used with the different meaning of non-selective or dual compounds, with the aim of describing multitarget agents able to interact with more than one biological macromolecules (i.e., receptor, enzyme, channel, etc.) (van Zwieten 1988, Di Marzo et al. 2001).

Moving toward the concept of hybrid compounds currently most used in drug design and medicinal chemistry, there are examples of molecular hybrids obtained by fermentation in enriched culture media or by genetic engineering. Feeding erythronolide B, an intermediate of erythromycin biosynthesis, to *Streptomyces antibioticus*, a strain able to produce oleandomycin (a 14-membered macrolide similar to erythromycin), a small series of new erythromycin/oleandomycin hybrid antibiotics was obtained (Spagnoli et al. 1983). As an alternative, isolation of genes that codify for isochromanequinone antibiotics and their transfer between different strains of *Streptomyces* allowed production of new hybrid compounds by integrated biosynthetic pathways derived from two different streptomycetes. Following this approach, new hybrid antibiotics were obtained by gene transfer between microorganisms able to produce different antibiotics (Hopwood et al. 1985).

Further approaching the hybrid compounds of the drug design process, studies performed in the early 80s led to a combination of α and β human chorionic gonadotropin subunits to produce a new pharmaceutical product able to induce gonadal stimulations (Rosemberg 1982). In a similar way, combination of the A chain of insulin and the B domain of insulin-like growth factor I yielded a hybrid peptide with insulin-like properties, although its activity profile was very weak in comparison to insulin (Joshi et al. 1985).

During the same years, computer-assisted drug design has made a breakthrough in the process of drug design and discovery. Many papers appeared at that time to describe research projects where dedicated computer softwares were used to increase the efficacy of drug identification steps. Part of these works was aimed at finding new hybrid compounds by merging already known active small molecules, under the assumption that such compounds acted with the same mechanism of action by interactions with the same site on their receptor. As an example, following a classical medicinal chemistry approach, the common pharmacophoric portions of known aldose reductase inhibitors were identified by SAR and merged together into new hybrid inhibitors which were further optimized by a molecular simplification approach (Butera et al. 1989). Computational resources were also applied to build hybrid compounds by combining or shuffling the building blocks of two or more known compounds into libraries of first generation daughter molecules. These methods were based on the attempt to convert biological evolution into chemical evolution and are known as genetic algorithms or drug evolution (Lazar et al. 2004).

In recent years, a huge amount of literature reports described new compounds that have been derived from molecular hybridization (Viegas-Junior et al. 2007, de Oliveira Pedrosa et al. 2017, Manssour Fraga 2009). Expectedly, our research group also designed new structures by merging portions of already known bioactive agents. As examples, suradista analogues (a hybrid class of compounds built with portions of suramin and distamycin) were studied as inhibitors of the bFGF (Manetti et al. 1998) or the HIV-1 entry on host cells (Manetti et al. 2000), WB4101/arylpiperazine hybrids (Barbaro et al. 2002) and trazodone-like arylpiperazines (Betti et al. 2002) were proposed as inhibitors of the α_1-adrenergic receptors, new antimycobacterial aminopyrroles were designed as hybrids between the antitubercular agents SQ109 and BM212 (Bhakta et al. 2016), and, finally, quercetin/oleic acid hybrids were found as insulin secretion modulators (Badolato et al. 2017).

The purpose of this chapter is to describe representative examples of molecular hybridization applied to the neglected tropical diseases. Alternative rational design tools, such as bioisosterism and molecular modifications (simplification and complication, rigidification and structural pruning, ring-chain transformation such as anelation and ring opening, homologation and branching, and salification) will not be considered.

In particular, we have taken into account the list of neglected tropical diseases (defined as "a diverse group of communicable diseases that prevail in tropical and subtropical conditions in 149 countries") reported by WHO (World Health Organization, Neglected Tropical Diseases 2018b). For each of them, the WHO web site reports a link to the PubMed references that cited the specific disease. Next, citations for each disease were pruned by keeping only those that deal with hybrid compounds. The resulting publications are reviewed here. A very recent survey on hybrid compounds designed against leishmaniasis and Chagas disease has been reported (Cardona-Galeano et al. 2018). However, several additional examples were found in the literature and described here.

In addition to neglected tropical diseases, tuberculosis and malaria, a mycobacterial and a parasitic disease, respectively, which are widely diffused within tropical regions, also deserve great attention for their re-emergence, and wide distribution and could be in principle considered as appropriate topics for this review. However, an article on recent advances in antitubercular molecular hybrids was published in 2017 (Singh et al. 2017) and no significant improvements were done in this field in the last year. For this reason, a survey of hybrid compounds to be used as antimycobacterial agents does not fall within the purpose of our bibliographic research. On the contrary, scientific reports dealing with antimalarial hybrid compounds are reviewed here.

Hybrid Derivatives Active against American Trypanosomiasis (Chagas Disease)

Chagas disease is a zoonotic disease caused by the protozoan parasite *Trypanosoma cruzi* that can be transmitted to humans by blood-sucking triatomine bugs (also known as the "kissing" bug) belonging to the genera *Triatoma*, *Rhodnius*, and *Panstrongylus* (Centers for Disease Control and Prevention 2018a). The parasite life cycle is divided in human (host) stages and triatomine bug stages. Chagas disease is currently treated with nifurtimox 1 and benznidazole 2 (Figure 1).

Antiparasitic treatment, however, has common side effects that become more frequent and severe in adults older than 50 years with chronic *T. cruzi* infection (Centers for Disease Control and Prevention 2018b). Efficacy limited to early stage disease, significant side effects, and access to drugs for less than 1% infected people are the major limitations of the current therapy that suggest the need for new drugs, as well as for more effective diagnostics and biomarkers for disease progression (Dumonteil and Herrera 2017, Reed and McKerrow 2018).

One of the first attempts to use hybrid molecules with the aim of affecting the cell cycle of *T. cruzi* was based on the pivotal evidence of the parasite ability to internalize IgG antibodies attached to the external surface of its membrane and that different stages of the parasite life depend on the availability of low density lipoproteins (LDL). A combination of these facts led to the rational design of immunotoxins (more recently referred to as antibody-drug conjugates, ADC), which are molecular constructs between an antibody (anti *T. cruzi* LDL receptor) and a small molecule or protein acting as cytotoxic agent. While these ADC were demonstrated to be excellent carriers to deliver drugs to specific target cells, they showed only partial success in parasite eradication. In fact, ADC with abrin and ricin (two plant protein toxins acting as type 2 ribosome-inactivating proteins) abrogated motility of parasite forms *in vitro*, without reducing parasitemia or increasing survival of infected mice (Santana and Teixeira 1989). When the drug was replaced by chlorambucil (that was already known to be efficiently delivered by ADC systems) (Ghose and Nigam

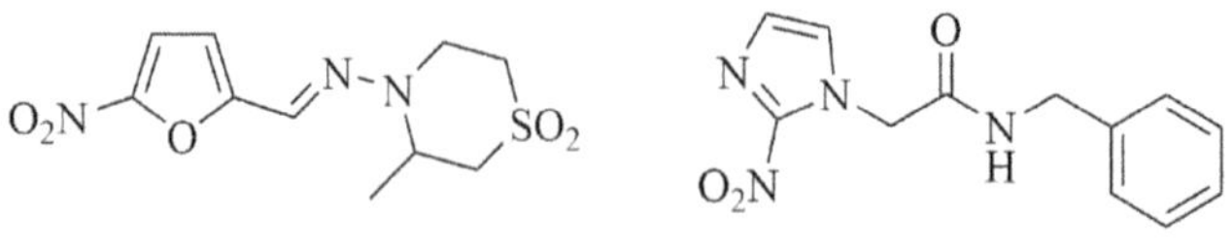

nifurtimox, **1**   benznidazole, **2**

Figure 1. Structure of active ingredients (nifurtimox and benznidazole) of drugs for Chagas disease.

1972), replication of the parasite was blocked (1 µM test concentration), the levels of parasitemia were reduced significantly (3–30-fold decrease), and consequently, treated mice survived 11 days post-infection in comparison to 55% of mice which died in untreated control group (Carvalhaes et al. 1998).

In recent years, there has been a recurrence of interest in studying natural compounds as a source of biologically active entities. As expected, chemical scaffolds mainly isolated by plants or microorganisms currently represent useful tools for the identification of new antitrypanosomal agents. Naphthoquinones are examples of naturally-occurring compounds characterized by a broad spectrum of action. On this basis, the naphthoquinone pharmacophore is considered as a privileged scaffold to obtain new classes of compounds with various biological activity. The main feature of the quinone system is its ability to be reduced chemically and, as a consequence, to be an oxidizing agent able to generate reactive oxygen species.

As an example of naphthoquinones, lapachol **3** and the isomeric tricyclic α- and β-lapachone (**4** and **5**) were extracted from the inner wood of various plants belonging to the Bignoniaceae family, such as *Tabebuia avellanedae* Lorentz ex Griseb (Figure 2). These compounds caused oxidative damage in trypanosomatids consequent to the release of peroxide and superoxide anions and radicals. Their major limitation was the inactivation in the presence of serum proteins, whose free amino groups can react with the quinone system. Fortunately, this reaction was avoided in the 3-allyl derivative of β-lapachone that proved effective toward trypomastigotes also in the presence of blood (Gonçalves et al. 1980).

Considering the antiparasitic activity of β-lapachone derivatives, their tricyclic naphthoquinone pharmacophore was chosen as the starting point to design new trypanocidal hybrid compounds. Considering that phenazines were known for their broad microbicidal activity, hybrids were synthesized by merging both the phenazine nucleus and the β-lapachone structure to obtain new polycyclic trypanocidal compounds. In particular, **6** (reminiscent of clofazimine, an antimycobacterial agent used toward non-tuberculous mycobacteria, such as *M. leprae*, in antileprosy drugs) was obtained following an original synthetic procedure using a quinone and a mono-amine instead of the usual synthesis based on quinone and 1,2-phenylenediamine (Neves-Pinto et al. 2002). In detail, the iminophenazine **6** resulted from reaction of β-lapachone (in turn obtained from lapachol extracted by natural sources) and aniline in the presence of HCl. Trypanocidal activity was better than that of crystal violet used as the reference compound (ED_{50} values after 24 h were 61 and 536 µM, respectively, toward bloodstream trypomastigote forms of *T. cruzi*, measuring the lysis of the parasites). Many additional lapachone hybrid derivatives were also designed and synthesized by changing the dione redox center of β-lapachone with various heterocycles known to have antibacterial or antiparasitic activity, such as indole, oxazole, and triazole rings (Pinto and de Castro 2009, de Moura et al. 2001). Among the resulting compounds, the arylimidazoles **7** and **8** (reminiscent of benznidazole) showed an enhancement in activity in comparison to the parent compound (15 and 37 µM) and were also effective toward intracellular forms of the parasite, with only moderate cytotoxicity to host (de Moura et al. 2001).

Moreover, the dihydropyran ring was also transformed into the corresponding dihydrofuran moiety by a ring contraction approach. Among the anilino derivatives of *nor*-β-lapachone, only the *m*-NO$_2$ and *p*-OMe substituents (as in **9** and **10**, respectively) resulted in IC_{50} values of 86 and 88 µM, respectively, toward the bloodstream trypomastigotes of the Y strain (measuring the lysis of the parasites as in the assay above), in comparison to a 103 µM found for benznidazole. No scientifically-compelling SAR considerations can be ruled for these compounds (da Silva et al. 2008a). Further hybridization of the *nor*-β-lapachone scaffold through 1,3-dipolar reaction led to 3-(1,2,3-triazol-1-yl) derivatives that showed the best activity with the 4-phenyl and 4-cyclohexyl substituents (17 and 58 µM found for **11** and **12**, respectively) or with the corresponding 3-azido precursor **13** (50 µM) (da Silva et al. 2008b). Very recently, additional 1,4-naphthoquinones were described to have trypanocidal activity toward both bloodstream and cultured trypomastigotes of *T. cruzi* Y strain (Lara et al. 2018). Compound **14** also showed an inhibitory profile better than or comparable to that of benznidazole toward trypomastigotes of different strains (Brazil— IC_{50} = 8 and 93 µM, respectively—and CL - IC_{50} = 54 and 69 µM, respectively) and clones (Dm28c-Luc, IC_{50} = 21 and 25 µM, respectively). A significant activity was also found toward the intracellular amastigotes of Dm28c-Luc clone and Y strain (IC_{50} = 9 and 4 µM, respectively). The same compound showed low toxicity for cardiac muscle cells, as also found for benznidazole (CC_{50} = 137 and > 500 µM, respectively, with a selectivity index of 44 and > 455, respectively).

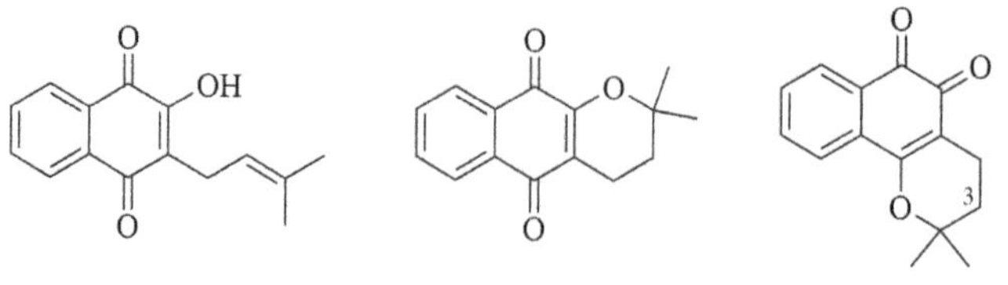

lapachol, **3**   α-lapachone, **4**   β-lapachone, **5**

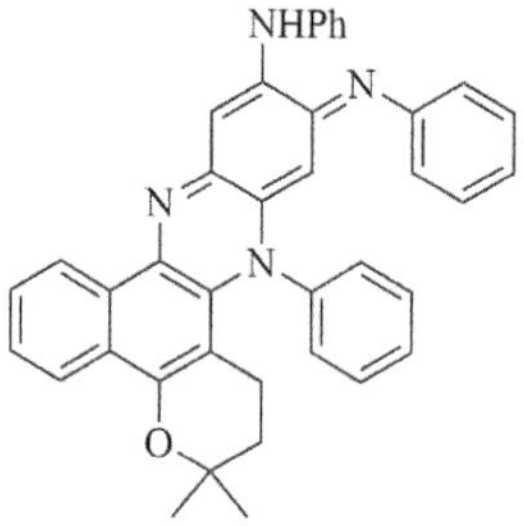

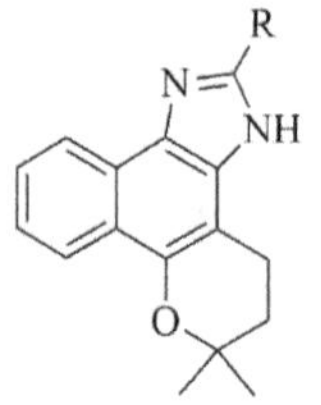

6
ED$_{50}$ = 61 μM

7: R = Ph, ED$_{50}$ = 37 μM
8: R = indol-3-yl, ED$_{50}$ = 15 μM

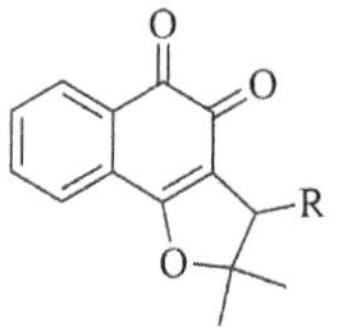

9: R = *m*-NO$_2$-anilino, IC$_{50}$ = 86 μM
10: R = *m*-OMe-anilino, IC$_{50}$ = 88 μM
11: R = 4-phenyl-1*H*-1,2,3-triazol-1-yl, IC$_{50}$ = 17 μM
12: R = 4-(1-hydroxycyclohexyl)-1*H*-1,2,3-triazol-1-yl, IC$_{50}$ = 58 μM
13: R = azido, IC$_{50}$ = 50 μM

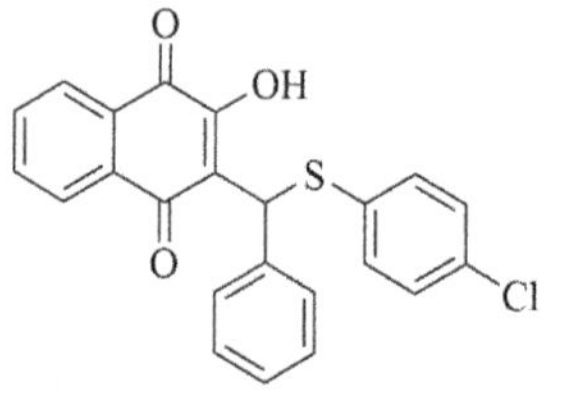

14
antitrypomastigotes IC$_{50}$ = 8-54 μM
antiamastigotes IC$_{50}$ = 9 μM
cytotoxicity CC$_{50}$ = 137 μM

Figure 2. Design and optimization of naphthoquinone-phenazine hybrids.

Another interesting example of anti *T. cruzi* hybrids is represented by compounds designed by merging a furoxan nucleus (a 1,2,5-oxadiazole *N*-oxide known to be a nitric oxide donor) with an *N*-acylhydrazone or thiosemicarbazone moiety that are chemical features found in several inhibitors of various parasitic enzymes, such as the major cysteine protease cruzain (Figure 3). The rational design of these compounds was based on the fact that nitric oxide is a cytotoxic and cytostatic agent for different parasites, including *T. cruzi*. On the other hand, cruzain, which can be inhibited by *N*-acylhydrazone or thiosemicarbazone derivatives, is a *T. cruzi* specific cysteine protease, whose inhibitors should not affect host cysteine proteases. Experimental data on the trypanocidal activity toward epimastigotes and amastigotes *in vitro* showed that two of the most active *N*-acylhydrazone derivatives (**15** and **16**) had the isoniazide moiety and showed

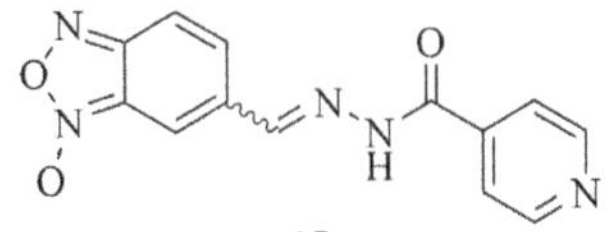

15

$IC_{50,\ epimast} = 33\ \mu M$
$IC_{50,\ amast} = 5.6\ \mu M$
$SI = 24$

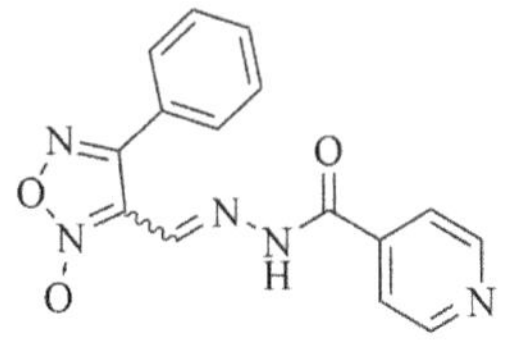

16

$IC_{50,\ epimast} = 11\ \mu M$
$IC_{50,\ amast} = 6.4\ \mu M$
$SI > 63$

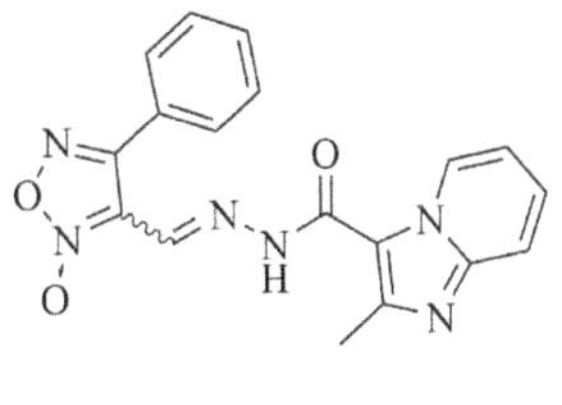

17

$IC_{50,\ epimast} = 5.0\ \mu M$
$IC_{50,\ amast} = 0.9\ \mu M$
$SI = 62$

Figure 3. Structure and activity of N-acylhydrazone-furoxan hybrids.

high selectivity index (> 63 and 24, respectively, determined as $IC_{50,macrophages}/IC_{50,amastigotes}$ and $IC_{50,VERO\ cells}/IC_{50,amastigotes}$) that indicated low cytotoxicity (Hernandez et al. 2013). An additional compound (**17**) bearing an imidazo-pyridine heterocycle instead of the pyridine nucleus was the most active compound reported, with submicromolar activity toward amastigotes and an $IC_{50} = 5\ \mu M$ toward epimastigotes.

In the attempt to generate retro-isosters of the *N*-acylhydrazone-furoxan derivatives, a series of 15 compounds was synthesized and tested (Figure 4) (Serafim et al. 2014). The most active compounds **18** and **19** possessed a *p*-nitro benzamide moiety, while decoration at the heterocyclic nucleus (in terms of substituents and position of the *N*-oxide moiety) seemed not to be important for activity. Moving the nitro group to the meta position as in **20** and **21**, activity underwent a reduction with IC_{50} values within the two-digit micromolar concentration (from 3 to 10 μM, and from 3 to 15 μM, respectively), while unsubstituted phenyl derivatives are inactive (see **22** as an example). These results supported the hypothesis of the importance of the nitro substituent as a "parasitophoric group" that may interfere with the redox machinery of the parasites (Serafim et al. 2014). Moreover, replacement of the phenyl moiety with a furan cycle led to **23** and **24** with significant activity (7 and 8 μM, respectively). Trypanocidal activity was not dependent on the amount of nitric oxide released, the most active compounds showing intermediate values of released NO. A cell-free assay to evaluate the ability of **18** and **19** to inhibit cruzain showed two-digit micromolar inhibition (11 and 15 μM, respectively). Moreover, Caco-2 permeability assay indicates good absorption for **18** and low permeability for **19**, without significant P-gp-mediated efflux transport.

Among (iso)thiosemicarbazone-furoxan hybrids, **25**–**27** showed an *in vitro* antiepimastigote activity toward two parasite strains (Tulahuen 2 strain and Brener clone) comparable to that of reference compounds nifurtimox and benznidazole (Figure 5) (Porcal et al. 2008). Cytotoxicity of **26** and **27** toward J-774 mouse macrophages was low (142 and 400 μM, respectively), with an important selectivity between 21 and 27. Unexpectedly, cruzain, which was predicted to be one of the possible targets of such compounds, was inhibited by **25** and **27** with IC_{50} values of 78 μM and 43 μM, respectively, thus suggesting that the mechanism of action was not based on the inhibition of this enzyme. Interestingly, ESR spectroscopy showed that **25** and **27** were metabolically instable in parasite microsomes, yielding *N*-oxide and hydroxyl radical. This result was consistent with the hypothesis that *N*-oxide moiety could affect the parasite redox system by generating oxidative stress.

The NO releasing furoxan pharmacophore was also used to design hybrid compounds together with the antimalarial drug amodiaquine (**28**, Figure 6) (Mott et al. 2012). The purpose of this strategy

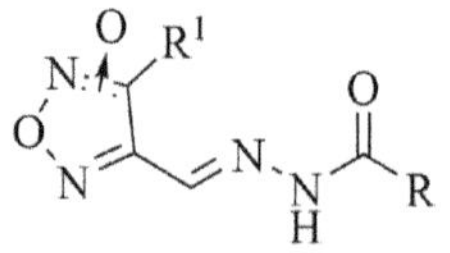

18: R = *p*-NO$_2$-Ph, R^1 = Me, 5-*N*-oxide, IC$_{50}$ = 3 μM
19: R = *p*-NO$_2$-Ph, R^1 = Ph, 2-*N*-oxide, IC$_{50}$ = 3 μM
20: R = *m*-NO$_2$-Ph, R^1 = Me, 5-*N*-oxide, IC$_{50}$ = 10 μM
21: R = *m*-NO$_2$-Ph, R^1 = Ph, 2-*N*-oxide, IC$_{50}$ = 15 μM
22: R = Ph, R^1 = Me, 5-*N*-oxide, IC$_{50}$ > 100 μM
23: R = fur-2-yl, R^1 = Me, 5-*N*-oxide, IC$_{50}$ = 7 μM
24: R = fur-2-yl, R^1 = Ph, 2-*N*-oxide, IC$_{50}$ = 8 μM

Figure 4. Structure and activity of N-acylhydrazone-furoxan hybrids.

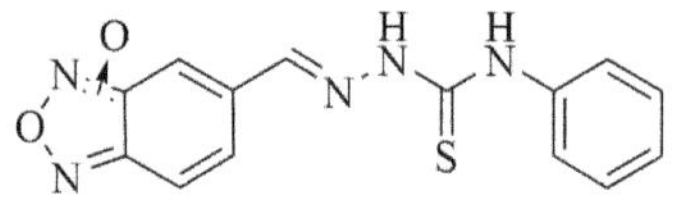

25: IC$_{50, \text{Tulahuen 2}}$ = 8.9 μM, IC$_{50, \text{Brener CL}}$ = 2.6 μM
CC$_{50, \text{J-774}}$ < 50 μM, SI < 6

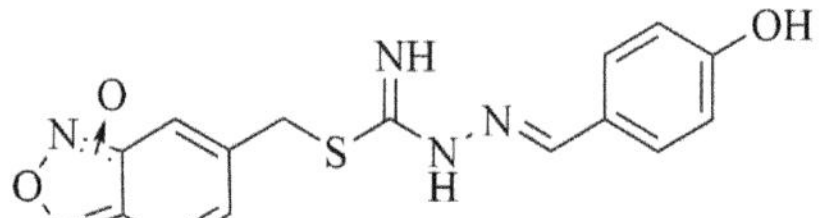

26: IC$_{50, \text{Tulahuen 2}}$ = 6.8 μM
CC$_{50, \text{J-774}}$ = 142 μM, SI = 21

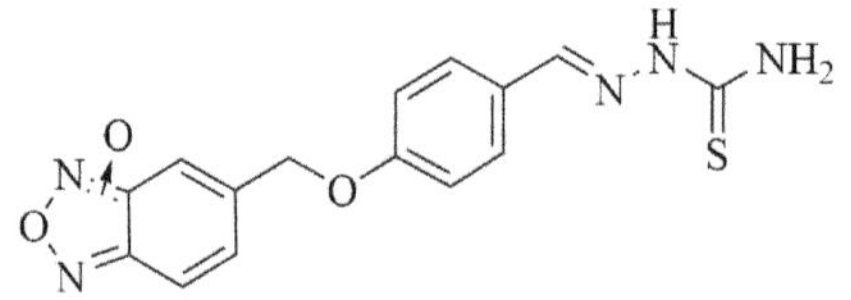

27: IC$_{50, \text{Tulahuen 2}}$ = 15 μM, IC$_{50, \text{Brener CL}}$ = 20 μM
CC$_{50, \text{J-774}}$ = 400 μM, SI = 27

Figure 5. Structure and activity of (iso)thiosemicarbazone-furoxan hybrids.

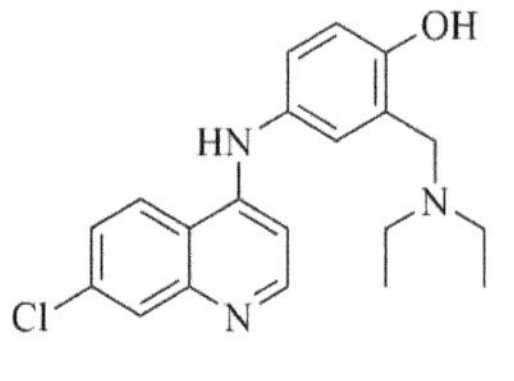

amodiaquine, **28** 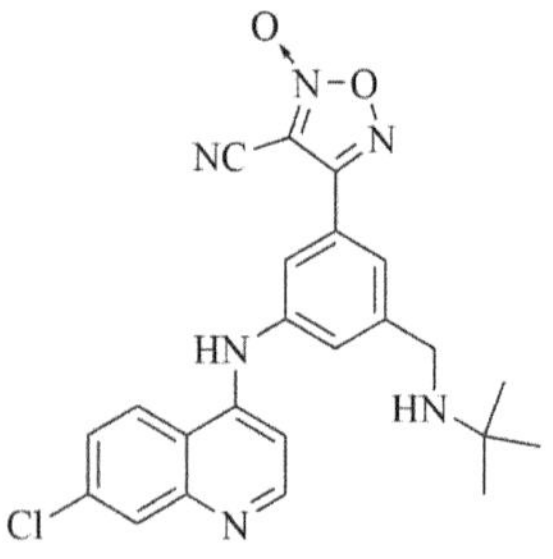   **29**

Figure 6. Amodiaquine and its hybrid derivative with a furoxan nucleus.

was the combination of different pharmacophores to enable hybrids to point toward different molecular targets. Hybridization between phenyl-furoxan (already known to affect life cycle of various parasites) and amodiaquine was planned in such a way to delete the phenolic hydroxyl substituent present in the *p*-aminophenol metabolite responsible for toxic side effects of amodiaquine. Moreover, resulting compounds were easily accessible (in terms of synthetic pathways) than amodiaquine itself. In particular, starting from 4,7-dichloroquinoline, an addition-elimination reaction was used to add a substituted anilino moiety in position 4 of the quinoline. In the next steps, the furoxan ring was obtained by cyclization of a cinnamyl ester yielded by the Heck reaction. Finally, che cyano group of the original phenyl-furoxan was added to the position 3 of the five-membered heterocyclic nucleus. Antimalarial activity of the resulting compounds was evaluated in infected human erythrocytes by monitoring short- and long-term (96 h) *P. falciparum* proliferation. The most active compound (**29**) showed a 40 and 630 nM IC_{50}, respectively. In addition, antischistosomal activity was evaluated in a cell-free assay (by monitoring the thioredoxin glutathione reductase activity that was known to be inhibited by furoxan-based NO release), as well as in an *ex vivo* worm (*S. mansoni*) killing assay. The hybrid compound **29** reduced enzyme activity by 80% at 10 µM, while worm survival was abrogated within 24 h (50 µM). Finally, an *ex vivo* worm survival assay was also performed to evaluate the nematicidal activity of **29** toward hookworm (*A. ceylanicum*). Percent survival of parasite was reduced to 40, 30, and 0 by 100 µM after 72, 96, and 120 h, respectively.

Antiprotozoal hybrid compounds, also characterized by antitrypanosomal activity, were designed starting from the structure of nitazoxanide **30** (Figure 7), the gold standard drug for the treatment of persistent diarrhea caused by parasites. The structure of this compound is made by merging the amino group of a 2-amino-5-nitro-thiazole moiety with the carboxy group of the acetylsalicylic acid in an amide bond. The major limitation of this drug is its solubility (7.6 mg/L) (The Human Metabolome Database 2018). In fact, it is classified as practically insoluble in water as a class IV drug (low solubility, low permeability), according to the biopharmaceutical classification system. In the attempt to enhance water solubility of the drug, hybrid compounds were generated replacing the acetylsalicylic portion of the molecule with structural portions of other non-steroidal antiinflammatory drugs (NSAIDs), such as diclofenac, ibuprofen, naproxen, clofibric acid, and indomethacin, thus leading to **31–35**, respectively (Colin-Lozano et al. 2017). A DCC-activated direct Steglich-type amidation of the NSAIDs drug with the amino-thiazole in the presence of DMAP as the basic catalyst led to the final hybrid compounds in low-medium yield (23–50%). Biological evaluation assays were performed toward a panel of protozoa including *T. cruzi*. IC_{50} values were in the range between 12 and 16 µM, about two-fold better than that of benznidazole (34 µM) and lower than that of nifurtimox (7 µM). Unfortunately, a significant cytotoxicity toward VERO cells was found (CC_{50} from 13 to 201 µM), that consequently led to very low selectivity index (the most favorable SI was 14

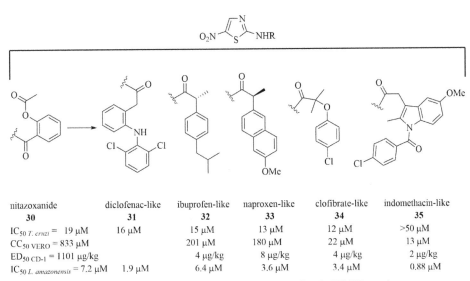

	nitazoxanide **30**	diclofenac-like **31**	ibuprofen-like **32**	naproxen-like **33**	clofibrate-like **34**	indomethacin-like **35**
$IC_{50\ T.\ cruzi}$ =	19 µM	16 µM	15 µM	13 µM	12 µM	>50 µM
$CC_{50\ VERO}$ =	833 µM		201 µM	180 µM	22 µM	13 µM
$ED_{50\ CD-1}$ =	1101 µg/kg		4 µg/kg	8 µg/kg	4 µg/kg	2 µg/kg
$IC_{50\ L.\ amazonensis}$ =	7.2 µM	1.9 µM	6.4 µM	3.6 µM	3.4 µM	0.88 µM

Figure 7. Nitazoxanide derivatives obtained by changing the NSAIDs portion.

for **33**). While the overall biological profile of these compounds as antitrypanosomal agents was not impressive, they showed *in vitro* nanomolar activity toward *Giardia intestinalis* and *in vivo* giardicidal effect from hundred- to thousand-fold better than that of metronidazole and nitazoxanide (ED_{50} ranged from 1.7 to 7.7 µg/kg, in comparison to 194 and 1100 µg/kg for the known drugs), respectively, in a CD-1 mouse model infected with trophozoites of the parasite. Interestingly, the antileishmanial activity of these compounds ranged within the single-digit micromolar concentrations (from 1.9 to 6.4 µM toward *L. amazonensis*), with **35** as the best active compound ($IC_{50} = 0.88$ µM).

As further examples of naturally-occurring compounds used to build nature-inspired hybrids, caffeic acid esters (Figure 8) are known for their ability to affect life cycle of *Leishmania* and *Trypanosoma* parasites, although they are generally toxic for mammalian cells. On the other hand, also triclosan **36** is able to inhibit *Leishmania* and *Plasmodium* by a competitive inhibition of enoyl-acyl carrier protein reductase. In the attempt to find new antiparasitic agents, the diphenyl ether scaffold of triclosan was combined with the caffeic acid structure through an alkyl spacer of variable length (Otero et al. 2017). Hybrid compounds were assayed on intracellular amastigotes of *T. cruzi* and *L. panamensis* to check for their ability to kill the parasites inside macrophages. Being macrophages the host cells that undergo infections, they were used to assess cytotoxicity of the new compounds. SAR analysis suggested that activity depended on the overall length of the alkyl spacer and the number of carbon atoms (even or odd). Most of the new compounds showed significant cytotoxicity and low selectivity index, although some of them had high activity. The butyl spacer was associated to the most active compound **37**, which showed a micromolar activity toward both parasites ($EC_{50} = 4$ and 8 µM, respectively) and a significant cytotoxicity ($LD_{50} = 12$ µM).

Other diphenyl ethers, which bear a biphosphonic moiety at the terminal edge, are important compounds for antiparasitic treatments. Many parasites, including *T. cruzi*, have the ability to import cholesterol from the host. *T. cruzi* is, however, obligated to synthesize endogenous sterols, such as ergosterol and other 24-alkyl sterols, through the mevalonate pathway that progresses *via* the squalene synthase enzyme. Since both biphosphonate compounds and the 4-phenoxyphenoxyethyl thiocyanate WC-9 (**38**, Figure 9) are reported as inhibitors of squalene synthase of *T. cruzi*, their hybrid compounds (**39–42**) (Chao et al.

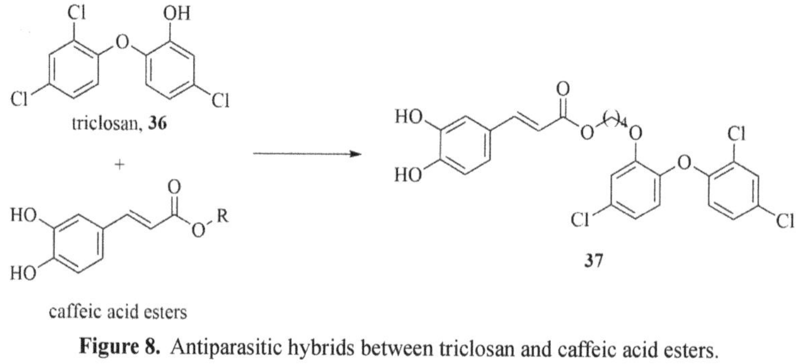

Figure 8. Antiparasitic hybrids between triclosan and caffeic acid esters.

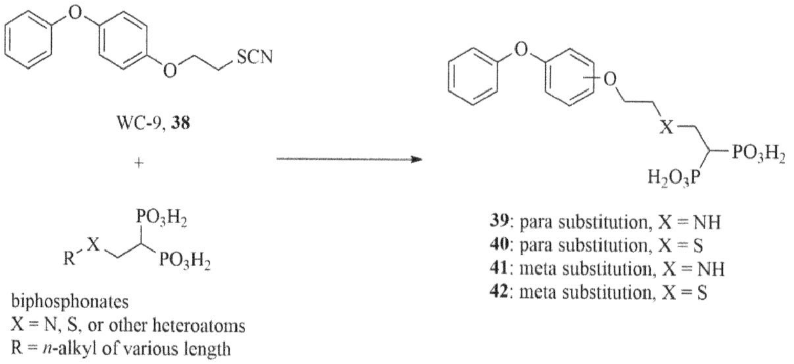

39: para substitution, X = NH
40: para substitution, X = S
41: meta substitution, X = NH
42: meta substitution, X = S

WC-9, **38**

biphosphonates
X = N, S, or other heteroatoms
R = *n*-alkyl of various length

Figure 9. Diphenyl ether-biphosphonate hybrids as inhibitors of *T. cruzi* amastigotes.

2016) were designed as putative antitrypanosomal agents with improved activity in comparison to the parent compounds. Unfortunately, they showed a weak activity toward *T. cruzi* amastigotes (EC_{50} values higher than 10 µM), although they are highly active toward *T. gondii* tachyzoite proliferation (EC_{50} values ranging from 0.67 to >10 µM).

Antimicrobial peptides are produced by living organisms as a defense mechanism against pathogens. Among the huge variety of antimicrobial peptides contained in amphibian skin secretions, temporins (isolated from the European red frog *Rana temporaria* L., Ranidae) are short polypeptide (10–13 residues) with activity toward trypanosomatidae family and low cytotoxicity in mammalian cells. To take advantage of temporin activity and, at the same time, to reduce mammalian toxicity, a hybrid peptide was built by linking the N-terminal portion of temporin A (responsible for the anchorage to the cell membrane), the sequence of gramicidin responsible for pore formation, and a C-terminal poly-Leu-Lys chain for overall stability (Souza et al. 2016). Such new peptide (referred to as temporizin) showed a dose-dependent ability to kill *T. cruzi* after 1 h. EC_{50} value was significantly improved in comparison to that of gramicidin (795 ng/mL vs 150 µg/mL, respectively). However, toxicity (in particular, membrane damage) was observed in J-744 macrophages (CC_{50} = 83 µg/mL), thus prompting the researchers to change the sequence of temporizin by shortening the temporin A-derived polypeptide for cell membrane insertion. The resulting temporizin-1 maintained an antitrypanosomal activity (887 ng/mL) comparable to that of temporizin but showed a lower cytotoxicity in mammals (CC_{50} = 123 µg/mL). Both the hybrid peptides were responsible for intracellular destruction, mitochondrial and chromatin disorders, without alterations of plasma membranes. More recently, additional temporin derivatives were disclosed with inhibition of *T. cruzi* epimastigotes in the two-digit micromolar concentration range (Raja et al. 2017).

Hybrid Derivatives Active against African Trypanosomiasis

The human African tripanosomiasis (the sleeping sickness) occurs in Sub-Saharan regions and is caused by *T. brucei gambiense* and *T. brucei rhodesiense* that are both transmitted by a blood-sucking insect of the genus *Glossina* (namely, the tsetse fly). Pentamidine, suramin, melarsoprol, and eflornithine are the sole drugs for the treatment of the disease, while nifurtimox is used in special cases. However, they suffer from complex administration (in particular eflornithine), some toxic effects, and potential parasite resistance. These reasons prompted the researchers worldwide to pursue the identification of new effective therapeutic agents for this disease.

Studies on naphthoquinones and naphthoquinones-coumarin hybrids led to discover dual-targeted compounds able to inhibit the enzymatic activity of both glyceraldehyde-3-phosphate dehydrogenase from *T. brucei* and trypanothione reductase from *T. cruzi* (Figure 10) (Uliassi et al. 2017). A structural comparison of these quinones (such as the 2-phenoxy derivative **43**) with naturally-occurring similar compounds led to focus attention to crassiflorone **44**, isolated from *Diospyros crassiflora* Hiern (Ebenaceae), a Central African ebony that has been continuously felled for the wood, and is now classified as endangered (The International Union for Conservation of Nature, Red List of Threatened Species 2018). Crassiflorone is characterized by a pentacyclic core where the naphthoquinone ring is condensed to a coumarin moiety through a furane ring. In other words, crassiflorone could be also considered as a hybrid compound between naphthoquinone and coumarin scaffolds. Taking into consideration the dual activity of both the original naphthoquinone and coumarin compounds, it was suggested that crassiflorone and its derivatives also could share the same type of activity. Unexpectedly, crassiflorone was not tested either in cell-free or in cell-based assay. Moreover, among a small series of its *des*-methyl derivatives (synthesized without the two methyl groups because of their synthetic accessibility), only one compound (**45**, corresponding to the *des*-methyl crassiflorone) showed "a balanced dual profile" toward both enzymes (about 60% inhibition of enzyme activity at 10 µM), although it showed a low aqueous solubility.

In another study, experimental evidence showing both benzoxaborole and chalcone derivatives as antitrypanosomal agents prompted the researchers to design, synthesize, and test toward bloodstream form of *T. brucei* many hybrid derivatives that contained the two moieties (Figure 11) (Qiao et al. 2012). The most simple (unsubstituted) benzoxaborole-chalcone derivative showed an IC_{50} = 89 ng/mL (that represented the ability to inhibit growth of the *T. brucei* 427 strain), and a selectivity index higher than

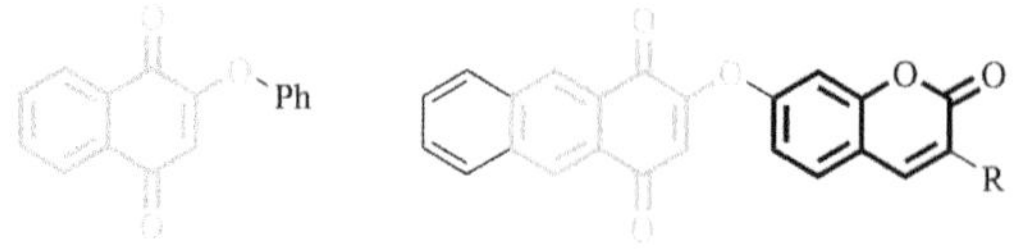

2-phenoxy-naphthoquinone, **43**   naphthoquinone-coumarin hybrids

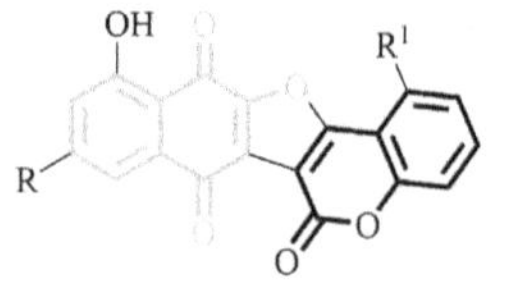

crassiflorone, **44**: R = R^1 = Me
des-methyl-crassiflorone, **45**: R = R^1 = H

Figure 10. Naphthoquinone-coumarin hybrids resembling crassiflorone.

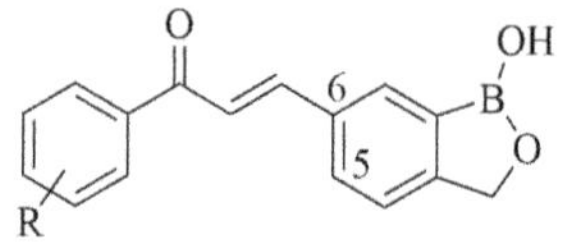

various derivatives: R = Me, Et, OMe, SMe, Cl, OH, 43 < IC$_{50}$ < 71 ng/mL
46: R = *p*-NH$_2$, IC$_{50}$ = 24 ng/mL, selectivity index > 400
47: R = *m*-OMe, IC$_{50}$ = 22 ng/mL, selectivity index > 450
48: R = *m*-OMe, *p*-NH$_2$, IC$_{50}$ = 10 ng/mL, selectivity index = 145

Figure 11. Benzoxaborole-chalcone hybrids as antitrypanosomal agents.

100 in mouse lung fibroblasts L929. Insertion of small substituents at the para position of the pendant phenyl ring resulted in improved activity in many cases. As examples, a Me, Et, OMe, SMe, Cl, and OH groups gave activity in the range between 43 and 71 ng/mL, with a primary amino group as in **46** being the most profitable substituent (24 ng/mL). Changing the substitution pattern at the phenyl ring yielded many compounds with IC$_{50}$ values lower than 60 ng/mL. A methoxy group in position 3 as in **47** was the best substituent (22 ng/mL with a selectivity index higher than 450). Fortunately, the obvious combination of the *p*-NH$_2$ with the *m*-OMe groups as in **48** led to a further improvement of activity (10 ng/mL), even if a higher cytotoxicity (1450 ng/mL) consequently resulted in a decrease of the selectivity index (145). Further attempts to modify the scaffold of the benzoxaborole-chalcone core (such as the reduction of the carbonyl group to an alcohol side chain, or replacement of the heterocyclic moiety with a phenyl ring) were unfruitful and yielded compounds with low or very low activity. A selection of 12 compounds active in *in vitro* assays was administered (50 mg/kg, twice a day, intraperitoneally) to female BALB/c mice infected with 600 *T. brucei* parasites. In agreement with *in vitro* results, **47** and **48** allowed eradication of parasites 30 days after infection and led to 100% survival. Although impressive *in vitro* and *in vivo* results were reached by these two compounds, their mechanism of action and cellular target were not further investigated. Very recently, benzoxaborole derivatives bearing simple substituent (such as a F in position 5) (Manhas et al. 2018), a substituted benzamide side chain or more complex appendages at position 6 (Wall et al. 2018) showed antiparasitic activity by targeting *L. donovani* leucyl-tRNA synthetase, or the *T. brucei* cleavage and polyadenylation specificity factor 3, respectively, laying the foundations for the discovery of molecular targets of these useful compounds.

Hybrid Derivatives Active against Schistosomiasis

Schistosomiasis is a poverty-related disease caused by the cercariae (larvae) of a helminth parasite of the genus *Schistosoma* present in fresh water in tropical and sub-tropical areas. Adult parasites of different species live in the urogenital or intestinal tract, thus causing urogenital and intestinal schistosomiasis. Praziquantel (**50**, Table 1), a condensed tetrahydro isoquinolino-piperazinyl tricyclic compound, is the only drug available that can be used in co-administration with albendazole and ivermectin. Unfortunately, praziquantel shows low solubility in water and can induce upregulation of the homologue protein of the mamalian P-gp, thus leading to parasite resistance.

In the attempt to find alternative chemical tools to affect *Schistosoma* life cycle, considering the activity of praziquantel toward all adult schistosomes and the ability of furoxan derivatives (such as the 3-cyano-4-phenyl furoxan, **49**) to inhibit parasite thioredoxin glutathione reductase (TGR) of all stages of *S. mansoni*, hybrid compounds were designed by inserting the furoxan moiety within the praziquantel scaffold (Guglielmo et al. 2014). A small series of hybrid compounds was generated and tested toward both the recombinant enzyme and *ex vivo* parasites. The most interesting compounds **51–54** showed a balanced activity comprised of reduction of parasite mobility and worm contraction (this is a property of praziquantel) combined to a micromolar inhibition of the enzyme (typical of furoxans). Moreover, the NO-releasing properties of furoxan derivatives seemed to be related to better worm-killing ability of the

Table 1. Praziquantel-furoxan derivatives acting as antischistosomal compounds.

An exemplificative furoxan, **49**
IC_{50} = 6 µM toward TGR of all forms of *S. mansoni*

praziquantel (**50**), **51-54**

Compound	R	R¹	TGR[a]	Worm mobility[b]	Worm death[c]	NO release[d]
Furoxan, **49**			6[e]	–	50 µM, 24 h	29
Praziquantel, **50**	H	cyclohex	NA[f]	+ (10 µM)	50 µM, 40%	
51	H		0.01	+ (10 µM)	50 µM, 80%	1.8
52	H		0.3	+ (50 µM)	50 µM, 72 h	56
53		cyclohex	0.3	+ (50 µM)	50 µM, 24 h	34
54		cyclohex	8.5	+ (50 µM)	50 µM, 24 h	16

[a] Inhibition of thioredoxin glutathione reductase activity, expressed as IC_{50} values in µM concentrations.

[b] -: no worm mobility up to a 50 µM compound concentration; +: worm contraction and low mobility at the test dose (10 or 50 µM).

[c] Compound concentration that provokes 100% parasite death at the time reported, or percent death at 144 h.

[d] Amount of NO released, measured as percent amount of nitrite ion formed.

[e] Active toward all forms of *S. mansoni* and adults of other schistosomes.

[f] NA: not active.

new compounds, as already reported (Mott et al. 2012). Interestingly, both compounds where the furoxan moiety was inserted instead of the praziquantel pendant cyclohexane ring (**51** and **52**) or with a furoxan substituent at the position 10 on the condensed phenyl ring (**53** and **54**) showed ability to inhibit the enzyme, reduce worm mobility, and kill the parasites.

Another intriguing approach to kill *S. mansoni* is based on its feature to be a hematophagous worm. The parasites digest human hemoglobin, leading to the formation of significant amounts of free heme that are in turn aggregated to give hemozoin crystals within the food vacuole. Hemozoin (also known as malaria pigment because *Plasmodium* follows the same catabolic pathway found in *S. mansoni*) can be considered as the result of a detoxification pathway that avoids iron ions to be involved in redox machinery that eventually yields reactive oxygen species, highly toxic to the parasites. With this in mind, compounds able to block heme polymerization to hemozoin could be of great interest as antischistosoma and antiplasmodial agents. Inhibition of hemozoin formation could be achieved by affecting monomer-monomer assembly by means of alkylating agents or heme-stacking compounds. For this purpose, chemicals bearing the 1,2,4-trioxane moiety are known to alkylate heme moieties, while compounds with a quinoline core are able to give stacking with the π-system of heme.

An analysis of these results led to the obvious suggestion to combine both chemical features into hybrid compounds (termed trioxaquines) that could be able to inhibit both *S. mansoni* and *P. falciparum*, as well as other parasites that produce hemozoin for heme detoxification. One of the hybrid compounds, disclosed as PA1259 (**55**, Figure 12), showed a very high activity both *in vitro* and *in vivo* toward *S. mansoni* (Portela et al. 2012).

In fact, treatment of the larval form with 5 μg/mL resulted in cercaria immobilization (for at least 30 seconds) in 60 min in comparison to 4 h required for praziquantel, used as the reference compound. Immobilization of 21-day and 49-day (adult) schistosomes was observed after 3 and 5 h, as well as after 2 and 3 h using praziquantel and PA1259, respectively (5 μg/mL in the first experiment, 50 μg/mL in the second experiment). Moreover, parasite population in infected mice treated with praziquantel and PA1259 (50 mg/kg, four doses in 9 h) was reduced by 41 and 86% (larval or adult stage, respectively) and 53 and 40%, respectively, without "visible adverse effect in mice". The ability of the trioxaquine derivatives to affect life cycle of hematophagous parasites such as *S. mansoni* and *P. falciparum* led to hypothesize that such compounds could be used as therapeutic agents in patients co-infected with both parasites. More interestingly, preliminary results on the use of trioxaquines did not show *Schistosoma* resistant strains after a two-year treatment (Portela et al. 2012), while disappointingly cross-resistance with artemisinin derivatives and selection of *P. falciparum* strains resistant to trioxaquine and artemisinin were very recently disclosed (Paloque et al. 2018).

Following a similar hybridization strategy, eight new compounds were synthesized by coupling praziquantel with artesunate-inspired trioxane or tetroxane moieties (Duan et al. 2012). Three compounds were particularly active toward both the larval and adult forms of *S. japonicum*, in *ex vivo* and *in vivo* assays (Figure 13). Sequential assays showed that **56–58** killed all adult worms at concentrations ranging from 10 to 15 μM, in comparison to a 63% mortality caused by 50 μM praziquantel. In a similar way, 5–15 μM of the same compounds reduced larval worm survival to less than 9% within 24 h. *In vivo* assays in mice infected with about 50 cercariae showed that **58** (200 mg/kg) led to a 56 and 70% worm reduction rate in adult and larval forms, respectively, in comparison to 67 and 20% found for praziquantel. Unfortunately, the

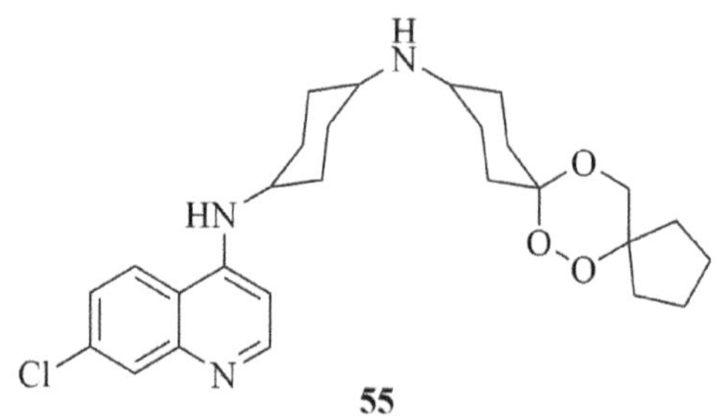

Figure 12. The trioxane-quinoline hybrid (trioxaquine) PA1259, **55**.

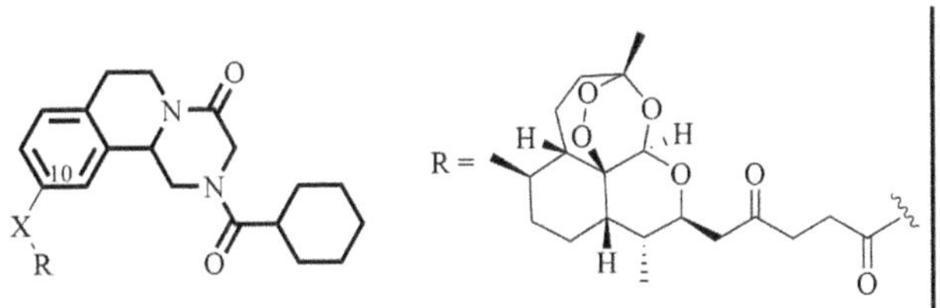

57, praziquantel-artesunate: X = NH
Adult worm survival: 0% at 15 μM
Larval worm survival: 9% at 5 μM

58, praziquantel-artesunate: X = O
Adult worm survival: 0% at 15 μM
Larval worm survival: 0% at 15 μM
Adult worm survival (ex vivo): 56%
Larval worm survival (ex vivo): 70%

56, 10-hydroxy praziquantel: X = O, R = H
Adult worm survival: 0% at 10 μM
Larval worm survival: 0% at 5 μM

Figure 13. Hybrids compounds bearing chemical portions taken from praziquantel and artesunate.

reduced number of compounds did not allow to rule SAR considerations, and doubt arose on the possibility that the praziquantel and the artesunate portions derived from *in vivo* hydrolysis could be responsible for activity, instead of the whole hybrid compounds.

Hybrid Derivatives Active against Leishmaniasis

Caused by *Leishmania* parasites, leishmaniasis is a mortal neglected tropical disease that can present cutaneous (CL), mucocutaneous (ML) or visceral (VL) forms depending on the specific *Leishmania* species involved (i.e., *L. aethiopica* and *L. amazonensis* are responsible for CL, while *L. donovani* is related to VL). More than 12 million people are affected by leishmaniasis with a high mortality level of around 50000 deaths each year in more than 90 countries (Maran et al. 2016). *Leishmania* are heteroxenous parasites involving an invertebrate and a vertebrate host in their lifecycle. In sandfly vector, the parasite is present in its extracellular promastigote form, while the intracellular amastigote form is the only one observed in the vertebrate host. Amastigotes are absorbed from a vertebrate infected host once a female sandfly bites it, and are transformed into promastigotes in the insect gut where they multiply by binary fission. Formed promastigotes transfer to the proboscis and are transferred by sandfly sting into the vertebrate host where they are phagocytized into macrophages to form amastigotes again. From macrophages, the parasites diffuse in internal organs, especially liver, spleen, lymph nodes, and bone marrow, where they can propagate and suppress the host immune system, thus generating a permanent, eventually lethal infection. Despite many efforts on developing new immunomodulators, immunosuppressive agents, and new antileishmanial compounds, there still is a real need for effective therapies. Pentavalent antimony was developed in 1959, but its current use is limited by its high toxicity. The first line drug is amphotericin B for LV, especially in Bihar State of India where several cases do not respond to antimonium anymore. Pentamidine is the second line treatment with many side effects observed, and it is not active by oral administration. Miltefosine can be considered as a very innovative drug in antileishmania therapy as it is the sole compound that is orally active, though teratogenic. This drug shows a long half-life with an easy induction of resistance.

The main limitations of all the current chemotherapy are represented by the high cost, toxicity, difficult administration, and resistant strains development. Most of the difficulties in developing effective therapies for *Leishmania* treatment are related to the poor information about the different mechanisms and pathways responsible for the parasite growth and replication. As a consequence, the hybridization approach was applied by different research groups to develop antileishmanial compounds, especially starting from natural products-based scaffolds. Many compounds active against leishmaniasis were discovered in the last years, but only a few of them are acting on well identified targets, thus limiting the development of hybrid molecules. Widely studied hybrids are the ones formed by β-carboline and quinazolinone scaffolds targeting *L. donovani* trypanothione reductase (*Ld*TR) that is a key enzyme for redox homeostasis in *Leishmania*. TR is a flavoenzyme directly involved in maintaining adequate levels of trypanothione by the NADH-mediated reduction of trypanothione disulfide dithiol, analogously to the transformation of glutathione disulfide into glutathione in mammal cells. TR is similar to glutathione reductase (GR), differing for the disulfide binding pocket that represents a good target for a selective chemotherapy (Dukhyil 2018, Rai et al. 2009, Krauth-Siegel et al. 2005). Natural products that contain β-carboline (such as buchtienine

59 and annomontine **60**) (Galarreta et al. 2008, Kumar et al. 2010) and quinazoline (such as tryptanthrin **61**) (Sharma et al. 2013, Ranieri Cortez et al. 2011, Chauhan et al. 2010) moieties are known to be very effective in inhibiting *Ld*TR. Moreover, hybrids with both functionalities, as rutacarpine (**62**), were isolated from *Phellodendron amurense* (Rutaceae, known as Amor cork tree) (Ikuta et al. 1998) (Figure 14).

On the basis of such considerations, many groups were inspired by nature to develop natural product-based hybrids to obtain more active compounds. The generation of hybrid *Ld*TR inhibitors was firstly studied by Chauhan and coworkers who reported compounds that contained a fully aromatic β-carboline moiety connected to C2 position of a quinazolinone ring (Chauhan et al. 2015). These compounds were prepared by using an effective 5-step synthesis involving a Pictet-Spengler cyclization on tryptophan to generate the tetrahydro-β-carboline nucleus **63** (Figure 15). The installation of the quinazoline ring occurred after an oxidation and deprotection process, reacting the obtained aldehyde **64** with 2-amino-alkylbenzamide and cyanuric chloride. Among the 15 compounds synthesized, six hits were demonstrated to inhibit TR with K_i in the range of 0.8–9.2 μM. The whole-cell screening assay highlighted that analogues **65–67** have IC_{50} values of 4.4, 6.0, and 4.3 μM, respectively, along with adequate selectivity index (SI) of > 91, 36, and 24, respectively, thus being considered as the most active compounds of this family (Table 2).

Both antipromastigote and antiamastigote activity were very promising in comparison to miltefosine and sodium stibogluconate (SSG), taken as the reference compounds.

Docking studies were performed to evaluate the free energy of binding of the new compounds within the active site of a *Ld*TR homology model. Considering **65** as a representative compound, the formation of a hydrogen bond with His46 and Glu466 in the active site seemed to be crucial for a good inhibitory activity. The clear correlation between K_i values and antileishmanial activity suggested that the compounds probably acted by inhibiting TR. Nevertheless, a direct evidence of the activity on the specific target was not confirmed by any biological data. Compounds **65–67** were evaluated as racemic mixture and the activity of the single enantiomers was not investigated.

More recently, Ramu and coworkers also reported a natural product-inspired diversity oriented synthesis (DOS) library of hybrids composed by β-carboline and quinazolinone scaffolds targeting *Ld*TR (Ramu et al. 2017). A 3-step synthesis starting from tryptophan methylester and involving a Pictet-Spengler reaction was reported (Figure 16), together with the evaluation of the inhibitory activity, without any consideration about the possible difference in the activity profile of the single stereoisomers. Six compounds showed anti-*Ld*TR activity in the nanomolar range.

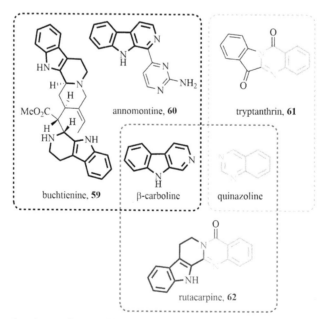

Figure 14. Natural products active as antileishmanial agents containing β-carboline and quinazoline moieties.

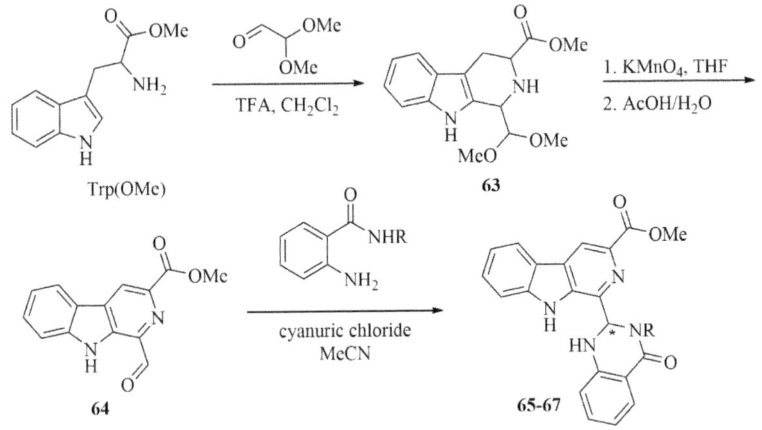

Figure 15. Synthesis of β-carboline-quinazolinone hybrids.

Table 2. [a]Antileishmanial activity of tetrahydro-β-carboline-quinazoline hybrids.

Compound	R	Antipromastigote IC$_{50}$	Antiamastigote IC$_{50}$	CC$_{50}$	SI
65	4-Cl-Ph	3.3 ± 0.7	4.4 ± 0.8	> 400	> 91
66	4-F-Ph	4.6 ± 0.6	6.0 ± 1.0	217 ± 13	36
67	3,4-Cl-Bn	4.8 ± 0.7	4.3 ± 0.5	104 ± 9	24
miltefosine		1.2 ± 0.4	8.1 ± 0.5	56 ± 4	7
SSG		not active	54 ± 2	> 400	7

[a] Activity is expressed in micromolar concentration.

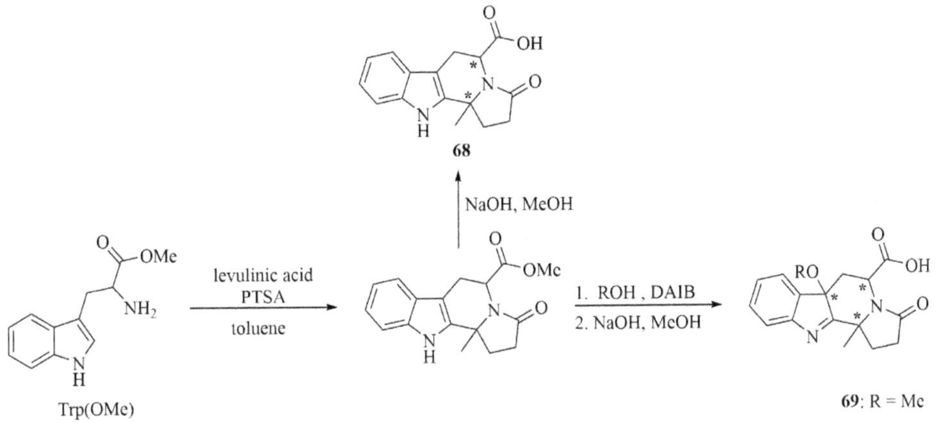

Figure 16. Diversity oriented synthesis of β-carboline hybrids.

Also in this case, docking simulations were used to explain the different binding mode. However, a direct correlation between free energy of binding and activity was not always found nor structure activity relationships can be extrapolated from the data reported. Compared with hybrids **65–67**, this class of compounds contains 2 (**68**) or 3 (**69–73**) stereogenic centers instead of just one, thus suggesting that the less planar conformation of the β-carboline nucleus could be crucial for a higher activity (in the nanomolar range). In this case, amphotericin B was used as the reference compound and the number of amastigotes was significantly reduced especially by **68** and **69** (Table 3).

Table 3. β-Carboline hybrids obtained by diversity-oriented synthesis.

Compound	IC$_{50}$ (nM)	CC$_{50}$ (HepG2, μM)	% infected macrophages
68	3.6	612	13 ± 3
69	19	218	19 ± 5
70	5.9	271	28 ± 5
71	16	151	27 ± 6
72	36	172	25 ± 6
73	14	269	21 ± 4
amphotericin B			14 ± 5
control			57 ± 6

The impact of the stereochemistry in the activity of **68** was also evaluated even if no indication was reported about the stereoselective synthesis and the purification of the racemic mixture. It is interesting to note that the stereochemistry affected toxicity, as **68a** was significantly more toxic than its diastereoisomer **68b** (Figure 17).

An extensive study on the effects of TR inhibition was also reported indicating that apoptosis occurred after *Ld*TR inhibition in *L. donovani* promastigotes. The mechanism of apoptosis was elucidated and directly related to an increase of ROS levels that trigged actin depolymerization and mitochondrial membrane alteration in a Ca^{2+}-independent manner. β-Carbolines were connected to 1,3,5-triazines in different positions to obtain hybrid, active antileishmanial agents whose molecular targets were not determined unambiguously in all the cases. The hybridization approach was not evidenced by Kumar and coworkers

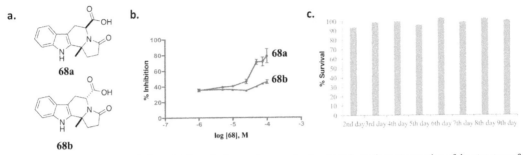

Figure 17. Cytotoxic effects of **68a** and **68b** on *L. donovani* promastigotes. (a) Schematic representation of the structure of the diastereomers. (b) (Adapted from Ramu et al. 2017). Compound **68a** exerted toxic effects on *L. donovani* promastigotes. Cytotoxic effect of **68a** and **68b** was evaluated using LDH Assay (post 72 h, conc.: 1–100 µM). Inhibition was calculated by taking the cytotoxicity of positive control (2.5 µg/mL amphotericin B) as 100% for normalization. (c) (Adapted from Ramu et al. 2017). Non-toxic effect of **68b** on *L. donovani* promastigotes. Long-term effect on promastigotes survival with **68b** exposure was examined by evaluation of cytotoxicity on parasites for 9 days following its addition.

in the first report where the triazine moiety was introduced on the N2 position of the β-carboline ring (Kumar et al. 2006). Only the cis or trans racemic mixtures were tested, but not the single enantiomers. Cis isomers of **74** and **75** (Figure 18) showed a 78 and 79% inhibition at day 7 in *in vivo* experiments. The percentage of inhibition was anyhow far away from the 90% shown by the reference compound SSG. *In vitro* experiments on these compounds were not reported.

Better results against *L. amazonensis* were obtained by adding a triazine ring in C3 position of a fully aromatic carboline moiety, thus eliminating stereochemical issues and introducing different spacers of 2, 6 or none carbon atoms in between the two cycles (**76–78**, Figure 19) (Bare et al. 2018). SARs suggested that a 3-nitrophenyl group in C1 was always present in the most active compounds, as well as a 2-carbon atom spacer. The substitution of a chlorine atom in the triazine ring with an amine generally produced a loss of activity, except for **76** that contained an *iso*-propylamine group and had a promising 6.2 µM and 1.2 µM IC$_{50}$ values toward promastigotes and amastigotes, respectively. This compound caused alterations in the cell cycle and an increased lipid storage responsible for cell death. Anyhow, the specific target has not been disclosed yet.

Very good results in term of both selectivity and activity were obtained when the triazine ring was hybridized with the quinazoline moiety (**79** and **80**, Figure 20) (Sharma et al. 2013). The preparation was a simple functionalization of a previously prepared quinazoline ring with cyanuric chloride, and a systematic substitution of the Cl atoms with different amines. The same quinazoline nucleus was hybridized with peptides thus obtaining 9 promising compounds. The triazine hybrids were both active as antipromastigotes and antiamastigotes with a low cytotoxicity and a very good SI. The hybrid peptide **81** bearing a ferrocene moiety was not active at all on promastigotes, while it strongly affected amastigote proliferation with a SI > 548. However, these hybrids, that were very promising even in *in vivo* studies in the golden hamster model, strongly reacted with blood proteins with a static and dynamic quenching of intrinsic fluorescence.

Interesting thiophene-indole based hybrids with lower toxicity with respect to reference drugs were also developed (Figure 21). In fact, thiophene derivatives had a documented antipromastigote activity in *L. amazonensis* (Takahashi et al. 1999), while indole-based alkaloids showed a promising antileishmanial activity (Staerk et al. 2000). Hybrids were synthesized using standard conditions for the 2-aminothiophene preparation followed by an imine formation by treatment with indole 3-carbaldehyde derivatives. Active compounds were found in all the classes synthesized. Most of the 32 compounds synthesized showed IC$_{50}$ values lower than 10 µg/mL, demonstrating higher activity than the reference drugs (penta- and trivalent antimonials). The most active compounds were **82–84** with IC$_{50}$ values of 2.1, 3.2, and 2.3 µg/mL, respectively, and activity in resistant mutant strains. All the active derivatives contained a 6-, 7-, or 8-membered ring fused with the thiophene moiety and a CN or methyl group in C5 position of the indole. These compounds were not toxic for blood cells as demonstrated by their activity on human erythrocytes, thus showing a high selectivity toward the parasite, sometimes higher than that of the reference

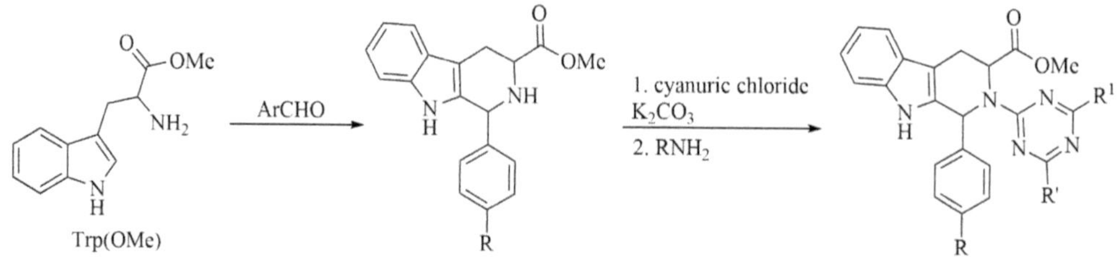

$(\pm)cis$ **74**: R = Me, R^1 = morpholine
$(\pm)cis$ **75**: R = Me, R^1 = NPh-piperidine

Figure 18. β-Carbolines with attached 1,3,5-triazine substituents.

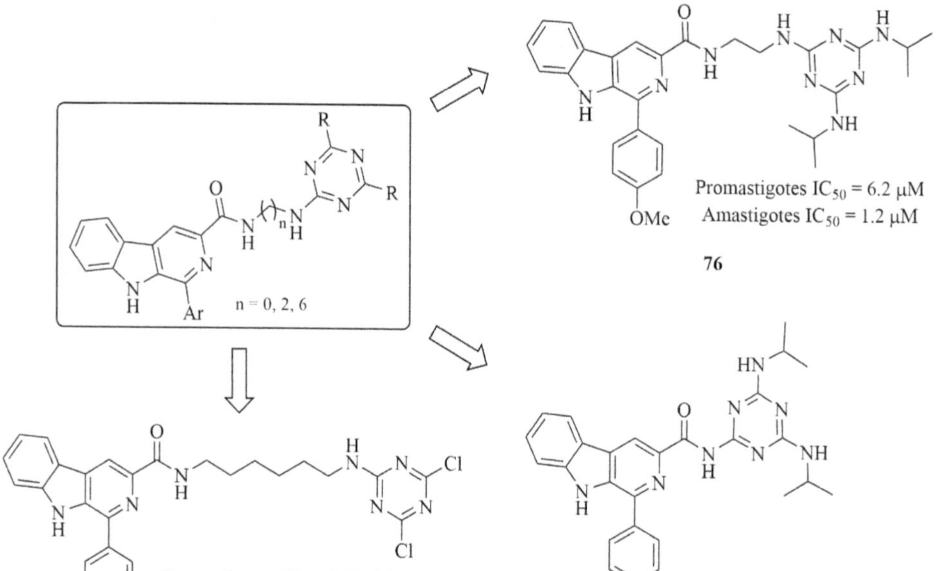

Promastigotes IC_{50} = 6.2 μM
Amastigotes IC_{50} = 1.2 μM

76

n = 0, 2, 6

Promastigotes IC_{50} >100 μM
Amastigotes IC_{50} >100 μM
77

Promastigotes IC_{50} >100 μM
Amastigotes IC_{50} >100 μM
78

Figure 19. Other β-carboline-triazine hybrids.

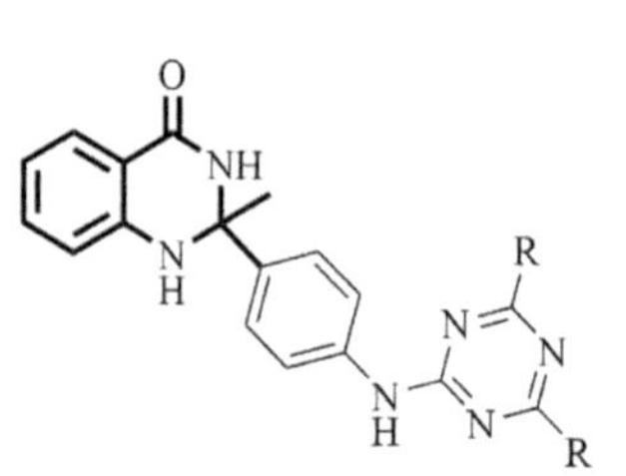

79: R = piperidine
amastigotes IC_{50} 3.9 ± 0.8 μM, SI > 101
in vivo % inhibition *L. donovani* 73 ± 12

80: R = tetrahydroisoquinoline
amastigotes IC_{50} 4.4 ± 1.4 μM, SI > 91
in vivo % inhibition *L. donovani* 81 ± 10

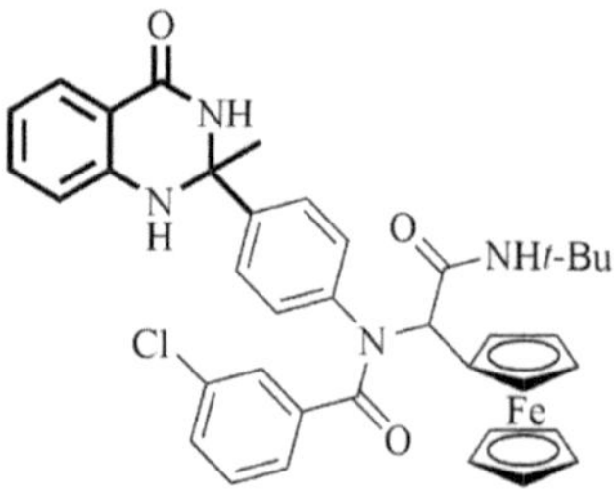

81
amastigotes IC_{50} 0.3 ± 0.2 μM, SI > 548
in vivo % inhibition *L. donovani* 51 ± 16

miltefosine: amastigotes IC_{50} 8.4 ± 2.1 μM, SI = 15

Figure 20. Tetrahydroquinazoline-triazine hybrid compounds.

drugs. Compound **82** had the best antileishmanial activity that seemed to be related to DNA damage. The authors also generated robust chemometric models with good statistical indices highlighting that the descriptors of hydrophobicity and molecular shape were closely related to the antileishmanial activity of these hybrids.

Indoles furnish interesting compounds even once hybridized with cumarin by using a chalcone-like linker (Sangshetti et al. 2016). The molecules obtained cannot probably be strictly defined as hybrids as their activity seemed to be exploited by interaction with pteridine reductase 1 (PTR1) and no data are available about the interaction of indole, cumarin, and chalcone derivatives with this specific target. PTR1 is a key NADPH dependent short-chain reductase responsible for the salvage of pterins in *Leishmania* by acting as a metabolic bypass for drugs targeting dihydrofolate reductase. On the basis of suggestions derived from the analysis of naturally occurring compounds active toward *Leishmania* promastigotes (Figure 22), a small library of PTR1 inhibitors has been synthesized by taking advantages from the catalytic activity of Ho^{3+}-doped $CoFe_2O_4$ nanoparticles in the final step of the synthesis, allowing the discovery of three promising products. The IC_{50} values toward *L. donovani* promastigotes were determined by using a modified MTT assay where the amount of formazan produced was considered as proportional to the number of

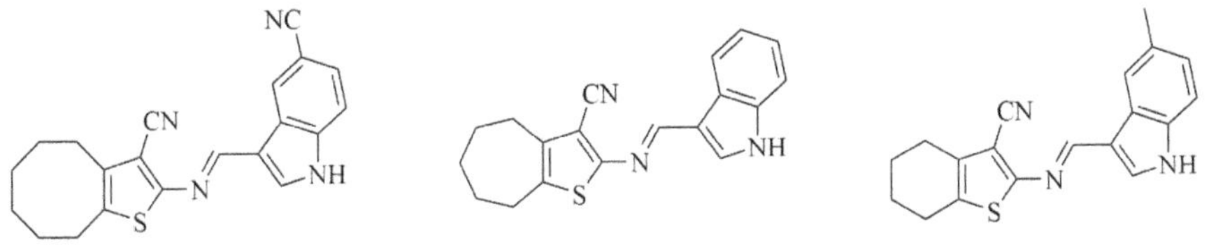

82: amastigotes IC_{50} 2.1 μM
SI > 193

83: amastigotes IC_{50} 3.2 μM
SI > 125

84: amastigotes IC_{50} 2.3 μM
SI > 173

amphotericine B: 0.2 μM, SI > 124
trivalent antimony: 9.0 μM, SI > 38

Figure 21. Thiophene-indole hybrids.

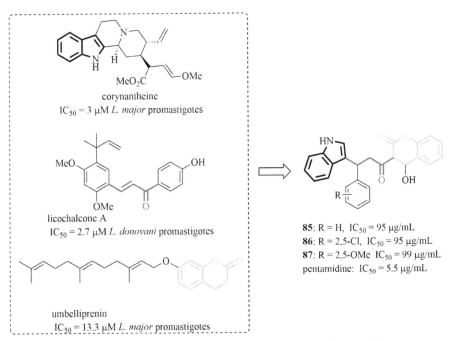

corynantheine
IC_{50} = 3 μM *L. major* promastigotes

licochalcone A
IC_{50} = 2.7 μM *L. donovani* promastigotes

umbelliprenin
IC_{50} = 13.3 μM *L. major* promastigotes

85: R = H, IC_{50} = 95 μg/mL
86: R = 2,5-Cl, IC_{50} = 95 μg/mL
87: R = 2,5-OMe IC_{50} = 99 μg/mL
pentamidine: IC_{50} = 5.5 μg/mL

Figure 22. Indole-coumarins designed by inspiration to natural compounds.

metabolically active cells. Compounds **85–87** were more potent than reference SSG but less active than pentamidine. The antioxidant activity was also evaluated, but results showed no direct correlation with the antileishmanial activity.

As shown above, the hybridization approach was widely applied to the development of antileishmanial agents by using different scaffolds and approaches. The main limitation on the application of this technology is still represented by the lack of a robust knowledge of the mechanisms and pathways involved in *Leishmania* infection, thus generating the random synthesis of compounds composed by potentially active scaffolds not always acting with the same mechanism of action. On the other hand, most of the hybrids evaluated in leishmaniasis are chiral molecules and only a few reports evaluated the possible impact of the stereochemistry on the activity of the single enantiomers on specific targets. This is probably the main issue to be approached for a fruitful investigation and development of new antileishmanial drugs.

Hybrid Derivatives Active against Malaria

Malaria is one of the most common tropical diseases with 216 million people infected in 2016 and 445 thousand deaths during the same year reported by WHO (World Health Organization 2018a). Malaria disease is caused by five different types of *Plasmodium* (*P. falciparum, P. vivax, P. ovale, P. malariae*, and *P. knowlesi*) that have different geographical distribution and aggressiveness. *P. falciparum* is common in African continent and is responsible for most of the deaths registered every year, while *P. vivax* is the most dominant parasite in all the other countries. Usually, the infection is transmitted to human by bites of female *Anopheles* mosquitoes. However, the transmission can occur even through exposure to infected blood. Female *Anopheles* containing *Plasmodium* injects 8 to 15 malarial sporozoites into the host during a bite. Sporozoites rapidly enter into hepatocytes where the asexual reproduction takes place generating pre-erythrocytic schizonts in an asymptomatic manner. Around 40 thousand merozoites are released into the bloodstream and enter into erythrocytes in a period of 7 to 30 days depending on the specific type of *Plasmodium*. From blood schizogony, trophozoites are formed thus evolving into schizonts that can release new merozoites that can infect other erythrocytes, continuing the cycle and generating recurring fever. Toxins release occurs after erythrocytes rupture inducing macrophages activity and the symptoms of malaria expression. At this point, some of the merozoites can mature into larger gametocytes that can undergo sexual replication once ingested by mosquitoes. The infective agent, the patient's age as well as his/her immunity level have a strong impact on the outcome of the infection. The best antimalarial treatment is nowadays represented by the artemisinin-based combination therapy (ACT). The application of a multidrug approach is crucial for malaria treatment, as resistance almost ordinarily occurs in infected patients, especially in the presence of *P. falciparum*. The first generation of antimalarial drugs, such as chloroquine and sulfadoxine-pyrimethamine, is actually almost useless because of resistance phenomena. The hybridization approach is thus widely applied to antimalarial drugs to minimize both resistance and side effects of ACT. The most representative hybrids in terms of efficacy on this infection are quinoline-based compounds (Nqoro et al. 2017, Agarwal et al. 2017). However, not all quinoline-based hybrids were included in this literature survey. We describe here the quinoline hybrids not previously reviewed or those that contain a chemical core different from quinoline.

Varotti and coworkers reported a very original antimalarial hybrid that is simply a salt of mefloquine and artesunic acid (MEFAS, Figure 23) (Penna-Coutinho et al. 2016, De Pilla Varotti et al. 2018). It represents a unique example because hybrid molecules known so far are usually composed of two molecules or fragment of molecules covalently linked. As an antimalarial drug needs to be not only active but even cheap to be accessible to the people in the malaria-affected countries, MEFAS represents an interesting opportunity. Mefloquine is a schizonticide, active toward *Plasmodium* species resistant to chloroquine, while artesunic acid has a not completely disclosed mechanism of action that affects somehow the EXP1 functionality. MEFAS acts as dual inhibitor with an unclear mechanism of action, impacting on calcium homeostasis by acting on the endoplasmatic reticulum, as well as on proton homeostasis. It is interesting to note that MEFAS is 280- and 15-fold more effective than the association of the two single molecules composing it, showing lower toxicity as well. MEFAS is a potential and less toxic alternative in resistant malarial treatment.

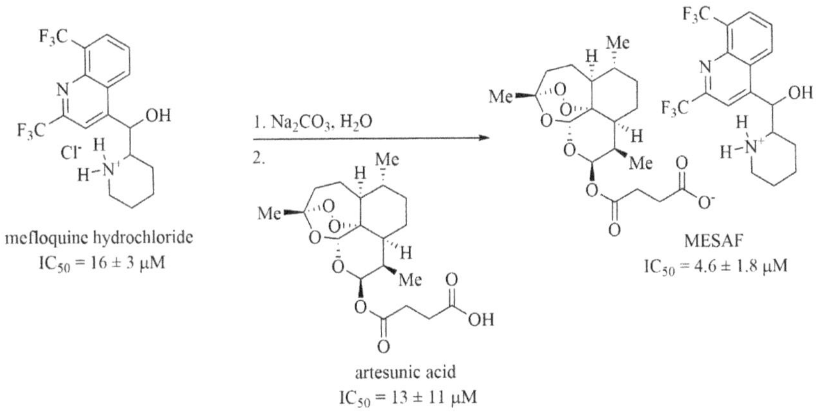

Figure 23. MEFAS is a hybrid compound derived from salification between mefloquine and artesunate.

Artemisinin is the core of different hybrid constructs. It has been hybridized with 1,2,4-trioxane ferrocene units showing an interesting antimalarial and antileukemia activity (Figure 24). The authors interestingly synthesized hybrids containing the 1,2,4-trioxane-ferrocene unit charged with just one or two artemisinin molecules and connecting them to the core in different manner. The two units are connected by an ester moiety directly involving the OH group of dihydroartemisinin (DHA) in **88** and **89**, or by introducing a 3-carbon atom spacer in the C10 deoxocarba analogue of DHA for **90** and **91**. The β-configuration of hybrid **88** has been determined by X-ray analysis while the α-configuration in **89** has been deduced by NMR analysis, as well as the β,β configuration assigned to **90** and **91**. All the hybrids are active toward *P. falciparum* 3D7 parasites with IC_{50} in the nanomolar range. Although **88–90** showed a better activity than that of reference chloroquine, they are less potent than DHA.

The same group reported ferrocene hybrids with the artemisinin derivative artesunic acid, as well as with egonol (Reiter et al. 2014). In this case, all hybrids showed a better activity against *P. falciparum* than that of the parent compounds. Particularly, artesunic acid homodimers **92** and **93** had an impressive 0.32 and 0.30 nM IC_{50} (Figure 25), thus suggesting a direct correlation between the number of endoperoxide bridges and the antimalarial activity. On the contrary, compounds comprising the egonol feature (**94** and **95**) were significantly less active.

Artemisinin has been used by Jones and coworkers in the generation of hybrids with acridine nucleus (Jones et al. 2009) (Figure 26). In this case, the hybridization did not have a very positive impact in terms of efficacy, as only **96** showed a 6.0 nM IC_{50} that was, however, higher than that of DHA.

More recently, the acridine moiety was hybridized with pyrrolidine derivatives, thus generating new compounds to be used alone or in combination with artemisinin (Pandey et al. 2016) (Figure 26). *In vivo* evaluation in MDR *P. yoelii nigeriensis* infected mice as well as pharmacokinetic properties demonstrated that **97** was a good candidate for malaria treatment alone or in combination with artemisinin. Despite the promising profile of this compound, further evaluation was not reported yet.

A small library of hybrid kaurenoid terpenes and 1,2,3-triazoles was prepared by using a convergent approach involving a Huisgen's reaction to generate regioselectively the triazole ring (de Oliveira Santos et al. 2016) (Figure 27). The modification of the natural kaurenoic acid derivatives yielded a more active analogue **98** that still had poor activity (micromolar range in W2 *P. falciparum*) and higher toxicity in Hep G2A16 cells with respect to chloroquine, taken as the reference compound. None of the hybrids prepared showed a promising antimalarial activity, even when a chloroquine moiety was introduced as in **99** and **101**. The best results in terms of potency were obtained by introducing a 3-pyridine ring on the triazole (**100** and **102**). In summary, the triazole moiety seemed to have a negative impact on the antimalarial profile of kaurenoic acid derivatives, as well as the introduction of other substituents in the skeleton, as demonstrated by **103**.

The most successful antimalarial hybrids reported so far still remain those containing chloro- or aminoquinoline functions. Once again, unbeaten hybrids are the ones designed by connecting moieties

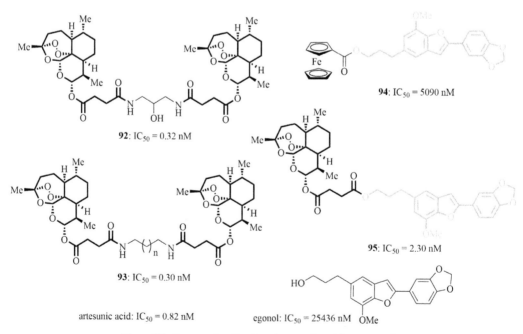

Figure 24. Artemisinin-ferrocene hybrids.

Color version at the end of the book

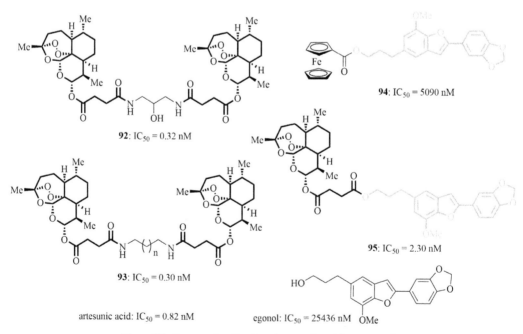

Figure 25. Compounds with artesunic, egonol, and ferrocene units.

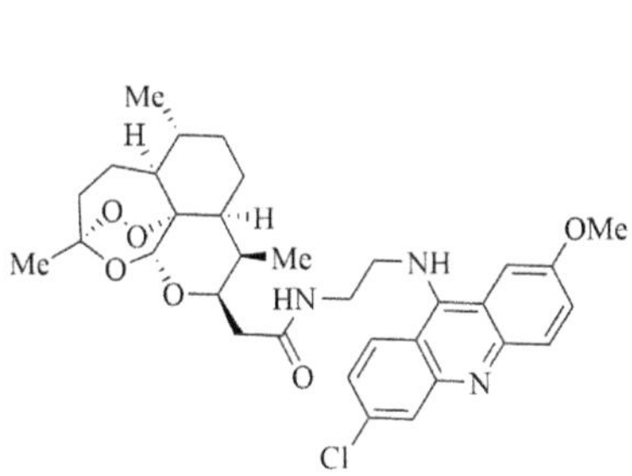

96: IC_{50} = 6.0 nM
DHA: IC_{50} = 2.3 nM

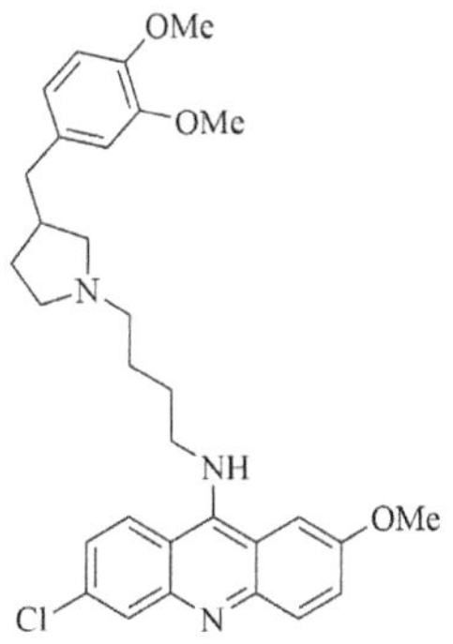

97: IC_{50} = 30 nM
chloroquine: IC_{50} = 6.3 nM

Figure 26. Acridine-based hybrid compounds.

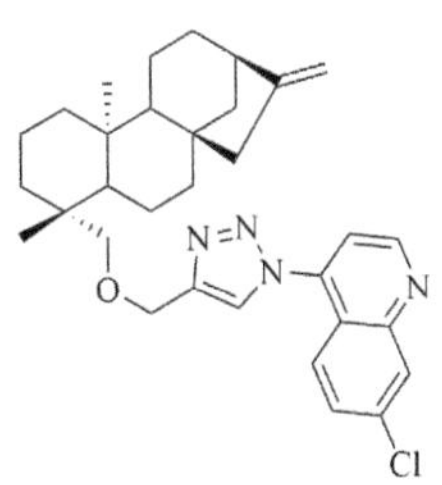

99: IC_{50} > 94 μM

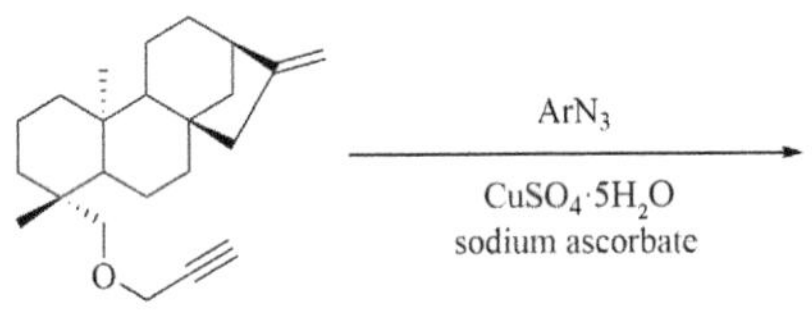

98: IC_{50} = 20 μM

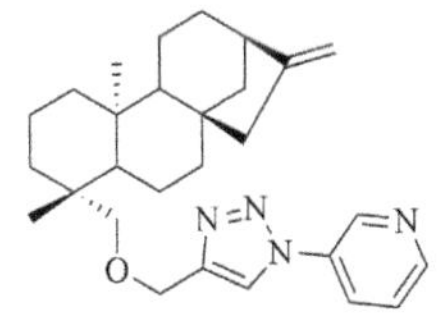

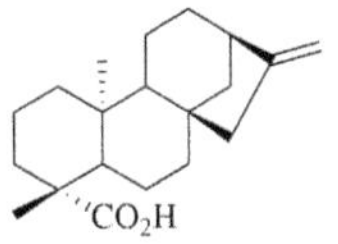

kaurenoic acid: IC_{50} = 21 μM

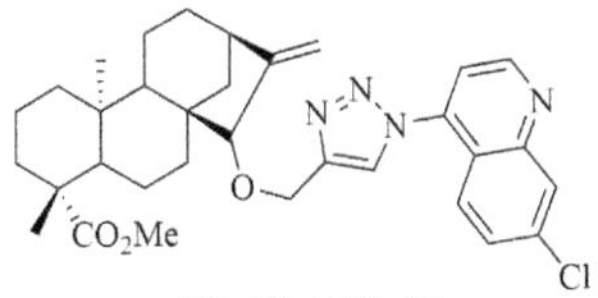

100: IC_{50} = 53 μM

101: IC_{50} > 87 μM

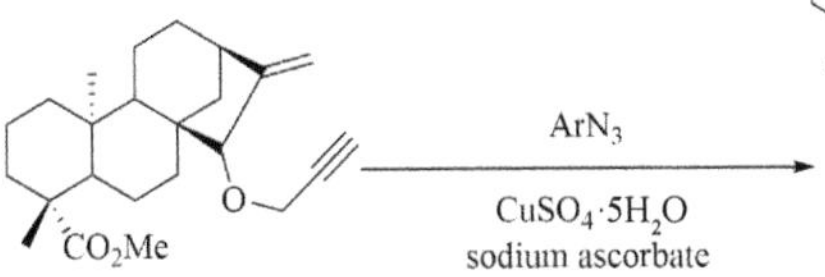

103: IC_{50} = 83.4 mM

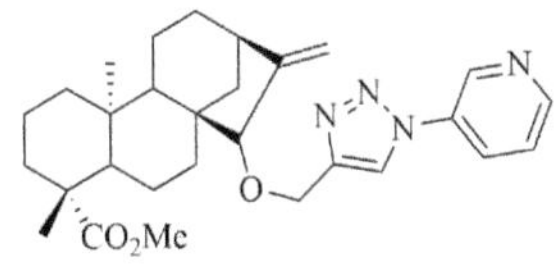

chloroquine: IC_{50} = 0.4 μM

102: IC_{50} = 56 μM

Figure 27. Kaurenoic acid-triazole hybrid compounds.

active against the same target. The main problem in malaria, as well as in many other tropical diseases here treated, is represented by a not completely disclosed mechanism of action of the current drugs or active molecules discover so far. This vague knowledge has a tremendous impact not only in hybrid design but also in the development of any effective therapy.

Conclusions

The major limitations of antiparasitic therapies comprise several issues that are well known within the drug design and optimization pipeline. In fact, some compounds show limited efficacy in post-marketing clinical phase (phase IV of clinical trials) or severe side effects and toxicity. Treatment duration and complexity of drug administration represent further difficulty to be dealt with by the researchers. Moreover, cases of parasites resistant to the drugs are also found, that nullify the current therapy. With this scenario in mind, the consequential countermeasures are based on the design of new compounds, with optimized pharmacokinetics and dynamics properties, to be administered in lower concentrations. For this purpose, the molecular hybridization approach combines known pharmacophoric portions present in different drugs in a single multipharmacophoric scaffold that could act as a multitarget agent or as a single target agent with better efficacy. However, even if the hybridization approaches often yield useful hit or lead compounds, or new drugs, the choice of appropriate pharmacophoric portions is a crucial step in designing new hybrids. In fact, many cases of hybrid compounds completely lack their biological activity, as the antiplasmodial hybrids that are generated without the quinoline scaffold.

References

Agarwal, D., R.D. Gupta and S.K. Awasthia. 2017. Are antimalarial hybrid molecules a close Reality or a distant dream? Antimicrob. Agents Chemother. 61: e00249–17.

Alighieri, D. 1304. And just as it often happens that a man goes looking for silver and apart from his intention finds gold. Alighieri, D. Il Convivio (The Banquet). Translated by Lansing, R. H. Garland Library of Medieval Literature, Ser. B. N, 1990. https://digitaldante.columbia.edu/text/library/the-convivio/book-02/#12, accessed 24 September 2018. E sì come essere suole che l'uomo va cercando argento e fuori de la 'ntenzione truova oro. Convivio, Trattato Secondo, Capitolo XII, 5.

Badolato, M., G. Carullo, M. Perri, E. Cione, F. Manetti, M.L. Di Gioia et al. 2017. Quercetin/oleic acid-based G-protein-coupled receptor 40 (GPR40) ligands as new insulin secretion modulators. Fut. Med. Chem. 9: 1873–1885.

Barbaro, R., L. Betti, M. Botta, F. Corelli, G. Giannaccini, L. Maccari et al. 2002. Synthesis and biological activity of new 1,4-benzodioxan-arylpiperazine derivatives. Further validation of a pharmacophore model for α_1-adrenoceptor antagonists. Bioorg. Med. Chem. 10: 361–369.

Bare, P., V. Aquilino Barbosa, D. Lazarin Bidoóia, J. Carreira de Paula, T. Fernandes Stefanello, W. Ferreira da Costa et al. 2018. Synthesis, antileishmanial activity and mechanism of action studies of novel β-carboline-1,3,5-triazine hybrids. Eur. J. Med. Chem. 150: 579–590.

Betti, L., M. Botta, F. Corelli, M. Floridi, P. Fossa, G. Giannaccini et al. 2002. α_1-adrenoceptor antagonists. Rational design, synthesis and biological evaluation of new trazodone-like compounds. Bioorg. Med. Chem. Lett. 12: 437–440.

Bhakta, S., N. Scalacci, A. Maitra, A.K. Brown, S. Dasugari, D. Evangelopoulos et al. 2016. Design and synthesis of 1-((1,5-bis(4-chlorophenyl)-2-methyl-1*H*-pyrrol-3-yl)methyl)-4-methylpiperazine (BM212) and *N*-Adamantan-2-yl-*N'*-((*E*)-3,7-dimethyl-octa-2,6-dienyl)-ethane-1,2-diamine (SQ109) pyrrole hybrid derivatives: discovery of potent anti-tubercular agents effective against multi-drug resistant mycobacteria. J. Med. Chem. 59: 2780–2793.

Butera, J., J. Bagli, W. Doubleday, L. Humber, A. Treasurywala, D. Loughney et al. 1989. Computer-assisted design and synthesis of novel aldose reductase inhibitors. J. Med. Chem. 32: 757–765.

Cardona-Galeano, W.I., A.F. Yepes and R.A. Herrera. 2018. Hybrid molecules: promising compounds for the development of new treatments against Leishmaniasis and Chagas disease. Curr. Med. Chem. 25: 3637–3679.

Carvalhaes, M.S., J.M. Santana, O.T. Nobrega, J.B. Aragao, P. Grellier, J. Schrevel et al. 1998. Chemotherapy of an experimental *Trypanosoma cruzi* infection with specific immunoglobulin-chlorambucil conjugate. Lab. Invest. 78: 707–714.

CDC, Centers for Disease Control and Prevention. Parasites—American trypanosomiasis (also known as Chagas disease), General Information. 2018a. https://www.cdc.gov/parasites/chagas/biology.html, accessed 9 August 2018.

CDC, Centers for Disease Control and Prevention. Parasites—American trypanosomiasis (also known as Chagas disease), Antiparasitic Treatment. 2018b. https://www.cdc.gov/parasites/chagas/health_professionals/tx.html, accessed 9 August 2018.

Chao, M.N., C. Li, M. Storey, B.N. Falcone, S.H. Szajnman, S.M. Bonesi et al. 2016. Activity of fluorine-containing analogues of WC-9 and structurally related analogues against two intracellular parasites: *Trypanosoma cruzi* and *Toxoplasma gondii*. ChemMedChem 11: 2690–2702.

Chauhan, S.S., L. Gupta, M. Mittal, P. Vishwakarma, S. Gupta and P.M. Chauhan. 2010. Synthesis and biological evaluation of indolyl glyoxylamides as a new class of antileishmanial agents. Bioorg. Med. Chem. Lett. 20: 6191–6194.

Chauhan, S.S., S. Pandey, R. Shivahare, K. Ramalingam, S. Krishna, P. Vishwakarma et al. 2015. Novel β-carboline-quinazolinone hybrid as an inhibitor of *Leishmania donovani* trypanothione reductase: synthesis, molecular docking and bioevaluation. Med. Chem. Comm. 6: 351–356.

Colin-Lozano, B., I. Leon-Rivera, M.J. Chan-Bacab, B.O. Ortega-Morales, R. Moo-Puc, V. Lopez-Guerrero, et al. 2017. Synthesis, *in vitro* and *in vivo* giardicidal activity of nitrothiazole-NSAID chimeras displaying broad antiprotozoal spectrum. Bioorg. Med. Chem. Lett. 27: 3490–3494.

da Silva, E.N. Jr., M.C.B.V. de Souza, M.C. Fernandes, R.F.S. Menna-Barreto, M.C.F.R. Pinto, F. de Assis Lopes et al. 2008a. Synthesis and anti-*Trypanosoma cruzi* activity of derivatives from nor-lapachones and lapachones. Bioorg. Med. Chem. 16: 5030–5038.

da Silva, E.N. Jr., R.F.S. Menna-Barreto, M.C.F.R. Pinto, R.S.F. Silva, D.V. Teixeira, M.C.B.V. de Souza et al. 2008b. Naphthoquinoidal[1,2,3]-triazole, a new structural moiety active against *Trypanosoma cruzi*. Eur. J. Med. Chem. 43: 1774–1780.

de Moura, K.C.G., F.S. Emery, C. Neves-Pinto, M.C.F.R. Pinto, A.P. Dantas, K. Salomao et al. 2001. Trypanocidal activity of isolated naphthoquinones from Tabebuia and some heterocyclic derivatives: a review from an interdisciplinary study. J. Braz. Chem. Soc. 12: 325–338.

de Oliveira Pedrosa, M., R. Marques Duarte da Cruz, J. de Oliveira Viana, R.O. de Moura, H. Mitsugu Ishiki, J.M. Barbosa Filho et al. 2017. Hybrid compounds as direct multitarget ligands: a review. Curr. Top. Med. Chem. 17: 1044–1079.

de Oliveira Santos, J., G.R. Pereira, G.C. Brandão, T.F. Borgati, L.M. Arantes, R.C. de Paula et al. 2016. Synthesis, *in vitro* antimalarial activity and *in silico* studies of hybrid kauranoid 1,2,3-triazoles derived from naturally occurring diterpenes. J. Braz. Chem. Soc. 27: 551–565.

De Pilla Varotti, F., A.C.C. Botelho, A.A. Andrade, R.C. De Paula, E.M.S. Fagundes, A. Valverde et al. 2008. Synthesis, antimalarial activity, and intracellular targets of MEFAS, a new hybrid compound derived from mefloquine and artesunate. Antimicrob. Agents Chemother. 52: 3868–3874.

Di Marzo, V., T. Bisogno, L. De Petrocellis, I. Brandi, R.G. Jefferson, R.L. Winckler et al. 2001. Highly selective CB_1 cannabinoid receptor ligands and novel CB_1/VR_1 vanilloid receptor "hybrid" ligands. Biochem. Biophys. Res. Commun. 281: 444–451.

Duan, W., S. Qiu, Y. Zhao, H. Sun, C. Qiao and C. Xia. 2012. Praziquantel derivatives exhibit activity against both juvenile and adult *Schistosoma japonicum*. Bioorg. Med. Chem. Lett. 22: 1587–1590.

Dukhyil, A.B. 2018. Targeting trypanothione reductase of *Leishmanial major* to fight against cutaneous leishmaniasis. Infect. Disord. Drug Targets (in press).

Dumonteil, E. and C. Herrera. 2017. Ten years of Chagas disease research: looking back to achievements, looking ahead to challenges. PLoS Negl. Trop. Dis. 11: e0005422.

Galarreta, B.C., R. Sifuentes, A.K. Carrillo, L. Sanchez, M.R.I. Amado and H. Maruenda. 2008. The use of natural product scaffolds as leads in the search for trypanothione reductase inhibitors. Bioorg. Med. Chem. 16: 6689–6695.

Ghose, T. and S.P. Nigam. 1972. Antibody as carrier of chlorambucil. Cancer. 29: 1398–13400.

Gonçalves, A.M., M.E. Vasconcellos, R. Docampo, F.S. Cruz, W. de Souza and W. Leon. 1980. Evaluation of the toxicity of 3-allyl-beta-lapachone against *Trypanosoma cruzi* bloodstream forms. Mol. Biochem. Parasitol. 1: 167–176.

Guglielmo, S., D. Cortese, F. Vottero, B. Rolando, V.P. Kommer, D.L. Williams et al. 2014. New praziquantel derivatives containing NO-donor furoxans and related furazans as active agents against *Schistosoma mansoni*. Eur. J. Med. Chem. 84: 135–145.

Hernandez, P., R. Rojas, R.H. Gilman, M. Sauvain, L.M. Lima, E.J. Barreiro et al. 2013. Hybrid furoxanyl *N*-acylhydrazone derivatives as hits for thedevelopment of neglected diseases drug candidates. Eur. J. Med. Chem. 59: 64–74.

Hopwood, D.A., F. Malpartida, H.M. Kieser, H. Ikeda, J. Duncan, I. Fujii et al. 1985. Production of "hybrid" antibiotics by genetic engineering. Nature. 314: 642–644.

Ikuta, A., T. Nakamura and H. Urabe. 1998. Indolopyridoquinazoline, furoquinoline and canthinone type alkaloids from *Phellodendron amurense* callus tissues. Phytochemistry. 48: 285–291.

Jones, M., A.E. Mercer, P.A. Stocks, L.J.I. La Pensée, R. Cosstick, B.K. Park et al. 2009. Antitumour and antimalarial activity of artemisinin–acridine hybrids. Bioorg. Med. Chem. Lett. 19: 2033–2037.

Joshi, S., G.T. Burke and P.G. Katsoyannis. 1985. Synthesis of an insulin-like compounds consisting of the A chain of insulin and a B chain corresponding to the B domain of human insulin-like growth factor I. Biochemistry. 24: 4208–4214.

Kumar, A., S.B. Katiyar, S. Gupta and P.M.S. Chauhan. 2006. Syntheses of new substituted triazino tetrahydroisoquinolines and β-carbolines as novel antileishmanial agents. Eur. J. Med. Chem. 41: 106–113.

Krauth-Siegel, R.L., H. Bauer and R.H. Schirmer. 2005. Dithiol proteins as guardians of the intracellular redox milieu in parasites: old and new drug targets in trypanosomes and malaria-causing plasmodia. Angew. Chem. Int. Chem. 44: 690–715.

Kubinyi, H. 1999. Chance favors the prepared mind—from serendipity to rational drug design. J. Recept. Signal Transduct. Res. 19: 15–39.

Kumar, R., S. Khan, A. Verma, S. Srivastava, P. Viswakarma, S. Gupta et al. 2010. Synthesis of 2-(pyrimidin-2-yl)-1-phenyl-2,3,4,9-tetrahydro-1*H*-β-carbolines as antileishmanial agents. Eur. J. Med. Chem. 45: 3274–3280.

Lara, L.S., C.S. Moreira, C.M. Calvet, G.C. Lechuga, R.S. Souza, S.C. Bourguignon et al. 2018. Efficacy of 2-hydroxy-3-phenylsulfanylmethyl-[1,4]-naphthoquinone derivatives against different *Trypanosoma cruzi* discrete type units: identification of a promising hit compound. Eur. J. Med. Chem. 144: 572–581.

Lazar, C., A. Kluczyk, T. Kiyota and Y. Konishi. 2004. Drug evolution concept in drug design: 1. Hybridization method. J. Med. Chem. 47: 6973–6982.

Manetti, F., V. Cappello, M. Botta, F. Corelli, N. Mongelli, G. Biasoli et al. 1998. Synthesis and binding mode of heterocyclic analogues of suramin inhibiting the human basic fibroblast growth factor. Bioorg. Med. Chem. 6: 947–958.

Manetti, F., F. Corelli, N. Mongelli, A. Lombardi Borgia and M. Botta. 2000. Research on anti-HIV-1 agents. Investigation on the CD4-Suradista binding mode through docking experiments. J. Comput. Aid. Mol. Des. 14: 355–368.

Manhas, R., S. Tandon, S.S. Sen, N. Tiwari, M. Munde, R. Madhubala et al. 2018. *Leishmania donovani* parasites are inhibited by the Benzoxaborole AN2690 targeting Leucyl-tRNA synthetase. Antimicrob. Agents Chemother. 62: e00079–18.

Manssour Fraga, C.A. 2009. Drug hybridization strategies: before or after lead identification? Expert Opin. Drug Discov. 4: 605–609.

Maran, N., P.S. Gomes, L. Freire-de-Lima, E.O. Freitas, C.G. Freire-de-Lima and A. Morrot. 2016. Host resistance to visceral leishmaniasis: prevalence and prevention. Exp. Rev. Anti-Infect. Ther. 14: 435–442.

Mott, B.T., K.C.-C. Cheng, R. Guha, V.P. Kommer, D.L. Williams, J.J. Vermeire et al. 2012. A furoxan-amodiaquine hybrid as a potential therapeutic for three parasitic diseases. MedChemComm. 3: 1505–1511.

Neves-Pinto, C., V.R.S. Malta, M.C.F.R. Pinto, R.H.A. Santos, S.L. de Castro and A.V. Pinto. 2002. A trypanocidal phenazine derived from *β*-lapachone. J. Med. Chem. 45: 2112–2115.

Nqoro, X., N. Tobeka and B.A. Aderibigbe. 2017. Quinoline-based hybrid compounds with antimalarial activity. Molecules. 22: 2268.

Otero, E., E. Garcia, G. Palacios, L.M. Yepes, M. Carda, R. Agut et al. 2017. Triclosan-caffeic acid hybrids: synthesis, leishmanicidal, trypanocidal and cytotoxic activities. Eur. J. Med. Chem. 141: 73–83.

Paloque, L., B. Witkowski, J. Lelièvre, M. Ouji, T. Ben Haddou, F. Ariey et al. 2018. Endoperoxide-based compounds: cross-resistance with artemisinins and selection of a *Plasmodium falciparum* lineage with a K13 non-synonymous polymorphism. J. Antimicrob. Chemother. 73: 395–403.

Pandey, S.K., S. Biswas, S. Gunjan, B.S. Chauhan, S.K. Singh, K. Srivastava et al. 2016. Pyrrolidine-acridine hybrid in artemisinin-based combination: a pharmacodynamic study. Parasitology. 143: 1421–2432.

Pasteur Vallery-Radot, J.L. 1939. Œuvres de Pasteur, Tome VII, Mélanges Scientifiques et Littéraires, pag. 215. Masson et Cᵢₑ, Éditeurs. Paris. https://gallica.bnf.fr/ark:/12148/bpt6k7363q/f221.image, accessed 24 September 2018.

Penna-Coutinho, J., M.J. Almelac, C. Miguel-Blancoc, E. Herrerosc, P.M. Sá, N. Boechatd et al. 2016. Transmission blocking potential of MEFAS, a hybrid compound derived from artesunate and mefloquine. Antimicrob. Agents Chemother. 60: 3145–3147.

Pinto, A.V. and S.L. de Castro. 2009. The trypanocidal activity of naphthoquinones: a review. Molecules. 14: 4570–4590.

Porcal, W., P. Hernandez, L. Boiani, M. Boiani, A. Ferreira, A. Chidichimo et al. 2008. New trypanocidal hybrid compounds from the association of hydrazone moieties and benzofuroxan heterocycle. Bioorg. Med. Chem. 16: 6995–7004.

Portela, J., J. Boissier, B. Gourbal, V. Pradines, V. Colliere, F. Cosledan et al. 2012. Antischistosomal activity of trioxaquines: *in vivo* efficacy and mechanism of action on *Schistosoma mansoni*. Plos Negl. Trop. Dis. 6: e1474.

Qiao, Z., Q. Wang, F. Zhang, Z. Wang, T. Bowling, B. Nare et al. 2012. Chalcone-benzoxaborole hybrid molecules as potent antitrypanosomal agents. J. Med. Chem. 55: 3553–3557.

Rai, S., U.N. Dwivedi and N. Goyal. 2009. *Leishmania donovani* trypanothione reductase: role of urea and guanidine hydrochloride in modulation of functional and structural properties. Biochim. Biophys. Acta Prot. Proteom. 1794: 1474–1484.

Raja, Z., S. André, F. Abbassi, V. Humblot, O. Lequin, T. Bouceba et al. 2017. Insight into the mechanism of action of temporin-Sha, a new broad-spectrum antiparasitic and antibacterial agent. PLosONE. 12: e0174024.

Ramu, D., S. Garg, R. Ayana, A.K. Keerthana, V. Sharma, C.P. Saini et al. 2017. Novel β-carboline-quinazolinone hybrids disrupt *Leishmania donovani* redox homeostasis and show promising antileishmanial activity. Biochem. Pharmacol. 129: 26–42.

Ranieri Cortez, L.E., I.C. Piloto Ferreira, M. Valdrinez Campana, A.G. Ferreira, P.C. Vieira, M.F. das Graças et al. 2011. Alkaloids and triterpene from *Almeidea coerulea* (Nees and Mart.) a. St.-Hil. and anti-leishmanial Activity. Arch. Biol. Technol. 54: 61–66.

Reed, S.L. and J.H. McKerrow. 2018. Why funding for neglected tropical diseases should be a global priority. Clin. Infect. Dis. 67: 323–326.

Reiter, C., A.C. Karagöz, T. Fröhlich, V. Klein, M. Zeino, K. Viertel et al. 2014. Synthesis and study of cytotoxic activity of 1,2,4-trioxane- and egonol-derived hybrid molecules against *Plasmodium falciparum* and multidrug-resistant human leukemia cells. Eur. J. Med. Chem. 75: 403–412.

Rosemberg, E. 1982. Biologic effect of a hybrid preparation of human chorionic gonadotropin in human subjects. Reproduction. 6: 117–132.

Sangshetti, J.N., F.A.K. Khan, A.A. Kulkarni, R.H. Patil, A.M. Pachpinde, K.S. Lohar et al. 2016. Antileishmanial activity of novel indolyl-coumarin hybrids: Design, synthesis, biological evaluation, molecular docking study and *in silico* ADME prediction. Bioorg. Med. Chem. Lett. 26: 829–835.

Santana, J.M. and A.L.R. Teixeira. 1989. Effect of immunotoxins against *Trypanosoma cruzi*. Am. J. Trop. Med. Hyg. 41: 177–182.

Serafim, R.A.M., J.E. Goncalves, F.P. de Souza, A.P. de Melo Loureiro, S. Storpirtis, R. Krogh et al. 2014. Design, synthesis and biological evaluation of hybrid bioisoster derivatives of *N*-acylhydrazone and furoxan groups with potential and selective anti-*Trypanosoma cruzi* activity. Eur. J. Med. Chem. 82: 418–425.

Sharma, M., K. Chauhan, R. Shivahare, P. Vishwakarma, M.K. Suthar, A. Sharma et al. 2013. Discovery of a new class of natural product-inspired quinazolinone hybrid as potent antileishmanial agents. J. Med. Chem. 56: 4374–4392.

Singh, P., B. Jaiyeola, N. Kerru, O. Ebenezer and A. Bissessur. 2017. A review of recent advancements in anti-tubercular molecular hybrids. Curr. Med. Chem. 24: 4180–4212.

Souza, A.L.A., B.X. Faria, K.S. Calabrese, D.J. Hardoim, N. Taniwaki, L.A. Alves et al. 2016. Temporizin and Temporizin-1 peptides as novel candidates for eliminating *Trypanosoma cruzi*. PLos ONE. 11: e0157673.

Spagnoli, R., L. Cappelletti and L. Toscano. 1983. Biological conversion of erythronolide B, an intermediate of erythromycin biogenesis, into new "hybrid" macrolide antibiotics. J. Antibiot. XXXVI: 365–375.

Staerk, D., E. Lemmich, J. Christensen, A. Kharazmi, C.E. Olsen and J.W. Jaroszewski. 2000. Leishmanicidal, antiplasmodial and cytotoxic activity of indole alkaloids from *Corynanthe pachyceras*. Planta Med. 66: 531–536.

Takahashi, H.T., C.R. Novello and T. Ueda-Nakamura. 1999. Synthesis and *in vitro* antiprotozoal activity of thiophene ring-containing quinones. Chem. Pharm. Bull. 47: 1221–1226.

The International Union for Conservation of Nature, Red List of Threatened Species, version 2018–1. http://www.iucnredlist.org/details/full/33048/0, accessed 4 October 2018.

The Human Metabolome Database, http://www.hmdb.ca/metabolites/HMDB0014649, accessed 4 October 2018.

Uliassi, E., G. Fiorani, R.L. Krauth-Siegel, C. Bergamini, R. Fato, G. Bianchini et al. 2017. Crassiflorone derivatives that inhibit *Trypanosoma brucei* glyceraldehyde-3-phosphate dehydrogenase (*Tb*GAPDH) and *Tryapnosoma cruzi* trypanothione reductase (*Tc*TR) and display trypanocidal activity. Eur. J. Med. Chem. 141: 138–148.

van Zwieten, P.A. 1988. Basic pharmacology of α-adrenoceptor antagonists and hybrid drugs. J. Hypertens. Suppl. 6: S3–11.

Viegas-Junior, C., A. Danuello, V. da Silva Bolzani, E.J. Barreiro and C.A. Manssour Fraga. 2007. Molecular hybridization: a useful tool in the design of new drug prototypes. Curr. Med. Chem. 14: 1829–1852.

Wall, R.J., E. Rico, I. Lukac, F. Zuccotto, S. Elg, I.H. Gilbert et al. 2018. Clinical and veterinary trypanocidal benzoxaboroles target CPSF3. Proc. Natl. Acad. Sci. U.S.A. 115: 9616–9621.

World Health Organization. 2018a. Malaria. http://www.who.int/malaria/en/, accessed 19 October 2018.

World Health Organization, Neglected Tropical Diseases. 2018b. http://www.who.int/neglected_diseases/diseases/en/, accessed 20 July 2018.

Chapter **4**

Current Inhibitors of Dengue Virus
An Overview

J. Jonathan Harburn[1],* *and G. Stuart Cockerill*[2]

Introduction

Currently, one of the globally most important neglected tropical infectious diseases is Dengue, a mosquito-borne viral disease which is widespread across tropical and sub-tropical countries. Dengue is considered a critical worldwide health concern with an estimated 3.6 billion people at risk of infection and approximately 390 million infected annually of which 96 million are present with clinically overt disease (Gubler 2012, Bhatt et al. 2013). It is now endemic in over 100 countries, with Africa, South-East Asia and Western Pacific regions most seriously affected. Furthermore, explosive outbreaks of the disease are frequent and there now exists a significant threat of an outbreak in Europe and North America. An estimated 500,000 people with severe dengue require hospitalisation each year, and about 2.5% of those affected currently die, putting a huge strain on health care systems during outbreaks (WHO 2012).

Most subjects recover from Dengue incurring asymptomatic or subclinical disease; however, progression can take the form of more dangerous dengue fever (DF), most severe dengue haemorrhagic fever (DHF) and dengue shock syndrome (DSS). There is currently no specific treatment for severe dengue which is managed by maintaining body fluid volume through fluid replacement and analgesia avoiding drugs that can increase bleeding complications.

Transmission of Dengue Virus

Dengue virus (DENV) belongs to the *Flaviviridae* family of single positive-stranded ribonucleic acid (RNA) viruses of the genus *Flavivirus*. The family also includes Zika virus (ZIKV), West Nile virus, yellow fever virus, Japanese encephalitis, hepatitis C virus (HCV) and tick-borne encephalitis virus, all of which share common characteristics. Many flaviviruses are transmitted by arthropod vectors, in particular *Aedes* mosquitos for transmission of DENV in a cycle involving humans and mosquitos, primarily *Aedes aegypti* and *Aedes albopictus* being the most prevalent vectors with tropical and subtropical geographic distribution.

[1] Newcastle University, Faculty of Medical Sciences, School of Pharmacy, Newcastle University, Newcastle-upon-Tyne, NE1 4LF, United Kingdom.
[2] ReViral Ltd, Stevenage Bioscience Catalyst, Gunnels Wood Road, Stevenage, Herts, SG1 2FX, United Kingdom.
* Corresponding author: jonathan.harburn@newcastle.ac.uk

Dengue viruses can be serologically classified into 4 major serotypes DENV (DENV1-4) on the basis of plaque reduction neutralisation assay and each generating a unique host immune response to the infection (Russel and Nisalak 1967). In 2013, a fifth serotype (DENV5) was classified emerging possibly from genetic recombination, natural selection and genetic bottlenecks (Mustafa et al. 2015). DENV1-4 are genetically similar and share approximately 65% of their genomes (Holmes 1998). DENV, being RNA viruses, display high mutation frequencies as a result of error-prone polymerase activity, with mutation rates being more than 100 times greater than the mutation rates of DNA genomes. The accumulation of mutations is a continuing and dynamic process in a state of flux, which, together with the possibility of intramolecular recombination due to simultaneous infections with different dengue virus serotypes, could lead to the emergence of a novel dengue virus serotype differing at one or more critical neutralising epitopes.

Genomic Organisation of Dengue Virus

The four main serotypes are enveloped, spherical viral particles with a diameter of approximately 500 angstrom. The DENV genome is a single stranded sense RNA molecule which is approximately 11 kilobases long containing a single open reading frame (ORF), flanked by non-translated regions (NTRs) or approximately 100 nucleotides at the 5' end and approximately 450 at the 3' end. The ORF encodes an approximately 3400 amino-acid residue long polyprotein which is subjected to a combination of host and virus NS3 proteases during and after translation, converting it into three structural proteins, the capsid (C), the membrane (M) and the envelope (E) and seven non-structural (NS) proteins, NS1, NS2a, NS2b, NS3, NS4a, NS4b and NS5. Some of the main features of the non-structural proteins are listed in Table 1.

The life cycle of DENV (Figure 1) has been extensively reviewed containing the following major events: viral entry, fusion and disassembly, viral genome replication, viral protein translation and processing, assembly, maturation, budding and release (Screaton et al. 2015).

Viral entry into a susceptible host starts through binding of the envelope (E) glycoprotein to unknown host cell-surface receptor and is achieved through receptor mediated endocytosis. The E protein is divided into three discrete domains, envelope domain I (EDI), EDII and EDIII of which EDIII controls receptor recognition (Smit et al. 2011). Once inside the host cell, the acidic pH of the endosome triggers conformational rearrangement of the E glycoprotein which facilitates fusion of the viral and endosomal membranes resulting in release of the nucleocapsid. The nucleocapsid disassembles to release capped viral genome into the cytoplasm which is then translated into a long polyprotein which is cleaved by non-structural 2B (NS2B) or N3 protease and host proteases into the ten viral proteins. The released NS proteins are targeted to the site of replication on endoplasmic reticulum(ER)-derived vesicle packets to initiate transcription where NS1 is expressed. The E protein and precursor membrane protein associate as heterodimers then embed into the ER membrane and enclose newly formed nucleocapsid budding into the ER lumen as an immature particle. This particle is trafficked through the secretory pathway under low pH of the trans-Golgi network causing structural rearrangement of the premembrane (prM) and E proteins allowing cleavage of prM by furin protease to form the mature M protein. The mature virion is released from the cell through release of the pr protein and exocytosis.

DENV Vaccine

Recently, a recombinant live-attenuated yellow fever-17D-DENV vaccine (Dengvaxia®, CYD-TDV) was developed by Sanofi Pasteur and was licensed for use in the Philippines, Brazil and Mexico (Vanice et al. 2016). The tetravalent vaccine consists of genes encoding prM and E proteins of DENV1-4 virus inserted into the live attenuated yellow fever virus 17 D genomic backbone. However, the serotype-specific efficacy of the DENV vaccine is varying with lower efficacy observed for DENV1 and 2 compared to DENV3 and 4 and the long-term protection and safety of this vaccine still need more investigation (Halstead and Russell 2016). Although a DENV vaccine with variable serotype efficacy is available, there is still an urgent need to develop small molecule inhibitors to support the treatment of DHF and DSS.

Table 1. DENV Genome (adapted from Guzman et al. 2016, Dung et al. 2014).

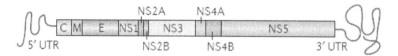

Name	Size (kDa)	Length (aa)	Key features	Functions
C		114	Highly basic. Contains bipartite nuclear location sequence that targets the protein to the nucleus. Binds RNA genome.	Nucleocapsid protein
M		166	Cleaved by furin in the Golgi to form mature membrane protein prior to virus release. Membrane remains associated with viron until virus leaves the cell by exocytosis.	Glycoprotein which protects envelope glycoprotein from low pH induced rearrangement and premature fusion during intracellular life cycle of the virus.
E		495	Dimerises with membrane protein in the immature virus or with second envelope molecule in the mature virus.	Envelope glycoprotein required for receptor-mediated endocytosis, antibody function and membrane fusion.
NS1	46	352	Can be endoplasmic reticulum-anchored, membrane associated or secreted (sNS1). Multiple oligomeric states, glycosylated secreted as hexamer.	Intracellular NS1 is involved in early viral RNA replication. sNS1 activates the innate immune system and is implicated in vascular cleavage.
NS2A	22	218	Hydrophobic integral membrane protein which forms part of the replication complex.	Involved in RNA replication and possible regulator of NS1 function.
NS2B	14	130	Small hydrophobic protein which forms part of the active site binding pocket of NS3.	Co-factor for NS3 protease. Mediates membrane association.
NS3	69	618	Multifunctional protein with several catalytic domains. Highly conserved and interacts with NS5. Involved in virus assembly and also interacts with NS4B.	Involved in nucleoside triphosphatase and helicase functions during RNA synthesis.
NS4A	16	150	Hydrophobic integral membrane protein binding to non-structural proteins in replication process.	Required for the formation of replication vesicles and postulated to play a role in protein targeting and anchoring.
NS4B	30	248	Small hydrophobic membrane protein like NS4A.	Supresses Interferon β and γ cytokine signalling
NS5	105	900	Largest and most highly conserved DENV protein which contains nuclear location sequence as both nuclear and cytoplasmic forms.	Involved in RNA synthesis and blockade of the Interferon system. The C-terminal RNA-dependent RNA polymerase is the viral replicase.

Animal Models in the Development of DENV Inhibitors

One of the main things hampering drug discovery for Dengue is that at present there is no existing animal model that approximates the human disease (Zompi and Harris 2012). The most widely used model to evaluate vaccines and antivirals is the AG129 mouse which is deficient in types I and II interferon receptors which would normally be required for an antiviral response (Schul et al. 2007). Recent examples of pitfalls of using this model was the clinical trials of repurposed Celgosivir (ER-associated α-glucosidase inhibitor) and Lovastatin (cholesterol synthesis inhibitor), both compounds showing reduction in viral load and increased survival rates in mice; neither compound met efficacy end point in clinical trials (Martinez-Guiterrez et al. 2014, Rathore et al. 2011). Drug dose timing could be a possible cause of inconsistency

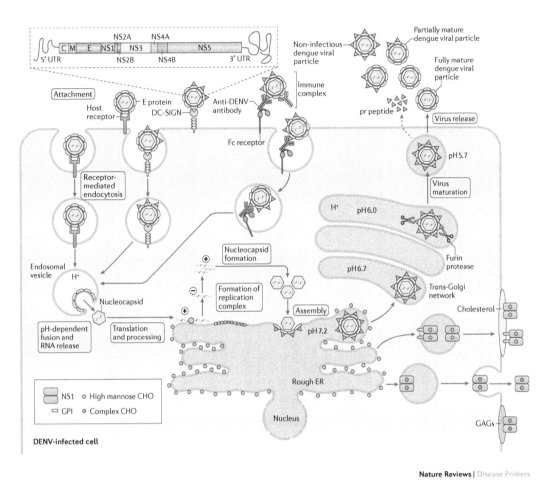

Figure 1. DENV lifecycle (printed with permission from Nature publishers, Guzman et al. 2016).

Color version at the end of the book

between animal studies versus clinical outcomes. Typically, in animal studies first dose begins at the point of detection of viremia whereas in clinical trials with patients the viral load is typically in decline due to presentation timings of the study. Although non-human primates (NHP, such as rhesus macaques) are natural hosts to DENV infection and develop viremia of similar time frame to humans, they rarely show clinical signs or symptoms (Halstead et al. 1973). NHP models addressing different DENV manifestations utility is limited to various factors (cost, scarce laboratory expertise); they could be invaluable as part of rational drug development for the advancement of novel drugs, especially direct-acting antiviral agents (Whitehorn et al. 2014).

Drug Repurposing in Anti-DENV Therapy

Drug repurposing involves the application of approved, marketed or failed compounds from previous drug discovery campaigns to a new disease indication (Corsello et al. 2017). Drug repurposing offers the possibility to reduce time and risks to the drug discovery process and to quickly advance a drug-candidate to late-stage development for new diseases or diseases for which a treatment is unavailable. Table 2 represents a summary of drugs repurposed as DENV inhibitors and even though most did not demonstrate substantial efficacy they represent a suitable and advanced starting point to develop new treatments (Botta et al. 2018). Currently, no licensed antiviral drugs are available to block DENV infection, and while vector control

Table 2. Repurposed drugs (adapted from Botta et al. 2018).

Drug class	Drug	Original activity	DENV activity	In vitro or In vivo assay
Antivirals	Nelfinavir	HIV-1 Protease Inhibitor	NS2B-NS3 protease inhibition	DENV2 EC_{50} = 3.5 ± 0.4 µM Vero cell based assay
	Balapavir	HCV RNA polymerase inhibitor	DENV polymerase	EC_{50} = 0.103 µM infected PBMC cells. DENV4 polymerase activity
	Mycophenolic acid and Ribavarin	Inosine Monophospahate Dehydogenase inhibitor and Human Respiratory Syncytial virus inhibitor	Guanosine depletion	IC_{50} = 0.4 ± 0.3 µM DENV2 monkey kidney cells
Antimalarics	**Chloroquine**	Increases the pH of acidic organelles	Inhibits low-pH dependent entry steps	Able to inhibit DENV2 replication in Vero cells at 5 µg/mL dose
	Amodiaquine	Postulated heme-polymerase inhibitor	unknown	DENV2 EC_{50} = 1.08 ± 0.9 µM plaque assay
Antidiabetics	Castanospermine	ER-glucosidase I inhibitor	Postulated glycoprotein processing inhibitor	DENV2 IC_{50} = 85.7 µM Huh-7 human hepatoma cells
	Celgosivir	ER-glucosidase I inhibitor	Accumulation of DENV NS1 in ER	DENV1 (EC_{50} = 0.65 µM), DENV2 (EC_{50} = 0.22 µM), DENV3 (EC_{50} = 0.68 µM), DENV4 (EC_{50} = 0.31 µM) cell-based flavivirus immune detection (CFI) assay
Anticancers	Dasatinib	Src and Abl kinase inhibitor for chronic myloid leukemia	Src Fyn kinase inhibitor	DENV2 IC_{90} = 132 µM Huh 7 cells
	Saracatinib	Src and Abl kinase inhibitor for chronic myloid leukemia	Src Fyn kinase inhibitor	DENV2 IC_{90} = 12.2 µM Huh 7 cells
	Bortezomib	Proteasome inhibitor	DENV egress inhibitor	DENV1–4 EC_{50} < 20 nM viral replication primary monocytes
Antipsychotics	Prochloroperazine	D2 receptor antagonist	DENV Binding and entry inhibition	DENV2 EC_{50} = 88 nM HEK293T infected cells
Antiparasitic	Ivermectin	Broad spectrum antiparasitic	NS3 helicase inhibitor	DENV2 helicase IC50 = 500 ± 70 nM
	Suramin	Antiparasitic	NS3 helicase inhibitor	DENV3 helicase IC_{50} = 0.6–0.8 µM, DENV4 helicase IC_{50} = 0.8 µM
	Nitazoxanide A	Antiprotozoal, Antibacterial	unknown	DENV2 IC_{50} = 0.1 µg/mL Vero cells

Table 2 contd. ...

...Table 2 contd.

Cholesterics	**Lovastatin**	HMG-CoA Reductase inhibitor	Cholesterol biosynthesis modulation	DENV2 IC_{50} = 38.4 µM Vero cells
Steroidal	Dexamethasone	Anti-inflammatory and immunosuppressant	Platelet count increase	Clinical data
	Prednisolone	Glucocorticoid	Anti-inflammatory anti-hemorrhagic	Clinical data
Antibiotic	Geneticin	80S ribosome interference	E protein inhibition	DENV2 EC_{50} = 3.0 ± 0.4 µg/mL BHK cells
	Narasin	Antiprotozoal	E and NS5 expression reduction	DENV1 (EC_{50} = 0.65 µM), DENV2 (EC_{50} = 0.39 µM), DENV3 (EC_{50} = 0.44 µM), DENV4 (EC_{50} = 0.05 µM) in HuH-7 cells
	Minocycline	Anti-inflammatory and immunosuppressant	ERK1/2 inhibition	DENV1-4 inhibition
Antiarrhytic	Lanatoside C	Na^+-K^+-ATPase pump inhibitor	Postulated post entry mechanism inhibition	DENV2 IC_{50} = 0.19 µM HuH-7

efforts remain the only means to stop the spread of the infection, they have not successfully inhibited annual epidemic outbreaks throughout the tropics.

Clinical Trial Status of Small Molecule Drugs Active against DENV

The clinical landscape for DENV is sparse with only five small molecule potential anti-DENV drugs- Balapiravir (ClinicalTrials.gov Identifier: NCT01096576), Chloroquine (NCT00849602), Celgosivir (NCT01619969, NCT02569827), Prednisolone (ISRCTN Registry No. 39575233) and UV-4B9 (NCT02061358, NCT02696291) have entered Phase I or Phase II clinical trials. These repurposed or off-patent drugs have been subjected to standard double-blinded, randomized trials with placebo-controlled design and showed good safety profiles in patients with acute dengue but failed to meet trial endpoints including reducing viral load. Future trials are recruiting for the use of the platelet activating factor Modipafant and the leukotriene antagonist Ketotefin to prevent vascular leakage in DHF and DSS.

General Medicinal Chemistry Properties for DENV Drug Discovery

Due to the complexity of the amelioration of DF, an effective antiviral should have an excellent safety profile and be active against all 4 serotypes of DENV (and ideally the recently discovered DENV5). Ideally an oral drug, due to expense of manufacture and distribution in resource-strained tropical countries, needs to be stable to heat and high humidity. The oral drug needs to be aqueous soluble due to the high paediatric disease burden and for possible once-daily dosing for good compliance. More acute DF may require up to four times a day to maintain drug concentration above a minimum concentration. Limits for oral bioavailability extend to approximately $MW \leq 1000$ Da, $-2 \leq cLogP \leq 10$, $HBD \leq 6$, $HBA \leq 15$, $PSA \leq 250$ Angstroms^2 and $NRotB \leq 20$.

Entry inhibitors

Viral entry inhibition is historically a logical approach to virus inhibition. Inhibitors act early in the life cycle of the virus and therefore find a role in treating infection early and subsequent re-infection as the virus life cycle continues. Initial entry inhibitors identified were based upon peptide sequences derived from the structure of the envelope E protein, a protein core to the fusion process of the virus with target cell and a protein that undergoes a significant conformational effect during the fusion process. Analogies with other virus fusion events are not unreasonable (Battles et al. 2016). Initial peptides screened were large, with 33 residues, and not potent (Hrobowski et al. 2005). Truncated and mutated forms of these peptides were identified, although still of significant size (Schmidt and Harrison 2010). A series of smaller tripeptides were found to be of low activity (Panya et al. 2014).

In the search for small molecule hits that could eventually lead to oral treatments, a range of approaches have been used: *de novo* design and *in silico* approaches, essentially pharmacophore analysis and docking to the reported structures of the E protein (1k4r.pdb and 4gsx.pdb). Fragment molecular orbital and molecular dynamics simulations have predicted hit molecules (Deasai et al. 2015, Gangopadhyay 2017), in addition to the use of publicly available databases (Zinc, ChemSpider and PubChem).

Structural diversity is clearly evident within the structures although the principles of drug likeness and potential development ability remain more elusive. Compound **2-1** certainly appears to hold the most promise from a structural perspective, although traditional solubility issues associated with such quinazoline based systems will undoubtedly form part of any optimization program. Additionally, from a mechanistic perspective, this compound was observed to act in the early stages of a whole virus assay, a biotinylated derivative was also observed to co-locate with E proteins (Wang et al. 2009).

Compound **2-2** was identified from a screen utilising an FP assay to identify inhibitors of peptide binding to the trimeric post-fusion complex of DENV2. 300,000 compounds were screened in a 384 well format assay and an SAR development follow program identified **2-2**, termed 3-11-22. In addition to low cell cytotoxicity, this compound is reported to exhibit IC_{90}s against DENV2 and 4 in plaque assays (0.74 μM and 2.3 μM) (Schmidt et al. 2012).

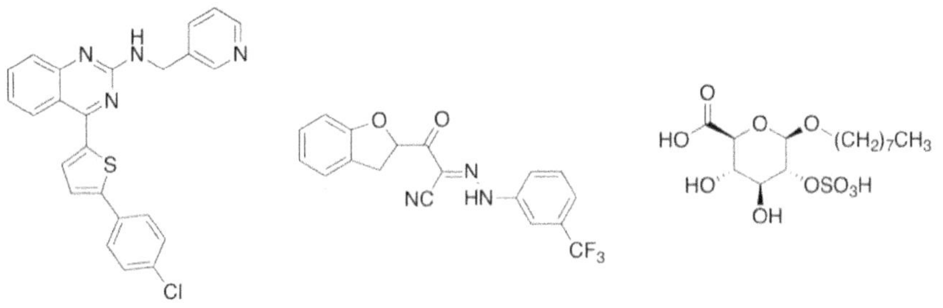

2-1	**2-2**	**2-3**
EC$_{50}$ 0.068 μM	EC$_{50}$ 0.74 μM	EC$_{50}$ 116 μM

Figure 2. Small molecule hits identified from screening approaches towards identification of entry inhibitors.

A fragment based molecular orbital based structural study was originally used for calculations on large molecules (Abe et al. 2014), starting with octyl-β-D-glucose identified compound **2-3**; however, activity remains poor for this series.

Polyprotein processing and translation inhibitors

Protease inhibitors play an important role as part of drug combinations against a number of viruses. The opportunity to target the DENV protease (NS2/NS3pro) and thereby halt its role in the processing of viral specific proteins has provided a number of lead compounds. The difficulty for inhibitor design for this target, however, is associated with an open and hydrophilic catalytic centre; the relevance of this is that historically protease inhibitors have utilised a covalent binding interaction driven by high affinity binding in viruses such as HCV and HIV. The hydrophilic nature of the active site predisposes inhibitors to mirror this property and although levels of potency (in this case moderate) may be achieved, the hydrophilic inhibitors identified suffer from issues created by their physicochemical nature, low permeability and metabolic stability. The crystal structure of a tetrapeptide bound to the protease (Figure 4) illustrates the nature of this active site and what they describe as binding channels. A complete structure containing both the protease and helicase domains has also been crystallised and shows distinct domains for both functionalities (Nitsche et al. 2014).

Thus far, following an exploration of peptide/pseudopeptide inhibitors, a number of inhibitors have been described with potency in the sub micromolar range (Figure 3).

In addition to the boronic acid warhead shown in Figure 3, a number of other classical warheads have been investigated and reviewed in detail (Nitsche et al. 2014). Of these, the trifluoroacetyl group was the only one to achieve sub-micromolar potency. The biggest issue with this type of compound was shown to be poor membrane permeability and metabolic instability. The permeability issue is certainly a well-known feature of previous generations of protease inhibitors stocked with single and multiple guanidine functionality (Kotthaus et al. 2011).

A number of peptide derived inhibitors have been described where by the C-terminal functionality has been modified (Nitsche et al. 2014 and references therein). Thiohydantoin and tyrophostin groups have been described; however, these compounds remain large, poorly permeable and with moderate potency (Figure 3). Compound **3–4** is the product of a programme looking at the applicability of cyclic peptides to the inhibition of the protease. An analysis of an early lead, residue by residue, resulted in the incorporation of a number of non-natural amino acid residues into the cyclic peptide structure with moderate whole virus activity and selectivity (Takagia et al. 2017).

The amphiphilic nature of these cyclic peptides is striking with positions P1–P4 occupied by hydrophilic residues and P1'–P4' by very hydrophobic residues which perhaps reflects the nature of the binding environment.

A number of molecules have been described as non-peptoid inhibitors of the protease. Typical of a target of this type with a relatively low level of industry interest, inhibitors remain diverse of structure with

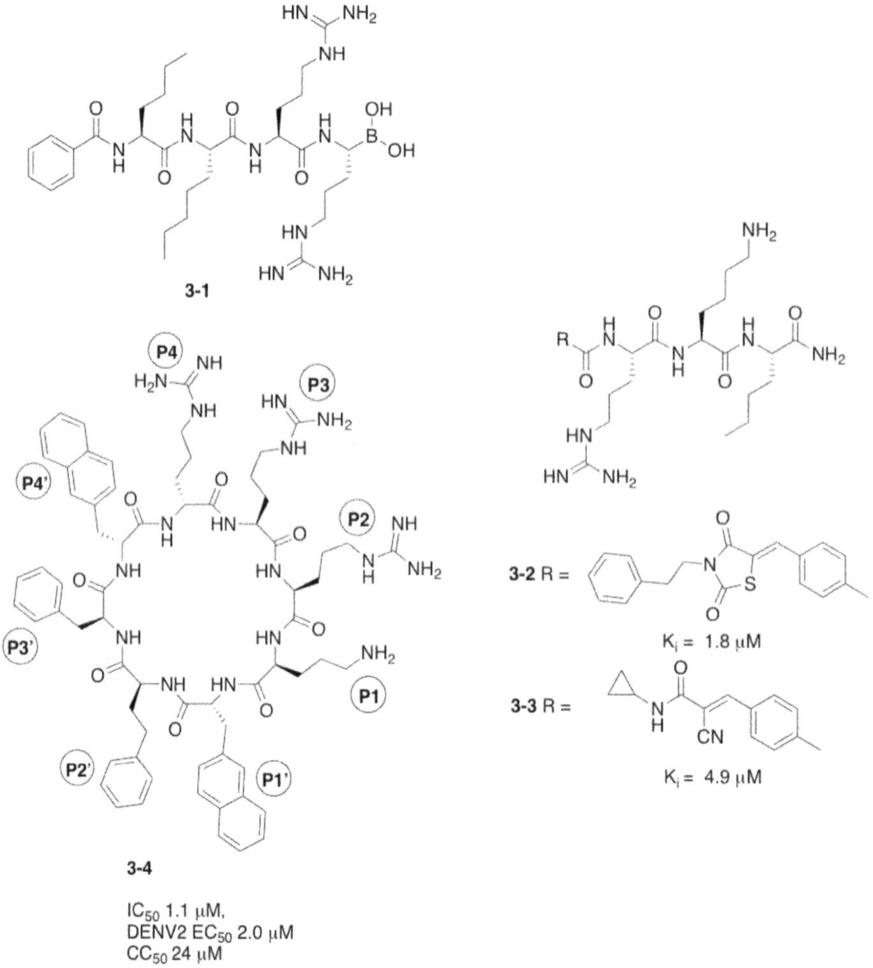

Figure 3. Peptide derived inhibitors of DENV2 Virus protease.

associated poor structural/development ability properties and moderate levels of potency. Tactics employed in the identification of hits have been to use the known structural information to target the catalytic centre and have invariably used the open form of the protease released in the crystallographic database. Issues that remain with these compounds typically are low permeability and the aforementioned poor drug like properties, e.g., metabolic instability. Perhaps the tractability of this approach can be contextualised by a retrospective view on the closely related Hepatitis C virus (HCV) protease; all protease inhibitors reaching the market in what was a heavily funded series of industry research programmes have been of peptide origin (de Leuw 2018).

Compounds worthy of note are shown in Figure 5. Benzothiazole **5-1** was identified from a programme looking for allosteric pocket binding inhibitors of the protease. Docking studies using the 3U1L structure of the protease were utilised to direct modifications that resulted in **5-1**. This series exhibited moderate levels of potency and showed a correlation in activity between whole virus and protease assays in cell culture (Wu et al. 2015) confirming NS3 as the mode of action.

Compound **5-2** was found from the virtual screening of the Molecular Operating Environment (MOE) lead like library; 661,417 structures in all using a virtual docking model of DENV 2 NS3/NS2B protease (PDB entry: 2FOM). The highest scoring 39 structures were evaluated in a cell based viral replication assay. Compound **5-2** was found to inhibit DENV1-4 from this assay and structural studies hypothesise that the compound binds to the NS2 binding site on the protease (Pambudi et al. 2013).

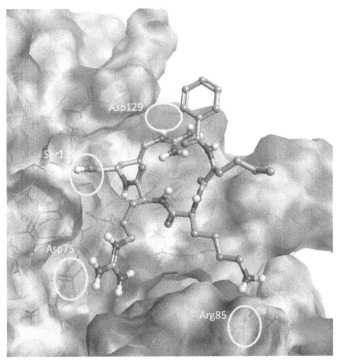

Figure 4. Tetrapeptide inhibitor shown as a ball and stick figure (Bz-*N*-Leu-Lys-Arg-Arg-H) covalently bound to the shallow and open binding pocket of DENV3 protease (3U1I). Key interactions are shown in yellow including the covalent link via the side chain of serine$_{135}$. The molecular surface is coloured by atom type; nitrogen in blue, oxygen in red and carbon in grey (Nitsche et al. 2014 and references therein).

Color version at the end of the book

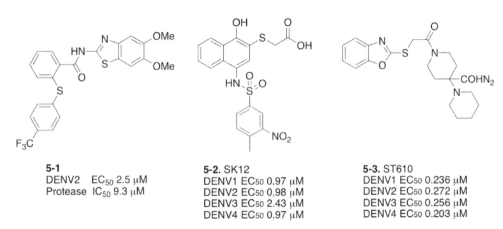

5-1
DENV2   EC$_{50}$ 2.5 µM
Protease IC$_{50}$ 9.3 µM

5-2. SK12
DENV1 EC$_{50}$ 0,97 µM
DENV2 EC$_{50}$ 0,98 µM
DENV3 EC$_{50}$ 2.43 µM
DENV4 EC$_{50}$ 0,97 µM

5-3. ST610
DENV1 EC$_{50}$ 0.236 µM
DENV2 EC$_{50}$ 0.272 µM
DENV3 EC$_{50}$ 0.256 µM
DENV4 EC$_{50}$ 0.203 µM

Figure 5. Non-peptoidal inhibitors of NS3-NS2 protease and helicase.

Compound **5-3** was identified from a screen of a 200,000 compounds diversity selection. Hits were evaluated in a cytopathic effect assay at 5 µM (Byrd et al. 2013). **5-3** was subsequently evaluated in a whole virus plaque assay and found to inhibit all 4 serotypes of the virus at sub micromolar levels and was also shown to be specific for flaviviruses. Moderate activity was observed for yellow fever virus (7.4 µM) and Venezuelan equine encephalitis virus (10.1 µM, of the family *Togaviridae*).

Time of addition studies indicated that the compound was most effective when added up to four hours post infection and resistance studies identified a point mutation (A263T) that mapped to the NS3 gene, specifically within the helicase component of this gene. The relatively quick onset of resistance (eight passages at 5 µM of compound), and fitness studies suggested that this mutant was as competent and functional as the wild type virus- an indicator of resistance as a therapeutic issue for this compound.

Replication inhibitors

The Novartis Institute for tropical disease has contributed a number of chemotypes to the investigation of inhibition of the DENV polymerase. The spiro-pyrazolopyridinones are our first example of this effort (Wang et al. 2015). This class of compound was discovered by a phenotypic screen of the Novartis library; specifically, the utilisation of a DENV2 sub-genomic replicon in A549 cells. Following an HCV replicon exclusion assay, hit compounds were evaluated in whole virus assays against all four serotypes and a representative group of other viruses (Figure 6). The spiro-pyrazolopyridinone **6-1** was identified from this screen and chiral resolution by chiral HPLC identified *R* stereoisomer as the active enantiomer with an approximate 200 fold differential over its *S* form. Lead optimisation identified the pyridyl variant **6-2** (Zou et al. 2015). This compound was sufficiently potent against DENV2 with improved solubility (504 µM) and bioavailability (63%) in rats, albeit with a somewhat compromised microsomal stability. Compound **6-2** was progressed into a mouse model of DENV2 viremia. The compound was dosed either once daily (QD at 100 mg/kg) or twice daily (BID at 50 mg/kg) and a 1.9 log reduction in viral titre could be observed relative to the control group.

Both the *R* form of **6-1** and **6-2** were active against DENV2 and 3 but not DENV1 or 4. Of other viruses evaluated, only moderate activity was observed for yellow fever virus for **6-2** (6.4 µM). *R* form **6-1** showed a 2 log suppression in viral titre up to 10 hours post infection and resistance studies located the V63 residue as the key point of mutation in the NS4B (polymerase) gene. Interestingly, this V63 mutation is conserved in DENV2 and 3 but not retained in DENV1 and 4. Direct interaction with this gene was demonstrated through the preparation of a ^{3}H labelled **6-2**, gel filtration of the labelled compound in combination with an NTD NS4b construct was observed. No co-elution with a V63I mutant construct was observed. Further publications on the expansion of this series into DENV1 and 4 inhibition are awaited.

An earlier series worthy of comment at this stage are the anthranillic sulfonamides discovered as inhibitors of DENV2 polymerase (Niyomrattanakit et al. 2010). These compounds were the product of a HTS of over one million compounds using a SPA based polymerase assay. Compound **6-3** is the product of a lead optimization program and displays a sub-micromolar IC_{50}. The compounds were shown to bind to the polymerase via a cross linked complex utilising a derivative of **6-3**. Mass spectral analysis of the cross-linked product led to the identification of methionine$_{343}$ as a residue close to the binding location of the inhibitor. The proposition that these compounds were RNA tunnel binders to the polymerase followed.

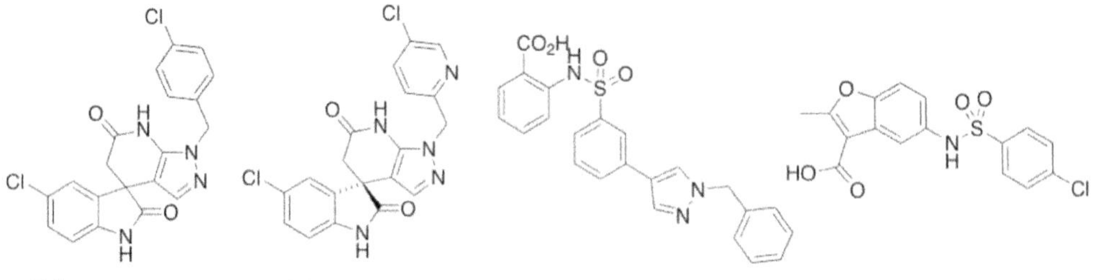

6-1
DENV2 EC_{50} 12 nM
DENV3 EC_{50} 32 nM

6-2
DENV2 EC_{50} 42 nM
DENV3 EC_{50} 76 nM

6-3
DENV2 RdRP IC_{50} 7.2 µM

6-4

Figure 6. Inhibitors of Dengue Virus Replication disclosed by Novartis.

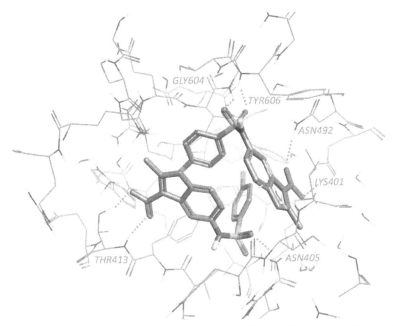

Figure 6a. Active site of Dengue polymerase (PDB accession number 3VWS) to 6A showing the binding of two molecules of Benzofuran **6-4**. Key hydrogen bond interactions are shown in green dotted lines and the relevant amino acids are labelled in green. The figure was generated using Flare™, Cressett Group UK.

Color version at the end of the book

The benzofuran **6-4** was identified from a high throughput screen utilising an RNA elongation assay of DENV4 RdRp (Noble et al. 2013). The compound was shown to be a weak binder to the polymerase by SPR but was successfully crystallised with DENV3 RdRp. The structure was refined to 2.1 angstom resolution. Curiously, two molecules of **6-4** were observed bound adjacent to one another within the RNA binding groove of the polymerase (Figure 6a). The sulfonamide and carboxylic acid groups make a number of hydrogen bonding and salt bridge interactions with lysine and threonine residues. The proposal was that the compound would provoke steric hindrance with the RNA template strand, essentially competing with the RNA substrate for binding. The size of the molecule (molecular weight 366) suggested it as a starting point for a fragment based optimization programme.

A series of indoles has been disclosed in the patent literature as replication inhibitors of DENV (Bardiot et al. 2013). These compounds exhibit pan-genotype activity, although there is a significant difference in potency between DENV2, against which the optimisation process was presumably carried out, and DENV4 as shown for **7-1** (Figure 7). Compounds were assayed against the whole virus in Vero cells with virus load assessed after four days post infection by viral RNA measurement utilising real time quantitative RT-PCR. Cell cytotoxicity was measured also in Vero cells using the metabolic stain MTS/PMS to assess cell viability (Xu et al. 2017). An example from this patent was evaluated in a mouse model *in vivo*, AG129 mice lacking α, β and χ interferon receptors that were inoculated with DENV2 and immediately treated with the compound; the route of administration was not stated. A significant delay in virus induced morbidity was claimed for the compound. Although no further progression of these compounds appears to have been reported, they remain some of the most potent, claimed inhibitors of the virus thus far.

Other compounds have been described as inhibitors of the polymerase of the virus and are shown in Figure 7. The active triphosphate metabolite of Sofosbuvir **7-2** has been shown to function via a chain termination mechanism as an inhibitor of the polymerase and additionally metal chelating agents have been identified, targeting catalytic site metal ions **7-3** (Xu et al. 2016). The tyrosine derivative **7-4** has been shown to bind at the site previously described for the anthranilic sulphonamides exemplified by **6-3**. Reported potencies for these compounds against DENV1-4 is moderate to poor (Tarantino et al. 2016).

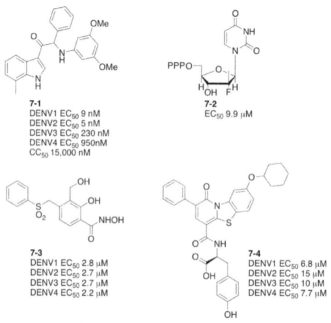

Figure 7. Reported polymerase inhibitors.

A 1.8 million compound screen at Novartis utilising a luciferase linked replicon screen of DENV2 identified **7-4**, an inhibitor that was subsequently shown to target the NS4B protein (Xie et al. 2011). The compound inhibited DENV1-4 ($EC_{50} < 4$ µM and $CC_{50} > 40$ µM), but did not inhibit closely related flaviviruses (West Nile virus and yellow fever virus) or non-flaviviruses (Western equine encephalomyelitis virus, Chikungunya virus, and vesicular stomatitis virus).

Mode of action studies suggested that the compound inhibits viral RNA synthesis. Generation and sequencing of replicons resistant to the inhibitor showed two mutations (P104L and A119T) in the viral NS4B protein that conferred additive resistance to the inhibitor. NS4B had been previously shown to interact with the viral NS3 helicase domain and one of the two NS4B mutations observed (P104L) prevented the NS3-NS4B interaction (Umreddy et al. 2007).

Miscellaneous inhibitors

A number of molecules have also been identified as either targeting host proteins, or essentially of unknown mechanisms. Known kinase inhibitors are prominent in this group of inhibitors, with inhibitors of the c-Src protooncogene and Bruton's tyrosine (BTK) at the forefront. Src family kinase inhibitors with activity against DENV were described in 2007 (Chu and Yang 2007). Both Dasatinib **8-1** and Saracatinib **8-2** have been identified with moderate levels of activity against DENV2 (Figure 8). The depletion of major kinases associated with these inhibitors utilising RNAi was used to identify the Src family kinase Fyn as the major mediator of the anti-viral effect (de Wispelaere et al. 2013). A study based upon utilising Src kinase inhibitors as the starting point was, after looking at a number of scaffolds, able to identify purine as **8-3** as a dual inhibitor of both the kinases Src/Fyn as well as being the first example of an inhibitor of a key NS5-NS3 interaction (Vincetti et al. 2015). Mutagenesis studies, involving amino acid residues contained within an allosteric pocket on the polymerase, had proposed this pocket as a key inhibitor binding pocket, disruption of this pocket being crucial to the inhibition of the initiation of RNA synthesis and the formation of a functional polymerase-helix complex. A design process utilising virtual screening of an in-house library was supported by an Alphascreen NS5-NS3 interaction assay to evaluate hit compounds. Induced fit docking was further used to confirm the binding mode for **8-3**. Anti-viral potency at micromolar level was achieved with a good selectivity index.

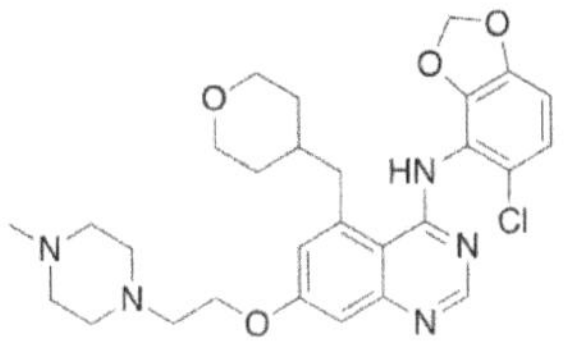

8-1 EC_{50} 12.2 μM

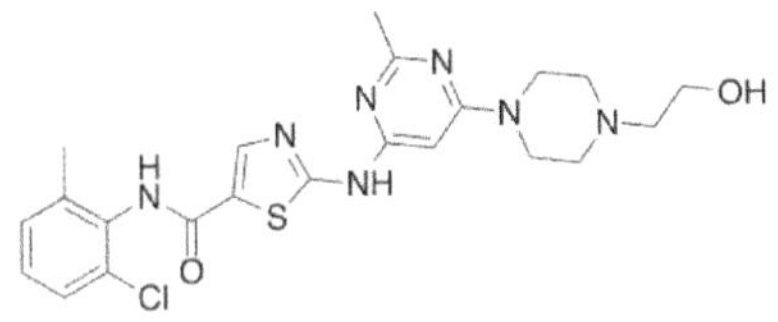

8-2 EC_{50} 4.7 μM

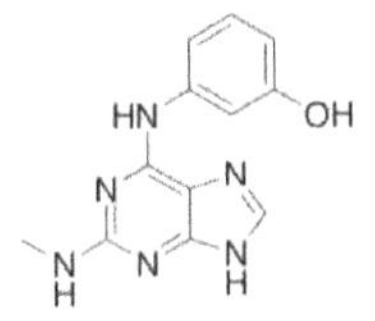

8-3 EC_{50} 5.3 μM

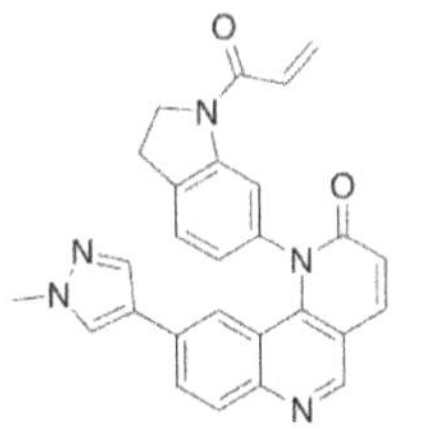

8-4
DENV2 IC_{90} 343 nM

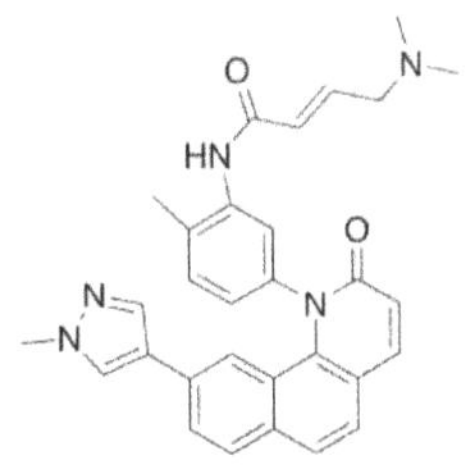

8-5
DENV2 IC_{90} 555 nM

Figure 8. Kinase and kinase derived inhibitors with activity against Dengue Virus.

A group based at the Dana Farber Institute and Harvard Medical School have reported an approach utilising a phenotypic screen of kinase inhibitors bearing cystine reactive covalent modifying groups (de Wispelare et al. 2017). This screening approach identified **8-4** (Figure 8), a known inhibitor of the Tec family kinase BTK as active against DENV2. The compounds were shown to block viral protein expression and subsequently repress the viral infectious cycle. Preliminary mechanistic studies of **8-4** suggested that its antiviral activity was correlated with effects on the steady-state abundance of viral proteins, likely due to an effect on translation of the viral RNA genome. The inhibition of Zika virus, West Nile virus, HCV and poliovirus was also observed. Subsequently, SAR studies were reported which produced **8-5**, YKL-04-085 (Liang et al. 2017). Compound **8-2** was shown to be active against DENV2 (IC_{90} = 555 nM) in Huh7 cells. Cell cytotoxicity in the same cell type was shown to be 20 μM (CC_{90}).

This compound did demonstrate a low level of oral absorption (12%) and reduced activity versus kinase targets (BTK IC_{50} = 911 nM). Further development of this series is described as being underway.

A disparate range of host target mechanisms and inhibitors have also been described in the last few years- Lactimidomycin binding to the E site of the host ribosome has been described to be active against DENV2 (EC_{50} = 0.4 μM) (Carocci and Yang 2016); the inhibition of sterol regulatory element-binding protein S1P has shown activity (EC_{50}=1.2 μM, DENV2) (Uchida et al. 2016); the possible complicity of host IMPDH in an anti-viral effect (Mazzucco et al. 2015); Heme oxygenase 1 (Tseng et al. 2016) and the HMG-CoA (Soto-Acosta et al. 2017) reductase pathway have received some attention. All of these proposed targets are at an early evaluation stage utilizing biochemical tool inhibitors or inducers.

Conclusion

Small molecule drug discovery for Dengue currently occupies a relatively immature position with regard to drug identification as no small molecules have reached clinical evaluation yet. Approaches to the identification of lead series have been supported by crystal structures of major viral targets (capsid, envelope, NS3 protease and helicase domains, methyltransferase and the polymerase have been solved) and several of the series described herein have made use of these structures, in terms of optimisation and hit identification. Despite this, no real progress even through the early development phase has been reported.

Approaches remain innovative and some targets have yielded compounds with potency and the dengue subtype coverage required for effective treatment of infection. Inhibition of host mechanism inhibition has provided some intriguing lead compounds although the number of potential mechanisms under evaluation is increasing. Whether any of these approaches create realistic anti-viral compounds is very much open to question. We have to remain hopeful that these approaches can yield leads that receive the appropriate support to break the current barrier and progress into clinical evaluation.

References

Abe, T.S., F. Teraoka, T. Otsubo, K. Morita, H. Tokiwa, K. Ikeda et al. 2014. Computational design of a sulfoglucuronide derivative fitting into a hydrophobic pocket of dengue virus E protein. Biochem. Biophys. Res. Commun. 449: 32–37.

Bardiot, D., G. Carlens, K. Dallmeier, S. Kaptein, N. McNaughton, A. Marchand et al. 2013. Viral replication inhibitors. WO 2013/045516 A1. 04.04.2013.

Battles, M.B., J.P. Langedijk, P. Furmanova-Hollenstein, S. Chaiwatpongsakorn, H.M. Costello, L. Kwanten et al. 2016. Molecular mechanism of respiratory syncytial virus fusion inhibitors. Nat. Chem. Biol. 12: 87–93.

Bhatt, S., P.W. Gething, O.J. Brady, J.P. Messina, A.W. Farlow, C.L. Moyes et al. 2013. The global distribution and burden of dengue. Nature. 496: 504–507.

Botta, L., M. Rivara, V. Zuliani and M. Radi. 2018. Drug repurposing approaches to fight Dengue virus infection and related diseases. Frontiers in Bioscience. 23: 997–1019.52.

Byrd, C.M.G., D.W. Berhanu, A. Dai, D. Jones, K.F. Cardwell, K.B. Schneider et al. 2013. Novel benzoxazole inhibitor of Dengue virus replication that targets the NS3 helicase. Antimicrob. Agents Chemother. 57: 1902–1912.

Carocci, M. and P.L. Yang. 2016. Lactimidomycin is a broad-spectrum inhibitor of dengue and other RNA viruses. Antiviral. Res. 128: 57–62.

Chu, J.H. and P.L. Yang. 2007. c-Src protein kinase inhibitors block assembly and maturation of dengue virus. PNAS. 104: 3520–3525.

Corsello, S.M., J.A. Bittker, Z. Liu, J. Gould, P. McCarren, J.E. Hirschman et al. 2017. The drug repurposing hub: a next-generation drug library and information resource. Nat. Med. 23: 405–408.

de Leuw, P. and C. Stephan. 2018. Protease inhibitor therapy for hepatitis C virus-infection. Expert. Opin. Pharmacother. 19: 577–587.

de Wispelaere, M., A.J. LaCroix and P.L. Yang. 2013. The small molecules AZD0530 and Dasatinib inhibit Dengue Virus RNA replication via Fyn kinase. J. Virol. 87: 7367–7381.

de Wispelaere, M., M. Carocci, L. Yanke, L. Qingsong, E. Sund, E. Vetter et al. 2017. Discovery of host-targeted covalent inhibitors of dengue virus. Antiviral. Res. 139: 171–179.

Desai, V.H.K., S.P. Pandya and H.A. Solanki. 2015. Receptor-guided de novo design of dengue envelope protein inhibitors. Appl. Biochem. Biotechnol. 177: 861–878.

Gangopadhyay, A., H.J. Chakraborty and A. Datta. 2017. Targeting the dengue β-OG with serotype-specific alkaloid virtual leads. J. Mol. Graph. Model. 73: 129–142.

Global Strategy for dengue prevention and control, 2012–2020. 2012. Accessed http://www.who.int/dengue control/9789241504034/en/ 08/0818.

Gubler, D.J. 2012. The economic burden of dengue. Am. J. Trop Med. Hyg. 86: 743–4.

Guzman, M.G., D.J. Gubler, A. Izquierdo, E. Martinez and S.B. Halstead. 2016. Dengue infection. Nat. Rev. Dis. Primers. 2: 16055.

Halstead, S.B., H. Shotwell and J. Casals. 1973. Studies on the pathogenesis of dengue infection in monkeys. II. Clinical laboratory responses to heterologous infection. J. Infect. Dis. 128: 7–14.

Halstead, S.B. and P.K. Russell. 2016. Protective and immunological behavior of chimeric yellow fever dengue vaccine. Vaccine. 34: 1643–7.

Holmes, E.C. 1998. Molecular epidemiology and evolution of emerging infectious diseases. Brit. Mel. Bull. 54: 533–543.

Hrobowski, Y.M., R.F. Garry and S.F. Michael. 2005. Peptide inhibitors of dengue virus and West Nile virus infectivity. J. Virol. 2.

Kotthaus, J., T. Steinmetzer, A. van de Locht and B. Clement. 2011. Analysis of highly potent amidine containing inhibitors of serine proteases and their N-hydroxylated prodrugs (amidoximes). J. Enzyme Inhib. Med. Chem. 26: 115–122.

Liang, Y., M. de Wispelaere, M. Carocci, Q. Liu, J. Wang, P.L. Yang et al. 2017. Structure–activity relationship study of QL47: A broad-spectrum antiviral agent. ACS Med. Chem. Lett. 8: 344–349.

Martinez-Gutierrez, M., L.A. Correa-Londono, J.E. Castellanos, J.C. Gallego-Gomez and J.E. Osorio. 2014. Lovastatin delays infection and increases survival rates in AG129 mice infected with dengue virus serotype 2. PLoS One. 9: e87412.

Mazzucco, M.B., L.B. Talarico, S. Vatansever, A.C. Carro, M.L. Fascio, N.B. D'Accorso et al. 2015. Antiviral activity of an N-allyl acridone against dengue virus. J. Biomed. Sci. 22: 29.

Mustafa, M.S., V. Rasotgi, S. Jain and V. Gupta. 2015. Discovery of fifth serotype of dengue virus (DENV-5): A new public health dilemma in dengue control. Med. J. Armed Forces India. 71(1): 67–70.

Nitsche, C., S. Holloway, T. Schirmeister and C.D. Klein. 2014. Biochemistry and medicinal chemistry of the dengue virus protease. Chem. Rev. 114(22): 11348–81.

Niyomrattanakit, P.C., Y.-L. Dong, H. Yin, Z. Qing, M. Glickman, F.J. Lin et al. 2010. Inhibition of dengue virus polymerase by blocking of the RNA tunnel. J. Virol. 84: 5678–5686.

Noble, C.G., S.P. Lim, Y.L. Chen, C.W. Liew, L. Yap, J. Lescar et al. 2013. Conformational flexibility of the Dengue virus RNA-dependent RNA polymerase revealed by a complex with an inhibitor. J. Virol. 87: 5291–5295.56.

Pambudi, S., N. Kawashita, S. Phanthanawiboon, M.D. Omokoko, P. Masrinoul, A. Yamashita et al. 2013. A small compound targeting the interaction between nonstructural proteins 2B and 3 inhibits dengue virus replication. Biochem. Biophys. Res. Commun. 440: 393–8.

Panya, A.B., K. Choowongkomon and P.-T. Yenchitsomanus. 2014. Peptide inhibitors against dengue virus infection. Chemical Biology and Drug Design. 84: 148–157.

Rathore, A.P., P.N. Paradkar, S. Watanabe, K.H. Tan, C. Sung, J.E. Connolly et al. 2011. Celgosivir treatment misfolds dengue virus NS1 protein, induces cellular pro-survival genes and protects against lethal challenge mouse model. Antivir. Res. 92: 453–460.

Russell, P.K. and A.J. Nisalak. 1967. Dengue virus identification by the plaque reduction neutralization test. J. Immunol. 88: 291–296.

Schmidt, A.G., P.L. Yang and S.C. Harrison. 2010. Peptide inhibitors of flavivirus entry derived from the E protein stem. J. Virol. 84: 12549–12554.

Schmidt, A.G., K.L. Priscilla, L. Yang and S.C. Harrison. 2012. Small-molecule inhibitors of dengue-virus entry. PLoS Pathog. 8(4): e1002627. Screaton, G., J. Mongkoisapaya, S. Yacoub and C. Roberts. 2015. New insights into the immunopathology and control of dengue virus infection. Nat. Rev. Immunol. 15: 745–759.

Schul, W., W. Liu, H.Y. Xu, M. Flamand and S.G. Vasudevan. 2007. A Dengue fever viremia model in mice shows reduction in viral replication and suppression of the inflammatory response after treatment with antiviral drugs. J. Infect. Dis. 95: 665–74.

Smit, J.M., B. Moesker, I. Rodenhuis-Zybert and J. Wilschut. 2011. Flavivirus cell entry and membrane fusion. Viruses. 3: 160–171.

Soto-Acosta, R., P. Bautista-Carbajal, M. Cervantes-Salazar, A.H. Angel-Ambrocio and R.M. del Angel. 2017. DENV up-regulates the HMG-CoA reductase activity through the impairment of AMPK phosphorylation: A potential antiviral target. PLOS Pathog. 13: e1006257.

Sung, C., G.B.S. Kumar and S.G. Vasudevan. 2014. Dengue drug development. pp. 293–321. *In*: D.J. Gubler et al. [eds.]. Dengue and Hemorrhagic Fever. 2nd Edition, CAB International.

Takagia, Y.M., K. Noboria, H. Maeda, H. Satoa, A. Kurosu, T. Orba et al. 2017. Discovery of novel cyclic peptide inhibitors of dengue virus NS2B-NS3 protease with antiviral activity. Bioorg. Med. Chem. Lett. 27: 3586–3590.

Tarantino, D., R. Cannalire, E. Mastrangelo, R. Croci, G. Querat, M.L. Berreca et al. 2016. Targeting flavivirus RNA dependent RNA polymerase through a pyridobenzothiazole inhibitor. Antiviral Res. 134: 226–235.

Tseng, C.-K., C.-K. Lin, Y.-H. Wu, Y-H. Chen, W.-C. Chen, K.-C. Young et al. 2016. Human heme oxygenase 1 is a potential host cell factor against dengue virus replication. Sci. Rep. 6: 32176.

Uchida, L., S. Urata, E.L.G. Ulanday, Y. Kamatsu, J. Yasuda, K. Morita et al. 2016. Suppressive effects of the site 1 Protease (S1P) inhibitor, PF-429242, on Dengue virus propagation. Viruses. 8(2): E46.

Umareddy, I., A. Chao, A. Sampath, F. Gu and S.G. Vasudevan. 2006. Dengue virus NS4B interacts with NS3 and dissociates it from single-stranded RNA. J. Gen. Virol. 87: 2605–2614.

Vanice, K.S., A. Durbin and J. Hombach. 2016. Status of vaccine research and development of vaccines for dengue. Vaccine. 34: 2934–8.

Vincetti, P.C., F. Kaptein, S. Gioiello, A. Mancino, V. Suzuki, Y. Yamamoto et al. 2015. Discovery of multitarget antivirals acting on both the Dengue virus NS5-NS3 interaction and the host Src/Fyn kinases. J. Med. Chem. 58: 4964–4975.

Wang, Q.-Y., S.J. Patel, E. Vangrevelinghe, H.Y. Xu, R. Rao, D. Jaber et al. 2009. A small-molecule dengue virus entry inhibitor. Antimicrob. Agents. Chemother. 53: 1823–1831.

Wang, Q.-Y., D. Hongping, B. Zou, R. Karuna, K.F. Wan, J. Zou et al. 2015. Discovery of Dengue virus NS4B inhibitors. J. Virol. 89: 8233–8244.

Whitehorn, J., S. Yacoub, K.L. Anders, L.R. Macareo, M.C. Cassetti, V.C.N. Van et al. 2014. Dengue therapeutics, chemoprophylaxis, and allied tools: State of the art and future directions. PLoS Neg. Trop. Dis. 8: e3025.

Wu, H., S. Bock, M. Snitko, T. Berger, T. Weidner, S. Holloway et al. 2015. Novel dengue virus NS2B/NS3 protease inhibitors. Antimicrob. Agents. Chemother. 59: 1100–9.

Xie, X., Q.-Y. Wang, H.Y. Xu, M. Qing, L. Kramer, Z. Yuan et al. 2011. Inhibition of Dengue virus by targeting viral NS4B protein. J. Virol. 85: 11183–11195.

Xu, H.-T., S.P. Colby-Germinario, S. Hassounah, P.K. Quashie, C. Fogarty, Y. Han et al. 2016. Identification of a Pyridoxine-derived small-molecule inhibitor targeting Dengue virus RNA-dependent RNA polymerase. Antimicrob. Agents Chemother. 60: 600–608.

Xu, H.-T., S.P. Colby-Germinario, S.A. Hassounah, C. Fogarty, N. Osman, N. Palanisamy et al. 2017. Evaluation of Sofosbuvir (β-D-2'-deoxy-2'-α-fluoro-2'-β-C-methyluridine) as an inhibitor of Dengue virus replication. Sci. Rep. 7: 6345–6356.

Zompi, D. and E. Harris. 2012. Animal models of dengue virus infection. Viruses. 4: 62–82.

Zou, B., W.L. Chan, M. Ding, S.Y. Leong, S. Nilar, P.G. Seah et al. 2015. Lead optimization of spiropyrazolopyridones: a new and potent class of dengue virus inhibitors. ACS Med. Chem. Letts. 6: 344–8.

Chapter **5**

Overview of Drugs used Against Zika Virus

Sinem Ilgın,* Özlem Atlı Eklioğlu, Begüm Nurpelin Sağlık
and *Serkan Levent*

Introduction

Zika virus (ZIKV) is a mosquito-borne pathogen belonging to Flaviviridae family whose primary transmission occurs via the infected *Aedes* sp mosquito (Esposito et al. 2018, Ioos et al. 2014, Koppolu and Shantha Raju 2018, Simanjuntak et al. 2018). Although it was first isolated from rhesus macaque monkey in 1947, there had been no ZIKV-related febrile disease reports until 1954 (Mourya et al. 2016, Plourde and Bloch 2016, Esposito et al. 2018).

ZIKV, like other flaviviruses, is a small enveloped virus which has icosahedral capsid structure and ~ 12 kb positive-sense RNA genome (Bollati et al. 2010, Wang et al. 2017, Esposito et al. 2018). ZIKV genome is a single stranded RNA consisting of two non-coding regions and one coding region. Coding region codes three structural (Capsid, Precursor-Membrane, Envelope) and seven non-structural proteins (NS1, 2A, 2B, 3, 4A, 4B, 5) (Göertz et al. 2017, Esposito et al. 2018). Phylogenetic analysis based on nucleotide and amino acid composition reveals that ZIKV genome is separated into two major lineages (Africa and Asia). It is accepted that both lineages can cause the same disease (Esposito et al. 2018). The structure of ZIKV is presented in Figure 1.

The feature that distinguishes this virus from other flaviviruses is related to its transmission. Especially, defining of sexual and transplacental transmission routes for ZIKV makes this virus unique (Hastings and Fikrig 2017). Other feature of ZIKV is viral persistence. The virus persistence between serum and genital fluids like cervical mucus and semen contributes to the blood, *in utero* and sexual transmission of ZIKV (Duggal et al. 2017, Esposito et al. 2018).

ZIKV infections generally remain asymptomatic while they can also cause mild febrile disease symptoms such as headache, myalgia, fever, rash and non-purulent conjunctivitis (Koppolu and Shantha Raju 2018, Mcdonald and Holden 2018, Simanjuntak et al. 2018). These symptoms usually disappear in a few days after onset of the disease (Koppolu and Shantha Raju 2018, Simanjuntak et al. 2018). However,

Anadolu University, Faculty of Pharmacy, Department of Pharmaceutical Toxicology, 26470, Eskisehir, Turkey.
* Corresponding author: silgin@anadolu.edu.tr

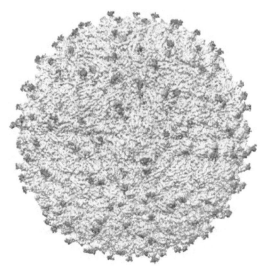

Figure 1. Overall structure of ZIKV (Sirohi et al. 2016).

Color version at the end of the book

during the spread of ZIKV through different geographical regions, the characteristics of ZIKV-originated infection appear to change in humans. The arboviral endemic infection which caused mild disease in equatorial Africa and Asia spreads worldwide and since 2007 ZIKV epidemics have then occurred in populations which were not exposed to virus before. In these populations, ZIKV has been linked to congenital abnormalities and neurological disorders including Guillain-Barré syndrome (GBS) since 2013 (Kindhauser et al. 2016). Congenital abnormalities observed in infants born from ZIKV-infected mothers during the outbreak in Brazil and the increased incidence of GBS in the territories with outbreaks accelerated the research efforts towards the identification of treatments against ZIKV (Passi et al. 2016, Plourde and Bloch 2016, Esposito et al. 2018). There has been a rapid increase in ZIKV-related research including ZIKV transmission routes, pathogenesis of infection, diagnosis, vaccines and treatment of infection when World Health Organization (WHO) declared it as a Public Health Emergency of International Concern (PHEIC) in 2016. It is noteworthy that the number of articles reached to 4019 after the year 2015 in Pubmed database while there were only 88 articles related to ZIKV until the year 2015.

ZIKV continues to affect the American, African, and Asian continents (Figure 2). About 75 countries/territories reported evidence of mosquito-borne ZIKV transmission since 2007 (Rana 2016).

Epidemiology

In 1948, a few months later than isolation of ZIKV from rhesus macaque monkey in 1947, the virus was isolated from *Aedes africanus* mosquitoes. However, only few studies on ZIKV were performed because of the local distribution and the low effects of the virus on human health (Esposito et al. 2018, Koppolu and Shantha Raju 2018, MacDonald and Holden 2018). First human cases of ZIKV infection were described in Uganda and United Republic of Tanzania in 1952. The geographical distribution of ZIKV expanded to Equatorial Asia, India, Indonesia, Malaysia, and Pakistan between the years 1969 and 1983 (WHO 2018a). Because of the high incidence of asymptomatic infection, the low burden of disease in Africa (ZIKV was endemic to the territories where the people were infected at their early stages of lives) and the limited opportunities for the detection of the virus, ZIKV infections did not gain any importance at that time (Esposito et al. 2018). Specially, there has been only 14 human cases reported until 2007 along with the identification of the virus in Africa and Asia (Ioos et al. 2014, WHO 2018a, MacDonald and Holden 2018). The ZIKV outbreak, which affected more than 5,000 people in Federated States of Micronesia in the year

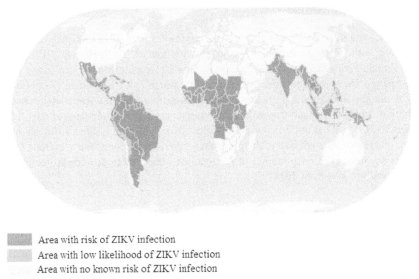

Area with risk of ZIKV infection
Area with low likelihood of ZIKV infection
Area with no known risk of ZIKV infection

Figure 2. World map of area with risk of ZIKV, according to the Centers for Disease Control and Prevention Centers for Disease Control and Prevention (CDC), 2018.

Color version at the end of the book

of 2007, was the first large outbreak drawing attention to ZIKV infections (WHO 2016, MacDonald and Holden 2018, Ventura and Ventura 2018). However, the outbreaks which caused ZIKV alert worldwide were the Pacific Island outbreaks in French Polynesia, Easter Island, the Cook Island, and New Caledonia between 2013 and 2014. French Polynesia outbreak was investigated in detail because of thousands of suspicious infection cases (WHO 2018a, MacDonald and Holden 2018, Ventura and Ventura 2018). It was estimated that there have been approximately 30,000 suspicious cases in these outbreaks (Esposito et al. 2018). Brazil notified WHO of an illness characterized by skin rash in northeastern states in 2015. Nearly 7,000 skin rash characterized cases were reported in Brazil. ZIKV infection was not suspected and no diagnostic tests were performed against the virus because of its mildly symptomatic status without any mortality (WHO 2018a). Nevertheless, the phylogenetic analysis carried out after confirming the relationship between ZIKV and the described status indicated that the virus was transferred to the northeastern region of Brazil by the travelers from French Polynesia or Southeast Asia during the Confederations Cup 2013. There have been approximately 270,000 ZIKV-suspected cases reported in Brazil until April 2017 (Esposito et al. 2018). The ZIKV infection and its link to microcephaly and other neurological diseases prompted WHO to declare spike ZIKV as PHEIC in February 2016 (Esposito et al. 2018, WHO 2018a, Koppolu and Shantha Raju 2018).

Routes of Transmission of ZIKV

ZIKV transmission is classified both as vector-borne and non-vector-borne. Vector-borne transmission develops via infected *Aedes* sp. mosquitoes. Besides, non-vector-borne transmission occurs via transplacental, blood and sexual routes in humans (Koppolu and Shantha Raju 2018, McDonald and Holden 2018, Simanjuntak et al. 2018). Also, ZIKV was isolated from urine, blood, semen, vaginal secretions, saliva, spinal fluid, amniotic fluid and breast milk in humans (McDonald and Holden 2018, Simanjuntak et al. 2018, Wikan and Smith 2016). A ZIKV sylvatic cycle of transmission is established between non-human primates and forest-dwelling mosquitoes (Althouse et al. 2016, Wikan and Smith 2016). At this point, it should be emphasized that the majority of ZIKV-related cases with vector-infected incidental hosts are associated with sylvatic cycle (Wikan and Smith 2016).

Mosquito-borne transmission

Zika virus was isolated from *Anopheles gambiae, A. coustani, Culex perfuscus,* and *Mansonia uniformis* mosquitoes along with 17 *Aedes* mosquito species (Epelboin et al. 2017, Hunter 2017). Amongst these species, only female *Aedes aegypti, A. albopictus, A. hensilli* (responsible for Yap Island outbreak), and *A. Polynesiensis* species were responsible for the transmission of ZIKV to humans (Koppolu and Shantha Raju 2018). *A. albopictus* mosquitoes are particularly responsible for ZIKV transmission because of their wide distribution over tropical, sub-tropical, and temperate regions (Caminade et al. 2017, Koppolu and Shantha Raju 2018). The most important way to protect from mosquito-borne transmission is to prevent exposure. For this reason, it is advised to the pregnant women to postpone their vacations to ZIKV-active regions. If it is essential, DEET-containing insect repellents are used to provide protection (Wylie et al. 2016, Koppolu and Shantha Raju 2018).

Transplacental transmission

It was demonstrated that ZIKV was capable of passing placental barrier and infecting the fetus (Noronha et al. 2016, Koppolu and Shantha Raju 2018). This transmission is also supported by the detection of ZIKV RNA and antigens in amniotic fluid, placenta and fetal brain tissue (Noronha et al. 2016, Sharma and Lal 2017, Koppolu and Shantha Raju 2018).

Sexual transmission

ZIKV transmits to couples during sexual intercourse (Zamani and Zamani 2017). The primary reason for the viral transmission to women is accepted as the sexual contact with the infected-men (Sharma and Lal 2017). Studies assert that virus stays alive for a long time in testicular cells and for this reason spreads the infection (Wong et al. 2017). Also, it is stressed that female genital cells are more sensitive to ZIKV infection. However, the cases related to different transmission routes such as men to men and women to men have drawn attention in the year 2016 (Koppolu and Shantha Raju 2018).

Several health organizations including WHO published guidelines to prevent sexual transmission because of the ZIKV-related congenital malformations in infants. Accordingly, unprotected sexual intercourse is not recommended at least 6 months after ZIKV diagnosis (Esposito et al. 2018).

Transmission by breastfeeding and blood transfusion

ZIKV RNA and particles were detected in infected mother's breast milk. However, the lack of infection reports in infants breastfed by infected mothers brings into mind that this route of transmission may be unimportant (Koppolu and Shantha Raju 2018, McDonald and Holden 2018). There have been also no reports showing ZIKV transmission via blood transfusion (Chen and Tang 2016, Sharma and Lal 2017). Therefore, WHO set up strict regulations regarding blood transfusion in ZIKV-endemic regions (Koppolu and Shantha Raju 2018).

Clinical Signs and Symptoms of ZIKV Infection

ZIKV infection generally remains asymptomatic or presents mild symptoms very similar to other flavivirus infections such as chikungunya and dengue, making ZIKV-related infections difficult to diagnose (Ioos et al. 2014, Esposito et al. 2018). The symptoms occur after an incubation period, 3–12 days after the bite of the infected mosquito (Ioos et al. 2014). Symptoms such as acute fever, maculopapular rash, myalgia, arthralgia, edema of extremities, headache, and conjunctivitis are observed in patients (Koppolu and Shantha Raju 2018, Mcdonald and Holden 2018, Simanjuntak et al. 2018). These symptoms generally subside in a few days/weeks and rarely severe clinical manifestations lead to a hospital stay (Koppolu and Shantha Raju 2018, Simanjuntak et al. 2018).

As a result of numerous ZIKV reports in 2015 and 2016, the undiagnosed diseases in previous outbreaks were associated with ZIKV infection (Esposito et al. 2018). The global alert which aroused from the clinical manifestations of Congenital Zika Syndrome (CZS) was related to *in utero* ZIKV exposure (Koppolu and Shantha Raju 2018, Simanjuntak et al. 2018). Apart from the birth defects, ocular impairments and GBS were also related to ZIKV infection (Esposito et al. 2018, Koppolu and Shantha Raju 2018, Simanjuntak et al. 2018). Recently, several thrombocytopenia reports attracted notice in ZIKV-infected patients (Sharp et al. 2016, Boyer Chammard et al. 2017).

CZS associated with ZIKA infection

Microcephaly, a clinical manifestation observed frequently in rare genetic diseases, may occur after some congenital infections (Araujo et al. 2016, Hanzlik and Gigante 2017). After the Brazil outbreak, the increased number of newborn babies with microcephaly has drawn attention to the association between ZIKV and microcephaly (Coelho and Crovella 2017, Esposito et al. 2018, Wheeler 2018). Even though retrospective studies indicated the association between the other ZIKV epidemics and microcephaly, scientific research exhibited the low incidence of microcephaly in Yap islands and French Polynesia outbreaks (Esposito et al. 2018). However, in the year 2016, after the detection of the virus in the fetal brain of an infected mother, *in utero* transmission was confirmed and the syndrome was accepted as an important public health concern (Sharma and Lal 2017, Esposito et al. 2018, Wheeler 2018). Also, CDC defined this clinical condition with neurological effects caused by ZIKV and different features in terms of systemic effects and malformations in infants as CZS (McDonald and Holden 2018, Ventura and Ventura 2018). This syndrome differs from the other congenital syndromes with the symptoms of severe microcephaly, and brain abnormalities, including thin cerebral cortices and subcortical calcifications, macular scarring and focal pigmentary retinal mottling, congenital contractures, early hypertonia and extrapyramidal involvement, and hearing loss (McDonald and Holden 2018, Pessoa et al. 2018, Ventura and Ventura 2018, Wheeler 2018). Although the most severe CZS was associated with the *in utero* exposures in the first trimester of the pregnancy, reports show that CZS may occur in case of any exposure during the three trimesters (Esposito et al. 2018, Wheeler 2018). It has to be stressed that CZS poses a danger to maternal and pregnant women living in or traveling to regions with ZIKV infection risk (Honein 2018). At this point, it has to be also underlined that there have not been any congenital malformation cases associated with ZIKV in Africa and Asia where ZIKV infection was accepted as endemic (Bailey and Ventura 2018, MacDonald and Holden 2018, Ventura and Ventura 2018).

GBS associated with ZIKV infection

GBS is an autoimmune demyelinating neurological disorder that mainly affects motor axons and may result in progressive muscle weakness and paralysis (Meena et al. 2011, Shrivastava et al. 2017). Some bacterial or viral infectious diseases increase the incidence of GBS (Styczynski et al. 2017, Tang et al. 2017, Esposito et al. 2018). The first case reports showing the relationship between GBS and ZIKV infection were published during the French Polynesia outbreak at the end of the year 2007 (Cao-Lormeau et al. 2016, Esposito et al. 2018, Koppolu and Shantha Raju 2018). The association between ZIKV infection and GBS was identified after the increase of GBS cases, which were reported by health officials during Brazil ZIKV outbreak (Araujo et al. 2016, Esposito et al. 2018).

Eye diseases associated with ZIKV infection

ZIKV may cause mild infections with symptoms such as conjunctivitis and uveitis in adults (Agrawal et al. 2018). However, ZIKV-related eye infections may also cause severe symptoms such as blindness with retina, optic nerve and retinal vessel degeneration, optic neuritis, chorioretinal atrophy, bilateral iris coloboma and intraretinal hemorrhages in infants (Koppolu and Shantha Raju 2018, Ventura and Ventura

2018). Furthermore, it is alleged that eyes may act as a reservoir for ZIKV following acute eye infection (Koppolu and Shantha Raju 2018).

Diagnosis of ZIKV

An accurate diagnosis at the right time is the key point to choose the treatment strategies against ZIKV infection (Ioos et al. 2014, Koppolu and Shantha Raju 2018). However, the clinical diagnosis of ZIKV is very difficult because of its symptoms similar to those of other flavivirus infections and the higher cross antibody reactivity with other flaviviruses in serum (Araujo et al. 2016, Esposito et al. 2018, Ioos et al. 2014, Koppolu and Shantha Raju 2018). Non-specific serological methods such as ELISA or immunofluorescent assay (IFA), which detect antibodies specific to viral antigen (IgM) in serum, are clinically used. However, virus neutralization assays and virus isolation from cell cultures should also be performed together with the previous assays to confirm the diagnosis (Ioos et al. 2014, Koppolu and Shantha Raju 2018). Fundamentally, the specific diagnosis in the acute phase of the disease can be done by using reverse transcriptase-polymerase chain reaction (RT-PCR) at an earlier onset of the symptoms or by the molecular detection of ZIKV RNA in urine (from the onset of the disease to the 14th day). However, this diagnostic approach is not always available in the developing countries (Araujo et al. 2016, Esposito et al. 2018).

Prevention and Treatment of ZIKV Infection

There are no FDA-approved treatments for ZIKV. However, there are various methods that have been adopted for the prevention of ZIKV infection and, perhaps, the most important of these is the prevention of mosquito bites. Insect repellents are often used by people for this purpose. Repellents do not kill the mosquitoes, but just make it harder for mosquitoes to find the human hosts to bite. Repellents generally consist of the following compounds: DEET (**1**), picaridin (**2**) and oil of lemon eucalyptus (**3**).

Repellents

DEET (*N,N*-diethyl-3-methylbenzamide) (**1**) prevents mosquitoes from finding a human host (Figure 3). It is recommended that people should use this repellent with a 10% to 30% concentration to skin and clothing. The concentration of this repellent is determined according to the desired duration of protection. The concentration used, and the duration of protection are parallel. High concentration should be preferred when prolonged protection is required. Also, people should be warned about this compound as it can be toxic and should be used only within limited concentrations when they are outside. DEET should never be used on the hands of young children or on infants younger than age 2 months (Zikavirusnet 2018).

Picaridin (**2**), a piperidine derivative, is also called KBR 3023. The prevention mechanism of this repellent is the same as DEET and this compound should be used in similar concentration. Picaridin has the advantage of being almost odorless. This increases the use of this compound in sensitive individuals (Zikavirusnet 2018).

The oil of lemon eucalyptus is a plant-based repellent which may provide protection at lower concentrations than DEET. It is not recommended to use it on children younger than 3 years (Zikavirusnet 2018).

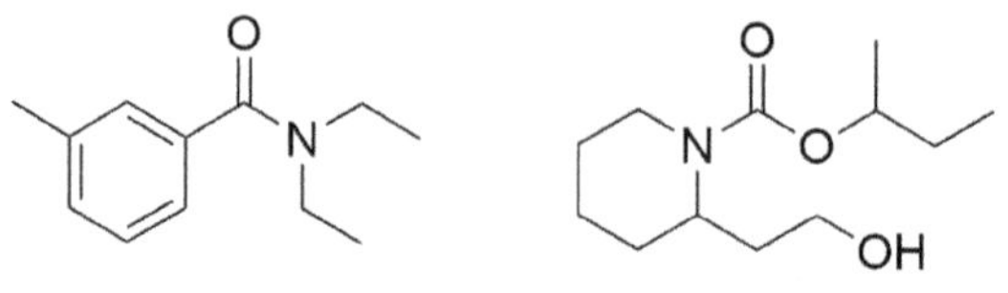

DEET (**1**)   Picaridin (**2**)

Figure 3. Structure of DEET (**1**) and Picaridin (**2**).

Antiviral drugs

Few antiviral drugs acting against Zika are currently under development. Revu et al. reported the synthesis of derivatives of the natural product (+)-trans-dihydronarciclasine (3). Anti-Zika virus activity was evaluated *in vitro* and the (+)-trans-dihydronarciclasine (3) was found to be the most potent derivative with an IC_{50} value of 0.1 μM (Revu et al. 2016) (Figure 4).

Pattnaik et al. have carried out a study by employing a structure-based approach targeting the ZIKV RNA-dependent RNA polymerase (RdRp). A library of 100,000 small molecules were chosen for *in silico* screening. According to the *in silico* results, top ten lead compounds were selected to test for their *in vitro* inhibitory activity against Zika virus. Compound (4) (TPB, Figure 5), a benzothiophene-2-carboxamide derivative, was found as the most potent derivative with IC_{50} and CC_{50} values of 94 nM and 19.4 μM, respectively. According to the molecular docking studies of this compound, TPB could bind to the catalytic active site of the RdRp. It has been suggested that TPB could block the viral RNA synthesis by an allosteric effect (Pattnaik et al. 2018).

In another *in silico* screening study carried out by Singh et al. new compounds were investigated for their docking profile to ZIKV RNA polymerase (RdRpC). Compound (5) was found to have a remarkable docking profile against the strictly conserved aspartate residues of the RdRpC active site (Singh et al. 2017).

Pitts et al. have shown that compound (6) could inhibit dengue virus 2 (DV2) and other flaviviruses by limiting the steady-state accumulation of viral RNA. From these findings, they have suggested that 4-HPR could inhibit ZIKV in mammalian cell culture and significantly reduce both serum viremia and brain viral burden in a murine model of ZIKV infection (Pitts et al. 2017).

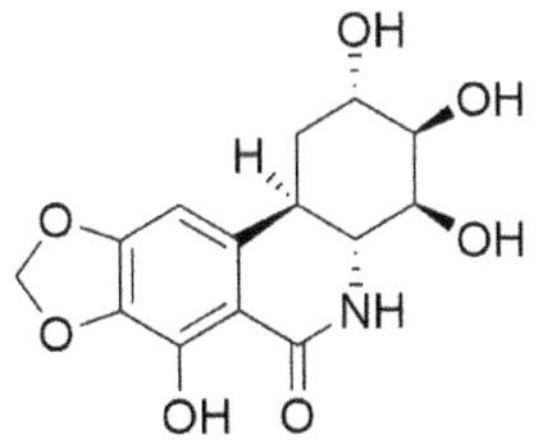

Figure 4. (+)-trans-Dihydronarciclasine (3).

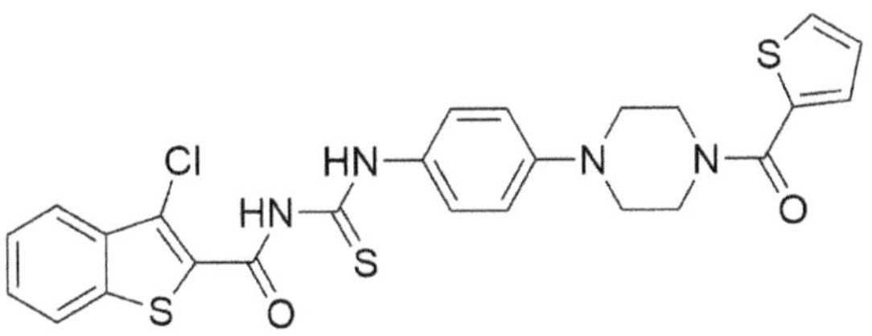

Figure 5. TPB (4).

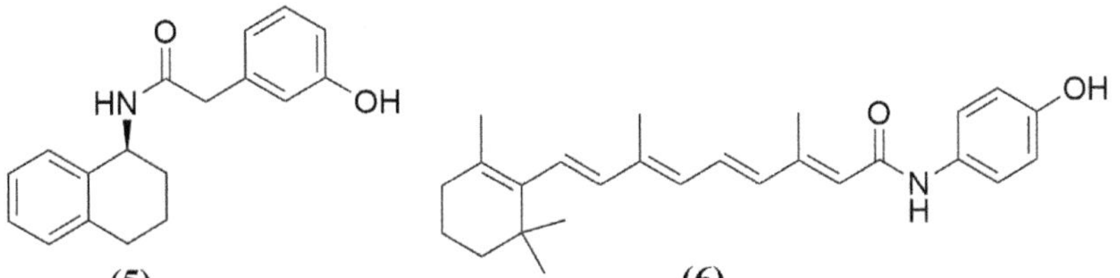

(5)   **(6)**

Figure 6. Structure of 2-(3-hydroxyphenyl)-*N*-(1,2,3,4-tetrahydronaphthalen-1-yl)acetamide (5) and *N*-(4-hydroxyphenyl) retinamide (fenretinide or 4-HPR) (6).

Vaccination

Currently, there is no FDA approved drug or treatment technique to stop or cure the disease caused by ZIKV. However, many research groups are focusing on treating the ZIKV-associated diseases. One of the major efforts is to identify a suitable vaccine. It is widely accepted that vaccines provide a cost-effective method of preventing infectious diseases (Levine and Sztein 2004). Given the rapid spread and severe outcomes associated with ZIKV infection, the development of a safe and efficacious vaccine is critical. The existence of successful vaccines against other flaviviral diseases (YFV, JEV, DENV, and TBEV) indicates that it is possible to develop a vaccine against ZIKV. Forty-five ZIKV vaccine candidates consisting of multiple vaccine platforms are currently under consideration and at various stages of development as summarized in the WHO vaccine pipeline tracker (WHO 2018a). Five candidate vaccines, including inactivated whole organism, DNA, synthetic peptide, and mRNA platforms are already in clinical trials (Table 1). In this section, some platforms as subtopics and some ongoing developed vaccines of ZIKV are presented.

According to data from WHO, vaccine pipeline tracker and vaccine trials continue on five different type platforms. Besides, there are several candidates in phase 1 and two candidates in phase 2 (WHO 2018b).

DNA-based vaccines

DNA based vaccine is a new fashion technology using genetically engineered DNA to take an immunologic response. To succeed this goal, the main strategy is to use DNA plasmids having antigens encoded on them. Cost, long term persistence of immunogenicity, stability properties and inducing protective humoral and cellular immune responses are some advantages of the DNA vaccination. However, it has some disadvantages like limited protein immunogens, inducing antibody production against DNA and inducing immunologic tolerance by antigens expressed inside host body (Khan 2013).

GLS-5700 is a candidate vaccine in phase I produced by VGXI Inc. It is a plasmid pGX7201 solution in sodium citrate buffer at a concentration of 10 mg/mL. The vaccine was studied in 40 participants split into two group and was given to recipients, either 1 mg or 2 mg intradermally, with each injection followed by electroporation at baseline, 4 wk and 12 wk. It has been reported that the trial shows the initial safety and immunogenicity of a DNA vaccine encoding consensus ZIKV premembrane and envelope antigens delivered by means of electroporation. Further studies will be needed to evaluate the efficacy of the vaccine and its long-term safety (Tebas et al. 2017).

VRC-ZKADNA090-00-VP (VRC320) is a Zika virus wildtype DNA vaccine developed by NIAID. The DNA vaccine is based on antigens PrM and E and is the only prospective Zika vaccine currently in Phase II trials. In phase I study, VRC320 was administrated to 45 participants (15 in each group) and two participants withdrew after one dose of vaccine. The vaccine was found safe and well tolerated. All local and systemic symptoms were reported as mild to moderate. In the study, pain and tenderness at the injection site were the most frequent local symptoms (36 of 45 [80%] in VRC320) and malaise and headache were the most frequent systemic symptoms (17 [38%] and 15 [33%], respectively, in VRC320). For VRC5283, 14 of 14 (100%) participants who received split-dose vaccinations by needle-free injection had detectable positive antibody responses, and the geometric mean titre of 304 was the highest across all groups. After all these findings, the vaccine advanced to phase II efficacy testing. Vaccine Research Center has developed another candidate named as VRC-ZKADNA085-00-VP (VRC319) by collaboration with NIAID. It is composed of a single closed-circular DNA plasmid that encodes the wild type precursor transmembrane M (prM) and envelope (E) proteins from the H/PF/2013 strain of ZIKV. Vaccine is supplied in single dose vials at a concentration of 4 mg/mL. ZIKV DNA vaccine dose will be 4 mg administered as an intramuscular (IM) injection in the deltoid muscle. Phase I trials were completed but results have not released yet (Gaudinski et al. 2017).

mRNA-based vaccines

The first successful application of mRNA vaccination was reported in 1990 (Wolff et al. 1990). Since that date, mRNA has become a promising therapeutic tool in the fields of vaccination. The mRNA-based vaccine uses the host cellular machinery to directly translate mRNA molecules into the viral proteins.

Table 1. ZIKV Vaccine candidates in Phase stages.

Pathogen	Candidate vaccine	Platform	Registry ID	Trial status	Sponsor name	Sponsor type	Phase	Study Start date	Completion date (anticipated or actual)	Age
ZIKV	GLS-5700	DNA	NCT02809443	Open, not recruiting	GeneOne Life Science, Inc./Inovio Pharmaceuticals	Industry	Phase I	1.07.2016	1.12.2017	Adult
ZIKV	GLS-5700	DNA	NCT02887482	Open, not recruiting	GeneOne Life Science, Inc./Inovio Pharmaceuticals	Industry	Phase I	1.08.2016	1.05.2018	Adult
ZIKV and others	AGS-v	Peptide	NCT03055000	Open, recruiting	NIH	Government	Phase I	9.02.2017	31.12.2019	Adult
ZIKV	MV-Zika	Recombinant viral vector	NCT02996890	Open, not recruiting	Themis Bioscience	Industry	Phase I	4.04.2017	1.08.2017	Adult
ZIKV	mRNA-1325	mRNA	NCT03014089	Open, recruiting	Moderna Therapeutics	Industry	Phase II	1.12.2016	1.09.2018	Adult
ZIKV	VRC-ZKADNA085-00-VP	DNA	NCT02840487	Open, not recruiting	NIAID	Government	Phase I	11.07.2016	28.12.2018	Adult
ZIKV	VRC-ZKADNA090-00-VP	DNA	NCT02996461	Open, not recruiting	NIAID	Government	Phase I	8.12.2016	28.12.2018	Adult
ZIKV	VRC-ZKADNA090-00-VP	DNA	NCT03110770	Open, recruiting	NIAID	Government	Phase II	29.03.2017	1.01.2020	Child/Adult
ZIKV	ZIKV PIV	Inactivated whole target organism	NCT02963909	Open, not recruiting	NIAID	Government	Phase I	1.11.2016	1.02.2019	Adult

Table 1 contd. ...

...Table 1 contd.

Pathogen	Candidate vaccine	Platform	Registry ID	Trial status	Sponsor name	Sponsor type	Phase	Study Start date	Completion date (anticipated or actual)	Age
ZIKV	ZIKV PIV	Inactivated whole target organism	NCT02952833	Open, not recruiting	NIAID	Government	Phase I	14.10.2016	5.02.2018	Adult
ZIKV	ZIKV PIV	Inactivated whole target organism	NCT02937233	Open, not recruiting	BIDMC	Academic	Phase I	1.10.2016	1.02.2018	Adult
ZIKV	ZIKV PIV	Inactivated whole target organism	NCT03008122	Open, recruiting	NIAID	Government	Phase I	24.02.2017	15.01.2020	Adult
ZIKV	PIZV or TAK-426	Inactivated whole target organism	NCT03343626	Open, recruiting	Takeda	Industry	Phase I	15.11.2017	23.05.2019	Adult

mRNA vaccines have some advantages compared to other vaccine types like safety, efficacy and production. Safety means that mRNA is a non-infectious, non-integrating platform and there is no potential risk of infection or insertional mutagenesis. mRNA is more stable and highly translatable and these features give the mRNA effective delivery capability. Production advantage is that mRNA vaccines have the potential for rapid, inexpensive and scalable manufacturing (Pardi et al. 2018).

Moderna Therapeutics announced that a new generation of transformative medicines for patients was created, demonstrating that its Zika mRNA vaccine prevented Zika virus transmission from pregnant mice to their fetuses. The study was designed to evaluate protection of fetuses during pregnancy in mice. Researchers gave a cohort of non-pregnant female mice (n = 20) a 10 µg intramuscular (IM) injection of the Zika mRNA vaccine followed by a boost at 28 d. An additional cohort of non-pregnant mice (n = 20) received placebo injections at the same time points. At day 49, the mice that received the mRNA vaccine produced high levels of neutralizing antibodies against Zika virus in their blood compared to placebo. Both cohorts were then mated and infected with the Zika virus. After 7 d, most fetuses in the vaccinated mice showed no evidence of having Zika virus transmitted to them from their pregnant mothers compared to placebo. In addition, vaccinated mice had significantly lower levels of Zika virus RNA in maternal, placental and fetal tissues compared to placebo-injected mice, resulting in protection against damage to the placenta and fetus (Richner et al. 2017). Moderna's Zika mRNA vaccine, mRNA-1325, is currently in Phase 1/2 clinical study in healthy volunteers.

Purified Inactivated Virus (PIV) vaccines

An inactivated virus vaccine is a virus that is grown in culture and then killed by methods such as heat or formaldehyde (Petrovsky and Aguilar 2014). Unlike vaccines with live attenuated viruses, inactivated vaccines negate the possibility of reactivation and replication and are thus not contraindicated in pregnant women or immunocompromised individuals. However, the attenuation also means that more immunization/ boosting strategies may be required to ensure long-term protection. The need for an adjuvant might be required, but it could complicate the use of a PIV in pregnancy (Makhluf and Shresta 2018). Several PIV vaccines are under development by different study groups.

The US Army tested a PIV vaccine based on the Puerto Rican isolate PRVABC59, which was inactivated with 0.05% formalin, purified, and formulated with alum for administration. A single immunization of BALB/c mice with the vaccine conferred protection against viremia upon challenge with ZIKV-BR strain 4 wk later. This ZIKV PIV vaccine was also tested for immunogenicity and protective efficacy in rhesus monkeys. Consistent with the mouse study, the vaccine induced ZIKV-specific neutralizing antibodies and protection against subsequent challenge with ZIKV-BR and ZIKV-PR strains. Virus was undetectable in blood, urine, or cerebrospinal fluid of the vaccinated monkeys (Abbink et al. 2016, Barouch et al. 2017).

ZIKV PIV (ZPIV) vaccines are currently being tested in four phase I clinical trials sponsored by the National Institute of Allergy and Infectious Diseases (NIAID) and Beth Israel Deaconess Medical Center. The trials are designed to evaluate their immunogenicity, reactogenicity, and safety in flavivirus-primed and -naïve healthy subjects (Table 1; NCT02963909, NCT02952833, NCT03008122, and NCT02937233). Modjarrad showed that a ZPIV candidate vaccine elicited robust neutralizing antibody titers in healthy human participants. About 55 healthy adults received two intramuscular injections of 5 µg of ZPIV with aluminum hydroxide adjuvant and 12 participants a placebo injection. An estimated 92% (52 out of 55) of these participants seroconverted by day 57 while no placebo participants changed titers. ZPIV was well tolerated, resulting in mild to moderate adverse effects such as pain at the injection site, malaise, headache and fatigue (Modjarrad et al. 2017).

Recombinant viral vector vaccine

The ZIKAVAX project, which possesses approximately 5 million Euros' budget, aims to construct and characterize recombinant measles vector (MV) expressing Zika virus proteins as soluble secreted antigens. In ZIKAVAX, immunization studies were conducted with the Zika vaccine candidate in mice and in a non-human primate challenge model that will be developed by the consortium. Phase I clinical trial of MV-ZIKA was completed but detailed report about the trial has not been released yet (Zikavax 2018).

Peptide vaccine

AGS-v was designed to protect against multiple mosquito-borne diseases, including Zika. The vaccine candidate has a double mechanism of action while preventing infection and also reducing mosquito survival. AGS-v was developed by the London-based pharmaceutical company SEEK, which has formed a joint venture with hVIVO in London. AGS-v is designed to trigger an immune response to mosquito salivary proteins rather than to a specific virus or parasite carried by mosquitoes. The test vaccine contains four synthetic proteins from mosquito salivary glands. The proteins are designed to induce antibodies in a vaccinated individual and to cause a modified allergic response that can prevent infection when a person is bitten by a disease-carrying mosquito. The AGS-v candidate is being evaluated in a Phase 1 clinical trial at the NIH Clinical Center in Bethesda, Maryland (Hvivo 2018).

Conclusion

In conclusion, the threatening information obtained after the rapid spread of ZIKV, which was initially accepted as an unimportant infectious agent, requires many efforts to develop preventive precautions against ZIKV and to reduce its transmission. The lack of data associated with the pathophysiology of neurological complications and congenital abnormalities related to ZIKV causes a limit in the fight against the ZIKV infection. Therefore, the elucidation of the pathophysiology of the symptoms will favor the development of treatment strategies against ZIKV-infections. Furthermore, chronic and regular follow-up of ZIK-infected patients will enable to determine the clinical outcomes and the duration of the disease. Since there is not any approved drug therapy against ZIKV, an immediate priority will be to develop new and effective therapeutic approaches for ZIKV treatment. It is important to emphasize that the development of drugs safe during pregnancy is of critical importance. The evaluation of the newborns in risky zones for ZIKV, including ZIKV-endemic regions in terms of congenital malformations, and the follow up of them in terms of neurological development, has to be of primary importance.

References

Abbink, P., R.A. Larocca, R.A. De La Barrera, C.A. Bricault, E.T. Moseley, M. Boyd et al. 2016. Protective efficacy of multiple vaccine platforms against Zika virus challenge in rhesus monkeys. Science. 353: 1129–1132.

Agrawal, R., H.H. Oo, P.K. Balne, L. Ng, L. Tong and Y.S. Leo. 2018. Zika Virus and the Eye. Ocul. Immunol. Inflamm. 26(5): 654–659.

Althouse, B.M., N. Vasilakis, A.A. Sall, M. Diallo, S.C. Weaver and K.A. Hanley. 2016. Potential for Zika virus to establish a sylvatic transmission cycle in the Americas. PLoS Negl. Trop. Dis. 10(12): e0005055.

Araujo, A.Q., M.T. Silva and A.P. Araujo. 2016. Zika virus-associated neurological disorders: a review. Brain. 139(Pt 8): 2122–30.

Aryamav, P., P. Nicholas, R.S. Bikash, Y. Zhe, H. Duoyi, S.A. Arun et al. 2018. Discovery of a non-nucleoside RNA polymerase inhibitor for blocking Zika virus replication through *in silico* screening. Antivir. Res. 151: 78–86.

Bailey, D.B. and L.O. Ventura. 2018. The likely impact of congenital Zika syndrome on families: Considerations for family supports and services. Pediatrics. 141(2): 180–187.

Barouch, D.H., S.J. Thomas and N.L. Michael. 2017. Prospects for a Zika Virus vaccine. Immunity. 46: 176–182.

Bollati, M., K. Alvarez, R. Assenberg, C. Baronti, B. Canard, S. Cook et al. 2010. Structure and functionality in flavivirus NS-proteins: perspectives for drug design. Antivir. Res. 87(2): 125–48.

Boyer-Chammard, T., K. Schepers, S. Breurec, T. Messiaen, A.L. Destrem, M. Mahevas et al. 2017. Severe thrombocytopenia after Zika virus infection, Guadeloupe, 2016. Emerg. Infect. Dis. 23(4): 696–698.

Caminade, C., J. Turner, S. Metelmann, J.C. Hesson, M.S. Blagrove, T. Solomon et al. 2017. Global risk model for vector-borne transmission of Zika virus reveals the role of El Niño 2015. Proc. Natl. Acad. Sci. U.S.A. 114(1): 119–124.

Cao-Lormeau, V.M., A. Blake, S. Mons, S. Lastere, C. Roche, J. Vanhomwegen et al. 2016. Guillain-Barré syndrome outbreak associated with Zika virus infection in French Polynesia: a case-control study. Lancet. 387(10027): 1531–1539.

CDC. 2018. https://wwwnc.cdc.gov/travel/page/world-map-areas-with-zika. Retrieved September 2018.

Chen, H.L. and R.B. Tang. 2016. Why Zika virus infection has become a public health concern? J. Chin. Med. Assoc. 79(4): 174–8.

Coelho, A.V.C. and S. Crovella. 2017. Microcephaly prevalence in infants born to Zika virus-infected women: A systematic review and meta-analysis. Int. J. Mol. Sci. 18(8): 1–10.

Duggal, N.K., J.M. Ritter, S.E. Pestorius, S.R. Zaki, B.S. Davis, G.J. Chang et al. 2017. Frequent Zika virus sexual transmission and prolonged viral RNA shedding in an immunodeficient mouse model. Cell Rep. 18(7): 1751–1760.

Epelboin, Y., S. Talaga, L. Epelboin and I. Dusfour. 2017. Zika virus: An updated review of competent or naturally infected mosquitoes. PLoS Negl. Trop. Dis. 11(11): e0005933.

Esposito, D.L.A., J.B. de Moraes and B. Antônio Lopes da Fonseca. 2018. Current priorities in the Zika response. Immunology. 153(4): 435–442.

Gaudinski, M.R., K.V. Houser, K.M. Morabito, Z. Hu, G. Yamshchikov, R.S. Rothwell et al. 2017. Safety, tolerability, and immunogenicity of two Zika virus DNA vaccine candidates in healthy adults: randomised, open-label, phase 1 clinical trials. Lancet. 391(10120): 552–562.

Göertz, G.P., S.R. Abbo, J.J. Fros and G.P. Pijlman. 2017. Functional RNA during Zika virus infection. Virus Res. 254: 41–53.

Hanzlik, E. and J. Gigante. 2017. Microcephaly. Children (Basel). 4(6): 47.

Hastings, A.K. and E. Fikrig. 2017. Zika virus and sexual transmission: A new route of transmission for mosquito-borne flaviviruses. Yale J. Biol. Med. 90(2): 325–330.

Honein, M.A. 2018. Recognizing the global impact of Zika virus infection during pregnancy. N. Engl. J. Med. 378(11): 1055–1056.

Hunter, F.F. 2017. Linking only aedes aegypti with Zika virus has world-wide public health implications. Front. Microbiol. 8: 1248.

Hvivo. 2018. AGS-v Zika Vaccine. http://hvivo.com/products/imutex-limited/ags-v. Retrieved April 2018.

Ioos, S., H.P. Mallet, I. Leparc Goffart, V. Gauthier, T. Cardoso and M. Herida. 2014. Current Zika virus epidemiology and recent epidemics. Med. Mal. Infect. 44(7): 302–307.

Khan, K.H. 2013. DNA vaccines: roles against diseases. Germs. 3(1): 26–35.

Kindhauser, M.K., T. Allen, V. Frank, R.S. Santhana and C. Dye. 2016. Zika: the origin and spread of a mosquito-borne virus. Bull. World Health Organ. 94(9): 675–686.

Koppolu, C.V. and T. Shantha-Raju. 2018. Zika virus outbreak: a review of neurological complications, diagnosis, and treatment options. J. Neurovirology. 24: 255–272.

Lagunas-Rangel, F.A., M.E. Viveros-Sandoval and A. Reyes-Sandoval. 2017. Current trends in Zika vaccine development. J. Virus Erad. 3(3): 124–127.

Levine, M.M. and M.B. Sztein. 2004. Vaccine development strategies for improving immunization: the role of modern immunology. Nat. Immunol. 5(5): 460–464.

Makhluf, H. and S. Shresta. 2018. Development of Zika virus vaccines. Vaccines (Basel). 6(1): 7.

Meena, A.K., S.V. Khadilkar and J.M. Murthy. 2011. Treatment guidelines for Guillain-Barré Syndrome. Ann. Indian Acad. Neurol. 14(Suppl. 1): S73–81.

Modjarrad, K., L. Lin, S.L. George, K.E. Stephenson, K.H. Eckels, R.A. De La Barrera et al. 2017. Preliminary aggregate safety and immunogenicity results from three trials of a purified inactivated Zika virus vaccine candidate: Phase 1, randomised, double-blind, placebo-controlled clinical trials. Lancet. 6736: 1–9.

Mourya, D.T., P. Shil, G.N. Sapkal and P.D. Yadav. 2016. Zika virus: Indian perspectives. Indian J. Med. Res. 143(5): 553–64.

Noronha, L.D., C. Zanluca, M.L. Azevedo, K.G. Luz and C.N. Santos. 2016. Zika virus damages the human placental barrier and presents marked fetal neurotropism. Mem. Inst. Oswaldo Cruz. 111(5): 287–293.

Pardi, N., M.J. Hogan, F.W. Porter and D. Weissman. 2018. mRNA vaccines—a new era in vaccinology. Nat. Rev. Drug Discov. 17: 261–279.

Passi, D., S. Sharma, S.R. Dutta and M. Ahmed. 2017. Zika virus diseases—the new face of an ancient enemy as Global Public Health Emergency (2016): Brief Review and Recent Updates. Int. J. Prev. Med. 8(1): 1–9.

Pessoa, A., V. van der Linden, M. Yeargin-Allsopp, M.D.C.G. Carvalho, E.M. Ribeiro, K. Van Naarden Braun et al. 2018. Motor Abnormalities and epilepsy in infants and children with evidence of congenital Zika virus infection. Pediatrics. 141(2): 167–179.

Petrovsky, N. and J.C. Aguilar. 2014. Vaccine adjuvants: Current state and future trends. Immunol. Cell Biol. 82(5): 488–496.

Pitts, J.D., P. Li, M. de Wispelaere and P.L. Yang. 2017. Antiviral activity of N-(4-hydroxyphenyl) retinamide (4-HPR) against Zika virus. Antivir. Res. 147: 124–130.

Plourde, A.R. and E.M. Bloch. 2016. A literature review of Zika virus. Emerg. Infect. Dis. 22(7): 1185–1192.

Rana, B.J. 2016. Zika virus situation update. The 8th Meeting of The Capsca Asia Pacific & The 6th Meeting of The Capsca Global Programme Coordination. 15–18 November 2016, Bangkok, Thailand.

Revu, O., C. Zepeda-Velázquez, A.J. Nielsen, J. McNulty, R.H. Yolken and L. Jones-Brando. 2016. Total synthesis of the natural product (+)-trans-Dihydronarciclasine via an asymmetric organocatalytic [3+3]-Cycloaddition and discovery of its potent anti-Zika Virus (ZIKV) Activity. Chemistry Select. 1: 5895–5899.

Richner, J.M., B.W. Jagger, C. Shan, C.R. Fontes, K.A. Dowd, B. Cao et al. 2017. Vaccine mediated protection against Zika virus-induced congenital disease. Cell. 170(2): 273–283.e12.

Sharma, A. and S.K. Lal. 2017. Zika virus: Transmission, detection, control, and prevention. Front. Microbiol. 8: 110.

Sharp, T.M., J. Muñoz-Jordán, J. Perez-Padilla, M.I. Bello-Pagán, A. Rivera, D.M. Pastula et al. 2016. Zika virus infection associated with severe thrombocytopenia. Clin. Infect. Dis. 63(9): 1198–1201.

Shrivastava, M., S. Nehal and N. Seema. 2017. Guillain-Barre syndrome: Demographics, clinical profile & seasonal variation in a tertiary care centre of central India. Indian J. Med. Res. 145(2): 203–208.

Simanjuntak, Y., J.J. Liang, S.Y. Chen, J.K. Li, Y.L. Lee, H.C. Wu et al. 2018. Ebselen alleviates testicular pathology in mice with Zika virus infection and prevents its sexual transmission. PLoS Pathog. 14(2): 1–23.

Singh, A. and N.K. Jana. 2017. Discovery of potential Zika virus RNA polymerase inhibitors by docking-based virtual screening. Comput. Biol. Chem. 71: 144–151.

Sirohi, D., Z. Chen, L. Sun, T. Klose, T.C. Pierson, M.G. Rossmann et al. 2016. The 3.8 Å resolution cryo-EM structure of Zika virus. Science. 352(6284): 467–70.

Styczynski, A.R., J.M.A.S. Malta, E.R. Krow-Lucal, J. Percio, M.E. Nóbrega, A. Vargas et al. 2017. Increased rates of Guillain-Barré syndrome associated with Zika virus outbreak in the Salvador metropolitan area, Brazil. PLoS Negl. Trop. Dis. 11(8): 1–13.

Tang, X., S. Zhao, A.P.Y. Chiu, X. Wang, L. Yang and D. He. 2017. Analysing increasing trends of Guillain-Barré Syndrome (GBS) and dengue cases in Hong Kong using meteorological data. PLoS One. 12(12): e0187830.

Tebas, P., C.C. Roberts, K. Muthumani, E.L. Reuschel, S.B. Kudchodkar, F.I. Zaidi et al. 2017. Safety and immunogenicity of an Anti–Zika virus DNA vaccine—Preliminary report. The N. Engl. J. Med. 1–9.

Ventura, C.V. and L.O. Ventura. 2018. Ophthalmologic manifestations associated with Zika virus infection. Pediatrics. 141(2): 161–166.

Wang, A., S. Thurmond, L. Islas, K. Hui and R. Hai. 2017. Zika virus genome biology and molecular pathogenesis. Emerg. Microbes Infect. 6(3): e13.

Wheeler, A.C. 2018. Development of infants with congenital Zika syndrome: What Do We Know and What Can We Expect? Pediatrics. 141(2): 154–160.

WHO. 2018a. http://www.who.int/news-room/fact-sheets/detail/Zika-virus. Retrieved May 2018.

WHO. 2018b. http://www.who.int/immunization/research/vaccine_pipeline_tracker_spreadsheet/en/Retrieved April 2018.

Wikan, N. and D.R. Smith. 2016. Zika virus: history of a newly emerging arbovirus. Lancet Infect. Dis. 16(7): e119–e126.

Wolff, J.A., R.W. Malone, P. Williams, W. Chong, G. Acsadi, A. Jani et al. 1990. Direct gene transfers into mouse muscle *in vivo*. Science. 247: 1465–1468.

Wong, G., S. Li, L. Liu, Y. Liu and Y. Bi. 2017. Zika virus in the testes: should we be worried? Protein & Cell. 8(3): 162–164.

Wylie, B.J., M. Hauptman, A.D. Woolf and R.H. Goldman. 2016. Insect repellants during pregnancy in the era of the Zika virus. Obstet. Gynecol. 128(5): 1111–1115.

Zamani, M. and V. Zamani. 2017. Sexual transmission of Zika virus: An assessment of the evidence. Iran J. Public Health. 46(9): 1305–1306.

Zikavax. 2018. Fast track development of a Zika vaccine based on measles vector. http://www.euvaccine.eu/portfolio/project-index/Zikavax. Retrieved April 2018.

Zikavirusnet. 2018. http://Zikavirusnet.com/mosquito-bites.html. Retrieved April 2018.

Chapter **6**

Chikungunya Virus Infection
A Review of its Control and Treatment

D. Velmurugan,* K. Manish and *D. Gayathri*

Introduction

Chikungunya fever is a viral disease transmitted to humans by the bites of infected *Aedes aegypti* mosquitoes. Chikungunya virus (CHIKV), which is a member of the genus alphavirus, in the family *Togoviridae*, is a re-emerging mosquito borne pathogen causing intense joint pain which can persist for weeks, months or even years in humans. The clinical features of CHIKV infection can be divided into three phases, namely, acute phase (less than three weeks), sub-acute phase (greater than three weeks, and up to three months) and chronic phase (more than three months). The common symptoms of CHIKV infection are fever, arthralgia/arthritis, backache, headache and skin rash/itching. In addition, symptoms like photophobia, retro-orbital pain, vomiting, diarrhea, meningeal syndrome and acute encephalopathy may also be seen rarely in adults and sometimes in children. Due to the poor understanding of the basic molecular underpinning of CHIKV infection and its replication cycles, there is no approved therapeutics against CHIKV. This chapter summarizes the history of CHIKV infection, describes its genome and the various protein targets for developing anti-CHIKV drugs, as well as the various new inhibitors designed so far through molecular modelling approaches and validated by molecular dynamics simulations.

History of CHIKV Infections

Chikungunya virus (CHIKV) infection is caused by an arboviral alphavirus transmitted to humans mainly by *Aedes aegypti* mosquitoes, as well as other mosquitoes of the genus *Aedes* like *Aedes albopictus* and *Aedes polynesienis*. CHIKV is an enveloped, spherical single-stranded positive-sense RNA alphavirus belonging to the family *Togoviridae*. CHIKV originates from sub-Saharan Africa but has spread to southeast Asia, Europe and more recently the Americas. An outbreak of CHIKV infection occurred in 2005

Centre of Advanced Study in Crystallography and Biophysics, University of Madras, Guindy Campus, Chennai - 600025, Tamil Nadu, India.
* Corresponding author: shirai2011@gmail.com

on the islands of Indian Ocean. CHIKV has the potential to cause infection in tens of millions of people (Weaver and Lecuit 2015). There is no approved therapeutics active against CHIKV, partly because of a poor understanding of the basic molecular underpinnings of its infection and replication cycle. High fever, headache, myalgia, arthralgia, poly-arthralgia, haemorrhage and rashes are the typical clinical signs of CHIKV fever. Occurrence of neurological complications is also reported as a consequence of CHIKV infection (Chandak et al. 2009, Bandeira et al. 2016, Murthy 2009).

CHIKV has spread to 100 countries and territories worldwide due to the presence of the vectors and their efficiency in transmitting the virus. Globally, there are an estimated 1 million cases per year including periodic large-scale epidemic outbreaks through the world and low level endemic transmission in Africa and southeast Asia (Morrison 2014). Travel patterns have increased the importation of the virus into new geographical regions via infected people. In Africa, CHIKV was first reported in Tanzania in 1952, whilst about half a million cases were reported in June 2004 in an outbreak that occurred in Kenya. After that, the infection migrated to nearby regions including Mauritius, Comoros and other places, until April 2005. Except Madagascar, many epidemics occurred on all the south western Indian Ocean islands during 2005 to 2007. Between 2006 and 2010, 106 probable cases of CHIKV were detected among travelers returning to the United States compared to only three cases reported between 1995 and 2005. In the Indian subcontinent, the first isolation of the virus was done in Kolkata in 1963. Later, several reports of CHIKV infection were reported from Pondicherry and Chennai in Tamil Nadu, Rajamundry, Vishakapatnam and Kakinada in Andhra Pradesh, Sagar in Madhya Pradesh and Nagpur in Maharashtra. CHIKV epidemics occurred in 2001, 2006, 2015 and 2016. In 2014, the total number of suspected chikungunya cases in India were 16049 and number of confirmed cases were 2571, but in the next year 2015, the number of suspected cases and confirmed cases increased to 27553 and 3342, respectively (National Health Mission 2016). The diagnosis of CHIKV infection is challenging as its clinical symptoms are similar to those of dengue. White blood cells count greater than or equal to 5.0×10^9 cells per liter, skin rash during fever and specific antigen testing form the basis of the differential diagnosis of CHIKV. The global expansion of CHIKV based on the mapping of 64 years history was reviewed by Wahid et al., in 2017.

It has been reported that over 60% of the people affected by CHIKV suffered from joint pain even three years after the infection. Chronic symptoms similar to those of seronegative rheumatoid arthritis, and often requiring long-term treatment using non-steroidal anti-inflammatory and immunosuppressive drugs have been also reported after CHIKV infection (Smalley 2016). Recently, CHIKV infection has been associated with neurological complications such as Guillain-Barre syndrome and meningoencephalitis. Other severe complications reported are conjunctivitis, myocarditis, pancreatitis and kidney failure (Morrison et al. 2016, Thiber Ville et al. 2013). Recently, the first case of neonatal CHIKV-induced encephalitis has been reported in Brazil (Bandeira et al. 2016). Most CHIKV infections that occur during pregnancy will not result in the virus being transmitted to the fetus. The highest transmission risk appears when women are infected during the intrapartum period wherein the vertical transmission rate is up to 49%. Infants are typically asymptomatic at birth and then develop fever, pain, rash, peripheral edema and may also develop neurological and myocardial diseases. Individuals above 65 years of age had a 50-fold higher mortality rate when compared to adults of less than 45 years.

Chikungunya (CHIK) must be distinguished from dengue fever, which has the potential for much worse outcomes, including death. Observations from previous outbreaks in Thailand and India have characterized the principle features distinguishing CHIK from dengue fever. In CHIK, shock or severe haemorrhage is very rarely observed; the onset is more acute and the duration of fever is much shorter. Maculopapular rash in CHIK is also more frequent than in dengue fever. The diffuse body pain is much more pronounced and localized to the joints and tendons in CHIK, in comparison to dengue fever. Even though an improvement in the general health and joint pain have been noted after 10 days of CHIKV infection, a relapse of symptoms can also occur with some patients complaining of various rheumatic symptoms. Some patients can also develop transient peripheral muscular disorders, depressive symptoms, general fatigue and weakness. These symptoms sometimes may persist for more than three months. Reports indicated that in India, 49% of CHIKV infected patients had persistent symptoms for 10 months and from

La Reunion as much as 80-to-93% of patients are reported to have persistent symptoms three months after disease onset and this decreased to 57% at 15 months and to 47% in 2 years.

CHIKV Genome

The genome size of CHIKV is approximately 12 kb and it consists of two open reading frames (ORF). The four non-structural proteins nsP1, nsP2, nsP3 and nsP4 and five structural proteins C, E1, E2, E3 and 6K cleave the CHIKV genome (Figure 1). The nsP1 contains methyltransferase and guanyltransferase activities and it is a membrane associated protein which is involved in the capping of the +RNA genome. The nsP2 is a helicase/protease enzyme which is made up of three domains, the first containing helicase RNA triphosphatase and nucleoside triphosphatase activities, whereas the second and third domains are papain-like protease and non-functional methyltransferase, respectively. Also, nsP2 contains a nuclear localization sequence allowing 50% of the translated nsP2 to be translocated into the nucleus, whereas nsP3 is an accessory protein involved in viral RNA synthesis. Although nsP3 protein is involved in the transcription process at an early stage of the infection, the functions, roles and activities of nsP3 are less well understood. nsP3 is made of two domains and the first one is a unique macrodomain located in the conserved N-terminal region. The less conserved C-terminal region is phosphorylated up to 16 positions on serines and threonines. The deletion of the phosphorylated residue decreases the RNA synthesis level. The first 160 residues of the N-terminal region of nsP3 are known as the macrodomain. This has sequence similarity with rubivirus, alphavirus and coronavirus. This domain is remarkably conserved in all kingdoms of life among the 1081 considered (Letunic et al. 2006). The nsP4 is the RNA dependent RNA polymerase enzyme involved in genome replication and transcription.

E1 and E2 are the glycoproteins and both play an important role in viral replication. E1 is important for membrane fusion and E2 allows the virus to enter the cell through endocytosis. The single stranded RNA molecule in CHIKV genome has a positive polarity with a 7 mG cap at the 5' end and a poly-tail at the 3' end. The 5' ORF directly translated from the genomic RNA encodes the above four nsP's that serve various functions that are essential for virus replications. The 3' ORF is translated from the 26S sub genomic RNA and encoded for viral structural proteins such as nucleocapsid C, viral glycoproteins E1 and E2 and small peptides E3 and 6K.

Rathore et al., in 2014, detailed the interaction of CHIKV nsP3 and nsP4 with human heat shock protein HSP-90 to promote virus replication. They have also proved through *in vivo* experiments that HSP90 inhibitors reduce CHIKV infection and inflammation. Ramakrishnan et al. (2017) have reviewed structure-function relationship of CHIKV-nsP2 protease and compared with the papain.

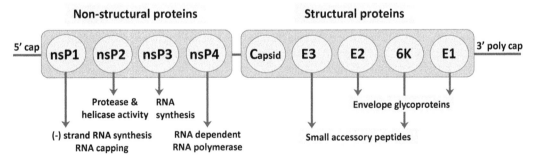

Figure 1. CHIKV genome.

Potential CHIKV Targets

CHIKV-nsP2 protease

The nsP2 protease domain belongs to the papain super-family of cysteine proteases (Lulla et al. 2006, Sourisseau et al. 2007). Among the CHIKV-encoded enzymes, nsP2 constitutes an attractive target for the development of antiviral drugs. nsP2 is a multifunctional protein of approximately 90 kDa with a helicase motif in the N-terminal portion of the protein while papain-like protease activity resides in the C-terminal portion. The nsP2 protease is an essential enzyme whose proteolytic activity is critical for virus replication. Biochemical characterization of nsP2 cysteine protease of CHIKV has been reported (Pastorino et al. 2008). As an insight into the protease catalytic mechanism, they have studied the effect of different protease inhibitors on the enzymatic activity of CHIKV-nsP2 protease by using the cost-effective BOC-AGG-MCA peptide as substrate. The enzyme was found to be completely resistant to the inhibitors of serine protease (aprotinin), aspartic proteases (pepstatin) and metallo-proteases (EDTA). It has also proven resistance to the cysteine protease inhibitor leupeptin. Based on these findings, nsP2 can be classified as a thiol protease of the papain super family. Pastorino also confirmed that the viral activity of CHIKV-nsP2 protease is contributed by the amino acids in the range 422 to 799 in the C-terminal region of protease-helicase complex. The amino acids in the N-terminal segment (166 to 630) show NTPase or helicase activity (Karpe and Lole 2010).

Cheung et al. (2011) first reported the crystal structure of CHIKV nsP2 protease, constituted mainly by 14 helices (H1-H14) and 3 sheets formed by 12 strands. The catalytic triad is formed by the active site amino acids Cys1013 and His1083. Cys1013 is held at the N-terminus by the H1 helix and His1083 is held by the linker region of first two strands. Before this, some studies on the structure function relationship of CHIKV-nsP2 protease were carried out taking into account the available structural information of the alphavirus nsP2 protease from *Venezuelan equine encephalitis virus* (VEEV) or the cysteine protease from papain.

Although crystal structures of many of alphaviruses are yet to be determined, the crystal structures of nsP2 protease belonging to VEEV are available (Russo et al. 2006, Hu et al. 2016). As the structure of VEEV-nsP2 protease showed 60% similarity to CHIKV-nsP2 protease, understanding the binding mode of the inhibitors of the VEEV nsP2 protease was useful in drug design. In 2012, Singh et al. developed a homology model of CHIKV-nsP2 protease based on the crystal structure of nsP2 protease of VEEV. The modeled protein was optimized using MD simulations. The studies shed light on the binding modes and the critical interactions with the junction peptides to provide insight into the chemical features needed to inhibit the CHIKV infection. Pharmacophore features for CHIKV-nsP2 were also proposed by these authors. Based on the docking studies with the public libraries of the compounds, the authors have proposed four compounds and suggested that the backbone structural scaffolds of these compounds could serve in the structure-based drug design of treatments against CHIKV (Figure 2).

Ramakrishnan et al. (2017) have discussed the alignment of nsP2 protease sequences belonging to different alphaviruses and had compared the structural behavior of CHIKV-nsP2 with papain proteases. These authors have also carried out molecular dynamics simulations to provide theoretical description on the molecular mechanism of native form of both CHIKV-nsP2 protease and papain. Root mean square deviation analysis confirms CHIKV-nsP2 to undergo more conformational changes compared to the papain and this is due to fact that the structure of CHIKV-nsP2 is constituted by the two domains connected by a long loop while there are no disulphide bridges. In the case of the structure of papain protease, secondary structural elements are rich and three disulphide bridges connect the flexible regions. The fluctuations in segment 1 of CHIKV-nsP2 protease are found to be slightly higher compared with its counterpart papain whereas they are considerably more in the case of segment 2 constituted by an anti-parallel beta sheet. The structural behavior of CHIKV-nsP2 protease differs from the papain due to the significant difference in the fluctuations of the segment 2. Even though CHIK-nsP2 undergoes more conformational changes, it does not make significant difference in forming ion pair interaction compared with the papain. Binding mode of the papain inhibitors with CHIKV-nsP2 protease was discussed. The results suggest the open-to-close and vice versa conformational change that is possible in CHIKV-nsP2 protease and this could be

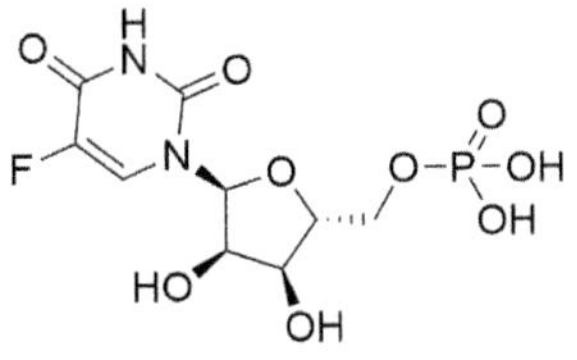

27943 (Binding Database)

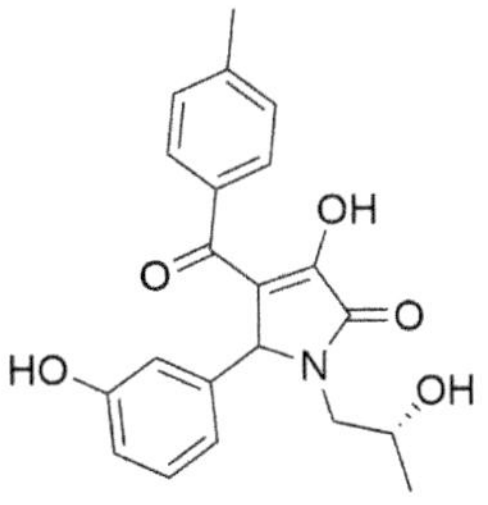

21362 (TosLab)

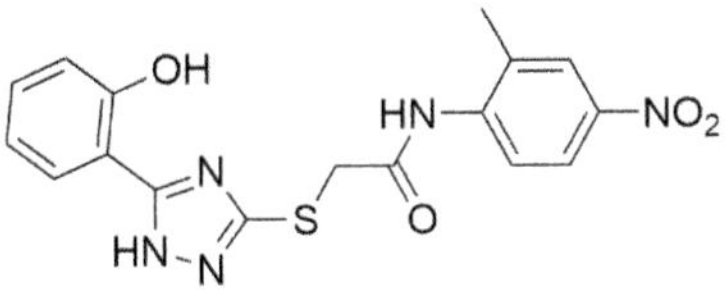

ASN 01107557 (Asinex)

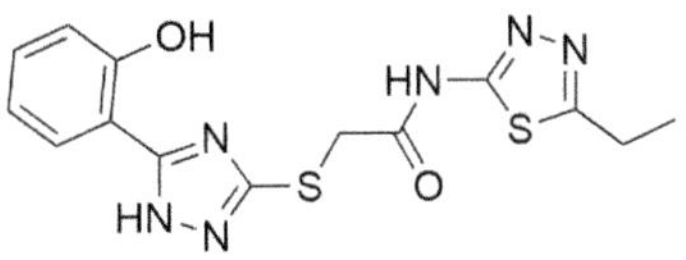

ASN 01541696 (Asinex)

Figure 2. Compounds identified as potential Chikungunya virus nsP2 protease inhibitors.

the reason to adopt the different scaffold of the active site to cleave the multiple sites in the polyprotein which promotes viral replication in the host cell.

CHIKV-VEEV nsP3

Helene et al. (2009) determined the crystal structures of CHIKV-nsP3 and VEEV-nsP3 macrodomains. These domains are found to be active as adenosine di-phosphoribose-1''-phosphate phosphatases. Both these macrodomains are ADP-ribose binding modules, as revealed by structural and functional analysis. A single aspartic acid was found to be conserved through all macrodomains, responsible for the specific binding of the adenine base. The crystal structure of CHIKV-nsP3 protease macrodomain with an RNA trimer reveals the binding mode that utilizes the same adenine-binding pocket as ADP-ribose but avoids the ADP-ribose 1''-phosphate phosphatase active site. Authors have concluded that the CHIKV macrodomain has a specificity for (i) an adenine rather than a guanine (ii) two phosphate groups rather than either one or three and (iii) a ribose at the distal position. Although CHIKV and VEEV macrodomains bind ADP-ribose, they exhibit a quite different thermal denaturation shift profile. CHIKV macrodomain was found to lose its stability to bind ADP-ribose when the D10 position was changed to alanine.

CHIKV-HSP-90

Rathore et al. (2014) determined the role of heat shock protein-90 (HSP-90) during CHIKV infection. The HSP-90 inhibitor geldanamycin was found to bind in the ATP binding site on HSP-90, rendering this protein in an open conformation. Geldanamycin treatment reduced CHIKV infection by nearly 2.5 log suggesting a significant involvement of HSP-90 during the CHIKV infection cycle. Their experiments with HSP-90 inhibitors on CHIKV replication suggest that blocking the chaperone function of HSP-90 did not affect its protein level or its transcription but resulted in a marked, early reduction in the levels of both viral RNA and protein.

nsP4

Rathore et al. (2013) proved the key interplay of viral nsP4 in modulating the post UPR (unfolded protein response) machinery. Two inhibitors of HSP-90, namely HS-10 and SNX-2112, are able to reduce CHIKV infection in a dose-dependent manner. In 2014, Rathore et al. showed that CHIKV nsP4 physically interacts with HSP-90 using the co-immunoprecipitation system. They identified CHIKV-nsP3 as a novel interacting partner of HSP-90 protein. The specificity in the interaction between nsP3 and HSP-90 beta or nsP4 and HSP-90 alpha shown using experimental data suggests an integral role of these interactions during CHIKV replication. As HSP-90 alpha is predominantly cytosolic, it may help in stabilization of CHIKV nsP4 and formation of the CHIKV replication complex (Strauss and Strauss 1994). Although the precise mechanism of interaction and immune-modulatory mechanism between HSP-90 and CHIKV remain to be seen in detail, the importance of HSP-90 protein during CHIKV replication and the reduction of CHIKV infection or inflammation by HSP-90 inhibitors are confirmed.

CHIKV Inhibitors

The development of CHIKV inhibitors is still in an early phase and only few examples have been reported in the last decade. In 2015, Ahola et al. constructed a CHIKV replicon system containing the virus replicase proteins together with puromycin acetyl transferase, EGFP and *Renilla luciferase* marker genes. The replicon was transfected into BHK21 cells to yield a stable cell line. Also, a non-cytopathic replication phenotype was achieved by combining nsP2 Pro718 to Gly substitution and a five amino acid insertion within CHIKV nsP2. The replicon cell line was characterized and adopted for anti-viral screening in 96 well plate formats. Assay experiments showed the suppression of CHIKV replicon expression levels when the flavonoids chrysin, naringenin and silybin were used.

Bhakat and Soliman (2015) reviewed several natural and semi-synthetic inhibitors with enhanced anti-viral activities. Epigallocatechin-3-gallate, quinine, trigocherrierin A, jatrophane ester, apigenin, chrysin, naringenin, silybin, cephalotaxine alkaloid, trigocherrin A/B/C, trigocherriolide A/B/C are few of the reported inhibitors of CHIKV / CHIKV pathway enzymes. Kaur et al. (2013) reported for the first

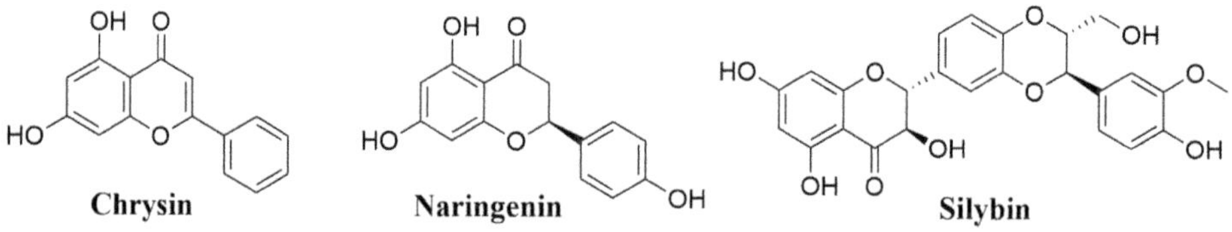

Figure 3. Structures of chrysin, naringenin and silybin.

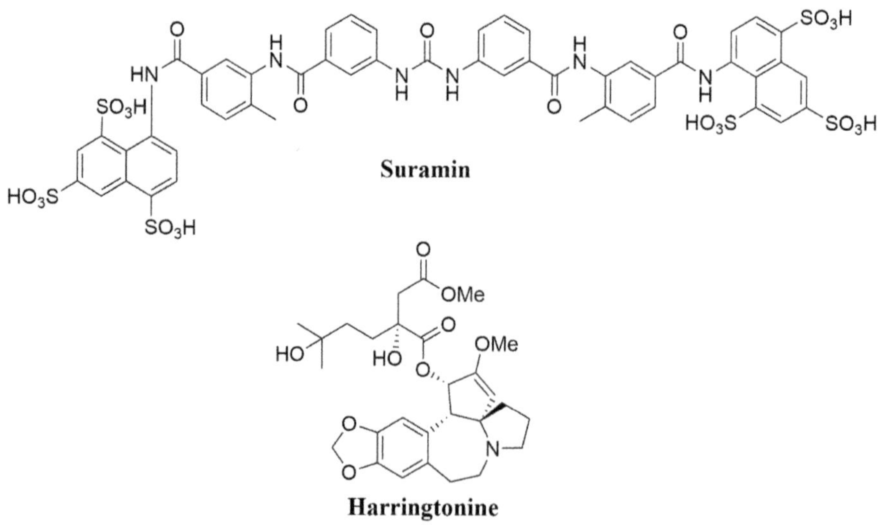

Figure 4. Structure of suramin and harringtonine.

time that harringtonine exerts its antiviral effects by inhibiting CHIKV viral protein synthesis. Mishra et al. (2016) reported the inhibition of CHIKV replication by 1-[(2-methylbenzimidazol-1-yl)-methyl]-2-oxo-indolin-3-ylidene]amino]-thiourea. Ho et al. (2015) demonstrated that suramin inhibits CHIKV entry and transmission through binding onto E1/E2 glycoproteins.

It has also been reported that suramin inhibits 3 clinical isolates including a 226 V mutant strain, Malaysia 0810bTw, with EC_{50} values ranging from 8.8 μM to 62.1 μM. Compound suramin shows potential effect as a novel anti-CHIKV agent targeting viral entry, extracellular transmission, and cell-to-cell transmission.

Das et al. (2016) designed and validated few inhibitors against CHIKV. It has been reported that compounds **1**, **2**, **3**, and **4** (Figure 5) suppress CHIKV RNA synthesis and infectious virus release. Among them, compound **4** was reported to be a very efficient inhibitor of viral RNA synthesis which was clearly translated into prominent suppression of progeny virus release. Compounds **5** and **3** were shown to be more potent inhibitors of virus replication (EC_{50}: 1.5 μM and 11 μM, respectively) than their potential to inhibit the protease activity of nsP2. Based on these results, it has been concluded that since the pronounced inhibitory effect of compound **3** was detected in experiments carried out using low MOI (multiplicity of infection) (virus inhibition) but not using a high MOI (positive-strand RNA synthesis), compound **3** might inhibit virus spread in cell culture which is crucial under low-MOI.

Recently, in our lab we carried out high throughput virtual screening of compounds of Asinex database against nsP3 macrodomain using Schrodinger suite in four stages. In the first three phases, rigid docking was performed with increasing accuracy in calculating binding free energy and for better conformational sampling efficiency of ligands. In each phase, 10% hit-list leads were filtered based on docking score, glide energy and good ADME properties and were used to redocking in a subsequent phase. In the last phase, 50 hit leads were retrieved from the high throughput virtual screening results and used for induced fit docking protocol where both ligand and receptor flexibility were incorporated. The known inhibitor harringtonine and the substrate compound ADP-ribose were also used in induced fit docking. Based on the docking score, glide energy, ADME properties and binding interactions with active site of nsP3, three best lead compounds were finally identified. The docking results suggest that the identified lead compounds have a better binding affinity (glide energy) compared to the known inhibitor as well as the substrate compound (Table 1).

These compounds also show similar binding mode and active site interactions with the inhibitor as well as the substrate (Figure 6).

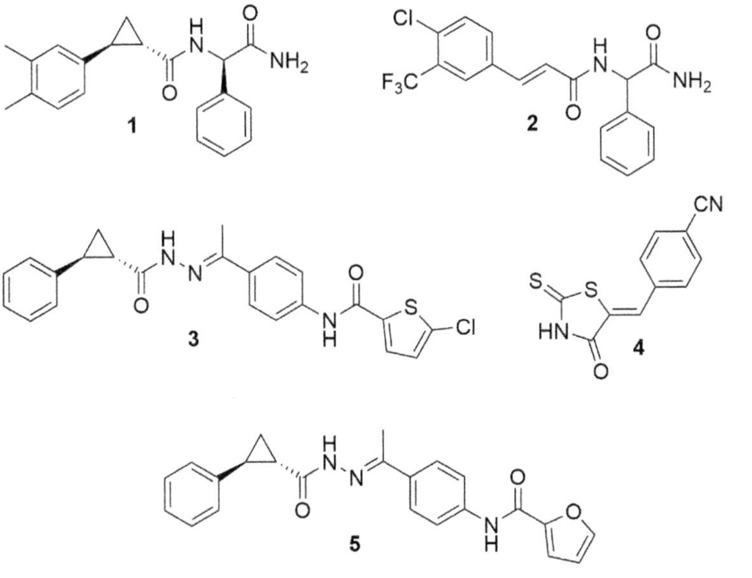

Figure 5. Structures of CHIKV inhibitors **1–5**.

Table 1. Docking score and Glide Energy of best-docked hit-lists from HTVS.

Compound-ID	Docking score (kcal/mol)	Glide energy (kcal/mol)	Interacting residues
ADP-ribose (Substrate)	−10.24	−75.30	Met9, Asp10, Ile11, Val33, Ser110, Gly112, Tyr114, Arg144
Harringtonine (Inhibitor)	−9.69	−59.98	Val33, Leu108, Gly112 , Val 113 , Tyr114, Try142, Arg144
Lead1 (Asn57310)	−11.86	−78.42	Asp31, Val33, Gly112, Leu108, Arg144
Lead2 (Asn01107557)	−8.59	−69.95	Leu108, Val113, Asp31, Arg144, Ser110
Lead3 (Asn131414)	−9.46	−86.22	Asp31, Val33, Ser110, Thr111, Gly112, Val113, Arg144

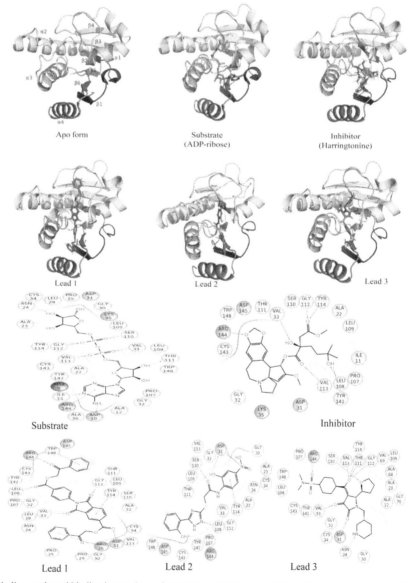

Figure 6. Binding mode and binding interactions of substrate (ADP ribose), inhibitor (harringtonine) and top identified lead compounds.

The central binding site for substrate binding is located at the top of the β2, β4 β5 strands and surrounded by the loops connecting β2-β1 and β5-β3. Binding mode of harringtonine inhibitor and identified lead complexes showed that these ligands orient towards the ribose binding site and phosphate binding site in the central crevice of binding pocket. In substrate binding, along with ribose binding site and phosphate binding site, ADP-ribose also orients in one additional binding pocket for adenine moiety towards α1 and β6 strand (Figure 6). Identified three compounds have also been found to have the most stable interactions with the active site residues of nP3 macrodomain of CHIKV comparable to the available inhibitor harringtonine. ADME properties were calculated for the identified leads and harringtonine. This analysis shows that for all the identified leads, the properties are similar to that of harringtonine (Table 2).

Table 2. ADME properties of Hit-list compounds and inhibitor.

Compound-ID	Molecular weight (Da)	Hydrogen bond donors	Hydrogen bond acceptors	QlogP o/w
Harringtonine	531.59	2	10	0.5
Lead 1	547.52	0	11	4.04
Lead 2	389.38	6	7.5	0.85
Lead 3	416.49	0	12	3.295

The three identified nsP3 complexes of the lead compounds, the inhibitor harringtonine, the substrate (ADP-ribose) and apo form of nsP3 were subjected to molecular dynamics simulations. To determine the stability of the system for the apo and complexes of nsP3, RMSD of the heavy atoms over 10 ns MD simulations with respect to their starting structures were plotted versus simulation time (Figure 7a).

It can be seen that the RMSD of apo proteins and complexes converged nicely [very small fluctuation (0.2–0.5Å)]. The radius of gyration (RGYR), which represents the compactness of internal structure, is almost constant and it means that the structure is properly folded during the simulations. The conformational changes in the nsP3 macro domain with respect to ligand binding (substrate and inhibitor) were analyzed in terms of fluctuations and deviations about backbone atoms (N, Cα, and C) and are represented in Figure 7b. Complexes of these docked compounds are stable during the simulation and show very least overall fluctuations in the binding pattern of active site residues. Due to ligand binding, conformations in alpha helix 1 and small loop (res 25–43 and res 106–120) are more arrested in substrate, inhibitor and identified lead bound complexes compared to apo form. Based on the overall binding contacts, binding free energy and electrostatic surface comparison in the central binding site, lead 1 and lead 3 are found to be more favorable and the conserved negative charge of the electrostatic surface in the active site also showed better binding affinity. These studies provide a clue for experimental studies aimed at understanding the binding mechanism of harringtonine inhibitor to nsP3 and viral replication. These studies identified two novel leads as anti-CHIK viral therapeutics which can be tested for experimental validation.

Prevention and Control of CHIKV Infections

Vector surveillance and control

In the absence of an effective CHIKV vaccine, the only tool available to prevent infection is detection of human-vector contact. *Aedes aegypti* is more closely associated with humans and their homes, and feeds preferentially on humans. Adult *Aedes aegypti* rest indoors and its larval habitats are most frequently containers in the household premises. On the other side, *Aedes albopictus* not only feeds on humans but also utilizes a broader range of blood meal hosts. Its larvae occur not only in heavy domestic habitats but also in the surrounding natural habitats. "*Aedes albopictus* can withstand in high temperature" compared to *Aedes aegypti*. The biology and control procedures for these two types of mosquitoes are similar. Successful control programs require well trained professional and technical staff with sufficient funding. An independent quality assurance program should also be incorporated into the integrated vector management (IVM)

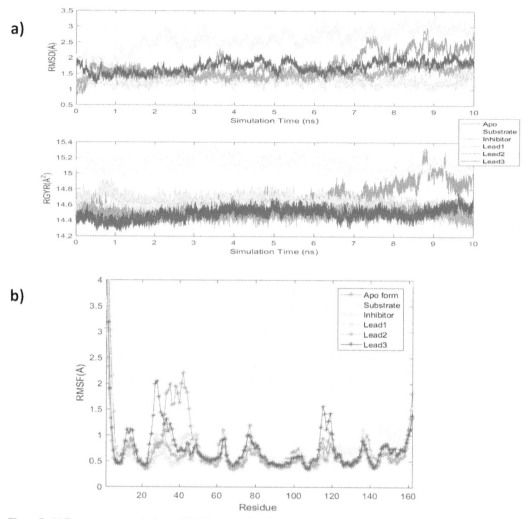

Figure 7. (a) Root mean square deviation (RMSD) and radius of gyration (RGYR) changes during simulation of the substrate (ADP ribose), inhibitor (harringtonine) and top identified lead compounds. (b) Root mean square fluctuation (RMSF) with respect to binding of the substrate (ADP ribose), inhibitor (harringtonine) and top identified lead compounds.

Color version at the end of the book

scheme. For a successful outcome during the outbreaks, the CHIKV IVM program needs collaboration at all levels of government among the health education, environment, social development and tourism agencies. Non-governmental organizations and private organizations could also come forward. Participation of communities is an essential component of IVM for effective implementation. IVM strategy must be well developed before the occurrence of CHIKV infection. Controlling or preventing CHIKV transmission in neighborhoods that traditionally have produced many cases of dengue should inhibit the virus amplification and its spread to other nearby neighborhood. Surveillance methods should include methods to monitor egg production, larval sites, pupil abundance and adult abundance. Septic tanks, storm drains, sump pumps and vacant plots are some of the cryptic locations to detect and identify the hidden and difficult larval sites. For the personal protection, individuals may reduce the likelihood of infection by the use of repellents on skin or clothing. *N,N*-diethyl-m-toluamide (DEET) and picaridin are some of the effective repellents widely available. Infants and others sleeping or resting during the day should use bed nets or insecticide coated bed nets to avoid the mosquito infection. Most importantly, the individuals who are potentially infected with

CHIKV during an outbreak should be more careful and follow the above precautions to avoid further spread of infection due to mosquito bites. For the household prevention, the use of intact screens indoors and on doors will reduce the entry of vectors into the home. Insecticide coated curtains will also reduce vector-human contact. Commercially available pyrethroid-based aerosol sprays and other products designed for the home, such as mosquito coils and electronic mat vaporizers may reduce the number of adult mosquitoes in the home. During the spraying of aerosol throughout the home, important areas like bedrooms, closets, clothing hampers, cooler areas and dark places must be taken into consideration. Unnecessary exposure to the pesticides should also be avoided. Vector control procedures should be followed, and any program should be managed by experienced professional vector control biologists to assure that the program uses current pesticide recommendation, incorporates new methods of vector control and includes resistance testing. The moment CHIKV infection has been confirmed in a region, the health department should inform the IVM program regarding the onset date and location of the case. Vector control procedures should be intensified in order to effectively reduce the abundance of infected vectors so that transmission in the area of occurrence can be halted. At the same time, at the local and national level, the emergency response committees should be informed of the situation and activated. Initial efforts should focus on controlling virus transmission and preventing expansion. Effective communication to the community and various stake holders are crucial to avoid confusion and mis-information and to engage people in steps to reduce the risk of CHIKV infection. The media, the public and many officials have to be educated about CHIKV infection, its mode of transmission, the lack of specific therapeutic treatment, means of symptomatic and supportive treatment and the adoption of control measures.

Laboratory diagnosis of CHIK fever

Laboratory diagnosis is critical to establish the cause of diagnosis and initiate specific public health response as the clinical manifestations of CHIK fever resemble those of dengue and other fevers caused by arthropod borne viruses. The three main laboratory tests to confirm CHIKV fever are the virus isolation, serological tests and molecular technique of polymerase chain reaction (PCR). Blood or serum can be used as the specimen. The most definitive diagnosis comes from the virus isolation even though it may take one to two weeks' time for completion. The diagnosis must be carried out in biosafety level 3 laboratories to reduce the risk of viral transmission. The degree of success depends on the time of collection, transportation, maintenance of cold chain, storage and processing of samples. ELISA assay is used in the serological diagnosis to measure chikungunya-specific IgM levels in the blood serum. The amount of 10 to 15 ml of whole blood is required to obtain the serum. Serum must be obtained twice, once immediately after the onset of illness and the other after 10 to 14 days. Results of MAC-ELISA can be available within the same day. In order to amplify several chikungunya-specific genes from the whole blood, RT-PCR technique can be used. CHIKV-RNA can be detected during the acute phase of illness, within a week after the symptom onset. The viral load in the blood can also be quantified using RT-PCR and within a day or two, the diagnostic results can be available. For the diagnosis of the CHIKV, nested primer pairs amplifying specific components of the three structural gene regions, Capsid (C), Envelope (E-2) and Envelope (E-1) are used in RT-PCR. Most of the countries have the directorate of national vector borne disease control program for surveillance of CHIKV fever cases across the country. Once epidemiological diagnosis of CHIKV fever is confirmed, symptomatic treatments should be started immediately. Confirmation of few cases would be enough to identify the cause of fever outbreak. Blood samples should be randomly collected for lab tests. Once a blood sample is found positive serologically for chikungunya IgM antibody, the respective area should be declared as having confirmed outbreak of chikungunya.

Progresses towards Therapy and Prevention of CHIKV

Drug repurposing

CHIKV fever is quite often accompanied by relapsing an incapacitating polyarthralgia. This may persist for several months. There are currently no recognized anti-viral therapies or human vaccines to control

CHIKV infections. Chloroquine was first reported to inhibit Sindbis virus (SINV) and Simian Foamy Virus (SFV) infections *in vitro* more than 35 years ago (Cassell et al. 1984, Inglot 1969). It has been later proved that the drug might enhance viral replication and aggravate the disease (Maheswari et al. 1991). Brighton (1984) used chloroquine phosphate to treat chronic CHIK arthritis by utilizing the anti-inflammatory properties of the molecule, rather than possible anti-viral effects. Cell culture results comparable with those of the SARS coronavirus were obtained. The experiments reported by De Lamballerie et al. (2008) did not justify the use of chloroquine to treat CHIKV infections. Quinine has an IC_{50} value much lower than that of chloroquine as an antiviral against CHIKV. Experiments proved quinine to be a good inhibitor for the alpha virus nsP1. Ribavarin acts mainly as an IMP dehydrogenase inhibitor against alpha viruses (Leyssen et al. 2005). Briolant et al. (2004) showed a synergistic effect on the *in vitro* inhibition of CHIKV when the combination of interferon-alpha and ribavin was used. Clinical tests are in progress in this direction. Ozden et al., in 2008, used furin inhibitors on CHIKV infected culture of human cells and had shown the inhibition by impairing the maturation of the CHIKV E2 surface glycoprotein. Evidence of inhibitory effects of carbodine was detected when it was administered up to four days post-infected period during VEEV infection. As VEEV-nsP2 protease structure has similarity with CHIKV-nsP2 protease, carbodine can also be studied for its anti-viral effects against CHIKV-nsP2. The protease domain of CHIKV-nsP2 is found to be the most promising target for rational inhibitor screening as this is responsible for non-structural polyprotein processing which is an essential function for virus replication.

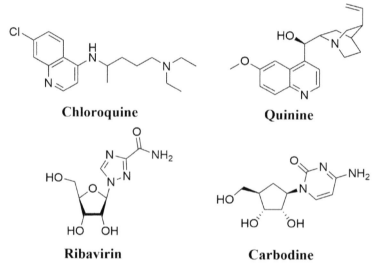

Figure 8. Structures of chloroquine, quinine, ribavirin, carbodine.

Finally, Chopra et al. (2014) have discussed in detail the effect of chloroquine and inflammatory cytokine in patients with early persistent musculo-skeleton pain and arthritis following CHIKV infection. Several inflammatory cytokines are reported to remain up regulated and persist despite clinical recovery.

Vaccine

Eckels et al. (1970) first attempted to develop inactivated vaccines against CHIKV but these early immunogens have not been developed as licensed vaccines. Although Edelman et al. (2000) developed a vaccine for CHIKV which proved highly immunogenic, some phase II volunteers developed transient arthralgia. Three suggested methods for safe and effective vaccines against CHIKV involved preparation of purified inactivated virus using the methods proposed by Pavlova et al. (2003) against tick-borne encephalitis virus, use of cDNA fragments representing the important immunogenic regions of CHIKV genome (Muthumani et al. 2008) and the procedures suggested by Wang et al. (2008). McPherson et al., in 2017, carried out extensive experiments and concluded that controlling the critical level of ADP-ribosylation may be at the fore front of the battle between the CHIKV and the host anti-viral response. Smalley et al. (2016) elaborated the status of research and development of vaccines for chikungunya and proposed the use of DNA vaccines against CHIKV.

Future Challenges

In spite of dramatic progress in the understanding of CHIKV infection, the research has to be continued into the pathogenesis of the long-lasting osteoarticular involvement. In search of efficient anti-viral drugs, new strategy must be developed with human anti CHIKV immunoglobulins. The most important challenge is the management of CHIKV infected patients. To overcome neuropathic pains in persistently symptomatic patients, specific pharmacological approach is required and the urgent need is to study the efficacy, safety and corticotherapy of some drugs to establish a strategy for the early treatment of destructive arthritis. When CHIKV infection is confirmed, rheumatologic assessment is essential and should always be initiated as early as possible to avoid delaying treatment. Staveness et al. (2016) reported a series of salicylate-based bryostatin analogues to inhibit the CHIKV replication in the low micromolar range. Varghese et al. (2016) reported berberine, a plant-derived alkaloid, to inhibit the *in vitro* replication of different CHIKV strains and to reduce the viral load and joints inflammation in CHIKV-infected mice. In this study, berberine was shown to reduce the activation of the major mitogen activated protein kinase (MAPK), signaling pathways in CHIKV-infected cells. MAPK signaling pathways were found to be activated during CHIKV infection and are important for the formation of infectious virus particles.

Conclusion

The identification of treatments against CHIKV is essential due to the worldwide re-emergence of CHIKV and the high morbidity rate associated with CHIKV infections. Vector control and prevention remain one of the action plans to control CHIKV spread but development of anti-viral compounds should be at a speedy rate due to the occurrence of acute CHIKV infection. Treatment for CHIKV infection should be started quickly after disease onset. Literature confirms CHIKV-nsP2 protease to be a relevant and excellent anti-viral target as nsP2 is involved in shutting of host-cell mRNA transcription and translation and inhibits cellular anti-viral response. Several numbers of classes of compounds have been reported to inhibit the *in vitro* CHIKV replication. Favipravir, the viral RNA polymerase inhibitor, licensed in Japan for the treatment of influenza virus infection, is found to inhibit CHIKV replication *in vitro* and in a mouse model. The potential use of this compound may also be studied in CHIKV-infected patients. Bindarit is a small molecule indazolic derivative that has anti-inflammatory properties and inhibits chemokine synthesis. As it is less immunosuppressive than the more widely used biological agents such as anti-TNF drug, it has the potential for a safe treatment to prevent viral-induced joint damage and bone loss. The main treatment for CHIKV rheumatism is with anti-inflammatory drugs, physiotherapy and short courses of oral steroids. Urate-lowering drugs can be effective and vitamin D can be used for bone strengthening. Although chloroquine has some anti-viral effect, other anti-inflammatory drugs like meloxicam can be used in acute and chronic CHIKV arthralgia. For patients with systemic polyarthritis due to CHIKV infection, methotrexate can be used, as literature shows 75% of patients to have positive clinical response to this drug. For good clinical efficacy, sulfasalazile can be combined with methotrexate. Biologic immuno-modulatory agents such as infliximab and etanercept are found to have successful effects in patients with severe disease symptoms. Since the initial description of CHIKV infection in 1950s, there were many CHIKV outbreaks worldwide. There is an increasing risk to the general population from *Ades-borne* viruses. The arthritis, which is an outcome of CHIKV infection, has often been treated as such with reasonable success rates. Although the mortality associated with CHIKV infection is small, the morbidity and burden of disease is quite large as it affects several million people worldwide. More research and awareness are necessary in order to develop better treatment strategies for CHIKV infected patients.

References

Ahola, T., T. Couderc, L.F. Ng, D. Hallengärd, A. Powers, M. Lecuit et al. 2015. Therapeutics and vaccines against chikungunya virus. Vector-Borne and Zoonotic Diseases. 15(4): 250–257.

Bandeira, A.C., G.S. Campos, V.F.D. Rocha, B.S. de Freitas Souza, M.B.P. Soares, A.A. Oliveira et al. 2016. Prolonged shedding of Chikungunya virus in semen and urine: A new perspective for diagnosis and implications for transmission. ID Cases. 6: 100–103.

Bhakat, S. and M.E.S. Soliman. 2015. Chikungunya virus (CHIKV) inhibitors from natural sources: a medicinal chemistry perspective. J. Nat. Med. 69: 451–462.

Brighton, S.W. 1984. Chloroquine phosphate treatment of chronic Chikungunya arthritis. An open pilot study. S. Afr. Med. J. 66(6): 217–218.

Briolant, S., D. Garin, N. Scaramozzino, A. Jouan and J.M. Crance. 2004. *In vitro* inhibition of Chikungunya and Semliki forest viruses replication by antiviral compounds: synergistic effect of interferon and ribavirin combination. Antivir. Res. 61(2): 111–117.

Cassell, S., J. Edwards and D.T. Brown. 1984. Effects of lysoso-motropic weak bases on infection of BHK-21 cells by Sindbis virus. J. Virol. 52(3): 857–864.

Chandak, N.H., R.S. Kashyap, D. Kabra, P. Karandikar, S.S. Saha, S.H. Morey et al. 2009. Neurological complications of Chikungunya virus infection. Neurol. India. 57(2): 177–180.

Chen, W., S.S. Foo, A. Taylor, A. Lulla, A. Merits, L. Hueston et al. 2015. Bindarit, an inhibitor of monocyte chemotactic protein synthesis, protects against bone loss induced by chikungunya virus infection. J. Virol. 89: 581–593.

Chopra, A., M. Saluja and A. Venugopalan. 2014. Effectiveness of chloroquine and inflammatory cytokine response in patients with early persistent musculoskeletal pain and arthritis following Chikungunya virus infection. Arthritis Rheumatol. 66(2): 319–326.

Das, P.K., L. Puusepp, F.S. Varghese, A. Utt, T. Ahola, D.G. Kananovich et al. 2016. Design and validation of novel Chikungunya virus protease inhibitors. Antimicrob. Agents Chemother. doi: 10.1128/AAC.01421-16.

De Lamballerie, X., V. Boisson, J.-C. Reynier, S. Enault, R.N. Charrel, A. Flahault et al. 2008. On Chikungunya acute infection and chloroquine treatment. Vector Borne Zoonotic Dis. 8(6): 837–839.

Eckels, K.H., V. R. Harrison and F.M. Hetrick. 1970. Chikungunya virus vaccine prepared by Tween-ether extraction. Appl. Microbiol. 19(2): 321–325.

Edelman, R., C.O. Tacket, S.S. Wasserman, S.A. Bodison, J.G. Perry and J.A. Mangiafico. 2000. Phase II safety and immuno-genicity study of live Chikungunya virus vaccine TSI-GSD-218. Am. J. Trop. Med. Hyg. 62(6): 681–685.

Gérardin, P., T. Couderc, M. Bintner, P. Tournebize, M. Renouil, J. Lémant et al. 2016. Chikungunya virus-associated encephalitis: A cohort study on La Réunion Island, 2005–2009. Neurology. 86(1): 94–102.

Hélène, M., C. Bruno, J. Saïd, D. Hélène, P. Nicolas, N. Maarit et al. 2009. The crystal structures of Chikungunya and *Venezuelan Equine Encephalitis* virus nsP3 Macro Domains Define a Conserved Adenosine Binding Pocket. J. Virol. 83(13): 6534–6545.

Ho, Y.-J., Y.-M. Wang, J.-W. Lu, T.-W. Wu, L-I. Lin, S.-C. Kuo et al. 2015. Suramin inhibits Chikungunya virus entry and transmission. PLoS ONE. 10(7): DOI: 10.1371/journal.pone.0133511.

Inglot, A.D. 1969. Comparison of the antiviral activity *in vitro* of some non-steroidal anti-inflammatory drugs. J. Gen. Virol. 4: 203–214.

Kaur, P., M. Thiruchelvan, R.C. Lee, H. Chen, K.C. Chen, M.L. Ng et al. 2010. Inhibition of chikungunya virus replication by harringtonine, a novel antiviral that suppresses viral protein expression. Antimicrob. Agents Chemother. 57(1): 155–167.

Letunic, I., R.R. Copley, B. Pils, S. Pinkert, J. Schultz and P. Bork. 2006. SMART 5: domains in the context of genomes and networks. Nucleic Acids Res. 34: D257–D260.

Leyssen, P., E. De Clercq and J. Neyts. 2006. The anti-yellow fever virus activity of ribavirin is independent of error-prone replication. Mol. Pharmacol. 69(4): 1461–1467.

Lulla, A., V. Lulla, K. Tints, T. Ahola and A. Merits. 2006. Molecular determinants of substrate specifity for Semliki Forest virus nonstructural protease. J. Virol. 80: 5413–5422.

Maheshwari, R.K., V. Srikantan and D. Bhartiya. 1991. Chloroquine enhances replication of Semliki Forest virus and encephalomy-ocarditis virus in mice. J. Virol. 65(2): 992–995.

McPherson, R.L., R. Abraham, E. Sreekumar, S.-E. Ong, S.-J. Cheng, V.K. Baxter et al. 2017. ADP-ribosylhydrolase activity of Chikungunya virus macrodomain is critical for virus replication and virulence. Proc. Natl. Acad. Sci. 114(7): 1666–1671.

Mishra, P., A. Kumar, P. Mamidi, S. Kumar, I. Basantray, T. Saswat et al. 2015. Inhibition of Chikungunya virus replication by 1-[(2-Methylbenzimidazol-1-yl) Methyl]-2-Oxo-Indolin-3-ylidene] Amino] Thiourea(MBZM-N-IBT). Scientific Reports. 6: 20122, DOI: 10.1038/srep20122.

Morrison, T., M.F. Julie, W.A. Alison, A.M. Nick, M.S. Kristin, M.T. Raul et al. 2016. Pathogenic Chikungunya virus evades B cell responses to establish persistence. J. Immunol. 196(1): 147–12.

Morrison, T.E. 2014. Reemergence of Chikungunya virus. J. Virol. 88(20): 11644–11467.

Murthy, J.M.K. 2009. Chikungunya virus: Neurology. 57(2): 113–115.

Muthumani, K., K.M. Lankaraman, D.J. Laddy, S.G. Sundaram, C.W. Chung, E. Sako et al. 2008. Immunogenicity of novel consensus-based DNA vaccines against chikungunya virus. Vaccine. 26(40): 5128–5134.

Ozden, S., M. Lucas-Hourani, P.-E. Ceccaldi, A. Basak, M. Valentine, S. Benjannet et al. 2008. Inhibition of Chikungunya virus infection in cultured human muscle cells by furin inhibitors: impairment of the maturation of the E2 surface glycoprotein. J. Biol. Chem. 283(32): 21899–21908.

Pastorino, B.A., C.N. Peyrefitte, L. Almeras, M. Grandadam, D. Rolland, H.J. Tolou et al. 2008. Expression and biochemical characterization of nsP2 cysteine protease of Chikungunya virus. Virus Res. 131(2): 293–298.

Pavlova, B.G., I.V. Stavitskaya, M.A. Gorbunov, O.V. Shtukaturova, A.P. Pomogayeva, O.V. Stronin et al. 2003. Immunization of children and adolescents with inactivated vaccines against tick-borne encephalitis. Biopreparations. 1: 24–28.

Ramakrishnan, C., N.H.V. Kutumbarao, S. Suhitha and D. Velmurugan. 2017. Structure–function relationship of Chikungunya nsP2 protease: A comparative study with papain. Chem. Biol. Drug Design. 89(5): 772–782.

Rathore, A.P., M.L. Ng and S.G. Vasudevan. 2013. Differential unfolded protein response during Chikungunya and Sindbis virus infection: CHIKV nsP4 suppresses eIF2α phosphorylation. Virol. J. 10(36): 1–15.

Rathore, A.P., T. Haystead, P.K. Das, A. Merits, M.L. Ng and S.G. Vasudevan. 2014. Chikungunya virus nsP3 & nsP4 interacts with HSP-90 to promote virus replication: HSP-90 inhibitors reduce CHIKV infection and inflammation *in vivo*. Antiviral. Res. 103: 7–16.

Russo, A.T., M.A. White and S.J. Watowich. 2006. The crystal structure of the Venezuelan equine encephalitis alphavirus nsP2 protease. Structure. 14: 1449–1458.

Singh, Kh. D., P. Kirubakaran, S. Nagarajan, S. Sakkiah, K. Muthusamy, D. Velmurgan et al. 2012. Homology modeling, molecular dynamics, e-pharmacophore mapping and docking study of Chikungunya virus nsP2 protease. J. Mol. Model. 18(1): 39–51.

Smalley, C., H.E. Jesse, B.C. Charles and W.C.B. David. 2016. Status of research and development of vaccines for Chikungunya. Vaccine. 34(26): 2976–2981.

Sourisseau, M., C. Schilte, N. Casartelli, C. Trouillet, F. Guivel-Benhassine, D. Rudnicka et al. 2007. Characterization of reemerging Chikungunya virus. PLoS Pathog. 3(6): e89.

Staveness, D., R. Abdelnabi, K.E. Near, Y. Nakagawa, J. Neyts, L. Delang et al. 2016. Inhibition of Chikungunya virus-induced cell death by salicylate-derived Bryostatin analogues provides additional evidence for a PKC-independent pathway. J. Nat. Prod. 79(4): 680–684.

Strauss, J.H. and E.G. Strauss. 1994. The alphaviruses: gene expression, replication, and evolution. Microbiol. Rev. 58(3): 491–562.

Thiberville, S.D., N. Moyen, L. Dupuis-Maguiraga, A. Nougairede, E.A. Gould, P. Roques et al. 2013. Chikungunya fever: epidemiology, clinical syndrome, pathogenesis and therapy. Antiviral. Res. 99(3): 345–370.

Varghese, F.S., B. Thaa, S.N. Amrun, D. Simarmata, K. Rausalu, T.A. Nyman et al. 2016. The antiviral alkaloid berberine reduces Chikungunya Virus-induced mitogen-activated protein kinase signaling. J. Virol. 90(21): 9743–9757.

Wahid, B., A. Ali, S. Rafique and M. Idrees. 2017. Global expansion of Chikungunya virus: mapping the 64-year history. Int. J. Infect. Dis. 58: 69–76.

Wang, E., E. Volkova, A.P. Adams, N. Forrester, S.Y. Xiao, I. Frolov et al. 2008. Chimeric alphavirus vaccine candidates for Chikungunya. Vaccine. 26(39): 5030–5039.

Weaver, S.C. and M. Lecuit. 2015. Chikungunya virus and the global spread of a mosquito-borne disease. N. Engl. J. Med. 372(13): 1231–1239.

Yogesh, A.K. and S.L. Kavita. 2010. NTPase and 5′ to 3′ RNA duplex-unwinding activities of the Hepatitis E virus helicase domain. J. Virol. 84: 73595–3602.

Chapter 7

Recent Advances in Repositioning Non-Antibiotics against Tuberculosis and other Neglected Tropical Diseases

M.M. Dorothy Semenya

Introduction: The Unrelenting Epidemic of Tuberculosis

Despite ongoing efforts to redress the research paucity associated with infectious diseases endemic in the tropics, many remain scourges that blight billions of lives annually. Tuberculosis (TB) presently leads the pack as the deadliest infectious disease worldwide with a disproportionately high incidence in tropical regions. Existing therapeutic options for TB are fraught with limitations including suboptimal efficacy, toxicity and inexorable emergence of drug-resistant strains. Inasmuch as the need for new medicines is paramount, their development is decelerated partly by the lack of commercial incentives in high disease burden regions which deter big pharma investments. Drug repositioning is among unconventional strategies being explored to streamline drug discovery and development, particularly for diseases endemic in resource-poor settings. Multiple TB drug development campaigns capitalize on drugs already approved by regulatory authorities including those originally indicated for diseases of a non-infectious aetiology but additionally exhibit antimicrobial properties, such drugs are referred to as non-antibiotics. This chapter highlights recent repositioning approaches for TB with emphasis placed on non-antibiotics as alternative therapeutics and starting points for lead discovery and optimization. These drugs carry appeal for diversifying the chemical space occupied by current antitubercular agents and also show potentiality against recalcitrant TB. Moreover, they hold promise as antimicrobials for some neglected tropical diseases (NTDs) prioritized by the World Health Organization (WHO).

Current Scenario and Available Chemotherapeutic Options

Antibiotics have been the panacea for TB since the advent of effective drug treatments including streptomycin **1** in the early 1940s (Figure 1). Nowadays, antibiotic therapies fall short of curtailing the

King's College London, School of Cancer and Pharmaceutical Sciences, 150 Stamford Street, SE1 9NH London, United Kingdom.
Emails: dorothy.semenya@kcl.ac.uk; dorothy.semenya@alumni.uct.ac.za

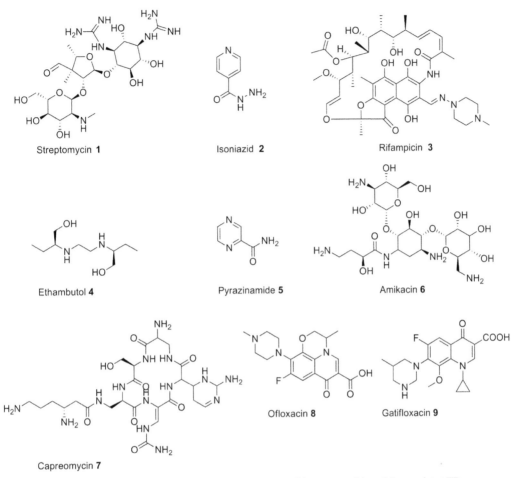

Figure 1. Examples of drugs employed in the treatment of drug-susceptible and drug-resistant TB.

global TB epidemic jeopardizing past gains. In 2016 alone, 6.3 million new cases of TB and 476,774 cases of HIV-positive TB were reported. Over half a million new drug-resistant TB cases were reported in the same year. Recent estimates indicate that over a million TB deaths occur annually. According to the WHO, the decrease in global TB incidence has to improve from 2% to about 4–5% annually and TB cases resulting in death have to fall from 16% to about 10% per year in order to reach the first milestones of the End TB Strategy by 2020 (WHO 2017a). As with NTDs prioritized by the WHO, progress against TB is stifled by research and development funding gaps, withering public health systems, limited accessibility to essential medicines and socioeconomic stagnation in high disease burden regions, among others (Molyneux et al. 2017, WHO 2017a). Although millions of deaths are averted annually through timely diagnosis and appropriate treatment, antimicrobial resistance remains a persistent impediment to the management of TB.

Many discoveries against TB pathogenesis were heralded by the identification of its principal causative bacterium, *Mycobacterium tuberculosis* (Mtb), over a century ago by Robert Koch (Gawad and Bonde 2018, Koul et al. 2011). TB is transmitted by inhalation of aerosolized droplets containing tubercle bacilli. Inhaled bacilli are phagocytosed primarily by alveolar macrophages which are subsequently subjected to apoptosis. Virulent strains may escape apoptosis by subversion of the immune system leading to prolonged survival in host cells. The dormant state of TB (latent TB) is asymptomatic and non-infectious. Mtb typically affects the lungs (pulmonary TB) but can also disseminate to other sites (extrapulmonary TB) (Ernst 2012, Koul et al. 2011, Martins 2011, WHO 2017a). The probability of TB infection progressing to active disease is inordinate among immunocompromised individuals (e.g., HIV co-infection) and it is also influenced by other risk factors including malnutrition and negative health practices (WHO 2017a). TB diagnosis and treatment monitoring are commonly conducted through sputum smear microscopy, a century-old technique. In settings with a more developed laboratory infrastructure, culture-based methods are used and results are normally provided within 3 mon. Rapid molecular tests are gaining popularity worldwide for diagnostic purposes. The WHO recommends Xpert® MTB/RIF assay (Cepheid) for the diagnosis of pulmonary TB in adults and also extrapulmonary TB in children. Rapid diagnostics are much more accurate than other methods and results can be obtained within hours (Wilson 2011, WHO 2017a).

TB chemotherapy is faced with formidable obstacles including rampant emergence of monodrug-resistant, multidrug-resistant (MDR) and extensively drug-resistant (XDR) Mtb strains (Dos Santos Fernandes et al. 2017, Gawad and Bonde 2018). At present, the treatment of drug-susceptible TB involves a decades-old and toxic drug regimen that is prone to poor patient compliance which may lead to drug-resistant cases. The intensive phase of treatment involves at least four first-line drugs (isoniazid **2**, rifampicin **3**, ethambutol **4** and pyrazinamide **5**) and lasts for 2 mon (Figure 1). A continuation phase including isoniazid and rifampicin follows for at least 4 mon, and a complete 6 mon course is about US$ 40 per person (Phillips et al. 2016, WHO 2017a). Around 90–95% cure rates can be achieved if the regimen is administered appropriately. However, patients usually fail to complete prescribed regimens due to prolonged duration of treatment that is necessitated by the complex nature of the physiological states in which Mtb exists (Tiberi et al. 2018). MDR TB which is resistant to both isoniazid and rifampicin requires a 9–12 mon treatment regimen involving second-line drugs (e.g., amikacin **6**, capreomycin **7**, ofloxacin **8** and gatifloxacin **9**) and costs about US$ 1000 per person (Figure 1) (WHO 2017a). Furthermore, MDR TB therapy consists mostly of drugs that are poorly tolerated, highly toxic and more expensive than those used for drug-susceptible TB. MDR TB therapy success rates are average, just over 50%. XDR TB, MDR TB resistant to at least one fluoroquinolone and one second-line injectable agent, is much more complex and expensive to treat. Recent statistics indicate that treatment success rates for XDR TB fall below 50% (D'Ambrosio et al. 2015, Tiberi et al. 2018, WHO 2017a). Reports of virtually untreatable TB that is resistant to all first- and second-line drugs (totally drug-resistant TB, TDR TB) aggravate the already onerous situation. TDR TB cases were recently detected in India, Iran and South Africa (Parida et al. 2015, Quan et al. 2017, Sharma et al. 2017).

In accordance with previous WHO guidelines, antitubercular drugs are categorized into five groups (in hierarchical order from group 1 to 5) based on factors such as efficacy, toxicity, mode of administration, structural identity and clinical evidence (Table 1) (Tiberi et al. 2017). A revised classification of agents that exclusively target the management of drug-resistant TB has recently been approved by the WHO. The updated guidelines classify the drugs into groups A–D (in hierarchical order) including fluoroquinolones as core drugs (Table 1) (Mafukidze et al. 2016, Tiberi et al. 2017, 2018).

Antitubercular drugs interfere with specific pathways or biomolecular targets that are crucial for the survival and persistence of Mtb. These include cell wall biosynthesis, DNA metabolism, transcription and translation processes and the cell membrane (Table 2) (Hoagland et al. 2016, Zhang 2005).

Mtb has nullified the effectiveness of the majority of drugs either through acquired resistance (e.g., modulation of drug targets by gene mutation) or intrinsic resistance which is conferred by its inherent structural or functional characteristics such as the highly impermeable lipid-rich cell wall composed of covalently linked mycolic acids, arabinogalactan and peptidoglycan or putative efflux pumps that extrude xenobiotics from the bacterial cytoplasm or periplasm (Hoagland et al. 2016, Kolyva and Karakousis 2012). Although research efforts against TB are constantly reinvigorated, therapeutic innovations to overcome Mtb drug tolerance remain insufficient.

Innovative Drug Discovery and Development against TB

TB is not as largely neglected in terms of policy, research and funding as most NTDs listed by the WHO, but it disproportionately affects many of the same marginalized populations plagued by NTDs. Funding for TB care and prevention has gradually increased over the years, about US$ 6.9 billion was available

Table 1. Classifications of drugs available for the treatment of TB.

TB drugs classification based on WHO guidelines				
Group 1	**Group 2**	**Group 3**	**Group 4**	**Group 5**
First-line drugs (*oral*)	Second-line drugs (*injectable*)	Second-line drugs[c] (*oral and injectable*)	Second-line drugs (*oral bacteriostatic*)	Miscellaneous roles[d]
Isoniazid Rifampicin Ethambutol Pyrazinamide Rifabutin	Streptomycin[a] Kanamycin[a] Amikacin[a] Capreomycin[b]	Levofloxacin Moxifloxacin Ofloxacin Gatifloxacin	Ethionamide or prothionamide Cycloserine/ terizidone *p*-Aminosalicylic acid	Linezolid Clofazimine Amoxicillin/ clavulanate Thioacetazone, Imipenem/ cilastatin High-dose isoniazid
Updated classification of TB drugs for the treatment of drug-resistant TB				
Group A	**Group B**	**Group C**	**Group D**	
Core drugs	Second-line drugs	Second-line drugs	Add-on drugs	
Levofloxacin Moxifloxacin Gatifloxacin	Amikacin Capreomycin Kanamycin	Ethionamide/ prothionamide Cycloserine/terizidone Linezolid Clofazimine	Pyrazinamide Ethambutol High-dose isoniazid Bedaquiline Delamanid *p*-Aminosalicylic acid (PAS) Imipenem-cilastatin Meropenem Amoxicillin-clavulanate	

Adapted from (Tiberi et al. 2017). [a]Aminoglycosides [b]Polypeptide [c]Fluoroquinolones [d]Drugs with sparse efficacy and toxicity data

Table 2. Biomolecular targets and/or mechanisms of action of established antitubercular drugs.

Drug	Chemical class	Effect on cell	Target/Mode of action
Isoniazid	Isonicotinic acid hydrazide	Bactericidal/bacteriostatic	Acyl carrier protein reductase (InhA) and other targets; Inhibits mycolic acid biosynthesis; Affects DNA, lipid, carbohydrate and NAD metabolism
Rifampicin	Rifamycin	Bactericidal	Inhibits RNA polymerase
Pyrazinamide	Pyrazine	Bacteriostatic/bactericidal	Disrupts cell membrane potential
Ethambutol	1,2-Aminoalcohol	Bacteriostatic	Inhibits arabinosyl transferase (arabinogalactan biosynthesis)
Streptomycin	Aminoglycoside	Bactericidal	Inhibits protein synthesis
Capreomycin	Polypeptide	Bactericidal	Inhibits protein synthesis
Kanamycin	Aminoglycoside	Bactericidal	Inhibits protein synthesis
Amikacin	Aminoglycoside	Bactericidal	Inhibits protein synthesis
Fluoroquinolones		Bactericidal	Inhibits DNA gyrase and topoisomerase IV
Ethionamide	Nicotinamide	Bacteriostatic	Inhibits InhA (mycolic acid biosynthesis)
Cycloserine	Isoxazolidinone	Bacteriostatic	Inhibits peptidoglycan biosynthesis
PAS	Aminobenzoic acid	Bacteriostatic	Inhibits folic acid biosynthesis and iron metabolism

Adapted from (Hoagland et al. 2016, Zhang 2005).

in 2017 compared to US\$ 3.3 billion in 2006. Despite these increments, the WHO revealed funding gaps of US\$ 2.3 billion in 2017 (WHO 2017a). With the global TB epidemic seemingly unabated, accelerating the development of novel diagnostics, drugs, treatment regimens and vaccines is becoming increasingly urgent. Adequate funding is key to incentivizing innovations in TB research and development.

Drug Candidates and Regimens under Clinical Development

Advances in TB research and development are continually made in spite of persistent funding gaps. A number of drugs, vaccine candidates and new combination regimens were in late-stage clinical development in 2017. A few diagnostic technologies are also on the horizon. There is a compelling need for effective vaccines given that bacille Calmette-Guerin (BCG) is the only licensed vaccine for prevention of severe TB forms in children, while none is available for preventing TB disease in adults. The 2017 global development pipeline for new antitubercular agents consists of 17 drugs in Phase I, Phase II or Phase III clinical trials including rifapentine **10**, bedaquiline **11** and delamanid **12** (Table 3) (Figure 2). The latter two drugs have already received accelerated or conditional regulatory approval for drug-resistant TB to improve therapy

Table 3. Drug candidates and regimens under advanced clinical development for the treatment of TB.

Drug	Chemical class	Target/Mode of action	Phase
GSK-3036656	Oxaborole[a]	Leucyl-tRNA synthetase (crucial for protein synthesis)	I
OPC-167832	Carbostyril[a]	DprE1 (flavoenzyme essential for cell wall biosynthesis)	I
Q203	Imidazopyridine[a]	ATPase (acts on qcrB subunit of the cytochrome bc_1 complex)	I
Delpazolid	Oxazolidinone	Targets protein synthesis (blocks the 23S rRNA)	II
PBTZ169	Benzothiazinone[a]	Interacts with active site residues in DprE1	II
SQ109	Ethylenediamine[a]	MmpL3 (mycolic acid transporter for cell wall assembly)	II
Sutezolid	Oxazolidinone	Inhibits protein synthesis (blocks the 23S rRNA)	II
Levofloxacin[b]	Fluoroquinolone	Type II and IV topoisomerases and DNA gyrase	II
Linezolid[b]	Oxazolidinone	Inhibits protein synthesis (blocks the 23S rRNA)	II
Nitazoxanide[b]	Nitrothiazole	Disrupts membrane potential and pH homeostasis	II
Rifampicin (high dose)	Rifamycin	Inhibits RNA polymerase	II
Rifapentine	Rifamycin	Inhibits RNA polymerase	II
Bedaquiline	Diarylquinoline	ATP synthase (inhibits the proton pumping mechanism)	III
Delamanid	Nitroimidazole	Inhibits mycolic acid synthesis and energy production	III
Pretomanid	Nitroimidazole	Inhibits mycolic acid synthesis and energy production	III
Clofazimine[b]	Riminophenazine	Releases reactive oxygen species	III
Rifampicin (high dose)	Rifamycin	Inhibits RNA polymerase	III
Rifapentine	Rifamycin	Inhibits RNA polymerase	III

Regimen	Phase
Bedaquiline and delamanid (ACTG5343 DELIBERATE trial)	II
Bedaquiline–Pretomanid–Pyrazinamide	II
Bedaquiline–Pretomanid–Moxifloxacin–Pyrazinamide	II
Delamanid–Linezolid–Levofloxacin–Pyrazinamide (MDR-END trial)	II
Bedaquiline–Pretomanid–Linezolid with/without moxifloxacin/clofazimine for MDR-/XDR-TB (TB PRACTECAL trial)	III
Bedaquiline–Pretomanid–Linezolid (NiX-TB trial)	III
Bedaquiline with two optimized background regimens (STREAM trial)	III
Bedaquiline–Linezolid with optimized background regimen for MDR-TB (NExT trial)	III
Bedaquiline–Delamanid with various existing regimens for MDR-TB and XDR-TB (endTB trail)	III
Rifapentine–Moxifloxacin for drug-susceptible TB (TB Trial Consortium Study 31/A54349)	III

Adapted from (WHO 2017a) (Quan et al. 2017) (Parida et al. 2015) (Gawad and Bonde 2018) (http://www.newtbdrugs. org/). [a]New chemical class [b]Repositioned drugs

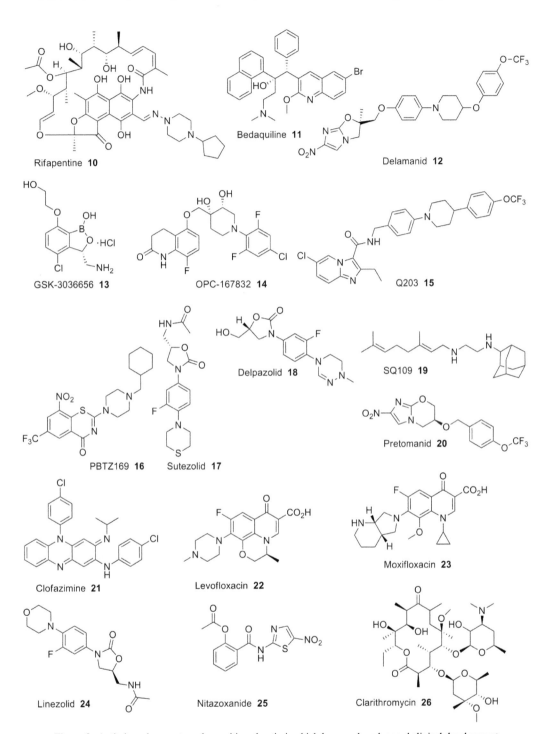

Figure 2. Antitubercular agents and repositioned antimicrobial drugs under advanced clinical development.

outcomes. Eight of the 17 drugs (GSK-3036656 **13**, OPC-167832 **14**, Q203 **15**, PBTZ169 **16**, sutezolid **17**, delpazolid **18**, SQ109 **19** and pretomanid **20**) are new compounds (Table 3) (Figure 2). Some of these represent a new chemical class or previously unexplored mechanisms (WHO 2017a).

GSK-3036656 is a new oxaborole candidate undergoing Phase I clinical development since March 2017. It potently and selectively inhibits Mtb leucyl-tRNA synthetase, a key enzyme for protein synthesis (Li et al. 2017). Q203 represents a new class of antitubercular imidazopyridines discovered through phenotypic screening against intracellular Mtb and subsequent lead optimization processes. It targets the cytochrome bc_1 complex which plays a central role in Mtb oxidative phosphorylation (Bald et al. 2017). The other candidates representing a novel class, OPC-167832 (carbostyril) and PBTZ169 (benzothiazinone), target cell wall biosynthesis by interacting with active site residues in DprE1, an enzyme crucial for arabinogalactan and arabinomannan biosynthesis (Bald et al. 2017, Parida et al. 2015, Quan et al. 2017). SQ109, also discovered by whole-cell screening, targets MmpL3 and interferes with ATP-dependent mycolate translocation which is essential for cell wall biosynthesis.

A few candidates clinically approved as antiparasitic, antiviral or antibacterial agents (clofazimine **21**, levofloxacin **22**, moxifloxacin **23**, linezolid **24** and nitazoxanide **25**) are also undergoing advanced development for TB therapy (Table 3) (Figure 2), illustrating the merit of drug repositioning in the search for new antitubercular agents (WHO 2017a). Clofazimine is a riminophenazine that is in clinical use for the treatment of leprosy. Prior to its approval as an antileprosy drug, it was being developed for TB therapy. However, the development was not pursued further due to inconclusive outcomes in animal models. It is now under re-development for the treatment of TB and has been recommended as a second-line agent for drug-resistant TB combination therapy. Fluoroquinolones (including levofloxacin and moxifloxacin) represent one of the most potent categories of antitubercular agents with favourable pharmacokinetic profiles. Levofloxacin is used for sinusitis and bronchitis therapy or as an alternative therapeutic for urinary tract infections whereas moxifloxacin is employed in the treatment of respiratory and enteric infections. Linezolid, an oxalidinone antibacterial normally used for the treatment of methicillin-resistant *Staphylococcus aureus* (MRSA) associated infections, forms a key component of emerging MDR/XDR TB treatment regimens. However, its higher rate of adverse effects raises red flags. Nitazoxanide, a broad-spectrum antiparasitic drug, is also showing promising prospects against Mtb. Other repositioned antibiotic drug classes including beta-lactams and macrolides are also under clinical development, some of which have been recommended by the WHO for the treatment of drug-resistant TB (Mafukidze et al. 2016, Quan et al. 2017, WHO 2017a). Clarithromycin **26** (a macrolide) has recently been withdrawn from drug-resistant TB treatment regimens recommended by the WHO due to limited efficacy against Mtb, severe hepatotoxicity and inducible resistance (Figure 2) (Mafukidze et al. 2016, Tiberi et al. 2018). Desirably, new treatments should exhibit effectiveness against every physiological state of Mtb including persistent or latent forms, reduce dosing frequency and pill burden, minimize drug-drug interactions and essentially shorten the duration of therapy (Quan et al. 2017).

Drug Repositioning as an Alternative to *de novo* Drug Discovery

The drug discovery and development landscape for infectious diseases is constantly changing with research interests shifting away from traditional approaches. *De novo* drug discovery and development is an exhaustive, time-consuming and costly multi-stage process that is faced with high attrition rates largely due to poor pharmacokinetics, toxicity and lack of efficacy in human subjects (Cook et al. 2014, Duran-Frigola et al. 2017, Hughes et al. 2011). Given the complexities associated with *de novo* approaches, alternative strategies that capitalize on past investments of such processes are gaining traction (Nwaka and Hudson 2006, Sharma et al. 2017, Zheng et al. 2018). Drug repositioning or repurposing is one such strategy that seeks new purposes for marketed or abandoned drugs. Other closely related strategies include drug reprofiling or redirecting (Ma et al. 2013, Persaud-Sharma and Zhou 2012). These terms are often used interchangeably as there is no consensus on terminology.

Drug repositioning is widely appreciated as a rational strategy towards accelerated development of much needed medicines particularly in instances where conventional drug discovery approaches run the risk of being unprofitable. Given that most research campaigns are profit-driven, repositioning approaches are seen as low-risk strategies that offer significant benefits such as potentially avoiding exorbitant costs and lengthy timelines by capitalizing on previous investments and established data (Chakraborty and Trivedi 2015, Duran-Frigola et al. 2017). Also, pharmacokinetic and toxicological profiles of repositioned drugs are validated; thus, chances of attrition in advanced clinical development are narrowed (Ma et al. 2013, Persaud-Sharma and Zhou 2012).

Advances in repositioning non-antibiotics for therapeutic effects against Mtb

Non-antibiotics are targeted in myriad drug discovery and development campaigns as potential novel therapeutics, adjuvants or adjuncts for TB chemotherapy. Repositioning strategies may involve advancing existing non-antibiotics with established antitubercular properties to clinical development or exploiting the privileged scaffolds as starting points for hit-to-lead optimization through iterative medicinal chemistry processes.

Antitubercular effects of psychotropic drugs

The clinical application of psychotropics in psychiatry spans over many decades (Carpenter 2012). In addition to neuropharmacological properties, sporadic reports have underscored their direct antimicrobial and antibiotic-potentiating effects pointing to their potentiality for the management of recalcitrant microbial infections (Amaral et al. 2001, Kristiansen et al. 2007, Varga et al. 2017, Wainwright 2012).

Antipsychotic phenothiazines: Phenothiazines are congeners of methylene blue **27**, a phenothiazinium dye whose therapeutic use was pioneered by Paul Ehrlich (Figure 3) (Kristiansen and Amaral 1997). The neuroleptic effects of these antipsychotics are exerted via a blockade of central nervous system (CNS) receptors including dopaminergic and serotonergic receptors (Jafari et al. 2012). Phenothiazines are amphiphilic in nature and obey a lipophilic chromophore/basic side chain paradigm. They are classified according to the type of terminal amine moiety, i.e., aliphatics, piperidines and piperazines. Specific structural traits and physicochemical properties facilitate blood-brain barrier penetration and promote their neuroleptic action including conformational resemblance to monoamine neurotransmitters, e.g., dopamine, a high degree of lipophilicity and the presence of a proton-accepting distal amine moiety (Feinberg and Snyder 1975, Jaszczyszyn et al. 2012, Pluta et al. 2011, Seelig et al. 1994). In recent decades, research efforts have brought to light their multiple non-neuroleptic properties especially antimicrobial effects which date back to antiquity (Amaral et al. 2004, Jaszczyszyn et al. 2012, Kristiansen and Amaral 1997, Varga et al. 2017). The effectiveness of phenothiazines against Mtb was first noted when patients treated with chlorpromazine **28** displayed alleviation of TB symptoms (Figure 3). As this observation was noted during the 'golden age' of antibiotics, there was no impetus for further assessment at the time (Amaral et al. 2004, Wainwright 2012). In the wake of antimicrobial resistance, phenothiazines have re-emerged as drugs of interest for the treatment of TB spurring numerous investigations that have revealed their efficacies against drug-susceptible and MDR strains of Mtb, minimum inhibitory concentration (MIC) range 4–32 µg/mL (Amaral et al. 1996, Bettencourt et al. 2000, Gadre and Talwar 1999, Ratnakar et al. 1995). Among the phenothiazines, thioridazine **29** has attracted substantial interest owing to its more superior therapeutic safety profile (Figure 3). It causes fewer extrapyramidal symptoms and has a low risk of severe side effects including QT interval prolongation and torsades de pointes (Amaral and Viveiros 2012, Ordway et al. 2003, Varga et al. 2017).

Thioridazine has shown activity against drug-susceptible and resistant forms of Mtb *in vitro* and *ex vivo*, with MICs against Mtb $H_{37}Rv$ ranging between 8 and 15 µg/mL (Amaral and Viveiros 2017). Recent preclinical investigations have demonstrated its *in vivo* efficacies in mono- or combination therapy against Mtb. Van Soolingen et al. demonstrated its efficacy in a BALB/c mouse model at a dose of 32 and 70 mg/kg/day for 2 mon which led to significant reduction in cfu of both susceptible and MDR TB bacilli. In addition, synergistic effects with isoniazid, rifampicin and pyrazinamide were observed (van Soolingen et al. 2010). Another study found that a human equivalent dose of the antipsychotic (25 mg/kg) was well tolerated in BALB/c mice and its accumulation in lung tissue was enhanced compared to serum. Moreover, its co-administration with isoniazid led to modest synergistic effects and decreased emergence of isoniazid-resistant mutants in murine lungs (Dutta et al. 2014). Conversely, an investigation of its

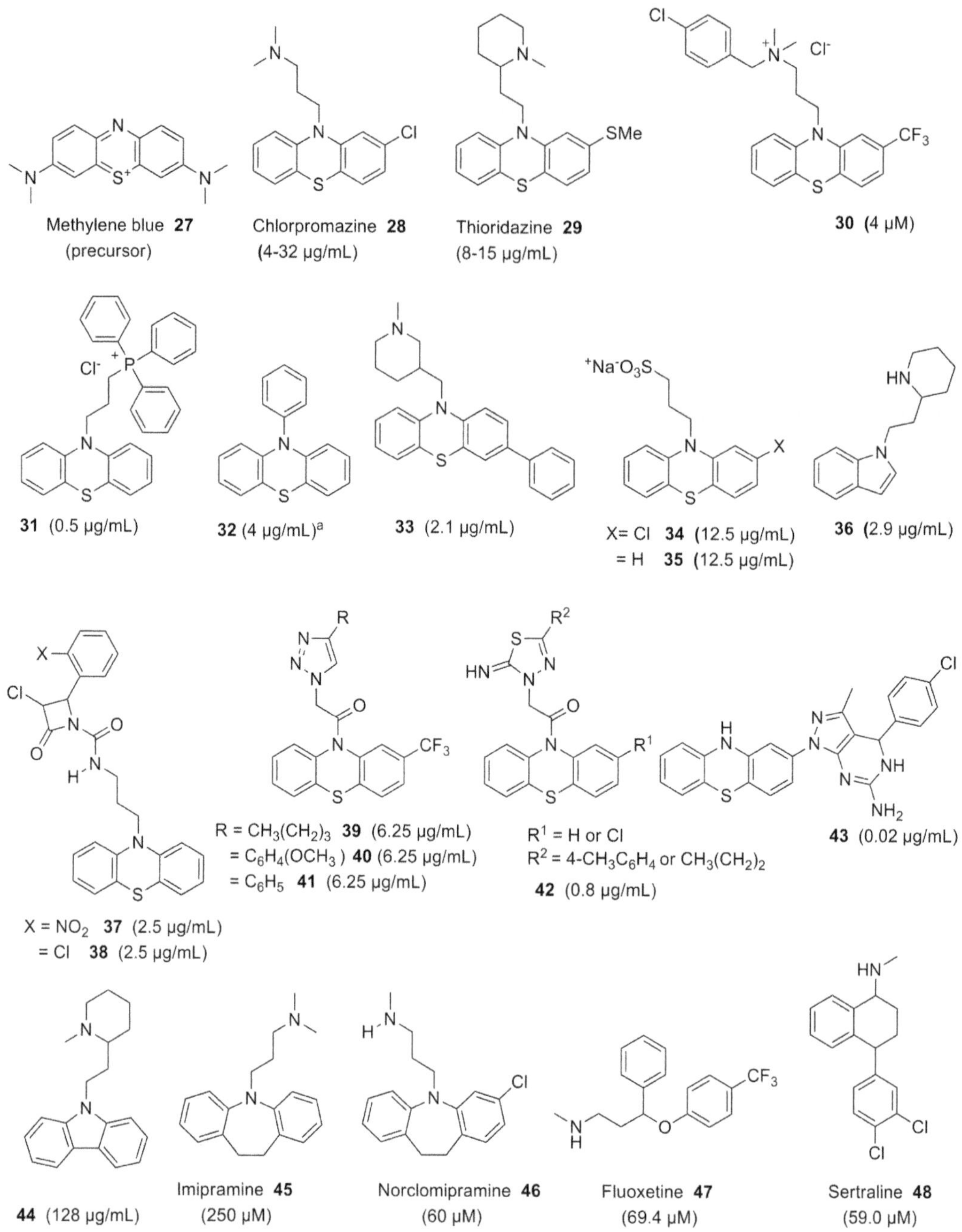

Figure 3. Structures and MICs of antitubercular antipsychotics, antidepressants and phenothiazine analogues [a]MIC$_{90}$.

bactericidal effect in guinea pigs suggested that it has limited efficacy against extracellular bacilli within necrotic granulomas (Dutta et al. 2013). Thioridazine has exhibited therapeutic efficacy against XDR TB in clinical settings with human subjects. A miniature clinical investigation in Buenos Aires (Argentina) reported successful therapy of 10 out 12 XDR TB patients using the antipsychotic in combination with antibiotics which XDR TB is normally resistant to. Also, its use as a salvage drug for XDR TB has been reported in Mumbai (India) (Amaral et al. 2010, Amaral and Viveiros 2012, Udwadia et al. 2011). The ability of Mtb to persist in non-replicating or dormant state presents hurdles to TB therapy. A study by Singh et al. revealed the antitubercular-potentiating effect of thioridazine with first-line drugs, isoniazid and rifampicin, against *in vitro* and murine model of latent Mtb, a finding which further accentuates prospects of phenothiazines for the management of TB (Singh and Sharma 2014).

Biological targets and/or mode of action: Phenothiazines interfere with multiple metabolic pathways that are crucial for the survival and persistence of pathogenic microorganisms (Varga et al. 2017). They show inhibitory effects on calcium-dependent enzyme systems including those catalyzing ATP hydrolysis for cellular energy. Moreover, phenothiazines have the propensity to concentrate in macrophages, an attribute that enhances their effects against phagocytosed bacteria. Inhibition of transport processes for Ca^{2+} or K^+ enhances retention of these ions in the cytoplasm of the macrophage which promotes acidification of the phagolysosome thereby activating cidal effects (Amaral and Molnar 2014, Kristiansen et al. 2007, Martins et al. 2008). It is known that overexpression of bacterial efflux pumps confers resistance to xenobiotics including drugs which are extruded from the periplasm or cytoplasm. Phenothiazines are said to supress the activity of these transporter proteins thereby hindering bacterial drug tolerance (Amaral et al. 2004, Kaatz et al. 2003, Kristiansen et al. 2015). Recent studies have indicated that phenothiazines are inhibitors of Mtb type II NADH:menaquinone oxidoreductase, a key enzyme of the respiratory chain that is implicated in Mtb persistence in dormancy (Bald et al. 2017, Teh et al. 2007, Warman et al. 2013, Yano et al. 2006). Another study revealed that phenothiazines inhibit Mtb RNase P RNA, an endoribonuclease involved in RNA cleavage (Wu et al. 2016). Others showed that thioridazine modifies the cell envelope permeability of Mtb which has implications for drug uptake (de Keijzer et al. 2016).

Potentiating antitubercular effects through structural remodelling: Numerous investigations have underscored the pharmaceutical relevance of phenothiazines. However, there is resistance to their extensive clinical application in non-neuroleptic indications owing to potential onset of adverse effects in addition to inherent neuroleptic effects at clinically relevant concentrations. Thus, many studies embark on structural remodelling experiments that exploit the synthetic tractability of the privileged phenothiazine structure for the discovery of novel therapeutics against Mtb. Phenothiazines are markedly promiscuous drugs that bind to a myriad of receptor types in different tissues. Given that they are potent dopamine antagonists, reducing their neuroleptic potential by deviating from the minimum structural requirements for antipsychotic activity has been a key remodelling strategy.

A quaternization strategy that targeted the distal amine moiety of trifluoperazine yielded an analogue **30** that inhibited non-replicating and actively growing Mtb $H_{37}Rv$ (MIC 4 µM) with no toxicity against Vero cells (Figure 3) (Bate et al. 2007). Since the presence of a protonatable amine species is known to favour CNS activity of phenothiazines, quaternized analogues could exhibit reduced neuroleptic potential. Employing a similar approach, Dunn et al. designed promazine analogues by incorporating a known intracellular delivery functionality, alkyl-triphenylphosphonium cation, to improve concentration and potency at the mycobacterial membrane. The antitubercular lead **31** (MIC 0.5 µg/mL) was reported to target NADH oxidation and oxygen consumption in a manner similar to native phenothiazines (Figure 3) (Dunn et al. 2014). Others identified an antitubercular promazine analogue **32** lacking the characteristic alkylamino side chain (Figure 3). The analogue displayed an MIC_{90} of 4 µg/mL and was less toxic to mammalian cells ($CC_{50} > 32$ µg/mL) in comparison to chlorpromazine (CC_{50} 8 µg/mL) (He et al. 2015). Madrid and co-workers demonstrated that it is possible to reduce the phenothiazine binding affinity for serotonin and dopamine receptors through structural remodelling and still retain antitubercular efficacy. The investigation led to the identification of a phenyl-substituted derivative **33** that exhibited an MIC of 2.1 µg/mL and showed reduced neuroleptic potential (Figure 3) (Madrid et al. 2007). Based on the same supposition, another study designed *N*-alkylsulfonates of phenothiazines (**34** and **35**) that displayed negligible dopamine and serotonin receptor binding activity whilst considerable *in vitro* and *ex vivo* antitubercular efficacies were retained (Figure 3). The active compounds (MIC 12.5 µg/mL) displayed no cytotoxicity in infected primary bone marrow-derived macrophages and also exhibited 40–60% inhibition of intracellular Mtb. Contrary to the study by Madrid et al. which reported phenothiazine derivatives with some degree of hydrophobicity, the remodelling strategy in this case relied on increasing polarity and altering charge at a critical receptor recognition site. Since the alkylamino species of phenothiazines is known to acquire a positive charge at physiological pH, substitution with an alkylsulfonate moiety not only imparts aqueous solubility but it is expected to exist as a negatively charged species (Salie et al. 2014).

More recently, Scalacci et al. generated distinctive series of thioridazine analogues by substitution of characteristic structural features including the tricyclic phenothiazine chromophore and piperidine moiety. The small library was first evaluated against a panel of non-pathogenic mycobacterium strains (*Mycobacterium smegmatis* mc^2155, *Mycobacterium bovis* BCG and Mtb mc^27000) which aided in triaging promising chemical entities for screening against Mtb $H_{37}Rv$, drug-susceptible CF73 clinical isolate and MDR clinical isolates (CF104 and CF81). This led to the identification of an indole bearing a demethylated piperidine moiety **36** that was more potent (Mtb $H_{37}Rv$ MIC 2.9 µg/mL, MRC-5 IC_{50} 15 µg/mL) and less toxic than thioridazine (MIC 10 µg/mL, IC_{50} 8.2 µg/mL) (Figure 3) (Scalacci et al. 2017).

Molecular hybridization of pharmacophoric subunits of phenothiazines and other known antibacterial structural motifs is another approach that has been employed to enhance antitubercular effects of phenothiazine drugs. A study by Sharma et al. identified 2-azetidinone promazine hybrids (**37** and **38**) that displayed an MIC of 2.5 µg/mL against Mtb $H_{37}Rv$ (Figure 3). Moreover, active compounds exhibited notable antifungal activity and activity against other bacteria such as *Escherichia coli* and *Staphylococcus aureus* (Sharma et al. 2012). Others reported hybrids of trifluoperazine and antitubercular clinical candidate I-A09 that were achieved using click chemistry. Three hybrids **39–41** showed significant activity (MIC 6.25 µg/mL) against Mtb $H_{37}Rv$ with selectivity index greater than 10 (Figure 3) (Addla et al. 2014). Ramprasad et al. reported antitubercular 1,3,4-thiadiazole phenothiazine hybrids which were non-toxic to a normal Vero cell line, the most active hybrid **42** displayed an MIC of 0.8 µg/mL (Figure 3). Moreover, delineation of structure-activity relationship revealed that the presence of alkyl or substituted phenyl moieties on the 1,3,4-thiadiazole ring enhanced antimycobacterial effects. Also, docking studies demonstrated strong π-π stacking interactions of active chemical entities with InhA and CYP121 (Ramprasad et al. 2015). Another study adapted a Biginelli multicomponent reaction to generate a series of pyrimidine derivatives bearing a phenothiazine nucleus, their evaluation against Mtb $H_{37}Rv$ led to the identification of a derivative **43** with pronounced *in vitro* activity (MIC 0.02 µg/mL), more potent than isoniazid (MIC 0.03 µg/mL) (Figure 3) (Siddiqui et al. 2014). In other reports, hybridization of thioridazine with a carbazole scaffold resulted in hybrid **44** with poor antimycobacterial activity (MIC 128 µg/mL) against Mtb $H_{37}Rv$ (Figure 3). However, the carbazole hybrid displayed a higher inhibitory activity of ethidium bromide (EtBr) efflux and less cytotoxicity in comparison to thioridazine, a known efflux pump inhibitor. Synergistic effects with isoniazid, rifampicin, amikacin and ofloxacin were also observed (Pieroni et al. 2015).

Tricyclic antidepressants and selective serotonin reuptake inhibitors: Antidepressant drugs are the mainstay for major depressive disorder and elicit their effects through blocking the reuptake of serotonin as well as norepinephrine. The majority of these antidepressants bear structural resemblance to phenothiazines (Krystal 2011). Godbole et al. docked libraries of FDA approved drugs into the homology model for Mtb topoisomerase I, an enzyme responsible for maintaining genome topology during DNA replication and transcription. From this *in silico* screening, compounds with a favourable docking score including imipramine **45** and norclomipramine **46** were selected for further evaluation against Mtb (Figure 3). Both drugs displayed some antimycobacterial activity against Mtb (MIC 250 µM and 60 µM, respectively) and also inhibitory effects against the topoisomerase enzyme. Moreover, imipramine acted synergistically with moxifloxacin, a well-known type II topoisomerase inhibitor (Godbole et al. 2015). The antitubercular effects of selective reuptake inhibitors, fluoxetine **47** (MIC 69.4 µM) and sertraline **48** (MIC 59.0 µM), have also been demonstrated (Figure 3). Both antidepressants displayed a dose-dependent growth restriction of Mtb after 72 hr treatment in resting primary murine macrophages. The study also showed that accumulation of protonatable forms of the drugs in macrophages is partially pH-dependent (Schump et al. 2017).

Recent formulation strategies: Another strategy to improve the effectiveness of drugs is through formulation or drug delivery approaches by addressing liabilities such as poor ADME properties and dose-related toxicities. Targeted pulmonary delivery by routes such as inhalation of dry powder drug formulations is an appealing strategy for TB therapy that offers advantages such as reduced dosing frequency and less systemic side effects. Also, using this pulmonary route minimizes drug degradation in the gut or drug biotransformation by first-pass metabolism in the liver (Patil and Sarasija 2012). A study by Parumasivam et al. assessed the *in vitro* aerosol performance, storage stability and *in vitro* antimycobacterial activities of novel inhalable powders composed of thioridazine and rifapentine, an antitubercular drug that has attracted research for pulmonary delivery. Both powders showed good aerosol performance and potent antimycobacterial activity against Mtb H_{37}Rv and Mtb H_{37}Ra. Moreover, the formulation of amorphous thioridazine and crystalline rifapentine was chemically more stable than that consisting of both drugs in an amorphous form (Parumasivam et al. 2016b). Others reported thioridazine encapsulated in biodegradable poly(lactic-*co*-glycolic) acid nanoparticles which showed modest bactericidal activity against Mtb and *M. bovis* BCG in macrophages. Compared with the free form, nanoparticle-loaded thioridazine was non-toxic in macrophages and zebrafish embryos and also potentiated rifampicin effects in a zebrafish model of TB (Vibe et al. 2015).

Antitubercular effects of non-steroidal anti-inflammatory drugs

Non-steroidal anti-inflammatory drugs (NSAIDs) are analgesic, anti-inflammatory and antipyretic medications that are used extensively worldwide. NSAIDs elicit their effects primarily via a blockade of cyclooxygenase enzymes, COX-1 and COX-2, which catalyze the formation of prostaglandins and other prostanoids. Classical NSAIDs inhibit both enzymes and are associated with adverse gastrointestinal effects when administered chronically. In contrast, selective COX-2 inhibitors have a reduced risk of gastric irritation but there are concerns over potential cardiovascular toxicity (Ong et al. 2007, Maitra et al. 2016).

NSAIDs have shown great potential as antitubercular agents and also as adjunctive therapy of TB to alleviate deleterious host inflammatory responses (Kroesen et al. 2017, Maitra et al. 2016). The antibacterial properties of anti-inflammatory drug diclofenac **49** against pathogenic microorganisms including *S. aureus*, *E. coli* and Mtb have long been established (Figure 4) (Mazumdar et al. 2009). *In vitro* and *in vivo* inhibitory effects of the NSAID have been shown against both drug-sensitive and drug-resistant clinical isolates of Mtb (Kumar et al. 2007, Dutta et al. 2004). Kumar et al. showed that diclofenac exhibits *in vitro* activity against Mtb H_{37}Rv (MIC 10 µg/mL) and was bactericidal at a concentration four times its MIC. The drug also inhibited MDR Mtb clinical strains, albeit at a higher concentration (25 µg/mL). Moreover, diclofenac acted synergistically with streptomycin *in vitro* (MIC lowered from 2 µg/mL to 0.25 µg/mL at 2.5 µg/mL diclofenac) and *in vivo* at a dose of 10 µg/g/day and 150 µg/g/day streptomycin (Kumar et al.

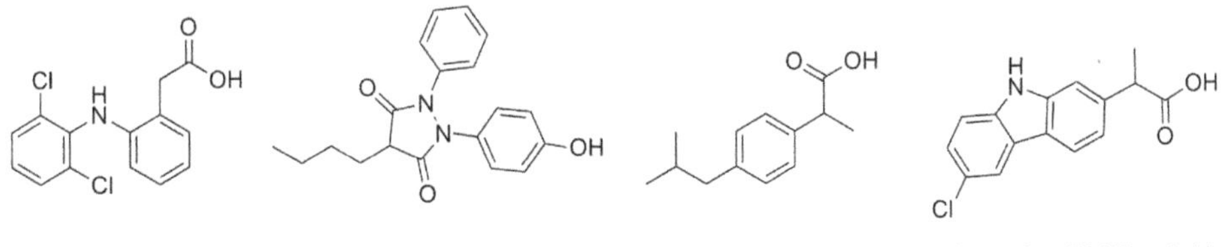

Diclofenac **49** (10 µg/mL) Oxyphenbutazone **50** (12.5 µM) Ibuprofen **51** (75 µg/mL) Carprofen **52** (40 µg/mL)

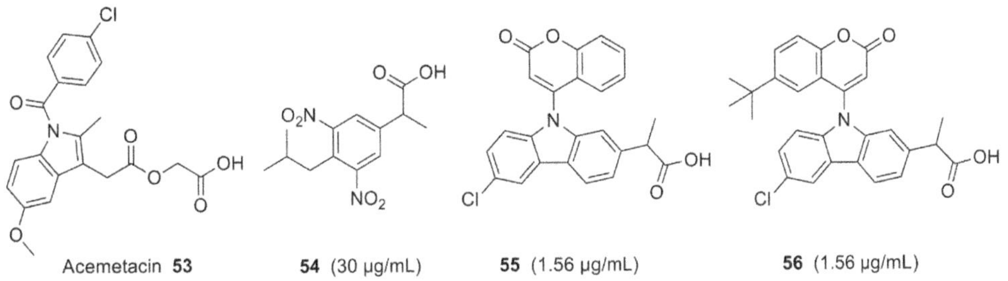

Acemetacin **53**   **54** (30 µg/mL)   **55** (1.56 µg/mL)   **56** (1.56 µg/mL)

Figure 4. Structures and MICs of antitubercular NSAID and their analogues.

2007). In another study, oxyphenbutazone **50** restricted the growth of non-replicating Mtb by 100% at 12.5 μM (Figure 4). The study further reported 4-hydroxylation of oxyphenbutazone fostered by mild acidity and reactive nitrogen intermediates under conditions that impose non-replication. The hydroxylated form was equipotent to oxyphenbutazone in inhibiting non-replicating Mtb but also displayed augmented cidal activity against replicating (25 μM) and drug-resistant Mtb. Furthermore, the modified form increased the sensitivity of Mtb to oxidants and exogenous antimicrobials (Gold et al. 2012). Guzman et al. evaluated the inhibitory effects of ibuprofen **51** and related 2-arylpropanoic acids against Mtb using a HT-SPOTi whole cell phenotypic assay. Inhibitory activity was observed against susceptible and multidrug-resistant Mtb clinical isolates as well as stationary phase *M. bovis* BCG. Ibuprofen and carprofen **52** exhibited inhibitory effects against MDR Mtb clinical isolates with MICs ranging between 20 and 50 μg/mL comparable to those obtained against $H_{37}Rv$ strain (75 and 40 μg/mL, respectively) (Figure 4) (Guzman et al. 2013).

Others reported the anti-inflammatory effects of ibuprofen in the treatment of Mtb-infected C3HeB/FeJ mice, a decrease in the number and size of lung lesions was evident post-treatment (Vilaplana et al. 2013). More recently, another NSAID, acemetacin **53**, and other FDA-approved drugs were reported to enhance the anti-persister activity of pyrazinamide, a first-line antitubercular agent with a requisite role in shortening TB therapy duration and minimizing relapse cases (Figure 4) (Niu et al. 2017).

Antitubercular activity of compounds bearing NSAID structural motifs: Guzman et al. designed and synthesized chemical entities using ibuprofen scaffold as a template for structural modifications including esterification, nitration and amide formation. A 3,5-dinitro-ibuprofen derivative **54** displayed more potent activity (MIC 30 μg/mL) against Mtb $H_{37}Rv$ than the parent ibuprofen and comparable activity against MDR Mtb clinical isolates (Figure 4) (Guzman et al. 2013). A more recent study inspired by diverse biological properties of coumarin and carbazole scaffolds generated a series of molecular hybrids through multi-step synthesis. The hybrids exhibited MICs against Mtb $H_{37}Rv$ in the range 1.56–50 μg/mL. Two hybrids **55** and **56** displayed *in vitro* antimycobacterial activity (MIC 1.56 μg/mL) more potent than standard antitubercular drugs pyrazinamide (3.125 μg/mL) and streptomycin (6.25 μg/mL) (Figure 4) (Pattanashetty et al. 2017).

Antitubercular effects of antihypertensives

Antihypertensive therapy aims to mitigate adverse cardiovascular events associated with high blood pressure such as stroke and myocardial infarction. Antihypertensives are categorized into various classes including beta-blockers, angiotensin-converting enzyme (ACE) inhibitors, calcium channel blockers, angiotensin-receptor blockers (ARBs) and diuretics (Aronow 2012). A number of cardiovascular agents including amlodipine **57**, dobutamine **58** and nifedipine **59** exhibit promising antimicrobial properties against a range of pathogenic microorganisms (Figure 5) (Mazumdar et al. 2010). Among calcium-channel blockers, verapamil **60**, a known mycobacterial efflux pump inhibitor with antitubercular-potentiating effects, holds great potential as adjunctive therapy of TB (Figure 5).

A recent study by Gupta et al. reported the ability of verapamil to sensitize both susceptible and drug-resistant clinical isolates of Mtb to bedaquiline and clofazimine (Gupta et al. 2014). A related study by the same group later demonstrated that at subinhibitory doses of bedaquiline, the adjunctive use of verapamil could augment the bactericidal activity of bedaquiline against Mtb in an *in vivo* mouse model, a finding which holds beneficial implications for TB therapy duration and dose-related issues (Gupta et al. 2015). Around the same time, findings reported by Adams et al. suggested that verapamil has inhibitory effects on Mtb macrophage-induced tolerance thereby potentiating the activity of antitubercular drugs including bedaquiline and moxifloxacin (Adams et al. 2014). More studies continue to emerge supporting the body of work that suggests antihypertensives, particularly verapamil, as antitubercular-potentiating adjuncts whose effects are widely attributed to inhibition of efflux pumps (Machado et al. 2016, Juarez et al. 2016, Jang et al. 2017). More recently, Chen et al. provided an alternate mechanistic basis for the potentiation of antitubercular agents by verapamil. Findings from the study suggested that verapamil disrupts membrane function and induces a membrane stress response in a manner that is similar to known membrane-targeting drugs (Chen et al. 2018).

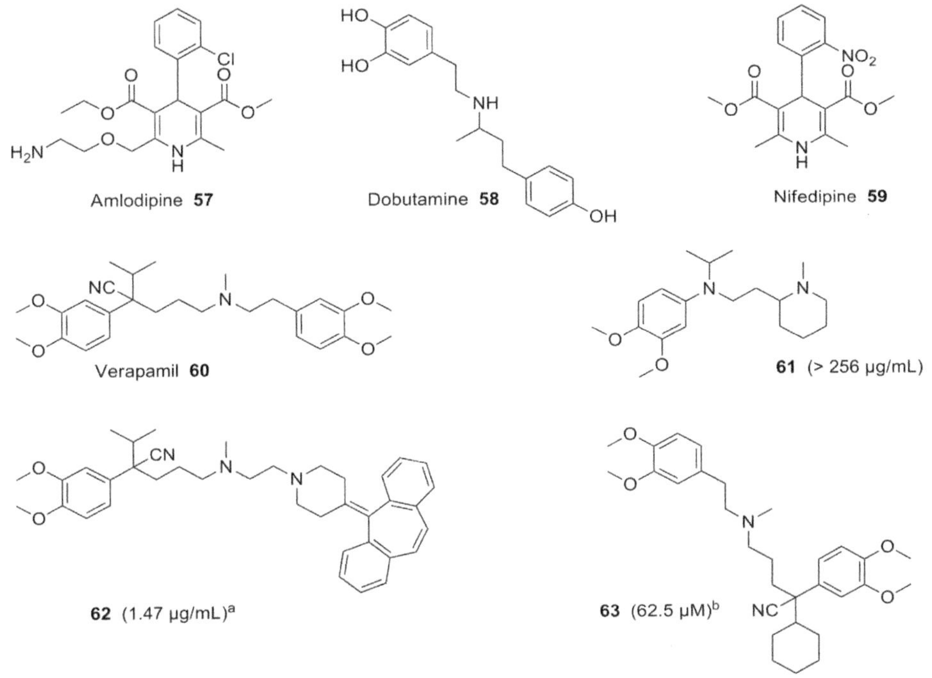

Figure 5. Examples of antimicrobial antihypertensives and MICs of antitubercular verapamil analogues [a]MIC_{90} [b]MIC_{99}.

Antitubercular activity of verapamil analogues: There is a growing interest in the rational design and synthesis of efflux pump inhibitors as a means to tackle Mtb drug resistance by reducing tolerance to already established drugs. Pieroni et al. reported verapamil and thioridazine hybrids and their evaluation for antimycobacterial and efflux inhibitory activities. Although some verapamil analogues displayed significantly poor antibacterial effects (MIC > 256 µg/mL) against Mtb *in vitro* and *ex vivo*, they showed considerable activity against EtBr efflux. A verapamil analogue **61** displayed an efflux inhibitory effect (RFF 0.84 ± 0.02) that was more potent than thioridazine (RFF 0.27 ± 0.02) but not verapamil (RFF 1.94 ± 0.005), RFF-relative final fluorescence based on accumulation of EtBr at 0.5 µg/mL (Figure 5) (Pieroni et al. 2015). Employing a similar approach, others designed a series of hybrids via fusion of verapamil substructure with various structural motifs. Hybrids were evaluated for antimycobacterial effects against Mtb and efflux pump inhibition activity. In addition to inhibitory effects against EtBr efflux, some hybrids showed intrinsic antimycobacterial activity, *ex vivo* activity as well as synergistic effects with first-line antitubercular drugs. A hybrid **62** with an MIC_{90} of 1.47 µg/mL displayed more than 40% inhibition of Mtb growth in macrophages at 12.5 µg/mL and potentiated rifampicin as well as isoniazid (Figure 5). It also showed inhibitory effects against EtBr efflux with an increase in fluorescence superior to that of verapamil (Kumar et al. 2016). Another study demonstrated antitubercular-potentiating effects as well as inhibitory effects of verapamil analogues against intracellular Mtb replication and EtBr efflux.

The most active analogue **63** (MIC_{99} 62.5 µM) displayed inhibitory effects against mycobacterial efflux equipotent to verapamil and also enhanced activity of isoniazid and rifampicin against intracellular Mtb (Figure 5). In contrast to verapamil and norverapamil (an N-demethylated form of verapamil), the analogue did not interfere with proliferation of Mtb-specific T cells which act against the progression of TB (Abate et al. 2016).

Recent formulation approaches: Efflux pump inhibitors hold great promise as antitubercular-potentiating agents that could circumvent Mtb drug resistance mechanisms. The efflux pump inhibitor verapamil is known to exhibit drug-drug interactions with rifamycins. Rifamycins such as rifampicin and rifapentine induce the hepatic CYP-3A4 enzyme system that metabolizes verapamil (Gupta et al. 2013). Since oral co-administration of verapamil with rifamycins leads to poor bioavailability, some studies have sought other routes of administration. In one particular study, an inhalable dry powder composed of amorphous verapamil and crystalline rifapentine with L-leucine as an excipient showed suitable properties for aerosol delivery with a respirable fraction greater than 70%. The drug combination displayed inhibitory effects against Mtb $H_{37}Rv$ and Mtb $H_{37}Ra$ that were comparable to rifapentine alone, enhanced inhibition of Mtb $H_{37}Ra$ growth in macrophages relative to either drug alone and also showed acceptable IC_{50} (62.5 µg/mL) on THP-1 and A549 cell lines. Moreover, anhydrous packaging conditions proved necessary for long-term storage stability (Parumasivam et al. 2016a).

Antitubercular effects of anticancer agents

Cancer is characterized by the disruption of mechanisms that regulate the normal functioning of the cell cycle. Drug classes in clinical use for cancer chemotherapy include alkylating agents, antimetabolites, antitumour antibiotics, topoisomerase inhibitors, mitotic inhibitors and corticosteroids. Cancer treatment is associated with a plethora of side effects including bone marrow suppression, hair loss and gastrointestinal tract lesions due to the inability of anticancer drugs to differentiate between healthy cells and tumour cells (Nussbaumer et al. 2011, Stewart et al. 2003).

Various anticancer agents have shown promising antibacterial effects. A recent study by Napier et al. demonstrated the antitubercular effects of imatinib **64**, an inhibitor of tyrosine kinases approved as a therapeutic for chronic myelogenous leukemia and other cancers (Figure 6). The study showed that imatinib reduces intracellular survival of Mtb in macrophages at 10 µM and bacterial load in mice infected with Mtb. Its synergistic effects with rifampicin were also reported. Moreover, this study also implicated host tyrosine kinases in entry and intracellular survival of mycobacteria including Mtb (Napier et al. 2011). Olakanmi et al. explored the antibacterial effects of gallium nitrate **65** against Mtb (Figure 6).

The study was based on the premise that disruption of iron acquisition is detrimental to metabolism and growth of Mtb, which has previously been correlated to antitubercular effects of gallium. To cope with iron scarcity, pathogenic microorganisms have developed efficient iron-uptake systems which involve the

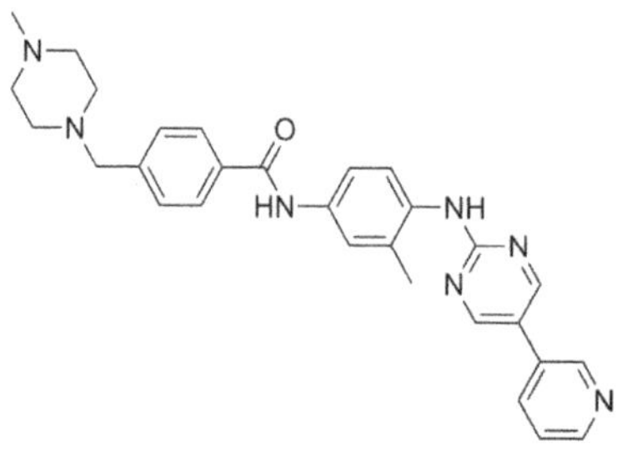

Imatinib **64** (10 µM) 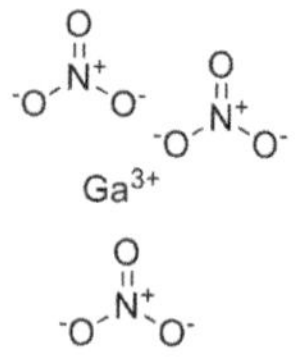   Gallium nitrate **65** (1.25-2.5 µM)[a] 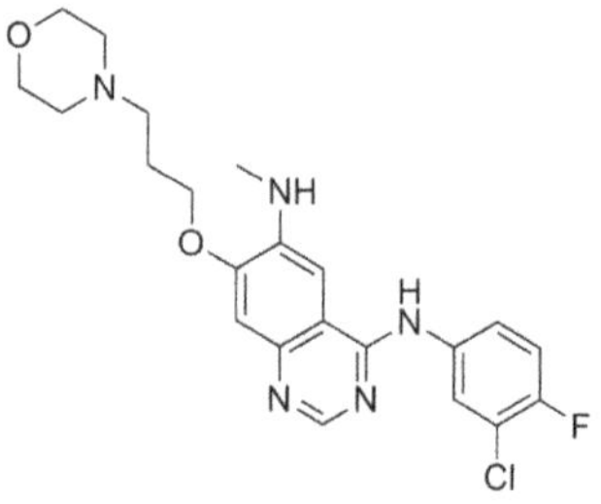   Gefitinib **66** (5 µM)[b]

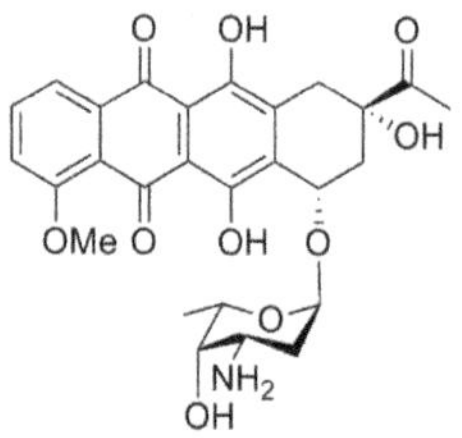

Daunorubicin **67** (1.25 µM) 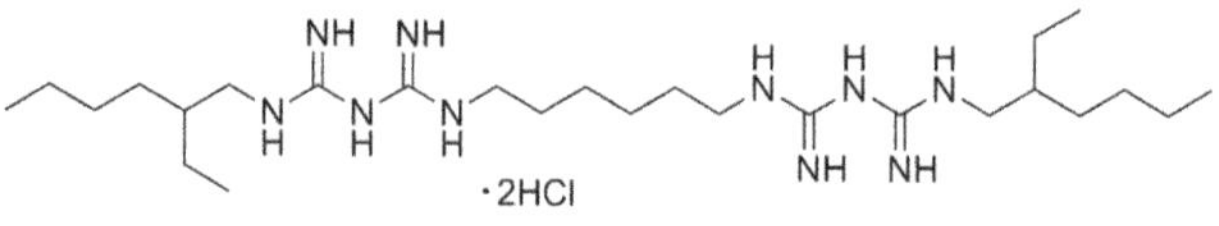   Bis-biguanide dihydrochloride **68** (0.05 µg/mL)

Figure 6. Structures and MICs of anticancer agents with antitubercular activity [a]MIC_{50} in the presence of 2 µM Fe [b]Concentration that inhibited Mtb growth in macrophages.

production of natural chelators such as siderophores. The study exploited the inability of biological systems to distinguish between Fe^{3+} from Ga^{3+} which displays binding affinity for ferric iron-binding proteins and chelators. In contrast to Fe^{3+}, Ga^{3+} is not reducible under physiological conditions; therefore its insertion at active sites of iron-dependent enzymes may block their activity. It has been previously shown that gallium nitrate has potent inhibitory effects (MIC_{50} 1.25–2.5 µM) against Mtb in the presence of 2 µM iron; however, its effects were restricted when iron was in excess. Also gallium inhibited Mtb growth within cultured human macrophages (Olakanmi et al. 2000). A subsequent investigation demonstrated that gallium is efficacious *in vivo* in a SCID or BALB/c mouse Mtb infection model. Moreover, gallium inhibited the activity of Mtb iron-dependent enzymes ribonucleotide reductase (crucial for DNA synthesis) and acotinase (involved in ATP production) (Olakanmi et al. 2013). Other authors reported the antitubercular efficacy of gefitinib **66**, an epidermal growth factor receptor inhibitor that is used for non-small cell lung cancer therapy (Figure 6). Gefitinib restricted growth of Mtb in both J774 murine macrophages and primary mouse bone marrow-derived macrophages at a concentration of 5 µM. Moreover, gefitinib inhibited bacterial replication in the lungs of Mtb-infected mice at a dose of 100 mg/kg/day for 6 d (Stanley et al. 2014). Gajadeera et al. investigated antitubercular effects of DNA intercalators including anthracyclines such as daunorubicin **67** which exhibited pronounced activity (Figure 6). Daunorubicin exhibited potent inhibition of *in vitro* growth of Mtb (MIC 1.25 µM) relative to other anthracyclines and also inhibited Mtb primase DnaG which is crucial for chromosomal DNA replication and cell division (Gajadeera et al. 2015). Another anticancer drug, bis-biguanide dihydrochloride **68**, has been shown to restrict extracellular and intracellular growth of *M. Smegmatis* and *M. bovis* BCG (Figure 6). The anticancer agent has also shown high potency against clinically isolated Mtb (MIC 0.05 µg/mL) and MDR TB strains ($\geq$ 0.05 µg/mL). Moreover, it reduced bacillary burden in the lung and spleen of Mtb-infected mice and also attenuated Mtb-induced lesions (Shen et al. 2016).

Non-antibiotics repositioned against various WHO-listed NTDs

Historically, NTDs prioritized by the WHO are associated with extreme paucity in terms of funded research and development and also policy and control measures. The socioeconomic and health burden of these diseases weighs heavily on poverty-stricken populations and belligerent nations in tropical regions where they thrive best. The treatment and prophylaxis of many NTDs rely solely on drugs. Although many of these diseases are amenable to chemotherapy, the provision of efficacious, safe and affordable medicines is still lacking (WHO 2017b). The majority of drugs that are available are rendered ineffective by antimicrobial resistance mechanisms and the monetary incentive for developing new ones is significantly low. Repositioning approaches thus carry great appeal for rejuvenating drug pipelines against NTDs.

Native phenothiazines and analogues have shown great promise as potential unconventional agents against NTDs with reported antileishmanial, antiplasmodial, antischistosomal and antitrypanosomal effects (Chan et al. 1998, Go 2003, Khan et al. 2000, Thanacoody 2007) More recently, Simanjuntak et al. have demonstrated the *in vitro* and *in vivo* efficacy of prochlorperazine **69**, an antiemetic phenothiazine drug, against dengue virus infection and the mode of action is said to implicate a dopamine D2 receptor and clathrin-associated mechanisms (Figure 7) (Simanjuntak et al. 2015). Another study has explored the effect of thioridazine for *in vivo* therapy of *Trypanosoma cruzi* infection which resulted in reduced abnormalities and improved survival rates of infected mice. Thioridazine is also reported to inhibit trypanothione reductase irreversibly, an enzyme crucial for maintaining redox balance in trypanosomatids (Lo Presti et al. 2015, Vazquez et al. 2017). Efficacies of tricyclic antidepressants (clomipramine **70** and amitriptyline **71**) and selective serotonin reuptake inhibitors (sertraline and paroxetine **72**) against human African trypanosomiasis (HAT) have also been previously demonstrated (Figure 7). Additionally, clomipramine, an inhibitor of trypanothione reductase, has also displayed antichagasic effects and was found to reduce myocardial fibrosis in *T. cruzi*-infected mice (Ferreira and Andricopulo 2016). Imipramine, also a trypanothione reductase inhibitor, and ketanserin **73** showed inhibitory effects against *Leishmania donovani* (Figure 7). Ketanserin is said to block 3-hydroxy-3-methylglutaryl coenzyme A reductase of *L. donovani*, an enzyme implicated in ergosterol biosynthetic pathway (Nagle et al. 2014, Singh et al. 2014).

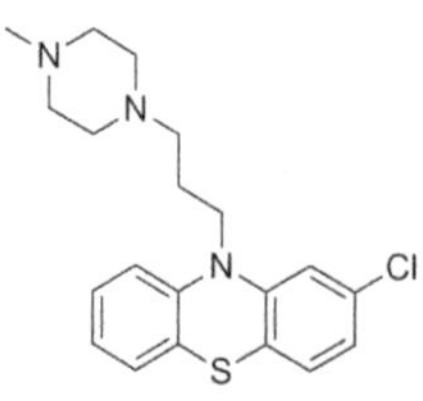

Prochlorperazine **69**
(Dengue)

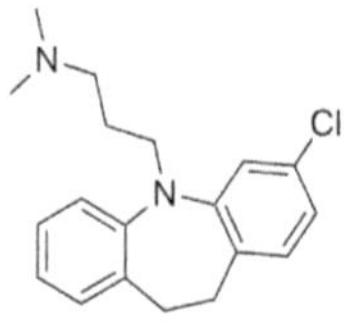

Clomipramine **70**
(HAT, Chagas disease)

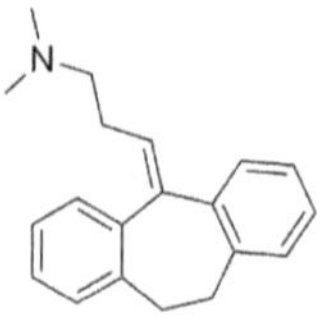

Amitriptyline **71**
(HAT)

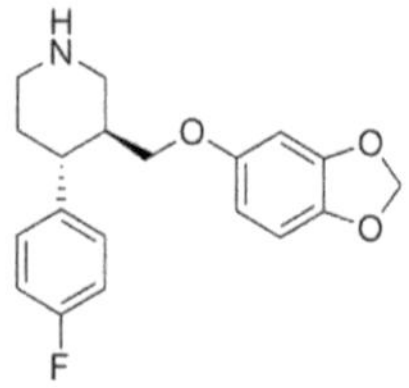

Paroxetine **72**
(HAT)

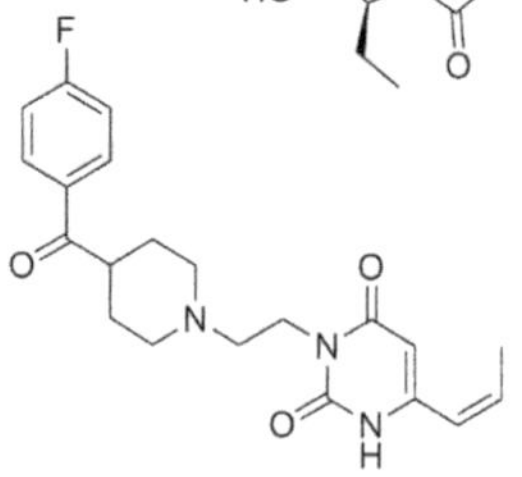

Ketanserin **73**
(Leishmaniasis)

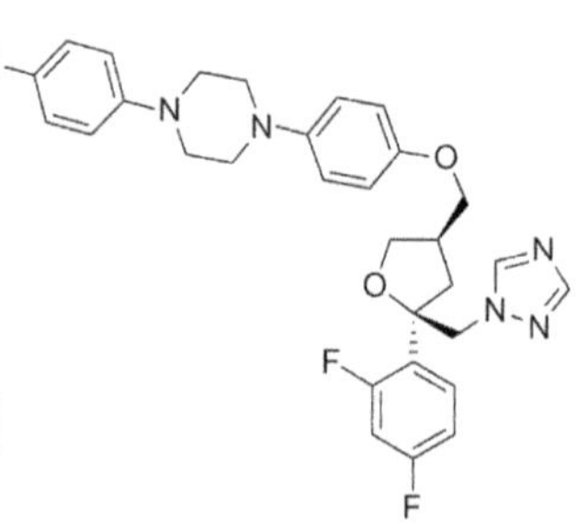

Posaconazole **74** (antifungal drug)
(Chagas disease)

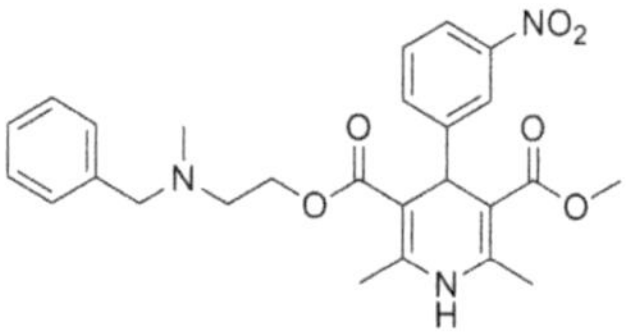

Nircadipine **75**
(Schistosomiasis)

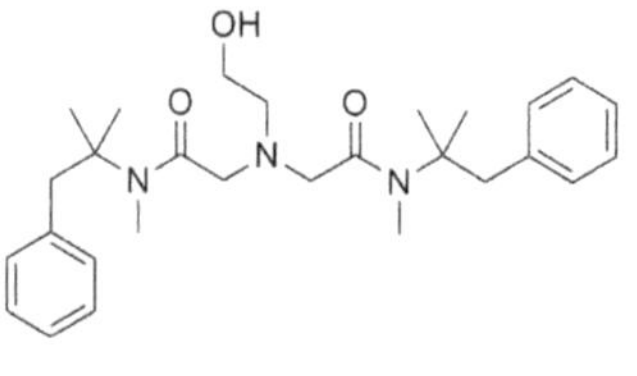

Oxethazaine **76**
(Schistosomiasis)

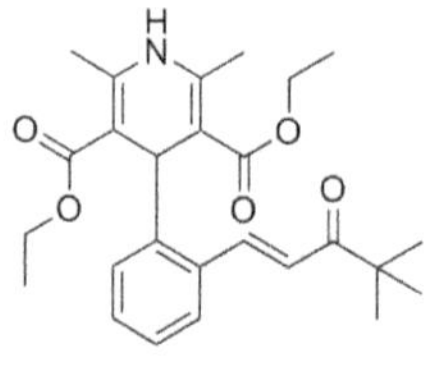

Lacidpine **77**
(Leishmaniasis)

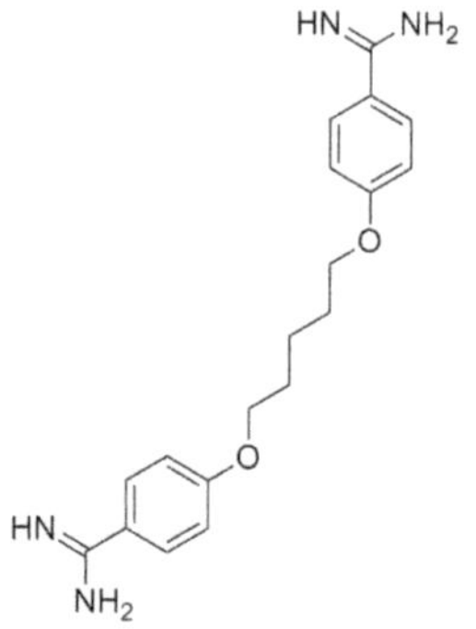

Pentamidine **78**
(antitrypanosomal drug)

Figure 7. Examples of non-antibiotics repositioned against NTDs that are prioritized by the WHO.

Antihypertensives have also been reported in drug repositioning approaches for the treatment of NTDs. Amlodipine, a calcium antagonist with known antibacterial effects against Gram-positive and Gram-negative bacteria, has shown inhibitory effects against mammalian stage *T. cruzi* parasites. Also, its combination with posaconazole **74** (an antifungal drug) proved effective at lowering parasitemia in *T. cruzi*-infected mice (Figure 7) (Mazumdar et al. 2010, Planer et al. 2014).

The antiparasitic activity of another calcium antagonist nicardipine **75** and local anaesthetic oxethazaine **76** have been shown against *Schistosoma mansoni* (Figure 7) (Panic et al. 2015). Others have reported the antileishmanial activities of amlodipine and lacidipine **77** *in vitro* and also in BALB/c mice when administered orally (Figure 7) (Palit and Ali 2008). Additionally, amlodipine has acted synergistically with pentamidine **78** and other drugs against visceral leishmaniasis (Figure 7) (Reimao and Tempone 2011).

Eflornithine **79** and miltefosine **80** are currently in clinical use for the treatment of HAT and visceral leishmaniasis, respectively, but were originally developed as anticancer agents (Figure 8) (Nagle et al. 2014).

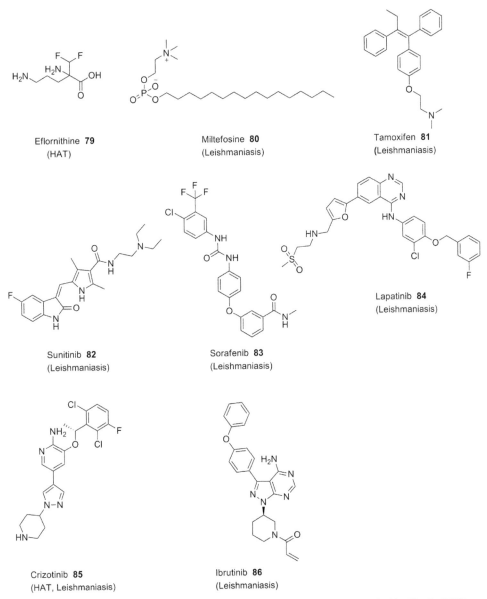

Figure 8. Further examples of non-antibiotics repositioned against NTDs that are prioritized by the WHO.

Anticancer tamoxifen **81** has shown efficacy against visceral and cutaneous leishmaniasis in rodent models (Figure 8) (Miguel et al. 2009). Sanderson et al. have recently evaluated anticancer protein kinase inhibitors against various Leishmania species. Some of the kinase inhibitors including sunitinib **82**, sorafenib **83** and lapatinib **84** displayed potent activity against *L. donovani* amastigotes in cultured murine macrophages, comparable to that of miltefosine (Figure 8) (Sanderson et al. 2017). Others found that *in vitro* imatinib treatment significantly changes the morphology and physiology of adult schistosomes. Also, imatinib blocked schistosomal tyrosine kinases (Buro et al. 2014). Several other human kinase inhibitors including crizotinib **85** (an anticancer agent used for non-small cell lung carcinoma) and ibrutinib **86** (anticancer agent in use for the treatment of mantle cell lymphoma and lymphoid leukemia) have shown promising prospects for drug development against trypanosomatid diseases (Figure 8) (Dichiara et al. 2017).

Overview and Perspectives

Decades on since TB was declared a health emergency by the WHO, the global scenario remains gravely dire. Even more worrisome, the burden of TB is felt inordinately among marginalized populations in low-income regions with an inadequacy of resources for the containment of this scourge. The high burden of TB is further exacerbated by the upsurge in antimicrobial resistance and co-epidemics such as HIV. Although existing antibiotic therapies have provided some relief over the years, their overuse and misuse including counterfeit or poor quality antibiotics has contributed largely to the propagation of antimicrobial resistance. Hence, innovative and intensified drug discovery efforts are essential to launch novel and efficacious drugs that represent new chemical scaffolds or previously unexplored mechanisms of action against Mtb. *De novo* drug discovery approaches are faced with bottlenecks including exorbitant research costs and high attrition rates. Newly developed bedaquiline and delamanid have only recently been introduced for TB therapy, more than half a century since the discovery of 'blockbuster antibiotics'. Given that, repositioning strategies are now increasingly utilized for replenishing antibiotic drug pipelines against TB. Repositioned antibiotics (e.g., clofazimine, linezolid, fluoroquinolones, etc.) currently under clinical development evince the value of such strategies and have shown promise for shortening treatment regimens for MDRTB and XDRTB. Arguably, with threatening antimicrobial resistance, the long term utility of these newly repositioned antibiotics may suffer limitations given their history of extensive application in the management of other microbial infections. On the other hand, repositioned non-antibiotics which are originally indicated for non-infectious diseases hold great potential in the context of diversifying the chemical space occupied by existing antitubercular drugs or possibly identifying unexplored drug targets to circumvent resistance mechanisms. A growing body of evidence suggests that such drugs have direct antimycobacterial efficacies and/or antitubercular-potentiating effects which have been demonstrated extracellularly, intracellularly and also in animal models. Among the non-antibiotics discussed in this chapter including NSAIDs, neuroleptics, antihypertensives and anticancer agents, antipsychotic phenothiazines take centre stage. Of note, thioridazine augments the effects of standard antitubercular drugs and also exhibits multiple mechanisms of action which have implications for Mtb drug tolerance. Additionally, this milder phenothiazine has also shown encouraging therapeutic prospects for combination therapy of XDR TB in clinical settings. Moreover, thioridazine and antihypertensive verapamil have displayed promising sensitizing effects against Mtb through inhibition of bacterial efflux pumps. The adjunctive use of these non-antibiotics particularly for host-directed TB therapy, especially in the case of NSAIDs, also shows great promise for improving therapy outcomes.

Although drug repositioning strategies offer significant benefits, they are not devoid of drawbacks. Repositioning approaches rely on the fact that clinically approved drugs carry immense privilege as they have undergone rigorous testing in human subjects. Reliance on previously validated data could avoid high costs incurred during drug development processes and narrow the chances of attrition in advanced clinical studies. Additionally, drugs that are off-patent and inexpensive may offer even more benefits for diseases endemic in resource-poor settings. Apart from intellectual property issues, one drawback of repositioning strategies is inherent effects of repositioned drugs which may become undesirable side effects in diseases of interest. Hence, structural remodelling is seen as a viable strategy to improve pharmacokinetics and pharmacodynamics post-repositioning. Such approaches have proven successful in enhancing activities of repositioned drugs; in some cases, new chemical entities were identified with antitubercular activities more potent than parent non-antibiotics or standard antitubercular drugs. Also, inherent effects of repositioned drugs could be abrogated to improve selectivity, particularly in the example of phenothiazines. Drug formulation is another medicinal chemistry approach that goes hand in hand with drug repositioning. As with examples provided herein, drug formulation offers advantages such as targeted drug delivery and minimized dose-related toxicities or drug metabolism.

Research investments for the development of new or better drugs against WHO-listed NTDs are extremely low. Given the significant dearth of effective and affordable drugs against these NTDs, repositioning approaches offer a cheaper, less resource consuming and time-efficient means for the discovery of new agents. Noteworthy, repositioning strategies targeting non-antibiotics have previously proven successful for NTDs prioritized by the WHO. Originally developed as anticancer agents, eflornithine and miltefosine are currently in clinical use for the treatment of HAT and visceral leishmaniasis, respectively.

Repositioning non-antibiotics appears to be a plausible alternative to *de novo* drug discovery approaches in efforts to replenish drug pipelines against infectious diseases, particularly those endemic in low-income regions. The challenge post-repositioning is optimizing drugs such that the desired biological effect is retained whilst enhancing pharmacokinetics and pharmacodynamics. Repositioning approaches unlock exciting possibilities not only for big pharma but also for other sectors to join in drug discovery innovations against pertinent public health issues.

Acknowledgements

A special thanks to Vernita Reed (Institute of Infectious Disease and Molecular Medicine, University of Cape Town, South Africa) for helping with proofreading.

References

Abate, G., P.G. Ruminiski, M. Kumar, K. Singh, F. Hamzabegovic, D.F. Hoft et al. 2016. New verapamil analogs inhibit intracellular mycobacteria without affecting the functions of mycobacterium-specific T cells. Antimicrob. Agents Chemother. 60: 1216–1225.

Adams, K.N., J.D. Szumowski and L. Ramakrishnan. 2014. Verapamil, and its metabolite norverapamil, inhibit macrophage-induced, bacterial efflux pump-mediated tolerance to multiple anti-tubercular drugs. J. Infect. Dis. 210: 456–466.

Addla, D., A. Jallapally, D. Gurram, P. Yogeeswari, D. Sriram and S. Kantevari. 2014. Rational design, synthesis and antitubercular evaluation of novel 2-(trifluoromethyl)phenothiazine-[1,2,3]triazole hybrids. Bioorg. Med. Chem. Lett. 24: 233–236.

Amaral, L., J.E. Kristiansen, L.S. Abebe and W. Millett. 1996. Inhibition of the respiration of multi-drug resistant clinical isolates of *Mycobacterium tuberculosis* by thioridazine: potential use for initial therapy of freshly diagnosed tuberculosis. J. Antimicrob. Chemother. 38: 1049–1053.

Amaral, L., J.E. Kristiansen, M. Viveiros and J. Atouguia. 2001. Activity of phenothiazines against antibiotic-resistant *Mycobacterium tuberculosis*: a review supporting further studies that may elucidate the potential use of thioridazine as anti-tuberculosis therapy. J. Antimicrob. Chemother. 47: 505–511.

Amaral, L., M. Viveiros and J. Molnar. 2004. Antimicrobial activity of phenothiazines. *In Vivo.* 18: 725–731.

Amaral, L., M.J. Boeree, S.H. Gillespie, Z.F. Udwadia and D. van Soolingen. 2010. Thioridazine cures extensively drug-resistant tuberculosis (XDR-TB) and the need for global trials is now! Int. J. Antimicrob. Agents. 35: 524–526.

Amaral, L. and M. Viveiros. 2012. Why thioridazine in combination with antibiotics cures extensively drug-resistant *Mycobacterium tuberculosis* infections. Int. J. Antimicrob. Agents. 39: 376–380.

Amaral, L. and J. Molnar. 2014. Mechanisms by which thioridazine in combination with antibiotics cures extensively drug-resistant infections of pulmonary tuberculosis. *In Vivo.* 28: 267–272.

Amaral, L. and M. Viveiros. 2017. Thioridazine: a non-antibiotic drug highly effective, in combination with first line anti-tuberculosis drugs, against any form of antibiotic resistance of *Mycobacterium tuberculosis* due to its multi-mechanisms of action. Antibiotics. 6: 1–14.

Aronow, W.S. 2012. Treatment of systemic hypertension. Am. J. Cardiovasc. Dis. 2: 160–170.

Bald, D., C. Villellas, P. Lu and A. Koul. 2017. Targeting energy metabolism in *Mycobacterium tuberculosis*, a new paradigm in antimycobacterial drug discovery. Am. Soc. Microbiol. 8: 1–11.

Bate, A.B., J.H. Kalin, E.M. Fooksman, E.L. Amorose, C.M. Price, H.M. Williams et al. 2007. Synthesis and antitubercular activity of quaternized promazine and promethazine derivatives. Bioorg. Med. Chem. Lett. 17: 1346–1348.

Bettencourt, M.V., S. Bosne-David and L. Amaral. 2000. Comparative *in vitro* activity of phenothiazines against multi-drug resistant *Mycobacterium tuberculosis*. Int. J. Antimicrob. Agents. 16: 69–71.

Buro, C., S. Beckmann, K.C. Oliveira, C. Dissous, K. Cailliau, R.J. Marhofer et al. 2014. Imatinib treatment causes substantial transcriptional changes in adult *Schistosoma mansoni in vitro* exhibiting pleiotropic effects. PLoS Negl. Trop. Dis. 8: e2923.

Carpenter, D.T. 2012. Another view of the history of antipsychotic drug discovery and development. Mol. Psychiatry. 17: 1168–1173.

Chakraborty, A. and V. Trivedi. 2015. Streamlining the drug discovery process through repurposing of clinically approved drugs. Austin J. Biotechnol. Bioeng. 2: 3–5.

Chan, C., H. Yin, J. Garforth, J.H. McKie, R. Jaouhari, P. Speers et al. 1998. Phenothiazine inhibitors of trypanothione reductase as potential antitrypanosomal and antileishmanial drugs. J. Med. Chem. 41: 148–156.

Chen, C., S. Gardete, R.S. Jansen, A. Shetty, T. Dick, K.Y. Rhee et al. 2018. Verapamil targets membrane energetics in *Mycobacterium tuberculosis*. Antimicrob. Agents Chemother. (in press).

Cook, D., D. Brown, R. Alexander, R. March and P. Morgan. 2014. Lessons learned from the fate of AstraZeneca's drug pipeline: a five-dimensional framework. Nat. Rev. Drug Discov. 13: 419–431.

D'Ambrosio, L., R. Centis, G. Sotgiu, E. Pontali, A. Spanevello and G.B. Migliori. 2015. New anti-tuberculosis drugs and regimens: 2015 update. ERJ Open Res. 1: 1–15.

de Keijzer, J., A. Mulder, P.E.W. de Haas, A.H. de Ru, E.M. Heerkens, L. Amaral et al. 2016. Thioridazine alters the cell-envelope permeability of *Mycobacterium tuberculosis*. J. Proteome Res. 15: 1776–1786.

Dichiara, M., A. Marrazzo, O. Prezzavento, S. Collina, A. Rescifina and E. Amata. 2017. Repurposing of human kinase inhibitors in neglected protozoan diseases. ChemMedChem. 12: 1235–1253.

Dos Santos Fernandes, G.F., C.M. Chin and J.L. Dos Santos. 2017. Advances in drug discovery of new antitubercular multidrug-resistant compounds. Pharmaceuticals. 10: 1–17.

Dunn, E.A., M. Roxburgh, L. Larsen, R.A.J. Smith, A.D. McLellan, A. Heikal et al. 2014. Incorporation of triphenylphosphonium functionality improves the inhibitory properties of phenothiazine derivatives in *Mycobacterium tuberculosis*. Bioorg. Med. Chem. 22: 5320–5328.

Duran-Frigola, M., L. Mateo and P. Aloy. 2017. Drug repositioning beyond the low-hanging fruits. Curr. Opin. Syst. Biol. 3: 95–102.

Dutta, N.K., K.A. Kumar, K. Mazumdar and S.G. Dastidar. 2004. *In vitro* and *in vivo* antimycobacterial activity of antiinflammatory drug, diclofenac sodium. Indian J. Exp. Biol. 42: 922–927.

Dutta, N.K., M.L. Pinn, M. Zhao, M.A. Rudek and P.C. Karakousis. 2013. Thioridazine lacks bactericidal activity in an animal model of extracellular tuberculosis. J. Antimicrob. Chemother. 68: 1327–1330.

Dutta, N.K., M.L. Pinn and P.C. Karakousis. 2014. Reduced emergence of isoniazid resistance with concurrent use of thioridazine against acute murine tuberculosis. Antimicrob. Agents Chemother. 58: 4048–4053.

Ernst, J.D. 2012. The immunological life cycle of tuberculosis. Nat. Rev. Immunol. 12: 581–591.

Feinberg, A.P. and S.H. Snyder. 1975. Phenothiazine drugs: structure-activity relationships explained by a conformation that mimics dopamine. Proc. Nat. Acad. Sci. USA. 72: 1899–1903.

Ferreira, L.G. and A.D. Andricopulo. 2016. Drug repositioning approaches to parasitic diseases: a medicinal chemistry perspective. Drug Discov. Today 21: 1699–1710.

Gadre, D.V. and V. Talwar. 1999. *In vitro* susceptibility testing of *Mycobacterium tuberculosis* strains to trifluoperazine. J. Chemother. 11: 203–206.

Gajadeera, C., M.J. Willby, K.D. Green, P. Shaul, S. Garneau-Tsodikova and J.E. Posey. 2015. Antimycobacterial activity of DNA intercalator inhibitors of *Mycobacterium tuberculosis* primase DnaG. J. Antibiot. (Tokyo). 68: 153–157.

Gawad, J. and C. Bonde. 2018. Current affairs, future perspectives of tuberculosis and antitubercular agents. Indian J. Tuberc. 65: 15–22.

Go, M.-L. 2003. Novel antiplasmodial agents. Med. Res. Rev. 23: 456–487.

Godbole, A.A., W. Ahmed, R.S. Bhat, E.K. Bradley, S. Ekins and V. Nagaraja. 2015. Targeting *Mycobacterium tuberculosis* topoisomerase I by small-molecule inhibitors. Antimicrob. Agents Chemother. 59: 1549–1557.

Gold, B., M. Pingle, S.J. Brickner, N. Shah, J. Roberts, M. Rundell et al. 2012. Nonsteroidal anti-inflammatory drug sensitizes *Mycobacterium tuberculosis* to endogenous and exogenous antimicrobials. PNAS. 109: 16004–16011.

Gupta, S., S. Tyagi, D.V. Almeida, M.C. Maiga, N.C. Ammerman and W.R. Bishai. 2013. Acceleration of tuberculosis treatment by adjunctive therapy with verapamil as an efflux inhibitor. Am. J. Respir. Crit. Care Med. 188: 600–607.

Gupta, S., K.A. Cohen, K. Winglee, M. Maiga, B. Diarra and W.R. Bishai. 2014. Efflux Inhibition with verapamil potentiates bedaquiline in *Mycobacterium tuberculosis*. Antimicrob. Agents Chemother. 58: 574–576.

Gupta, S., S. Tyagi and W.R. Bishai. 2015. Verapamil increases the bactericidal activity of bedaquiline against *Mycobacterium tuberculosis* in a mouse model. Antimicrob. Agents Chemother. 59: 673–676.

Guzman, J.D., D. Evangelopoulos, A. Gupta, K. Birchall, S. Mwaigwisya, B. Saxty et al. 2013. Antitubercular specific activity of ibuprofen and the other 2-arylpropanoic acids using the HT-SPOTi whole cell phenotypic assay. BMJ OPen. 3: 1–14.

He, C.-X., H. Meng, X. Zhang, H.-Q. Cui and D.-L. Yin. 2015. Synthesis and bioevaluation of phenothiazine derivatives as new anti-tuberculosis agents. Chinese Chem. Lett. 26: 951–954.

Hoagland, D.T., J. Liu, R.B. Lee and R.E. Lee. 2016. New agents for the treatment of drug-resistant *Mycobacterium tuberculosis*. Adv. Drug. Deliv. Rev. 102: 55–72.

Hughes, J.P., S.S. Rees, S.B. Kalindjian and K.L. Philpott. 2011. Principles of early drug discovery. Br. J. Pharmacol. 162: 1239–1249.

Jafari, S., F. Fernandez-Enright and X.F. Huang. 2012. Structural contributions of antipsychotic drugs to their therapeutic profiles and metabolic side effects. J. Neurochem. 120: 371–384.

Jang, J., R. Kim, M. Woo, J. Jeong, G. Kim and V. Delorme. 2017. Efflux attenuates the antibacterial activity of Q203 in *Mycobacterium tuberculosis*. Antimicrob. Agents Chemother. 61: 1–8.

Jaszczyszyn, A., K. Gasiorowski, P. Swiatek, W. Malinka, K. Cieslik-Boczula, J. Petrus et al. 2012. Chemical structure of phenothiazines and their biological activity. Pharmacol. Reports. 64: 16–23.

Juarez, E., C. Carranza, G. Sanchez, M. Gonzalez, J. Chavez, C. Sarabia et al. 2016. Loperamide restricts intracellular growth of *Mycobacterium tuberculosis* in lung macrophages. Am. J. Respir. Cell Mol. Biol. 55: 838–847.

Kaatz, G.W., V.V. Moudgal, S.M. Seo and J.E. Kristiansen. 2003. Phenothiazines and thioxanthenes inhibit multidrug efflux pump activity in *Staphylococcus aureus*. Antimicrob. Agents Chemother. 47: 719–726.

Khan, M., S.E. Austin, C. Chan, H. Yin, D. Marks, S.N. Vaghjiani et al. 2000. Use of an additional hydrophobic binding site, the Z site, in the rational drug design of a new class of stronger trypanothione reductase inhibitor, quaternary alkylammonium phenothiazines. J. Med. Chem. 43: 3148–3156.

Kolyva, A.S. and P.C. Karakousis. 2012. Old and new TB drugs: mechanisms of action and resistance. pp. 209–232. *In*: P.-J. Cardona [ed.]. Understanding Tuberculosis—New Approaches to Fighting against Drug Resistance. InTech.

Koul, A., E. Arnoult, N. Lounis, J. Guillemont and K. Andries. 2011. The challenge of new drug discovery for tuberculosis. Nature. 469: 483–490.

Kristiansen, J.E. and L. Amaral. 1997. The potential management of resistant infections with non-antibiotics. J. Antimicrob. Chemother. 40: 319–327.

Kristiansen, J.E., O. Hendricks, T. Delvin, T.S. Butterworth, L. Aagaard, J.B. Christensen et al. 2007. Reversal of resistance in microorganisms by help of non-antibiotics. J. Antimicrob. Chemother. 59: 1271–1279.

Kristiansen, J.E., S.G. Dastidar, S. Palchoudhuri, D.S. Roy, S. Das, O. Hendricks et al. 2015. Phenothiazines as a solution for multidrug resistant tuberculosis: From the origin to present. Int. Microbiol. 18: 1–12.

Kroesen, V.M., M.I. Groschel, N. Martisnson, A. Zumla, M. Maeurer, T.S. van der Werf et al. 2017. Non-steroidal anti-inflammatory drugs as host-directed therapy for tuberculosis: A systematic review. Front. Immunol. 8: 1–9.

Krystal, A.D. 2011. Antidepressant and antipsychotic drugs. Sleep Med. Clin. 5: 571–589.

Kumar, M., K. Singh, K. Naran, F. Hamzabegovic, D.F. Hoft, D.F. Warner et al. 2016. Design, synthesis, and evaluation of novel hybrid efflux pump inhibitors for use against *Mycobacterium tuberculosis*. ACS Infect. Dis. 2: 714–725.

Kumar, N., K. Mazumdar, S.G. Dastidar and J.-H. Park. 2007. Activity of diclofenac used alone and in combination with streptomycin against *Mycobacterium tuberculosis* in mice. Int. J. Antimicrob. Agents. 30: 336–340.

Li, X., V. Hernandez, F.L. Rock, W. Choi, Y.S.L. Mak, M. Moham et al. 2017. Discovery of a potent and specific *M. tuberculosis* leucyl-tRNA synthetase inhibitor (S)-3-(aminomethyl)-4-chloro-7-(2-hydroethoxy)benzo[c][1,2] oxaborol-1(3H)-ol (GSK656). J. Med. Chem. 60: 8011–8026.

Lo Presti, M.S., P.C. Bazan, M. Strauss, A.L. Baez, H.W. Rivarola and P.A. Paglini-Oliva. 2015. Trypanothione reductase inhibitors: Overview of the action of thioridazine in different stages of Chagas disease. Acta Trop. 145: 79–87.

Ma, D.-L., D.S.-H. Chan and C.-H. Leung. 2013. Drug repositioning by structure-based virtual screening. Chem. Soc. Rev. 42: 2130–2141.

Machado, D., D. Pires, J. Perdigao, I. Couto, I. Portugal, M. Martins et al. 2016. Ion channel blockers as antimicrobial agents, efflux inhibitors, and enhancers of macrophage killing activity against drug resistant *Mycobacterium tuberculosis*. PLoS One. 11: 1–28.

Madrid, P.B., W.E. Polgar and M.J. Tanga. 2007. Synthesis and antitubercular activity of phenothiazines with reduced binding to dopamine and serotonin receptors. Bioorg. Med. Chem. Lett. 17: 3014–3017.

Mafukidze, A., E. Harausz and J. Furin. 2016. An update on repurposed medications for the treatment of drug-resistant tuberculosis. Expert Rev. Clin. Pharmacol. 9: 1–10.

Maitra, A., S. Bates, M. Shaik, D. Evangelopoulos, I. Abubakar, T.D. McHugh et al. 2016. Repurposing drugs for treatment of tuberculosis: a role for non-steroidal anti-inflammatory drugs. Br. Med. Bull. 118: 145–155.

Martins, M., S.G. Dastidar, S. Fanning, J.E. Kristiansen, J. Molnar, J.-M. Pages et al. 2008. Potential role of non-antibiotics (helper compounds) in the treatment of multidrug-resistant Gram-negative infections: mechanisms for their direct and indirect activities. Int. J. Antimicrob Agents. 31: 198–208.

Martins, M. 2011. Targeting the human macrophage with combinations of drugs and inhibitors of Ca2+ and K+ transport to enhance the killing of intracellular multi-drug resistant *M. tuberculosis* (MDR-TB)- a novel, patentable approach to limit the emergence of XDR-TB. Recent Pat. Antiinfect. Drug Discov. 6: 1–8.

Mazumdar, K., S.G. Dastidar, J.H. Park and N.K. Dutta. 2009. The anti-inflammatory non-antibiotic helper compound diclofenac: an antibacterial drug target. Eur. J. Clin. Microbiol. Infect. Dis. 28: 881–891.

Mazumdar, K., K. Asok Kumar and N.K. Dutta. 2010. Potential role of the cardiovascular non-antibiotic (helper compound) amlodipine in the treatment of microbial infections: scope and hope for the future. Int. J. Antimicrob. Agents. 36: 295–302.

Miguel, D., R.C. Zauli-Nascimento, J.K. Yokoyama-Yasunaka, C.L. Barbieri and S.R. Uliana. 2009. Tamoxifen as a potential antileishmanial agent: efficacy in the treatment of *Leishmania braziliensis* and *Leishmania chagasi* infections. J. Antimicrob. Chemother. 63: 365–368.

Molyneux, D.H., L. Savioli and D. Engels. 2017. Neglected tropical diseases: progress towards addressing the chronic pandemic. Lancet. 389: 312–325.

Nagle, A.S., S. Khare, A.B. Kumar, F. Supek, A. Buchynskyy, C.J.N. Mathison et al. 2014. Recent developments in drug discovery for leishmaniasis and human African trypanosomiasis. Chem. Rev. 114: 11305–11347.

Napier, R.J., W. Rafi, M. Cheruvu, K.R. Powell, M.A. Zaunbrecher, W. Bornmann et al. 2011. Imatinib-sensitive tyrosine kinases regulate mycobacterial pathogenesis and represent therapeutic targets against tuberculosis. Cell Host Microbe. 10: 475–485.

Niu, H., C. Ma, P. Cui, W. Shi, S. Zhang, J. Feng et al. 2017. Identification of drug candidates that enhance pyrazinamide activity from a clinical compound library. Emerg. Microbes Infect. 6: 1–3.

Nussbaumer, S., P. Bonnabry, J.-L. Veuthey and S. Fleury-Souverain. 2011. Analysis of anticancer drugs: a review. Talanta. 85: 2265–2289.

Nwaka, S. and A. Hudson. 2006. Innovative lead discovery strategies for tropical diseases. Nat. Rev. Drug Discov. 5: 941–955.

Olakanmi, O., B. Britigan and L. Schlesinger. 2000. Gallium disrupts iron metabolism of mycobacteria residing within human macrophages. Infect. Immun. 68: 5619–5627.

Olakanmi, O., B. Kesavalu, R. Pasula, M.Y. Abdalla, L.S. Schlesinger and B.E. Britigan. 2013. Gallium nitrate is efficacious in murine models of tuberculosis and inhibits key bacterial Fe-dependent enzymes. Antimicrob. Agents Chemother. 57: 6074–6080.

Ong, C.K., P. Lirk, C.H. Tan and R.A. Seymour. 2007. An evidence-based update on nonsteroidal anti-inflammatory drugs. Clin. Med. Res. 5: 19–34.

Ordway, D., M. Viveiros, C. Leandro, R. Bettencourt, J. Almeida, M. Martins et al. 2003. Clinical concentrations of thioridazine kill intracellular multidrug-resistant *Mycobacterium tuberculosis*. Antimicrob. Agents Chemother. 47: 917–922.

Palit, P. and N. Ali. 2008. Oral therapy with amlodipine and lacidipine, 1, 4-dihydropyridine derivatives showing activity against experimental visceral leishmaniasis. Antimicrob. Agents Chemother. 52: 374–377.

Panic, G., M. Vargas, I. Scandale and J. Keiser. 2015. Activity profile of an FDA-approved compound library against *Schistosoma mansoni*. PLoS Negl. Trop. Dis. 9: e0003962.

Parida, S.K., M.V. Rao, N. Singh, I. Master, A. Lutckii, S. Keshavjee et al. 2015. Totally drug-resistant tuberculosis and adjunct therapies. J. Int. Med. 277: 388–405.

Parumasivam, T., J.G.Y. Chan, A. Pang, D.H. Quan, J.A. Triccas, W.J. Britton et al. 2016a. *In vitro* evaluation of inhalable verapamil-rifapentine particles for tuberculosis therapy. Mol. Pharm. 13: 979–989.

Parumasivam, T., J.G.Y. Chan, A. Pang, D.H. Quan, J.A. Triccas, W.J. Britton et al. 2016b. *In vitro* evaluation of novel inhalable dry powders consisting of thioridazine and rifapentine for rapid tuberculosis treatment. Eur. J. Pharm. Biopharm. 107: 205–214.

Patil, J.S. and S. Sarasija. 2012. Pulmonary drug delivery strategies: a concise, systematic review. Lung India. 29: 44–49.

Pattanashetty, S.H., K.M. Hosamani, P. Satapute, S.D. Joshi and K. Obelannavar. 2017. Discovery of new drugs and computational studies of coumarin-carprofen scaffolds as a novel class of anti-tubercular, anti-inflammatory and anti-bacterial agents. Eur. J. Pharm. Med. Res. 4: 486–498.

Persaud-Sharma, V. and F. Zhou. 2012. Drug Repositioning: a faster path to drug discovery. Adv. Pharmacoepidem. Drug Safety. 1: 1–3.

Phillips, P.P.J., K.E. Dooley, S.H. Gillespie, N. Heinrich, J.E. Stout, P. Nahid et al. 2016. A new trial design to accelerate tuberculosis drug development: the Phase IIC Selection Trial with Extended Post-treatment follow-up (STEP). BMC Med. 14: 1–11.

Pieroni, M., D. Machado, E. Azzali, I. Couto, G. Costantino and M. Viveiros. 2015. Rational design and synthesis of thioridazine analogues as enhancers of the antituberculosis therapy. J. Med. Chem. 58: 5842–5853.

Planer, J., M.A. Hulverson, J.A. Arif, R.M. Ranade, R. Don and F.S. Buckner. 2014. Synergy testing of FDA-approved drugs identifies potent drug combinations against Trypanosoma cruzi. PLoS Negl. Trop. Dis. 8: e2977.

Pluta, K., B. Morak-Mlodawska and M. Jelen. 2011. Recent progress in biological activities of synthesized phenothiazines. Eur. J. Med. Chem. 46: 3179–3189.

Quan, D., G. Nagalingam, R. Payne and J.A. Triccas. 2017. New tuberculosis drug leads from naturally occurring compounds. Int. J. Infect. Dis. 56: 212–220.

Ramprasad, J., N. Nayak and U. Dalimba. 2015. Design of new phenothiazine-thiadiazole hybrids via molecular hybridization approach for the development of potent antitubercular agents. Eur. J. Med. Chem. 106: 75–84.

Ratnakar, P., S.P. Rao, P. Sriramarao and P.S. Murthy. 1995. Structure-antitubercular activity relationship of phenothiazine-type calmodulin antagonists. Int. Clin. Psychopharmacol. 10: 39–44.

Reimao, J.Q. and A.G. Tempone. 2011. Investigation into *in vitro* antileishmanial combinations of calcium channel blockers and current anti-leishmanial drugs. Mem. Inst. Oswaldo Cruz. 106: 1032–8.

Salie, S., N.-J. Hsu, D. Semenya, A. Jardine and M. Jacobs. 2014. Novel non-neuroleptic phenothiazines inhibit *Mycobacterium tuberculosis* replication. J. Antimicrob. Chemother. 69: 1–8.

Sanderson, L., V. Yardley and S.L. Croft. 2017. Activity of anti-cancer protein kinase inhibitors against leishmania spp. J. Antimicrob. Chemother. 69: 1888–1891.

Scalacci, N., A.K. Brown, F.R. Pavan, C.M. Ribeiro, F. Manetti, S. Bhakta et al. 2017. Synthesis and SAR evaluation of novel thioridazine derivatives active against drug-resistant tuberculosis. Eur. J. Med Chem. 127: 147–158.

Schump, M.D., D.M. Fox, C.R. Bertozzi and L.W. Riley. 2017. Subcellular partitioning and intramacrophage selectivity of antimicrobial compounds against *Mycobacterium tuberculosis*. Am. Soc. Microbiol. 61: 1–12.

Seelig, A., R. Gottschlich and R.M. Devant. 1994. A method to determine the ability of drugs to diffuse through the blood-brain barrier. Proc. Nat. Acad. Sci. USA. 91: 68–72.

Sharma, D., Y.K. Dhuriya, N. Deo and D. Bisht. 2017. Repurposing and revival of the drugs: A new approach to combat the drug resistant tuberculosis. Front. Microbiol. 8: 1–5.

Sharma, R., P. Samadhiya, S.D. Srivastava and S.K. Srivastava. 2012. Synthesis and pharmaceutical importance of 2-azetidinone derivatives of phenothiazine. J. Chem. Sci. 124: 633–637.

Shen, H., F. Wang, G. Zeng, L. Shen, H. Cheng and D. Huang. 2016. Bis-biguanide dihydrochloride inhibits intracellular replication of *M. tuberculosis* and controls. Nat. Sci. Reports. 6: 1–10.

Siddiqui, A.B., A.R. Trivedi, V.B. Kataria and V.H. Shah. 2014. 4,5-Dihydro-1H-pyrazolo[3,4-d]pyrimidine containing phenothiazines as antitubercular agents. Bioorg. Med. Chem. Lett. 24: 1493–1495.

Simanjuntak, Y., J.-J. Liang, Y.-L. Lee and Y.L. Lin. 2015. Repurposing of prochlorperazine for use against dengue virus infection. J. Infect. Dis. 211: 394–404.

Singh, A. and S. Sharma. 2014. Chemotherapeutic efficacy of thioridazine as an adjunct drug in a murine model of latent tuberculosis. Tuberculosis. 94: 695–700.

Singh, S., N. Dinesh, P.K. Kaur and B. Shamiulla. 2014. Ketanserin, an antidepressant, exerts its antileishmanial action via inhibition of 3-hydroxy-3-methylglutaryl coenzyme A reductase of *Leishmania donovani*. Parasitol. Res. 113: 2161–2168.

Stanley, S.A., A.K. Barczak, M.R. Silvis, S.S. Luo, K. Sogi, M. Vokes et al. 2014. Identification of host-targeted small molecules that restrict intracellular Mycobacterium tuberculosis growth. PloS Pathog. 10: 1–16.

Stewart, Z.A., M.D. Westfall and J.A. Pietenpol. 2003. Cell-cycle dysregulation and anticancer therapy. Trends Pharmacol. Sci. 24: 139–145.

Teh, J.S., T. Yano and H. Rubin. 2007. Type II NADH: menaquinone oxidoreductase of *Mycobacterium tuberculosis*. Infect. Disord. Drug Targets. 7: 169–181.

Thanacoody, H.K.R. 2007. Thioridazine: resurrection as an antimicrobial agent? Br. J. Clin. Pharmacol. 64: 566–574.

Tiberi, S., A. Scardigli, R. Centis, L. D'Ambrosio, M. Munoz-Torrico, M.A. Salazar-Lezama et al. 2017. Classifying new anti-tuberculosis drugs: rationale and future perspectives. Int. J. Infect. Dis. 56: 181–184.

Tiberi, S., M. Munoz-Torrico, R. Duarte, M. Dalcolmo, L. D'Ambrosio and G.-B. Migliori. 2018. New drugs and perspectives for new anti-tuberculosis regimens. Pulmonology. 24: 86–98.

Udwadia, Z.F., T. Sen and L.M. Pinto. 2011. Safety and efficacy of thioridazine as salvage therapy in Indian patients with XDR-TB. Recent Pat. Antiinfect. Drug Discov. 6: 88–91.

van Soolingen, D., R. Hernandez-Pando, H. Orozco, D. Aguilar, C. Magis-Escurra, L. Amaral et al. 2010. The antipsychotic thioridazine shows promising therapeutic activity in a mouse model of multidrug-resistant tuberculosis. Plos One. 5: 1–6.

Varga, B., A. Csonka, A. Csonka, J. Molnar, L. Amaral and G. Spengler. 2017. Possible biological and clinical applications of phenothiazines. Anticancer Res. 37: 5983–5993.

Vazquez, K., M. Paulino, C.O. Salas, J.J. Zarate-Ramos, B. Vera and G. Rivera. 2017. Trypanothione reductase: A target for the development of anti-*Trypanosoma cruzi* drugs. Mini Rev. Med. Chem. 17: 939–946.

Vibe, C.B., F. Fenaroli, D. Pires, S.R. Wilson, V. Bogoeva, R. Kalluru et al. 2015. Thioridazine in PLGA nanoparticles reduces toxicity and improves rifampicin therapy against mycobacterial infection in zebrafish. Nanotoxicology. 10: 680–688.

Vilaplana, C., E. Marzo, G. Tapia, J. Diaz, V. Garcia and P.-J. Cardona. 2013. Ibuprofen therapy resulted in significantly decreased tissue cacillary loads and increased survival in a new murine experimental model of active tuberculosis. J. Infect. Dis. 208: 199–202.

Wainwright, M. 2012. The evolution of antimycobacterial agents from non-antibiotics. Open J. Pharmacol. 2: 1–11.

Warman, A.J., T.S. Rito, N.E. Fisher, D.M. Moss, N.G. Berry, P.M. O'Neill et al. 2013. Antitubercular pharmacodynamics of phenothiazines. J. Antimicrob. Chemother. 68: 869–880.

WHO. 2017a. Global tuberculosis report, World Health Organization. http://www.who.int/tb/publications/global_report/en/.

WHO. 2017b. Integrating neglected tropical diseases into global health and development, World Health Organization. http://www.who.int/neglected_diseases/resources/97892415654.

Wilson, M.L. 2011. Recent advances in the laboratory detection of *Mycobacterium tuberculosis* complex and drug resistance. Clin. Infect. Dis. 52: 1350–1355.

Wu, S., G. Mao and L.A. Kirsebom. 2016. Inhibition of bacterial RNase P RNA by phenothiazine derivatives. Biomolecules. 6: 1–16.

Yano, T., L. Lin-Sheng, E. Weinstein, J.S. Teh and H. Rubin. 2006. Steady-state kinetics and inhibitory action of antitubercular phenothiazines on *Mycobacterium tuberculosis* type-II NADH-menaquinone oxidoreductase (NDH-2). J. Biol. Chem. 281: 11456–11463.

Zhang, Y. 2005. The magic bullets and tuberculosis drug targets. Annu. Rev. Pharmacol. Toxicol. 45: 529–564.

Zheng, W., W. Sun and A. Simeonov. 2018. Drug repurposing screens and synergistic drug-combinations for infectious diseases. Br. J. Pharmacol. 175: 181–191.

Chapter 8

Prospects of Pre-clinical [6.6.0] Bicyclic Nitrogen Heterocycles in the Treatment of Tuberculosis

Neha P. Agre,[1,2] *Mariam S. Degani*[2] *and Sanjib Bhakta*[1,*]

Introduction

Tuberculosis (TB), caused by *Mycobacterium tuberculosis* (Mtb), is the leading cause of death by a single infectious agent and ranks above HIV/AIDS. In 2017, there were an estimated 10.0 million new cases and 1.3 million mortalities among HIV-negative people and an additional 300,000 deaths amongst HIV-positive people due to TB worldwide. The emergence of multi-drug resistant (MDR-TB) and extensively drug resistant (XDR-TB) strains of tubercle bacilli is a major hurdle in the successful treatment of TB. MDR-TB is defined as strains of Mtb that have developed resistance against isoniazid (**1**) and rifampicin (**2**), two of the most important drugs in the frontline therapy for TB. The more extensively resistant forms of TB (XDR-TB) are resistant to both of these drugs as well as fluoroquinolones and one of the three injectable drugs- capreomycin (**3**), kanamycin (**4**) or amikacin (**5**), leaving virtually no effective antibiotics to treat such cases in the clinic. In 2017, there were 558,000 new cases with resistance to rifampicin (**2**) (RR-TB), the most effective first-line drug, of which 82% cases had multidrug-resistant TB (MDR-TB). Drug resistance surveillance data showed that 3.5% of new and 18% of previously treated TB cases were MDR/RR-TB cases and 8.5% of MDR-TB cases were XDR-TB cases worldwide (WHO 2018).

TB is the leading cause of death amongst patients living with AIDS. Due to the severely compromised immune system, the body fails to contain the actively replicating TB pathogen. Hence, the probability of developing active TB is 20 to 30 times higher in AIDS patients than in people not suffering from AIDS. The high mortality rate amongst AIDS patients is due to the atypical symptoms that TB exhibits during a co-infection, resulting in delayed diagnosis of TB; also, difficult to treat resistant forms of TB are more prevalent in AIDS patients (Kwan and Ernst 2011). 78% of TB patients living with AIDS are on highly

[1] Department of Biological Sciences, Birkbeck, University of London, Malet Street, Bloomsbury, London WC1E 7HX, United Kingdom.
[2] Department of Pharmaceutical Sciences and Technology, Institute of Chemical Technology, Nathalal Parekh Marg, Matunga, Mumbai 400019, India.
* Corresponding author: s.bhakta@bbk.ac.uk; sanjib.bhakta@ucl.ac.uk

active anti-retroviral therapy (HAART) (WHO 2017). The success rate of the treatment for HIV-associated TB (2015 cohort) and for XDR-TB (2014 cohort) were 78% and 30%, respectively. Treatment for AIDS (HAART) should be started 2–8 wk after starting TB treatment. However, there is a conflict between anti-TB drugs and HAART, which often complicates the treatments against the co-infection.

Development and Evolution of Anti-microbial Resistance (AMR) in *Mycobacterium tuberculosis*

One of the major challenges in the successful treatment of TB infection is the emergence of anti-microbial resistance (AMR) in Mtb, which is one of the major contributing factors in TB infection reaching its current pandemic scale (Ventola 2015). Without effective antibiotics, infections that were once simple and treatable are becoming extremely challenging to tackle resulting in prolonged illness, disability, and death. The alarming rate at which bacteria are becoming resistant has driven the selection pressure that facilitates mutated or resistant bacteria to survive and spread. Drug resistance evolves in Mtb by complex and varied mechanisms; one or more of the following factors are involved such as (a) compartmentalisation of infection *in vivo*, (b) presence of pre-existent resistant forms of disease-causing organism, (c) DNA mutations in the pathogens with high mutation rate and frequency (10^{-7} to 10^{-9} mutations per bacterium per cell-division), (d) acquisition of plasmid, or by mutation of chromosomal gene (Gillespie 2002). The occurrence of drug resistance is often the result of sub-optimal therapy that could be due to non-compliance, poor access to treatment, and incomplete treatment. Intrinsic drug resistance in Mtb is contributed structurally by its uniquely impermeable cell-wall and functionally by producing enzymes that inactivate drugs (Nasiri et al. 2017). Tubercle bacilli also possess varied classes of energy-dependent or energy-independent efflux pumps that can expel drugs out of the cell before they can achieve their required therapeutic concentrations to inhibit the cell function. These multidrug resistance efflux pumps fall into two categories: (1) secondary multidrug transporters (influx/efflux pumps), that use electrochemical gradient for the drug expulsion; (2) ABC-type multidrug transporter, that requires energy in the form of ATP for the drug expulsion (Louw et al. 2009). Acquired drug resistance in Mtb occurs through genetic modifications or mutations that can alter the drug targets. Horizontal transfer of genetic elements (*via* transposons, plasmids or integrons) is common in other bacteria and rare in fast growing mycobacteria but is an unlikely event in the slow growing TB-causing bacilli (Da Silva and Palomino 2011, Viveiros et al. 2003).

Furthermore, the tubercle bacilli are capable of developing cross-resistance among various structurally similar compounds. The best example is represented by the cross resistance between rifampicin (**2**) and rifabutin (**6**) (Senol et al. 2005). A key solution to tackle the growing AMR in Mtb is to discover and design new chemical agents that target novel, previously unchallenged, endogenous molecular machineries or metabolic pathways which are essential for the intracellular survival of the TB causing bacilli, avoiding the likelihood of cross-resistance to existing chemotherapy.

Quinolines Containing Anti-tuberculosis Agents

Quinoline is a bicyclic [6.6.0] nitrogen heterocyclic scaffold, which is the core of a number of anti-TB drugs, pre-clinical and clinical candidates. Bedaquiline (**7**) (Figure 1), a diarylquinoline, is the newest member of the class of anti-TB drugs and has been recently launched in the market for the treatment of MDR-TB infections (Fox and Menzies 2013). The quinoline scaffold is also present in fluoroquinolones (Figure 1), the largest class of second line TB drugs (Asif 2013). The agent TBAJ-587 (**8**) (Figure 1), a quinoline containing pre-clinical candidate, is a next-generation diarylquinoline derivative designed to possess bedaquiline's impressive anti-TB activities with improved pharmacological properties. The compound OPC-167832 (under patent, complete structure not disclosed) is a quinoline containing phase-I clinical trial candidate and an inhibitor of decaprenylphophoryl-β-D-ribose 2'-oxidase (DprE1), an enzyme involved in the cell-wall metabolism. The newest member of the fluoroquinolone class showing promising anti-TB activity is DC-159a (**9**) (Figure 1), which is currently undergoing pre-clinical trials (Dhiman and Singh 2018). Furthermore, the TB alliance pipeline has three new drug combinations in clinical trials,

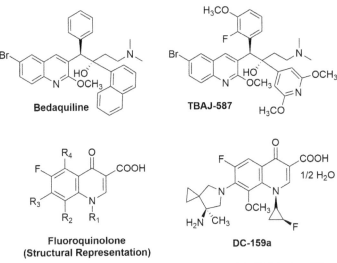

Figure 1. Quinoline containing anti-TB drugs and pre-clinical/clinical candidates.

all containing bedaquiline together with an additional fluoroquinolone: bedaquiline (**7**) + pretonamid (**10**) + pyrazinamide (**11**); bedaquiline (**7**) + pretonamid (**10**) + moxifloxacin (**12**) + pyrazinamide (**11**) (phase II advanced), and bedaquiline (**7**) + pretonamid (**10**) + linezolid (**13**) (phase 3) (Li et al. 2017). Some attempts have been made to repurpose already available non-toxic drugs in order to circumvent the time and investment required to discover and develop new drugs (Maitra et al. 2018, Maitra and Bhakta 2014). Anti-malarials constitute one such therapeutic class explored for their anti-tuberculosis potential. Mefloquine (**14**) has shown to have a good anti-TB potential (Bermudez and Meek 2014). Derivatives of mefloquine (Mao et al. 2010), primaquine (**15**) (Pavić et al. 2018) and quinine (**16**) (Tukulula et al. 2012) have also shown to possess some promising anti-TB activity.

Bioisosterism represents an approach used by medicinal chemists for the rational modification of lead compounds into safer and clinically more potent anti-infectives (Patani and LaVoie 1996). Quinoline is the most widely explored scaffold of the [6.6.0] nitrogen bicyclic class for its anti-TB potential, partly due to the promise shown by bedaquiline (**7**). This chapter focuses on deciphering the anti-TB prospects of derivatives of the lesser explored bioisosteres of quinoline: quinoxaline, quinazoline, 1,8-naphthyridine, deazapteridine, and pteridine in terms of their whole cell activity against Mtb, structure activity relationship (SAR), drug-likeness predicted based on pharmacokinetic/ADME (Absorption, Distribution, Metabolism, and Excretion) properties and the relevant medicinal chemistry properties to assess the drug-likeness of the most potent derivatives, calculated by SWISSADME (Daina et al. 2017).

Quinoxaline Containing Anti-tuberculosis Agents

Quinoxaline is a bioisostere of quinoline, containing additional nitrogen at the position 4 of the ring, depicted in Figure 2.

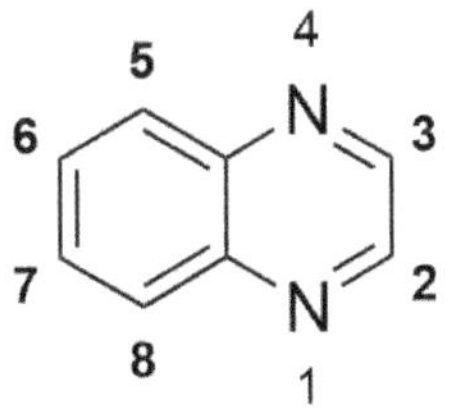

Figure 2. Structural representation of the quinoxaline scaffold.

Quinoxaline-1,4-di-N-oxide derivatives

Several derivatives of quinoxaline-2-carbonitrile 1,4-di-*N*-oxide developed by Ortega et al. were evaluated for their anti-TB potential under the Tuberculosis Antimicrobial Acquisition and Coordinating Facility (TAACF) screening program. The compounds showed high level of inhibition against Mtb H37Rv. The most potent compound was found to be compound **17** (Table 1) with a minimum inhibitory concentration (MIC) of < 0.2 µg/mL (Ortega et al. 2001). Several analogues of quinoxaline-1,4-di-*N*-dioxide with different substituents in positions 3, 6, 7, and 8 were synthesized by Ortega et al. and evaluated against Mtb H37Rv at 6.25 µg/mL concentration using the Microplate Alamar Blue Assay (MABA) with the BACTEC 12B medium as the primary anti-TB screening. Compounds that demonstrated at least 90% inhibition in BACTEC 460 radiometric assay were re-evaluated in the MABA assay at lower concentrations to determine the actual MIC. The most potent analogue of the series was found to be compound **18** (Table 1) with a MIC of 0.39 µM. The 1,4-*N*-dioxide group led to increase in anti-TB activity whereas the compounds without the *N*-oxide moiety showed little or no activity. The type of basic chain in position 3 of the ring did not influence the anti-TB potential. Substitution on positions 6 and 7 did not appear to determine activity, regardless of being monosubstituted or disubstituted with electron-donating or electron-withdrawing groups. The presence of two moderately withdrawing groups such as chlorine on the ring seems to exert a great influence on the anti-TB activity causing 99% growth inhibition. The derivatives with no substituents in positions 6 and 7 were also found to be active. Disubstitution with both electron donating and electron-

Table 1. Structures and anti-TB activities of the most active compounds of the several quinoxaline series.

Compound	Substitution	MIC**
17	R_2 = CN; R_3 = 4-(4-nitrophenylpiperazinyl; R_6, R_7 = CH_3	< 0.2 µg/mL^a
18	R_2 = CN; R_3 = NH_2; R_6 = F; R_7 = Cl	0.39 µM^a
19	R_2 = $COOCH_3$; R_3 = CH_3; R_7 = Cl	0.78 µM^a
20	R_2 = $COOCH_3$; R_7 = Cl	0.78 µM^b
21	R_2 = $COOCH_3$; R_3 = benzyl; R_7 = H	0.1 µg/mL^a
22	R_2 = $COOCH_3$; R_3 = benzyl; R_7 = Cl	0.1 µg/mL^a
27	R_2 = COOEt; R_3 = CH_3; R_7 = Cl	0.78 µg/mL^a
28	R_2 = CN; R_3 = 4-fluorophenyl; R_7 = CH_3	< 0.2 µg/mL^a
29	R_2 = COOEt; R_3 = 4-fluorophenyl	0.39 µg/mL^a
30	R_2 = $CONH(CH_2)$-phenyl; R_6 = Cl; R_7 = Cl	< 0.2 µg/mL^a
31	R_2 = $CONH(CH_2)_2$-phenyl; R_6 = H; R_7 = Cl	< 0.2 µg/mL^a
32	R_2 = COOEt; R_3 = CH_3; R_6, R_7 = Cl	< 12.5 µg/mL^b
33	R_2 = CN; R_3=$NHCOCH_3$; R_6, R_7 = Cl	12.5 µg/mL^b
34	R_3 = 4-acetoxybenzylcarboxy	6.25 µg/mL^a
35*	R_2,R_3 = C = O; R_4 = (3-methyl-5-oxo-pyrazol-4-yl)methyl-	8.012 µg/mL^a
36	R_2 = phenyl-CH =; R_3 = 2-(4-methylaminophenyl)-4-thiazolidinonyl)-phenyl-N=	0.67 µg/mL^a

Compounds 1–12 are derivatives of quinoxaline 1,4-di-*N*-oxide (N$^+$-O$^-$); *quinoxaline-2,3(1H,4H)-dione derivative; **all MICs are against Mtb H37Rv; Method of MIC determination: ^{a}MABA, ^{b}BACTEC 460 radiometric assay

withdrawing groups resulted in compounds with good Mtb growth inhibition and derivatives with 6 or 7 mono substitution were also found to be active (Ortega et al. 2002). It is plausible to conclude that steric, rather than electronic parameters are responsible for effects at 6 and 7 positions.

The anti-TB activity of 2-acetyl and 2-benzoyl-6(7)-substituted quinoxaline-1,4-di-*N*-oxide derivatives that were developed by Jaso et al. was determined using BACTEC 460 radiometric and MABA assays against Mtb H37Rv. The results showed that unsubstituted and 2-acetyl-3-methyl quinoxaline-1,4-di-*N*-oxide derivatives with chlorine, methyl, or methoxy group in position 7 of the ring exhibited good anti-TB activity with MIC between 0.78–3.13 μM. The most potent compound was the derivative with 7-chloro substitution, **19** (Table 1) with MIC of 0.78 μM. Introduction of an electron-withdrawing group in positions 6 and 7 of the ring reduced the MIC, whereas an electron-releasing group increased the MIC value. The replacement of the methyl of the acetyl group with phenyl at position 2 of the ring could be detrimental for the anti-TB activity (Jaso et al. 2003).

As a continuation of the aforementioned work, Zarranz et al. developed a series of quinoxaline-2-carboxamide-1,4-di-*N*-oxides which were evaluated for their potential to inhibit Mtb H37Rv using BACTEC-460 radiometric method. The compound **20** (Table 1) with a chloro in position 7 on the ring showed a MIC of 0.78 μM. As in the previous series, the 1,4-di-*N*-oxide group was found to be essential for the anti-TB activity of the compounds. The *N*-arylcarboxamide group in position 2 led to compounds which showed 98% to 100% growth inhibition against H37Rv. No activity was shown by piperazinyl carbonyl substituted quinoxaline derivatives. Compounds with a chloro in the positions 6 or 7 of the ring and the corresponding unsubstituted derivatives showed the best activity. The reduction of activity was seen by the introduction of an electron-releasing group (i.e., methyl) on the ring (Zarranz et al. 2003).

Analogues of esters of 6(7)-substituted quinoxaline-2-carboxylate-di-1,4-*N*-oxide developed by Jaso et al. were evaluated against Mtb H37Rv *in vitro*. Compounds **21** and **22** (Table 1) were the most active compounds of the series, showing a MIC of 0.1 μg/mL against Mtb H37Rv. The introduction of chloro, methyl, or methoxy in position 7 of the ring decreased the MIC value. The activity improved based on the substitution of the ester group at position 2 of the ring in the order: benzyl > ethyl > 2-methoxyethyl > allyl > tert-butyl. Moreover, the ethyl and benzyl esters of 3-methylquinoxaline-2-carboxylate di-*N*-1,4-oxide derivatives with the chloro group in position 7 of the ring and the unsubstituted derivatives showed good activity against Mtb H37Rv (Jaso et al. 2005).

The *in vitro* efficacies of the aforementioned 1,4-di-*N*-oxide quinoxaline ester derivatives against Mtb H37Rv were further explored by Villar et al. They were evaluated against a panel of single drug resistant (SDR) tuberculosis bacterial strains. The most active compound of the series, **21**, exhibited a MIC of 0.2 μg/mL against SDR strains resistant to isoniazid (**1**), rifampicin (**2**), thiacetazone (**23**), and *p*-aminosalicylic acid (**24**). Besides, it showed MICs of 0.1 μg/mL and 0.4 μg/mL against ciprofloxacin (**25**) and ethambutol (**26**) resistant strains, respectively (Villar et al. 2008). This was indicative of the fact that the molecule possesses a mechanism of action different from the current drugs due to the comparable susceptibility of these strains and H37Rv to the compound. Few analogues were evaluated in *in vivo* assays including evaluations of the maximum tolerated doses, the levels of oral bioavailability and the efficacies in a low-dose aerosol model of tuberculosis in mice. Following an oral administration, compound **27** was found to reduce the CFU counts in spleen and lung of infected mice. Also, it was found to be highly potent against dormant bacteria and active against PA-824 resistant *Mycobacterium bovis* which is indicative of the fact that the bio-reduction/activation pathway was unrelated to the one of PA-824 (Vicente et al. 2008). The compound **27** showed a MIC of 0.78 μg/mL against Mtb H37Rv and kanamycin (**4**) resistant strains, 1.56 μg/mL against isoniazid (**1**) resistant and ciprofloxacin (**25**) resistant strains, and ≤ 0.39 μg/mL against rifampicin (**2**) resistant and ethambutol (**26**) resistant strains. It exhibited a minimum bactericidal concentration (MBC) of 0.78 μg/mL against Mtb H37Rv and rifampicin (**2**) resistant strains, and 0.5 μg/mL against isoniazid resistant strains. Compound **27** was found to be orally active in a murine model of TB, bactericidal, active against NRP bacteria and active on MDR-TB and poly drug-resistant clinical isolates (resistant to 3–5 anti-TB drugs), indicating that activation occurred in both growing and non-replicating bacteria leading to cell death (Villar et al. 2008).

For the improvement of the anti-TB potential, the solubility and the selectivity, structural modifications were carried out using isosteric and homologous strategies on the lead compounds described by Ortega

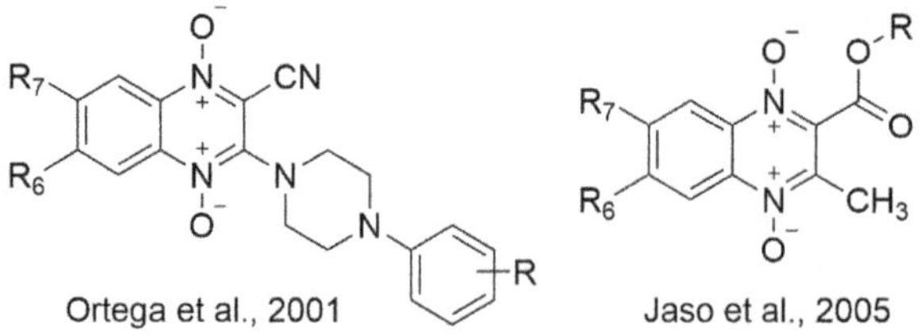

Ortega et al., 2001   Jaso et al., 2005

Figure 3. Structural representation of the Ortega et al. (2001), Jaso et al. (2005) series.

et al., in 2001 and Jaso et al., in 2005. The structural representation of these series is reported in Figure 3. The modified series of 3-phenylquinoxaline 1,4-di-*N*-oxide derivatives was further synthesized and evaluated by Vicente et al., in 2009 explored the relevance of molecular volume and hybridisation of C-atom (from sp species to sp^2 species) at position 2 of the quinoxaline scaffold, replacing the carbonitrile group with an ester group. Homologation of the substituents at position 3 of the scaffold was done by replacing the methyl with a phenyl group for the ester analogues and by eliminating the piperazine ring for the carbonitrile analogues. Several functional groups with variable electronic properties were substituted on the phenyl group. These modifications were done to comprehend the electronic and steric contributions in activity. The best compounds of the carbonitrile and ester series were **28**, with a MIC < 0.2 μg/mL, and **29** with a MIC of 0.39 μg/mL (Table 1), respectively. The quinoxaline-2-carbonitrile derivatives were found to be more potent than the ester derivatives against Mtb. In particular, the electronic profile of the substituent on the phenyl ring did not appear to influence the anti-TB activity as both electron-donating groups and electron-withdrawing groups led to compounds with the same MIC. Finally, fluorinated derivatives exhibited higher selectivity to Mtb than Vero cell-line (Vicente et al. 2009).

Amide derivatives of quinoxaline 1,4-di-*N*-oxide developed by Ancizu et al. were evaluated against Mtb H37Rv in BACTEC 12B medium using the MABA assay. Compounds exhibiting more than 90% inhibition in the BACTEC were re-evaluated to determine MIC in the MABA assay. Compounds **30** and **31** (Table 1) have a MIC of < 0.2 μg/mL. The introduction of an electron-withdrawing group on the quinoxaline ring led to increase in anti-TB activity, whereas introduction of an electron-donating group reduced the activity. The substitution of a *para* methoxy group on the benzene ring (present on the position 2 side chain) and the increase of the length of the aliphatic chain (linker between the quinoxaline ring and benzene ring at position 2) caused an increment in the cytotoxicity of the molecules. The most suitable linker was established to be a single methylene group between the carboxamide and the benzene ring (Ancizu et al. 2010).

Quinoxaline 1,4-di-*N*-oxides derivatives with diverse substituents in 2, 3, 6 and 7 positions developed by Sainz et al. were evaluated against Mtb H37Rv in BACTEC 12B medium using the BACTEC 460 radiometric system at 12.5 μg/mL. Out of the 10 compounds evaluated, 6 showed a MIC < 12.5 μg/mL, and compounds **32** and **33** (Table 1) showed 100% inhibition. The most promising compounds were the 6,7-dichloro substituted derivatives which were found to be better than 6,7-difluoro substituted compounds in terms of activity. The substituents in positions 6 and 7 increased the % inhibition in the 3-amino-2-quinoxaline carbonitrile 1,4-di-*N*-oxides. Also, the (6)7-chloro substitution was a better choice than (6)7-methyl substitution (Sainz et al. 2011).

Other quinoxaline derivatives

Seitz et al. evaluated for their anti-TB potential seven esters along with one 2-carboxamide and one 2-hydrazide derivative of 2-quinoline carboxylic acids. The determination of MIC was carried out against Mtb H37Rv in BACTEC 12B medium. Compound **34** (Table 1) showed the best activity in the series with a MIC of 0.5 μg/mL against Mtb H37Ra and MIC of 6.25 μg/mL against Mtb H37Rv (Seitz et al. 2002).

The derivatives of 1-((Substituted)methyl) quinoxaline-2,3(1H,4H)-diones and 1-((substituted) acryloyl) quinoxaline-2,3(1H,4H)-diones developed by Ramalingam et al. were also evaluated for their anti-TB potential using MABA assay. The most active compound of this series **35**, showed a MIC of 8.012 µg/mL (Ramalingam et al. 2010).

Puratchikody et al. developed a series of quinoxaline derivatives which were evaluated using MABA assay for their activity against Mtb H37Rv. The most potent compound of the series, **36** (Table 1) showed a MIC of 0.67 µg/mL. For the substituents of the phenyl ring on azetidin-2-one/thiazolidin-4-one ring, the anti-TB activity may be attributed to the introduction of electron withdrawing groups on the aromatic ring, but a moderate anti-TB activity was also observed by the introduction of electron releasing groups like methoxy and *para*-hydroxy. The introduction of a hydroxyl group in the ortho position led to complete loss of activity, whilst replacing it with a methyl group resulted in compounds with mild activity. Compounds bearing a five membered furan instead of a phenyl group did not show any considerable activity (Puratchikody et al. 2011).

Iron complexes quinoxaline derivatives

In addition to the derivatives mentioned above, iron complexes [Fe(L–H)$_3$], which have 3-aminoquinoxaline-2-carbonitrile-1,4-di-*N*-oxide derivatives (L) as ligands, were explored for their anti-TB potential (Figure 4). The L1 complex showed low activity, whereas L2, L3 and L4 complexes showed more activity compared to free ligand, indicating that metal coordination can change the anti-TB activity of 3-aminoquinoxaline-2-carbonitrile 1,4-di-*N*-oxide derivatives. The complexes L3 and L4 exhibited a MIC of 0.78 µg/mL (REMA assay) making them equivalent or more active than most second-line drugs (Tarallo et al. 2010).

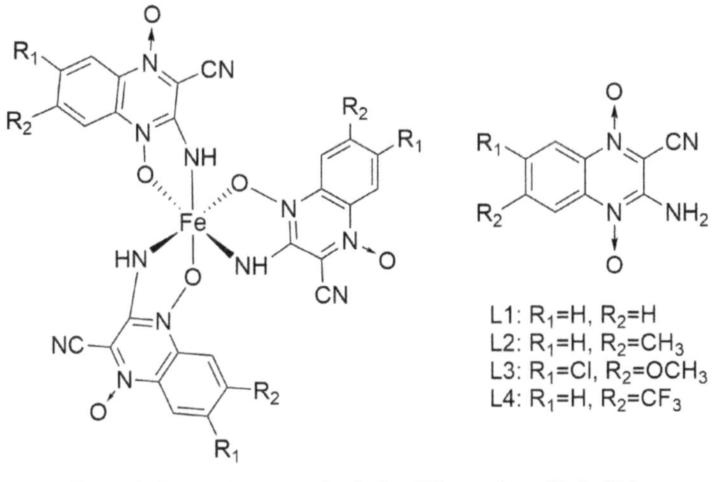

Figure 4. Proposed structure for the iron(III) complexes [Fe(L–H)$_3$].

ADME properties of quinoxaline derivatives

The ADME and medicinal chemistry properties of the 10 most potent compounds containing the quinoxaline scaffold are depicted in Table 2. The properties were predicted using SWISSADME program of Swiss Institute of Bioinformatics (Daina et al. 2017). The important pharmacokinetic parameters like GI absorption, BBB permeation, and CYP inhibition as well as relevant medicinal chemistry properties like Lipinski's rule of 5 (Ro5) (Lipinski et al. 2012), PAINS (Baell and Holloway 2010), and Brenk (Brenk et al. 2008) and Lead-likeness (Teague et al. 1999) that determine the drug-likeness of the molecules were predicted. A compound, to have the ideal pharmacokinetics and medicinal chemistry properties, should exhibit a high GI absorption, no BBB permeation (for molecules not targeted for CNS diseases, to avoid CNS side effects), no CYP enzyme inhibition and comply with Lipinski's Ro5. Moreover, it should show 0 alert in PAINS (pan assay interference compounds) filter, 0 alert in Brenk filter (structural fragments identified to be putatively toxic, chemically reactive, metabolically unstable or to bear properties responsible

Table 2. Pharmacokinetic (ADME) and medicinal chemistry properties of the most potent quinoxaline derivatives.

Compound	GI absorption	BBB permeant	CYP inhibition	Lipinski's rule of 5	PAINS	Brenk	Lead-likeness
17	High	No	Yes (2C19, 2C9)	Yes	1 alert	4 alerts	No, 1 violation
18	High	No	No	Yes	0 alert	2 alerts	Yes
19	High	No	No	Yes	1 alert	2 alerts	Yes
21	High	No	No	Yes	1 alert	2 alerts	Yes
22	High	No	Yes (2C19, 2C9)	Yes	1 alert	2 alerts	Yes
27	High	Yes	No	Yes	1 alert	2 alerts	Yes
28	High	Yes	Yes (1A2)	Yes	1 alert	2 alerts	Yes
29	High	Yes	Yes (2C19)	Yes	1 alert	2 alerts	Yes
30	High	No	Yes (2C19)	Yes	0 alert	2 alerts	No, 1 violation
31	High	No	Yes (2C19)	Yes	1 alert	2 alerts	Yes

for poor pharmacokinetics) and should comply with the lead-likeness filter ($250 \leq$ molecular weight $\leq$ 350, XLOGP ≤ 3.5, rotatable bonds ≤ 7).

Based on the SWISSADME predictions, compound **18** was predicted to be most prospective in terms of drug-likeness amongst the 10 most potent molecules of this class. It was predicted to have high GI absorption, no BBB permeation, and no CYP inhibition. It was also compliant with Lipinski's rule of 5, 0 alerts in PAINS filter, and compliant with the lead-likeness filter. It was predicted to have 2 alerts in the Brenk filter, which were shown by all the molecules. The other prospective compounds based on the SWISSADME predictions were compounds **19** and **21** (which had 1 alert in PAINS filter, in addition to the 2 Brenk alerts). These compounds need to be studied further to confirm their experimental drug-likeness and their prospects as anti-TB hits/leads. The insight provided could be further used for designing newer molecules and/or optimising the design of the current quinoxaline containing molecules having anti-TB potential.

Quinazoline Containing Anti-tuberculosis Agents

Quinazoline is a bioisostere of quinoline with additional nitrogen in position 3 of the ring, as depicted in Figure 5.

Quinazolin-4(3H)-one derivatives

2-Phenyl-3-(5-mercapto-1,3,4-thiadiazol-2-yl)-quinazolin-4(3H)-one derivatives developed by Kumar et al. were screened for their potential activity against Mtb H37Rv using serial dilution tube technique. Compounds **37** and **38** (Table 3) showed MIC of 10 µg/mL. The derivatives unsubstituted at position 6 of the quinazoline scaffold showed the best activity, whereas derivatives with 6-bromo or 6-iodo substitution

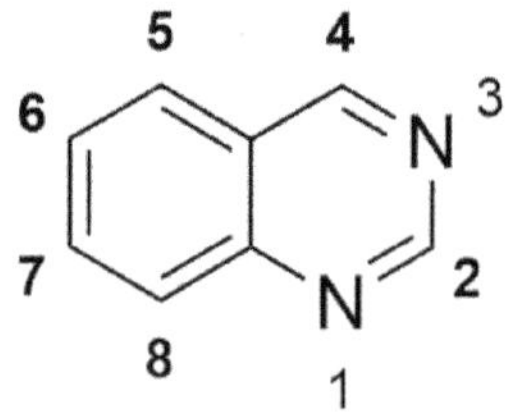

Figure 5. Structural representation of the quinazoline scaffold.

Table 3. Structures and anti-TB activities of the most active compounds of the several quinazoline series.

Compound	Substitution	MIC
37	R_2 = phenyl; R_3 = 5-mercapto-1; 3,4-thiadiazol-3-yl; R_4 = C=O	10 µg/mL[a]
38	R_2 = phenyl; R_3 = 5-carboxymethy mercapto-1,3,4-thiadiazol-3-yl; R_4 = C=O; R_6 = I	10 µg/mL[a]
39	R_2 = phenyl; R_3 = 2-methyl-imidazol-1-yl-acetamido; R_6, R_8 = Br; R_4 = C=O	0.4 µg/mL[b]
41	R_2 = $CH_2CH_2CH_3$; R_3 = 5-nitrofuran-2-yl-CH=N-; R_4 = C=O; R_6, R_8 = Br	0.2 µg/mL[b]
42	R_2 = phenyl; R_3 = 5-nitrofuran-2-yl-CH=N-; R_4 = C=O; R_6, R_8 = Br	0.78 µg/mL[b]
43	R_2 = CH_3; R_3 = 5-nitrofuran-2-yl-CH=N-; R_4 = C=O; R_6 = Br	0.78 µg/mL[b]
44	R_2 = C_3H_7; R_3 = 5-nitrofuran-2-yl-CH=N-; R_4 = C=O; R_6, R_8 = Br	0.78 µg/mL[b]
45	R_2 = CH_3; R_3 = 3;5-dimethoxyphenyl-sulfonylamino; R_4 = C=O; R_6 = pyrazine-2-yl-oxymethylcarbonylhydrazinosulfonyl-	23 µg/mL[a]
46	R_2 = [(4'-Oxo-3'-chloro-2'-{p-nitrophenyl}-azetidin-1'-ylamino)-methyl]-; R_3 = [N-isonicotin-amide-yl]; R_4 = C=O	50 µg/mL[a]
47	R_2 = 2-chlorophenyl; R_3 = (((3-(pyridin-4-yl)-1-(p-tolyl)-1H-pyrazol-4-yl) methylene) amino)-; R_4 = C=O	< 3.125 µg/mL[a]
48	R_2 = 4-chlorophenyl; R_3 = (((3-(pyridin-4-yl)-1-(p-tolyl)-1H-pyrazol-4-yl) methylene) amino)-; R_4 = C=O	< 3.125 µg/mL[a]
49	R_2 = 2-methylphenyl; R_3 = (((3-(pyridin-4-yl)-1-(p-tolyl)-1H-pyrazol-4-yl) methylene) amino)-; R_4 = C=O	< 3.125 µg/mL[a]
50	R_2 = 2-methoxyphenyl; R_3 = (((3-(pyridin-4-yl)-1-(p-tolyl)-1H-pyrazol-4-yl) methylene) amino)-; R_4 = C=O	< 3.125 µg/mL[a]
51	R_2 = 3-nitrophenyl R_3 = (((3-(pyridin-4-yl)-1-(p-tolyl)-1H-pyrazol-4-yl) methylene) amino)-; R_4 = C=O	< 3.125 µg/mL[a]
52	R_2 = CH_3; R_3 = phenylaminocarbonylmethyl; R_4 = C=O; R_6 = Cl	4.76 µM[b]
54	R_2 = 4-chlorophenyl; R_4 = C=O	31.5 µg/mL[c]
55	R_3 = phenyl; R_4 = C=O	31.5 µg/mL[c]
56	R_4 = $S(CH_2)_3CH_3$	63 µg/mL[a] CNCTC TBC 1/47
57	R_2 = CH_3; R_3 = 4-OCH_3; R_4 = C=S; R_6 = Cl	31 µmol/dm[3a] CNCTC My 331/88
58	R_2 = CH_3; R_3 = 4-iPr; R_4 = C=S; R_6 = Cl	31 µmol/dm[3a] CNCTC My 331/88

Method used for MIC determination: [a]serial broth dilution (visual turbidity observation), [b]agar-based spot-culture inhibition, [c]REMA; if strain not specified: Mtb H37Rv

resulted in lower activity. The mercaptoetherification (–SR) at the position 5 of the thiadiazole ring, where R on the mercapto group is allyl or epoxypropyl group, resulted in loss of activity against Mtb H37Rv, whereas when R is CH_2COOH, it improved the activity (Kumar et al. 1983).

Raghavendra et al. developed a series of 2-Imidazolyl-*N*-(4-oxo-quinazolin-3(4*H*)-yl)-acetamide analogues which were evaluated for their anti-TB potential against Mtb H37Rv using agar dilution method. The plates were incubated at 37°C for 4 wk. The most potent molecule of this series was compound **39** (Table 3) with a MIC of 0.4 µg/mL, which is equipotent with gatifloxacin (**40**). The phenyl substitution at position 2 of the scaffold was found to improve the activity compared to propyl and methyl substitution. Methyl substituted azoles attached to acetamido side chain (at position 3 of the scaffold) showed better activity compared to unsubstituted azoles while substitution of H by bromo in position 6 and 8 of the scaffold favoured the anti-TB activity (Raghavendra et al. 2007a).

A further modification of the aforementioned series was carried out by Raghavendra et al., where the acetamido side chain was modified into a methylene-amino and the azole with a furan. The most potent molecule of the series is compound **41** (Table 3) which showed a MIC of 0.2 µg/mL. Three other compounds of the series, namely **42**, **43** and **44**, were also found to be quite potent against Mtb with MIC of 0.78 µg/mL. Unsubstituted furan or furan with electron-withdrawing group like nitro was more potent than furans having electron-donating group, like methyl, at position 3 of the quinazolinone scaffold. An electron-withdrawing group like bromo on the aromatic portion of quinazolinone led to an increase in the anti-TB activity while alkyl substitutions rather than aryl substitution at position 2 of the scaffold favoured the anti-TB activity (Raghavendra et al. 2007b).

A series of aryl sulphonamide substituted quinazolines was evaluated by Bonde et al. against Mtb H37Rv using test tube dilution technique with modified Kirchner's culture medium containing 0.5% sterilized horse serum incubated at 37°C for 14 d. The best molecules of the series, compound **45** (Table 3), showed a MIC of 23 µg/mL (Bonde et al. 2010).

Myangar et al. evaluated a series of quinazolin-4-one hybrids against Mtb H37Rv using Lowenstein Jensen MIC method. The tubes were initially incubated at 37°C for 24 hr followed by streaking of Mtb H37Rv (5×10^4 bacilli per tube). The tubes were then incubated at 37°C and the growth of bacilli was observed after 12, 22 and 28 d. The concentration at which no or < 20 colonies developed was considered the MIC of the molecule. The best molecule of the series, compound **46** (Table 3) showed a MIC of 50 µg/mL (Myangar and Raval 2012).

Quinazolin-4(3H)-one analogues were evaluated against Mtb H37Rv by Pandit et al. Determination of MIC was done using radiometric BACTEC and broth dilution assay techniques. Five molecules of the series, compounds **47–51** (Table 3), exhibited MIC of < 3.125 µg/mL. The phenyl group at position 2 of the scaffold, when substituted with chloro, methyl and methoxy groups at *ortho* position, chloro at *para* position and nitro at *meta* position, resulted in active compounds (Pandit and Dodiya 2013).

Pedgoankar et al. developed 2-(4-Oxoquinazolin-3(4H)-yl)acetamide derivatives which were evaluated against both drug sensitive and resistant TB strains. A bacterial suspension (5 mL, approx. 10^7 cfu per mL) was spotted onto 7H11 agar tubes containing different concentrations of the molecules and incubated at 37°C and observation done after 28 d. The overall most promising molecule of the series was compound **52** (Table 3) which showed MIC of 4.76 µM (Mtb H37Rv), 2.38 µM (Mtb H37Rv, in presence of efflux pump inhibitor piperine (**53**, 8 µg/mL)) and 19.06 µM (XDR-TB) (Pedgaonkar et al. 2014).

Finally, few compounds, designed as Mtb dihydrofolate reductase (DHFR) inhibitors, contained a quinazoline scaffold and were evaluated against Mtb H37Rv using Resazurin microtitre plate (REMA) broth microdilution method by Shelke et al. Compounds **54** and **55** (Table 3) exhibited MIC values of 31.5 µg/mL (Shelke et al. 2016).

Other quinazoline derivatives

A series of 4-alkylthioquinazolines were evaluated by Kuneš et al. for their anti-TB potential using Mtb CNCTC TBC 1/47 strain. The MIC was determined using the Šula semisynthetic medium (Sevapharma, Prague), with incubation at 37°C for 14 d. Compound **56** (Table 3) along with other 4-phenethyl substituted derivatives showed a MIC of 63 µg/mL. It has been observed that for unbranched alkyl substitutions at position 4 of the ring, the length of the chain affected the activity. The best activity was observed with four-carbon residue while any further lengthening of the chain depreciated the activity. The branching of the chain at the α-carbon rather than at the β-carbon can increase the anti-TB potential while unsaturated alkyl groups decreased the anti-TB potential (Kuneš et al. 2000).

Few 2,2-dimethyl-3-phenyl-1,2-dihydroquinazoline-4(3*H*)-thione and 2-methyl-3-phenylquinazoline-4(3*H*)-thione analogues were evaluated for their anti-TB activity by Kubicová et al. using Mtb CNCTC My 331/88 strain inoculated into a Petri dish containing Lowenstein Jensen medium and incubated at 37°C. The determination of MIC was done after 14 and 21 d. The compounds of the 2,2-dimethyl-3-phenyl-1,2-dihydroquinazoline-4(3*H*)-thione series showed MIC values between > 31 to > 125 µg/mL, whereas 2 molecules of the 2-methyl-3-phenylquinazoline-4(3*H*)-thione series **57** and **58** (Table 3) exhibited MIC of 31 µmol/dm^3 at 14 and 21 d (Kubicová et al. 2003).

The selenium derivative 1,2-di(quinazolin-4-yl)diselane (DQYD, **59**) (Figure 6) was evaluated by Tang et al. for its anti-TB potential using serial 2 fold dilution in medium using H37Rv bacterial cultures diluted to 1×10^6 cells per ml and plates incubated at 37°C for 21 d. DQYD (**59**) was found to have MIC of 1 µg/mL. The activity of DQYD against Mtb is associated with intracellular ATP homeostasis. Meanwhile, mycobacterium DNA damage level increased after DQYD (**59**) treatment. But there was no correlation between survival of mycobacteria in the presence of DQYD (**59**) and intercellular reactive oxygen species (Tang et al. 2017).

A series of cationic fullerene derivatives bearing substituted-quinazolin-4(3H)-one moiety as side chain was evaluated by Patel et al. for their anti-TB activity against Mtb H37Rv using Lowenstein Jensen MIC method. The test tubes were incubated at 37 ± 1°C and observed at 12, 22 and 28 d to note MIC. The spheroidal fullerene when attached to the quinazolinone moiety improved the anti-TB activity. It was proposed by the authors that the quinazolinone moiety alone cannot permeate the waxy cell wall of the tubercle bacteria. The small amount of activity, i.e., 200/250 µg/mL which was observed may be due to permeation through the porin channels. The attachment of the fullerene to the molecule facilitated its permeation and potentiated its inhibitory properties. The MIC of one of the molecules decreased to 6.25 µg/mL. It was hypothesized that the introduction of a cationic charge allows the compound to better interact with the Mtb cell wall mycolic acids, leading to a decrease of the MIC of the derivatives. The most potent molecule (**60**) of the series with MIC of 1.562 µg/mL is depicted in Figure 7. The fullerene increased the permeability of the quinazolinone containing molecule into the cytoplasm by disrupting Mtb cell wall (Patel et al. 2013). The prospects of this molecule are highly debatable due to the presence of the C$_{60}$ fullerene group, which though is reported to exhibit no acute or sub-acute toxicity

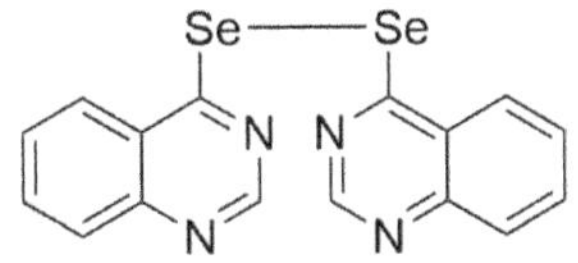

Figure 6. Structure of 1,2-di(quinazolin-4-yl)diselane (**DQYD, 59**).

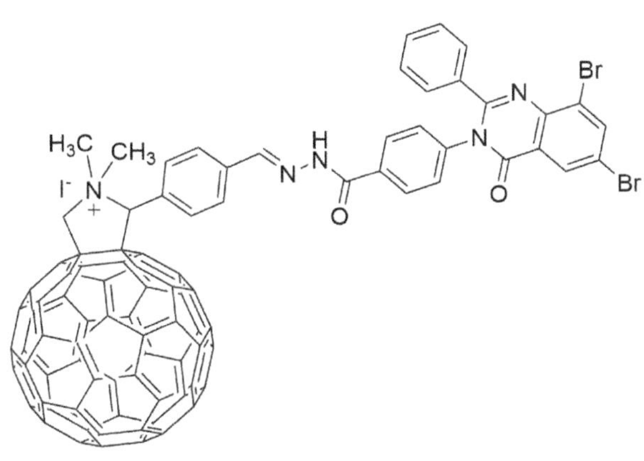

Figure 7. Most potent molecule (**60**) of the quinazolinone-fullerene series.

in a large variety of living organisms, bacteria, fungi, leukocytes, drosophila, mice, rats and guinea pigs (Kolosnjaj et al. 2007), can still be associated with formation of reactive oxygen species that may cause inflammation and genetic damage. The beneficial or adverse effects were found to be dose-dependent (Nielsen et al. 2008).

ADME properties of quinazoline derivatives

The ADME and medicinal chemistry properties of the 5 most potent molecules containing the quinazoline scaffold are depicted in Table 4. All the compounds showed high GI absorption, same level of CYP inhibition and none showed any PAINS alerts. Hence, these criteria could not be considered for selection of the most prospective molecule. Two compounds with better druglike prospects on a comparative basis were **39** and **41**. Compound **39** was predicted to show no BBB permeation and had 0 alerts in Brenk filter but did not comply with Lipinski's RO5. On the other hand, compound **41** was predicted to comply with Lipinski's Ro5 but could permeate the BBB barrier and showed 1 Brenk alert. Thus, further structural modification of the compounds could be proposed to make these molecules more compliant with respect to pharmacokinetics and drug-likeness, with little effect on the anti-TB potency, or a possible improvement in the anti-TB activity.

Table 4. Pharmacokinetic (ADME) and medicinal chemistry properties of the most potent quinazoline derivatives.

Compound	GI absorption	BBB permeant	CYP inhibition	Lipinski's rule of 5	PAINS	Brenk	Lead-likeness
39	High	No	Yes (1A2, 2C9, 2C19)	No, 1 violation	0 alert	0 alert	No, 2 violations
41	High	Yes	Yes (1A2, 2C9, 2C19)	Yes	0 alert	1 alert	No, 2 violations
42	High	No	Yes (1A2, 2C9, 2C19)	No, 2 violations	0 alert	3 alerts	No, 2 violations
43	High	No	Yes (1A2, 2C9, 2C19)	Yes	0 alert	3 alerts	No, 1 violation
44	High	No	Yes (1A2, 2C9, 2C19)	Yes	0 alert	3 alerts	No, 2 violations

1,8-Naphthyridine Containing Anti-tuberculosis Agents

1,8-Naphthyridine is a bioisostere of quinoline with additional nitrogen in the position 8 of the ring, as depicted in Figure 8.

Nalidixic acid (**61**) is known for its outstanding anti-bacterial potential, particularly towards Gram negative organisms, and it contains the 1,8-naphthyridine scaffold which made it worthwhile to explore for its anti-mycobacterial properties.

1-Substituted 1,4-Dihydro-7-[2-(5-nitro-2-furyl)vinyl]-4-oxo-1,8-naphthyridine derivatives were explored for their anti-TB potential by Nagasaki et al. The determination of the MIC of the compounds against Mtb H37Rv was done by two-fold serial dilution in Kirchner medium, and was recorded after 3 wk of incubation at 37°C. Molecules with 1-substitution as methyl, ethyl or *n*-propyl and a 3-carboxylic acid group, namely compounds **62**, **63** and **64** (Table 5), exhibited MIC of 1.6 µg/mL. These molecules were not specific against tuberculosis and showed broad spectrum anti-bacterial activity (Nagasaki et al. 1972).

4-Phenyl-1,8-naphthyridines with 2- and/or 7-piperazino substitution were evaluated for their tuberculostatic activity by Ferrarini et al. against Mtb H37Rv. Six molecules were found to possess more than 50% inhibition against Mtb H37Rv at a concentration of 12.5 µg/mL. The best compound of the series, **65** (Table 5) exhibited 77% inhibition. No structure activity relationship could be inferred as activity did

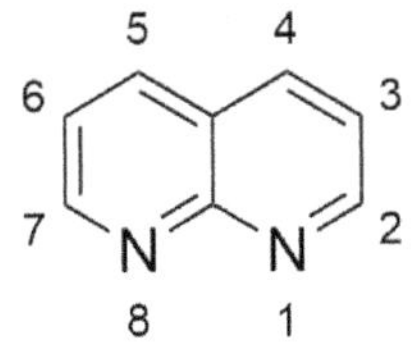

Figure 8. Structural representation of 1,8-naphthyridine.

Table 5. Structures of the most active compounds of the several 1,8-naphthyridine series.

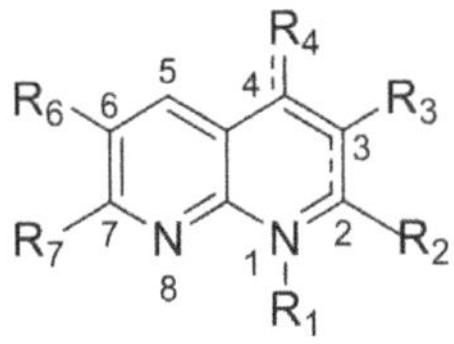

Compounds	Substitutions	MIC
62	R_1 = CH$_3$, Et n-Pr; R_3 =COOH; R_4 = C=O; R_7 = -CH=CH-(5-nitrofuran-2-yl)	1.6 µg/mL[a]
63	R_1 = CH$_3$, Et n-Pr; R_3 = COOH; R_4 = C=O; R_7 = -CH=CH-(5-nitrofuran-2-yl)	1.6 µg/mL[a]
64	R_1 = CH$_3$, Et n-Pr; R_3 = COOH; R_4 = C=O; R_7 = -CH=CH-(5-nitrofuran-2-yl)	1.6 µg/mL[a]
65	R_2 = OCH$_3$; R_4 = phenyl; R_7 = 4-ethhoxycarbonylpiperazino	77% inhibition at 12.5 µg/mL[b]
66	R_2 = piperazino; R_3 = benzyl; R_4 = piperazino; R_7 = CH$_3$	96% inhibition at 6.25 µg/mL[b]
67	R_2 = piperazino; R_4 = phenyl; R_7 = piperazino	99% inhibition at 6.25 µg/mL[b]
68	R_2 = piperazino; R_3 = phenyl; R_7 = phenyl	99% inhibition at 6.25 µg/mL[b]
69	R_1 = tert-butyl; R_3 = COOH; R_4 = C=O; R_6 =NO$_2$; R_7 = 4,4-dimethyloxazolidin-3-yl	0.1 µM[c]
70	R_1 = 4-fluorophenyl; R_3 = COOH; R_4 = C=O; R_6 = NO$_2$; R_7 = 4-thiomorpholino	0.44 µM[c]
71	R_1 = 4-fluorophenyl; R_3 = COOH; R_4 = C=O; R_6 = NO$_2$; R_7 = 2,6-dimethylmorpholino	0.43 µM[c]
72	R_1 = 4-fluorophenyl; R_3 = COOH; R_4 = C=O; R_6 = NO$_2$; R_7 = 2-carboxy-5,6-dihydroimidazo[1,2-*a*]pyrazin-7(8*H*)-yl	0.38 µM[c]
73	R_1 = tert-Butyl; R_3 = COOH; R_4 = C=O; R_6 = NO$_2$; R_7 = 2-carboxy-5,6-dihydroimidazo[1,2-*a*]pyrazin-7(8*H*)-yl	0.42 µM[c]
74	R_1 = 4-fluorophenyl; R_3 = COOH; R_4 = C=O; R_6 = NO$_2$; R_7 = 4,4-dimethyloxazolidin-3-yl	0.21 µM[c]

Method of MIC determination: [a]serial broth dilution (visual turbidity observation), [b]BACTEC 460 radiometric, [c]agar-based spot-culture growth inhibition

not seem to be related directly to substitutions present in various positions on the 1,8-naphythridine ring (Ferrarini et al. 1998).

Various substitutions on the 2, 3, 4 and 7 positions on the 1,8-naphthyridine nucleus were explored by Badawneh et al. as a continuation of the above work. The compounds were screened at 6.25 µg/mL against Mtb H37Rv using BACTEC 460-radiometric system. Three molecules showed an inhibition of more than 50%. The best molecule of the series, compound **66** (Table 5), showed 96% inhibition. It was found that

3-benzyl group was more effective than a 3-methyl group as substituent while the introduction of hydroxy group on positions 2, 4 or 7 of the ring yielded inactive compounds. The influence of 7-amino group on the anti-TB activity was unclear and piperidinyl group was found to be the most effective substituent in the positions 2, 4 or 7 of the ring (Badawneh et al. 2002).

A series of derivatives containing various substitutions at 2, 6 and 7 positions of 3-phenyl or 4-phenyl 1,8-naphthyridine scaffold was explored by Badawneh et al. for their anti-TB potential. Six compounds of the series had an inhibition of 91–99% against Mtb H37Rv at a concentration of 6.25 µg/mL. The two best compounds of the series, **67** and **68** (Table 5), showed 99% inhibition. The piperidinyl substituent in positions 2 and/or 7 was found to increase the activity, also the ethylcarbethoxypiperazinyl, ethylpiperazinyl and phenylpiperazinyl groups in positions 2 and/or 7 favoured the activity. Amino, chloro or methoxy groups in position 7 of the scaffold enhanced the activity while the introduction of a morpholinyl group either in position 2 or 7 of the scaffold caused a decrease in potency. The 6-amino or 6-nitro groups on 2,7-dipiperidinyl-3-phenyl-1,8-naphthyridines led to a fall in the anti-TB, and the presence of 7-hydroxy group on the ring yielded inactive compounds. Finally, a phenyl group (large lipophilic group) at position 3 or 4 of the ring was found to be paramount for activity (Badawneh et al. 2003).

Analogues of 1,8-naphthyridine-3-carboxylic acid were evaluated by Sriram et al. against Mtb H37Rv and MDR-TB. All compounds exhibited MIC of < 12 µM in the *in vitro* agar dilution method against Mtb. Eleven compounds of the series having MIC < 1 µM were found to be more potent than gatifloxacin (**40**) and two were found to be more potent than isoniazid (**1**). All 33 compounds screened inhibited MDR-TB with an MIC ranging from 0.08 to 6.19µM. The most potent compound against Mtb H37Rv and MDR-TB was compound **69** (Table 5) with MIC of 0.1 µM against Mtb H37Rv and MDR-TB and 3 to 455 times more potent than isoniazid (**1**) against Mtb and MDR-TB, respectively. For these analogues, the following activity trend was observed: for substituents at position 1 (R_1) tert-butyl > 4-F phenyl > cyclopropyl; for substituent at position 7 (R_7) oxazolidine > fused piperazines and piperidines > (thio)morpholine > substituted piperazines and piperidines. Contribution of R_7 in anti-TB activity is dependent on R_1. In fact, when R_1 is a cyclopropyl, the trend in R_7 is oxazolidines > fused piperazines and piperidines > substituted piperidines > substituted piperazines > (thio)morpholine. When R_1 is a 4-F phenyl, the trend in R_7 is oxazolidines > (thio)morpholine > substituted piperazine > substituted piperidines > fused piperazines and piperidines. Finally, when R_1 is a *tert*-butyl, the trend in R_7 is oxazolidines > substituted piperazines and piperidines > (thio) morpholine >> fused piperazines and piperidines (Sriram et al. 2007).

ADME properties of 1,8-naphthyridine derivatives

The ADME and medicinal chemistry properties of the 5 most potent compounds containing 1,8-naphthyridine scaffold against Mtb are depicted in Table 6. All the compounds did not penetrate the BBB, all show some degree of CYP inhibition. None showed any alerts in the PAINS filter whereas all showed 2 alerts in Brenk filter and none were lead-like. The parameters for selecting the most prospective molecule were a high GI absorption and complying with the Lipinski's rule of 5. Amongst these compounds, compounds **69**, **71** and **74** were predicted to have better parameters in this class, but further structural modifications may be needed to make these compounds more druglike and in turn more prospective.

Table 6. Pharmacokinetic (ADME) and medicinal chemistry properties of the most potent 1,8-Naphthyridine derivatives.

Compound	GI absorption	BBB permeant	CYP inhibition	Lipinski's rule of 5	PAINS	Brenk	Lead-likeness
69	High	No	Yes (1A2, 2C9, 2C19)	Yes	0 alert	2 alerts	No, 1 violation
71	High	No	Yes (2C9)	Yes	0 alert	2 alerts	No, 2 violations
72	Low	No	Yes (2C19, 2C9)	No	0 alert	2 alerts	No, 1 violation
73	Low	No	Yes (2C19)	No	0 alert	2 alerts	No, 1 violation
74	High	No	Yes (2C19, 2C9)	Yes	0 alert	2 alerts	No, 2 violations

Deazapteridine and Pteridine Containing Anti-tuberculosis Agents

1-/3-/5-Deazapteridine is a bioisostere of quinoline with 2 additional nitrogen as depicted in Figure 9.

Deazapteridine and pteridine scaffolds have been explored majorly as inhibitors of dihydrofolate reductase (DHFR) in several organisms including mycobacteria. DHFR is an established chemotherapeutic target (Lele et al. 2016) as it catalyses the last step in the biosynthesis of tetrahydrofolate (THF) which acts as a crucial co-enzyme for transferring one carbon unit in the synthesis of purines, thymidylate and amino acids like glycine, serine and methionine. DHFR is the most explored enzyme of this pathway and its inhibitors have been successfully used in treatment of cancer and in a variety of bacterial infections, though not yet in mycobacterial infections (Dias et al. 2014). Nevertheless, DHFR is a promising target for designing TB drugs, and for this reason many deazapteridine and pteridine derivatives have been investigated for their anti-TB potential.

Suling et al. evaluated analogues of 2,4-diamino-5-methyl-5-deazapteridine for their potential to inhibit TB and six of these compounds exhibited MIC of 6.25 μg/mL or below. The most promising compound of the series was compound **75** (Table 7), with MIC 3.13 μg/mL. The data showed that 2,4-diamino-5-methyl-5-deazapteridines which had a 6-arylaminomethyl substituents exhibited a potential to inhibit the tubercle bacillus with good level of selectivity and this selectivity can be varied by changing the aryl group as well as by methylation of the bridge (Suling et al. 1998).

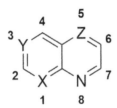

1-Deazapteridine: X: CH; Y: N; Z: N
3-Deazapteridine: X: N; Y: CH; Z: N
5-Deazapteridine: X: N; Y: N; Z: CH
Pteridine: X: N; Y: N; Z: N

Figure 9. Structural representation of the various deazapteridine scaffolds and the pteridine scaffold.

Table 7. Structure and anti-TB activities of the most potent deazapteridine and pteridine derivatives.

Compound	Substitution	MIC
75	X, Y = N; Z = C; R_2, R_4 = NH_2; R_5 = CH_3; R_6 = CH_2NH-(2,5-dimethoxyphenyl)	3.13 μg/mL[a]
76	X = CH; Y, Z = N; R_2 = $NHCOOCH_2Ph$; R_4 = NH_2; R_6 = Ph; R_7 = CH_3; R_8 = H	1.3-≤ 12.8 μg/mL[a] (H37Ra)
77	X, Y, Z = N; R_2, R_4 = NH_2; R_6 = CH_2S-(1-naphthyl)	58% inhibition at 6.25 μg/ mL[b]
78	X, Y, Z = N; R_2 = $NHCOOCH_2CH_3$; R_3 = $NHCH(CH_3)(CH_2)_3NEt_2$; R_6, R_7 = Ph	2 μg/mL[a] (H37Ra)
79	X, Z = N; Y = CH; R_2 = $NHCOOCH_2CH_3$; R_3 = $NHCH(CH_3)(CH_2)_3NEt_2$; R_6, R_7 = Ph	0.25 μg/mL[a] (H37Ra)

Method to determine MIC: [a]MABA, [b]BACTEC 460 radiometric, if strain unspecified: Mtb H37Rv

1-Deazapteridine-7,8-dihydropteridine derivatives were evaluated against Mtb H37Ra strain by Suling et al. using MABA assay. Ten analogues had an activity between 1.28–12.8 μg/mL against Mtb H37Ra One of the best molecules of this series was **76** (Table 7). In many instances, substitution at position 2 of the ring is alkoxycarbonyl and was not essential for anti-TB activity. The activity was found to be dependent on the substitutions on the phenyl ring at position 6 and on the presence of a 7-alkyl group. When the acetoxy carbonyl group and substituents on the phenyl ring were varied, it was observed that the molecule showed an activity of ≤ 12.8 μg/mL. Hence, the substitutions on the phenyl ring were not relevant for the anti-TB activity till there was an alkyl group present on position 7 or 8. Only 4-chlorophenyl and 3,4-dichlorophenyl substitutions did not need the presence of an alkyl group on the 1-deazapteridine ring for activity against Mtb H37Ra (Suling and Maddry 2001).

2,4-Diaminopyrido[2,3-d]pyrimidine derivatives having an aryl group linked via a 6-methylthio bridge were evaluated by Gangjee et al. against *Pneumocystis carinii* (pc) and *Toxoplasma gondii* (tg) DHFR. Compound **77** (Table 7), showing the highest selectivity ratio against pcDHFR and tgDHFR, was compared with rat liver DHFR. This molecule was evaluated *in vitro* for its potential to inhibit the growth of Mtb H37Rv cells, and showed 58% inhibition at a concentration of 6.25 μg/mL (Gangjee et al. 2001).

The protein FtsZ, homolog of bacterial tubulin, is a new target being explored for mycobacterial and other bacterial infections. FtsZ has a GTPase site characteristic of eukaryotic tubulins but exhibits low sequence similarity and differs in function. Its principal role is contractile Z ring formation which is vital for septation of bacteria, and like its mammalian couterpart it is not involved in chromosomal separation during mitosis. Reynolds et al. explored the potential of 2-carbamoyl analogues of pteridine and 3-deazapteridine as prospective FtsZ and TB inhibitors. The MIC of the 2-carbamoyl pteridine analogue **78** (Table 7) against Mtb H37Ra was found to be 2 μg/mL and the 3-deazapteridine analogue **79** (Table 7) had MIC of 0.25 μg/mL, determined using MABA assay. The pteridine analogue was as potent as the 3-deazapteridine in inhibiting FtsZ polymerisation but was a less potent inhibitor of GTP hydrolysis. Though GTP hydrolysis and FtsZ polymerisation were interconnected, the reason for this is not known. The pteridine scaffold was an acceptable substitution in terms of the FtsZ polymerisation but as far as the *in vitro* anti-tuberculosis activity is concerned, it is 8-fold less potent than the 3-deazapteridine analogue (Reynolds et al. 2004).

ADME properties of deazapteridine and pteridine derivatives

The ADME and medicinal chemistry properties of the 5 most active molecules containing the deazapteridine or the pteridine scaffolds are depicted in Table 8. All the 5 molecules showed high GI absorption, no BBB permeation, 0 alerts in PAINS filter and 0 alerts in BRENK filter. Amongst this class, compounds **50** and **52** seem prospective as they comply with Lipinski's rule of 5 and are lead-like. These compounds could be further modified structurally to yield more druglike and more potent anti-TB molecules.

Table 8. ADME and medicinal chemistry properties of the most potent deazapteridine and pteridine derivatives.

Compound	GI absorption	BBB permeant	CYP inhibition	Lipinski's rule of 5	PAINS	Brenk	Lead-likeness
75	High	No	Yes (1A2, 2D6, 3A4)	Yes, 0 violation	0 alert	0 alert	Yes
76	High	No	Yes (1A2, 2C19, 2C9, 2D6, 3A4)	Yes, 0 violation	0 alert	0 alert	No, 2 violations
77	High	No	Yes (1A2, 2C19, 2C9, 2D6, 3A4)	Yes, 0 violations	0 alert	0 alert	Yes
78	High	No	Yes (1A2, 2C19, 2C9, 2D6, 3A4)	No, 1 violation	0 alert	0 alert	No, 3 violations
79	High	No	Yes (1A2, 2C19, 2C9, 2D6, 3A4)	No, 1 violation	0 alert	0 alert	No, 3 violations

Conclusion

The [6.6.0] bicyclic nitrogen heterocycles include important scaffolds that possess anti-infective potential. Several marketed drugs for the treatment of tuberculosis such as bedaquiline (**7**) (treatment of MDR-TB) and fluoroquinolones (second line drugs for TB treatment) contain the quinoline scaffold, which falls under this class of nitrogen heterocycles. Due to the emergence of drug resistant strains of tuberculosis bacteria coupled with the inability of the current anti-tuberculosis drugs to cure such variants of TB and the development of cross-resistance, the discovery of new drugs that can treat drug resistant tuberculosis has become an urgent need. In order to design or identify new drugs for effectively treating the drug resistant forms of tuberculosis and/or shortening the existing chemotherapy that does not exhibit any cross resistance with the current drugs, there is an urgent need to explore drugs that are structurally different from the current ones. This chapter has discussed the potential of anti-TB molecules containing the nitrogen containing bioisosteres of quinoline such as quinoxaline, quinazoline, 1,8-naphthyridine, deazapteridine and pteridine, in terms of anti-TB activity and structure-activity relationship (SAR), where applicable. Furthermore, the most active molecules containing these aforementioned scaffolds were compared based on their predicted pharmacokinetic and medicinal chemistry properties with the aim to select the most prospective molecules on the basis of their drug-likeness. The insights given by the chapter could be effectively used to design newer derivatives containing these scaffolds with improved drug-likeness and anti-TB potential.

References

Ancizu, S., E. Moreno, B. Solano, R. Villar, A. Burguete, E. Torres et al. 2010. New 3-Methylquinoxaline-2-Carboxamide 1,4-di-N-Oxide derivatives as anti-*Mycobacterium tuberculosis* agents. Bioorg. Med. Chem. 18(7): 2713–2719.

Asif, M. 2013. Antimicrobial and anti-tubercular activity of quinolone analogues. Sci. Int. 1: 336–349.

Badawneh, M., C. Manera, C. Mori, G. Saccomanni and P.L. Ferrarini. 2002. Synthesis of variously substituted 1,8-Naphthyridine derivatives and evaluation of their antimycobacterial activity. Farmaco. 57(8): 631–639.

Badawneh, M., L. Bellini, T. Cavallini, J. Al Jamal, C. Manera, G. Saccomanni et al. 2003. Synthesis of 3- or 4-Phenyl-1,8-Naphthyridine derivatives and evaluation of antimycobacterial and antimicrobial activity. Farmaco. 58(9): 859–866.

Baell, J.B. and G.A. Holloway. 2010. New substructure filters for removal of pan assay interference compounds (PAINS) from screening libraries and for their exclusion in bioassays. J. Med. Chem. 53(7): 2719–2740.

Bermudez, L.E. and L. Meek. 2014. Mefloquine and its enantiomers are active against *Mycobacterium tuberculosis in vitro* and in macrophages. Tuberc. Res. Treat. 530815: 1–5.

Bonde, C.G., A. Peepliwal and N.J. Aikwad. 2010. Synthesis and antimycobacterial activity of Azetidine-, Quinazoline-, and Triazolo-Thiadiazole-containing pyrazines. Arch. Pharm. (Weinheim). 343(4): 228–236.

Brenk, R., A. Schipani, D. James, A. Krasowski, I.H. Gilbert, J. Frearson et al. 2008. Lessons learnt from assembling screening libraries for drug discovery for neglected diseases. ChemMedChem. 3(3): 435–444.

Daina, A., O. Michielin and V. Zoete. 2017. SwissADME: A free web tool to evaluate pharmacokinetics, drug-likeness and medicinal chemistry friendliness of small molecules. Sci. Rep. 7(42717): 1–13.

Da Silva, A., P. Eduardo and J.C. Palomino. 2011. Molecular basis and mechanisms of drug resistance in *Mycobacterium tuberculosis*: Classical and new drugs. J. Antimicrob. Chemother. 66(7): 1417–1430.

Dhiman, R. and R. Singh. 2018. Recent advances for identification of new scaffolds and drug targets for *Mycobacterium tuberculosis*. IUBMB Life. 70: 905–916.

Dias, M.V.B., P. Tyrakis, R.R. Domingues, A.F.P. Leme and T.L. Blundell. 2014. *Mycobacterium tuberculosis* dihydrofolate reductase reveals two conformational states and a possible low affinity mechanism to antifolate drugs. Structure. 22(1): 94–103.

Ferrarini, P.L., C. Manera, C. Mori, M. Badawneh and G. Saccomanni. 1998. Synthesis and evaluation of antimycobacterial activity of 4-Phenyl-1,8-Naphthyridine derivatives. Farm. 53(12): 741–746.

Fox, G.J. and D. Menzies. 2013. A review of the evidence for using bedaquiline (TMC207) to treat multi-drug resistant tuberculosis. Infect. Dis. Ther. 2(2): 123–144.

Gangjee, A., O. Adair and S.F. Queener. 2001. Synthesis of 2,4-Diamino-6-(thioarylmethyl)pyrido[2,3-d]pyrimidines as dihydrofolate reductase inhibitors. Bioorg. Med. Chem. 9(11): 2929–2935.

Gillespie, S.H. 2002. Evolution of drug resistance in *Mycobacterium tuberculosis*: Clinical and molecular perspective. Antimicrob. Agents Chemother. 46(2): 267–274.

Jaso, A., B. Zarranz, I. Aldana and A. Monge. 2003. Synthesis of new 2-Acetyl and 2-Benzoyl Quinoxaline 1,4-Di-N-oxide derivatives as anti-*Mycobacterium tuberculosis* agents. Eur. J. Med. Chem. 38(9): 791–800.

Jaso, A., B. Zarranz, I. Aldana and A. Monge. 2005. Synthesis of new Quinoxaline-2-Carboxylate 1,4-Dioxide derivatives as anti-*Mycobacterium tuberculosis* agents. J. Med. Chem. 48(6): 2019–2025.

Kolosnjaj, J., H. Szwarc and F. Moussa. 2007. Toxicity studies of fullerenes and derivatives. Adv. Exp. Med. Biol. 620: 168–180.

Kubicová, L., M. Šustr, K. Kráľová, V. Chobot, J. Vytlačilová, L. Jahodář et al. 2003. Synthesis and biological evaluation of Quinazoline-4-Thiones. Molecules. 8: 756–769.

Kumar, P., K.N. Dhawan, S. Vrat, K.P. Bhargava and K. Kishore. 1983. Synthesis of 6-Substituted 2-Phenyl-3-(5-Substituted Mercapto-1,3,4-thiadiazol-2-yl)quinazolin-4-(3H)-ones as antitubercular agents. Arch. Pharm. (Weinheim). 316(9): 759–763.

Kuneš, J., B. Jaroslav, M. Pour, K. Waisser, M. Iosárek and J. Janota. 2000. Quinazoline derivatives with antitubercular activity. Farmaco. 55(11-12): 725–729.

Kwan, C.K. and J.D. Ernst. 2011. HIV and tuberculosis: a deadly human syndemic. Clin. Microbiol. Rev. 24(2): 351–76.

Lele, A.C., D.A. Mishra, T.K. Kamil, S. Bhakta and M.S. Degani. 2016. Repositioning of DHFR inhibitors. Curr. Top. Med. Chem. 16(19): 2125–2143.

Li, S., R. Tasneen, S. Tyagi, H. Soni, P.J. Converse, K. Mdluli et al. 2017. Bactericidal and sterilizing activity of a novel regimen with bedaquiline, pretomanid, moxifloxacin, and pyrazinamide in a murine model of tuberculosis. Antimicrob. Agents Chemother. 61(9): e00913–e00917.

Lipinski, C.A., F. Lombardo, B.W. Dominy and P.J. Feeney. 2012. Experimental and computational approaches to estimate solubility and permeability in drug discovery and development settings. Adv. Drug Deliv. Rev. 64(SUPPL.): 4–17.

Louw, G.E., R.M. Warren, N.C. Gey van Pittius, C.R.E. McEvoy, P.D. Van Helden and T.C. Victor. 2009. A balancing act: Efflux/influx in mycobacterial drug resistance. Antimicrob. Agents Chemother. 53(8): 3181–3189.

Maitra, A. and S. Bhakta. 2014. TB Summit 2014. Virulence. 5(5): 638–644.

Maitra, A., S. Bates, T. Kolvekar, P.V. Devarajan, J.D. Guzman and S. Bhakta. 2018. Repurposing-a ray of hope in tackling extensively drug resistance in tuberculosis. Int. J. Infect. Dis. 32: 50–55.

Mao, J., H. Yuan, Y. Wang, B. Wan, D. Pak, R. He et al. 2010. Synthesis and antituberculosis activity of novel mefloquine-isoxazole carboxylic esters as prodrugs. Bioorg. Med. Chem. Lett. 20(3): 1263–1268.

Myangar, K.N. and J.P. Raval. 2012. Design, synthesis, and *in vitro* antimicrobial activities of novel Azetidinyl-3-Quinazolin-4-one hybrids. Med. Chem. Res. 21(10): 2762–2771.

Nagasaki, S., N. Nakazawa, Y. Osada, T. Hashizume and Y. Ôshima. 1972. Studies on the antibacterial activity of 1-Substituted 1, 4-Dihydro-7-[2-(5-nitro-2-furyl) vinyl]-4-oxo-1, 8-Naphthyridine derivatives. Chem. Pharm. Bull (Tokyo). 20(4): 639–649.

Nasiri, M.J., M. Haeili, M. Ghazi, H. Goudarzi, A. Pormohammad, A.A. Imani Fooladi et al. 2017. New insights in to the intrinsic and acquired drug resistance mechanisms in mycobacteria. Front. Microbiol. 8(681): 1–19.

Nielsen, G.D., M. Roursgaard, K.A. Jensen, S.S. Poulsen and S.T. Larsen. 2008. *In vivo* biology and toxicology of fullerenes and their derivatives. Basic Clin. Pharmacol. Toxicol. 103(3): 197–208.

Ortega, M.A., M.E. Montoya, A. Jaso, B. Zarranz, I. Tirapu, I. Aldana et al. 2001. Antimycobacterial activity of new Quinoxaline-2-Carbonitrile and Quinoxaline-2-Carbonitrile 1,4-Di-N-oxide derivatives. Pharmazie. 56(3): 205–207.

Ortega, M.A., Y. Sainz, M.E. Montoya, A. Jaso, B. Zarranz, I. Aldana et al. 2002. Anti-*Mycobacterium tuberculosis* agents derived from Quinoxaline-2-Carbonitrile and Quinoxaline-2-Carbonitrile 1,4-Di-N-Oxide. Arzneimittelforschung. 52(2): 113–119.

Pandit, U. and A. Dodiya. 2013. Synthesis and antitubercular activity of novel pyrazole-quinazolinone hybrid analogs. Med. Chem. Res. 22(7): 3364–3371.

Patani, G.A. and E.J. LaVoie. 1996. Bioisosterism: A rational approach in drug design. Chem. Rev. 96(8): 3147–3176.

Patel, M.B., U. Harikrishnan, N.N. Valand, N.R. Modi and S.K. Menon. 2013. Novel cationic Quinazolin-4(3H)-one conjugated fullerene nanoparticles as antimycobacterial and antimicrobial agents. Arch. Pharm. (Weinheim). 346(3): 210–220.

Pavić, K., I. Perković, Š. Pospíšilová, M. Machado, D. Fontinha, M. Prudêncio et al. 2018. Primaquine hybrids as promising antimycobacterial and antimalarial agents. Eur. J. Med. Chem. 143: 769–779.

Pedgaonkar, G.S., J.P. Sridevi, V.U. Jeankumar, S. Saxena, P.B. Devi, J. Renuka et al. 2014. Development of 2-(4-Oxoquinazolin-3(4H)-yl)acetamide derivatives as novel enoyl-acyl carrier protein reductase (InhA) inhibitors for the treatment of tuberculosis. Eur. J. Med. Chem. 86(1): 613–627.

Puratchikody, A., R. Natarajan, M. Jayapal and M. Doble. 2011. Synthesis, *in vitro* antitubercular activity and 3D-QSAR of novel quinoxaline derivatives. Chem. Biol. Drug Des. 78(6): 988–998.

Raghavendra, N.M., P. Thampi, P.M. Gurubasavarajaswamy and D. Sriram. 2007a. Synthesis, antitubercular and anticancer activities of substituted Furyl-Quinazolin-3(4H)-ones. Arch. Pharm. (Weinheim). 340(12): 635–641.

Raghavendra, N.M., P. Thampi, P.M. Gurubasavarajaswamy and D. Sriram. 2007b. Synthesis and antimicrobial activities of some novel substituted 2-Imidazolyl-N-(4-Oxo-Quinazolin-3(4H)-yl)-Acetamides. Chem. Pharm. Bull. 55(11): 1615–1619.

Ramalingam, P., S. Ganapaty and C.B. Rao. 2010. *In vitro* antitubercular and antimicrobial activities of 1-Substituted Quinoxaline-2,3(1H,4H)-diones. Bioorg. Med. Chem. Lett. 20(1): 406–408.

Reynolds, R.C., S. Srivastava, L.J. Ross, W.J. Suling and E.L. White. 2004. A new 2-Carbamoyl pteridine that inhibits mycobacterial FtsZ. Bioorg. Med. Chem. Lett. 14(12): 3161–3164.

Sainz, Y., M.E. Montoya, F.J. Martinez-Crespo, M.A. Ortega, A.L. de Ceráin and A. Monge. 2011. New Quinoxaline 1,4-Di-N-Oxides for treatment of tuberculosis. Arzneimittelforschung. 49(1): 55–59.

Seitz, L.E., W.J. Suling and R.C. Reynolds. 2002. Synthesis and antimycobacterial activiy of pyrazine and quinoxaline derivaitves. J. Med. Chem. 45(25): 5604–5606.

Senol, G., A. Erbaycu and A. Ozsoz. 2005. Incidence of cross resistance between rifampicin and rifabutin in *Mycobacterium tuberculosis* strains in Izmir, Turkey. J. Chemother. 17(4): 380–384.

Shelke, R.U., M.S. Degani, A. Raju, M.K. Ray and M.G.R. Rajan. 2016. Fragment discovery for the design of nitrogen heterocycles as *Mycobacterium tuberculosis* dihydrofolate reductase inhibitors. Arch. Pharm. (Weinheim). 349(8): 602–613.

Sriram, D., P. Senthilkumar, M. Dinakaran, P. Yogeeswari, A. China and Valakunja, Nagaraja. 2007. Antimycobacterial activities of novel 1-(Cyclopropyl/tert-butyl/4-Fluorophenyl)-1,4-Dihydro- 6-Nitro-4-Oxo-7-(Substituted Secondary Amino)-1,8-Naphthyridine-3-Carboxylic acid. J. Med. Chem. 50(24): 6232–6239.

Suling, W.J., R.C. Reynolds, E.W. Barrow, L.N. Wilson, J.R. Piper and W.W. Barrow. 1998. Susceptibilities of *Mycobacterium tuberculosis* and *Mycobacterium avium* complex to lipophilic deazapteridine derivatives, inhibitors of dihydrofolate reductase. J. Antimicrob. Chemother. 42(1998): 811–815.

Suling, W.J. and J.A. Maddry. 2001. Antimycobacterial activity of 1-Deaza-7,8-dihydropteridine derivatives against *Mycobacterium tuberculosis* and *Mycobacterium avium* complex *in vitro*. J. Antimicrob. Chemother. 47(4): 451–454.

Tang, B., M. Wei, Q. Niu, Y. Huang, S. Ru, X. Liu et al. 2017. Antimicrobial activity of quinazolin derivatives of 1,2-Di(Quinazolin-4-yl)Diselane against mycobacteria. BioMed. Res. Int. 5791781: 1–7.

Tarallo, M.B., C. Urquiola, A. Monge, B.P. Costa, R.R. Ribeiro, A.J. Costa-Filho et al. 2010. Design of novel iron compounds as potential therapeutic agents against tuberculosis. J. Inorg. Biochem. 104(11): 1164–1170.

Teague, S.J., A.M. Davis, P.D. Leeson and T. Oprea. 1999. The design of leadlike combinatorial libraries. Angew Chemie-Int. Ed. 38(24): 3743–3748.

Tukulula, M., S. Little, J. Gut, P.J. Rosenthal, B. Wan, S.G. Franzblau et al. 2012. The design, synthesis, *in silico* ADME profiling, antiplasmodial and antimycobacterial evaluation of new arylamino quinoline derivatives. Eur. J. Med. Chem. 57: 259–267.

Ventola, C.L. 2015. The antibiotic resistance crisis: Part 1: Causes and threats. Pharm. Ther. 40(4): 277–283.

Vicente, E., R. Villar, A. Burguete, B. Solano, S. Pérez-Silanes, I. Aldana et al. 2008. Efficacy of quinoxaline-2-Carboxylate 1,4-Di-N-Oxide derivatives in experimental tuberculosis. Antimicrob. Agents Chemother. 52(9): 3321–3326.

Vicente, E., S. Pérez-Silanes, L.M. Lima, S. Ancizu, A. Burguete, B. Solano et al. 2009. Selective activity against *Mycobacterium tuberculosis* of new quinoxaline 1,4-Di-N-Oxides. Bioorg. Med. Chem. 17(1): 385–389.

Villar, R., E. Vicente, B. Solano, S. Pérez-Silanes, I. Aldana, J.A. Maddry et al. 2008. *In vitro* and *in vivo* antimycobacterial activities of ketone and amide derivatives of quinoxaline 1,4-Di-N-Oxide. J. Antimicrob. Chemother. 62(3): 547–554.

Viveiros, M., C. Leandro and L. Amaral. 2003. Mycobacterial efflux pumps and chemotherapeutic implications. Int. J. Antimicrob. Agents. 22(3): 274–278.

WHO. 2018. WHO Global Tuberculosis Report 2018.

Zarranz, B., A. Jaso, I. Aldana and A. Monge. 2003. Synthesis and antimycobacterial activity of new quinoxaline-2-Carboxamide 1,4-Di-N-Oxide derivatives. Bioorg. Med. Chem. 11(10): 2149–2156.

Chapter 9

Progress in Antimalarial Drug Discovery and Development

Anna C.C. Aguiar,[1,#] Wilian A. Cortopassi[2,#] and Antoniana U. Krettli[3,*]

Introduction

Malaria is among the most important parasitic diseases in humans. In 2016, 216 million cases of malaria occurred worldwide, with an estimated 445,000 deaths globally in 91 countries (Figure 1). Malaria is transmitted by female *Anopheles* mosquitoes. Out of more than 400 *Anopheles* species, around 30 are considered important malaria vectors. Five species of *Plasmodium* cause malaria in human beings: *P. falciparum*, *P. vivax*, *P. malarie*, *P. ovale* and *P. knowlesi*. Most of the lethal cases are caused by *P. falciparum*, especially in sub-Saharan Africa. *P. vivax* is the predominant parasite outside Africa and represents 64% of malaria cases in South and Central Americas, more than 30% in Southeast Asia and 40% in the Eastern Mediterranean regions (Mol et al. 2003).

Malaria is usually classified as asymptomatic, uncomplicated or severe. The typical initial symptoms are nonspecific and include intermittent fever every two or three days, moderate-to-severe shaking chills, profuse sweating, headache, nausea, vomiting, diarrhea and anemia. The symptoms may appear suddenly (paroxysms), after hemolysis of the infected red blood cells (RBC), and then progress to drenching sweats, high fever and exhaustion. Severe malaria is often fatal and may be related to severe anemia and manifestations of multi-organ damage, including cerebral malaria. Severe disease is usually caused by infection with *P. falciparum*, and less frequently by *P. vivax* or *P. knowlesi* (Barber et al. 2013, Elizalde-Torrent et al. 2018, Saharan et al. 2009). The severity of *P. falciparum* is linked to sequestration of infected RBC (iRBC) within the microvasculature of various organs including the brain (Wassmer et al. 2017).

Uncomplicated *P. falciparum* malaria is treated with artemisinin (**1**)-based combination therapies (ACT). In low-transmission areas, an additional single dose (0.25 mg/kg) of primaquine (PQ, **2**) is administered to patients (except pregnant women, infants aged < 6 mon and women breastfeeding infants

[1] Instituto de Física de São Carlos, Avenida Joao Dagnone, 1100, Jardim Santa Angelina, São Carlos, SP, 13563-120, Brazil.
[2] Department of Pharmaceutical Chemistry, University of California, San Francisco, CA, 94158, USA.
[3] Laboratorio de Malaria, Instituto Rene Rachou, FIOCRUZ Minas, Belo Horizonte, 30130-100 MG, Brazil.
* Corresponding author: akrettli@minas.fiocruz.br
# These authors equally contributed for this Chapter

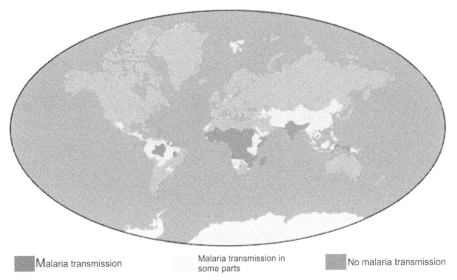

| | Malaria transmission in | |
| Malaria transmission | some parts | No malaria transmission |

Figure 1. Populations at risk of malaria. Source: Centers for Disease Control and prevention (CDC)—https://www.cdc.gov/malaria/about/distribution.html. Used with permission.

Color version at the end of the book

< 6 mon old) to reduce malaria transmission. Non-*P. falciparum* malaria in areas with chloroquine (CQ, **3**)-susceptible parasites is treated with either ACT (except pregnant women in the first trimester) or CQ (**3**). To prevent late relapse in *P. vivax* and *P. ovale* infections, a 14 d course (0.25–0.5 mg/kg daily) of PQ (**2**) is recommended. However, in areas where patients may be glucose-6-phosphate dehydrogenase (G6PD) deficient, this status has to be evaluated before starting PQ (**2**) treatment (Peters et al. 2009). The severe cases of malaria (including infants, pregnant women in all trimesters and lactating women) are treated with intravenous or intramuscular artesunate (ART, **4**) for at least 24 hr or until patients tolerate oral medication after which a complete ACT treatment within 3 d has to be undertaken (WHO 2018).

In spite of the recent introduction of ACT, *P. falciparum* has developed resistance, as evidenced since 2008 when the first case was detected in Cambodia. This resistance is now spread in the Southeast Asia region causing high treatment failure of ACT (Woodrow et al. 2017, Dondorp et al. 2009, Noedl et al. 2009).

The early diagnosis and treatment of malaria reduce disease symptoms, prevent deaths and contribute to reducing malaria transmission. Vector control strategies, including insecticide-impregnated bed nets and localized spraying, have been deployed with success (Mol et al. 2003). If coverage of vector control interventions within a specific area is high enough, it results in reduction of malaria transmission across the community. Nonetheless, treatment remains a vital component of malaria control. The current malaria elimination strategies include: early diagnosis followed by an effective treatment of malaria within 24–48 hr of symptoms onset; a rational use of antimalarials to reduce the spread of drug resistance; combination therapy to prevent resistance; and appropriate weight-based dosing to prolong useful therapeutic life and ensure that all patients have an equal chance of being cured (WHO 2018). Specific treatments are administered depending on the results of a parasitological test including species identification and level of parasitemia (Figure 2). Rapid diagnostic tests that detect *P. falciparum* antigens in human blood are sometimes the only alternative outside endemic areas or in remote areas with limited access to good quality microscopy services (Malaria rapid diagnostic tests 2018).

Human *Plasmodium* Life Cycle

Plasmodium spp parasites have a complex life cycle, which initiates when highly motile sporozoite forms are inoculated into the dermis of the mammalian host during the mosquito bite (Figure 3). A proportion

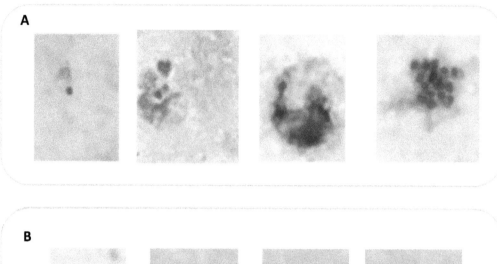

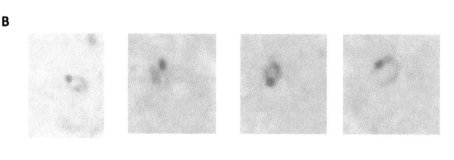

Figure 2. *P. vivax* (A) and *P. falciparum* (B) forms found on thick slides.

Color version at the end of the book

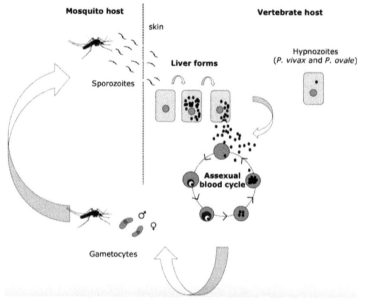

Figure 3. *Plasmodium* spp. life cycle.

Color version at the end of the book

of the parasites enters blood capillaries, relying on gliding motility, a random process enabling them to reach and penetrate blood vessels in the bloodstream (Frenal et al. 2017). Other sporozoites are drained in the lymphatic system and reach the lymph node where most are degraded by dendritic leucocytes. Some sporozoites partially differentiate into exoerythrocytic stages in the skin (Amino et al. 2008). The parasites migrating through Kupffer cells avoid phagocytosis by these resident macrophages and are retained in hepatocytes, then differentiate and divide thereby originating thousands of new cells, the merozoits (Tavares et al. 2013). The migration through the hepatocytes is an essential step of the *Plasmodium* life cycle, after exocytosis of the sporozoite apical organelles, a prerequisite for infection (Mota et al. 2001). In addition, prior to hepatocyte invasion, the sporozoites must leave the circumsporozoite (CSP), a multifunctional protein that is involved in the mosquitoes' sporogonic cycle, including invasion of the salivary glands. The specific arrest of sporozoites in the liver sinusoid depends on their gliding motility and the hepatocyte recognition and entry (Sultan 1999).

Once the tissue merozoites differentiate, they detach from their host hepatocytes, followed by the budding of parasite-filled vesicles, named merosomes, into the sinusoid lumen (Sturm et al. 2006). The released free merozoites will invade erythrocytes via a complex, multistep process involving a series of distinct receptor-ligand binding events (Miller et al. 1976, Weiss et al. 2015). The parasites develop into ring forms named trophozoites, and then to schizont stages, which, within 48 hr, start to release merozoites into the host's plasma to initiate a new cycle in the erythrocytes. Merozoites release coincides with periodic fever every 2 d in *P. falciparum* and *P. vivax* malaria, and every 72 hr in *P. malariae* (Figure 3) (Gerald et al. 2011, Miller et al. 2002).

The transmission of malaria from humans to mosquitoes is dependent on development of sexual stages in the bloodstream, the male and female gametocytes. At each round of schizogony, ~ 1% of merozoites differentiate into gametocytes (Baker 2010). If ingested by susceptible *Anopheles* mosquitos, the male gametocyte exflagelates and the female gamete leaves the RBC, then a sexual cycle begins. The zygote is formed by fertilization of a female macrogamete by a male microgamete in the mosquito's midgut lumen, leading to an ookinete—the only invasive stage that is not preceded by a replication step. The ookinete is motile and will develop further if it traverses the midgut epithelial cell layer to reach the basal lamina (Vinetz 2005). This invasion step is accompanied by a severe reduction in ookinete numbers due to the intervention of mosquito host protective mechanisms (Han et al. 2000). The surviving ookinetes become sessile and transform into oocysts. The oocyst is the only parasite developmental stage that grows extracellularly and results in the formation of sporozoites. Free sporozoites are released into the mosquito body cavity and invade the salivary glands, to be transmitted to the human host during the next mosquito blood meal and initiate liver infection (Aly et al. 2009).

Most antimalarial drugs currently in use target blood-stage parasites, which are responsible for the malaria pathologies including fatal disease. Compounds that act on other stages are needed. Compounds that act against the liver stages would offer protection from infection and may, in addition, be active against the cryptic hypnozoite formed by *P. vivax* and *P. ovale*, which are responsible for late malaria relapses in the infected hosts. A second bottleneck occurs during sexual development, thus compounds against male and female gametocytes could block malaria transmission. Following fertilization, the zygote differentiates into a motile and invasive ookinete. These processes occur within an environment almost totally derived from host blood, which provides a novel and ideal conduit for the delivery of drugs that inhibit parasite transmission to the mosquito. Compounds such as PQ (2) that act against intracellular stages in the liver stage, with the indication to prevent the late relapses, will block parasite development offering protection from malaria infections. However, in order for an antimalarial to have a curative effect, it should completely inhibit pre-erythrocytic stage formation because a single successful sporozoite can develop into over 10,000 liver merozoites and lead to malaria (Figure 3).

Antimalarial Drugs: Discovery and Development of the First Treatments

Ancient Chinese medical records, e.g., the Canon of Internal Medicine, show that malaria has affected the human society since the era Before Christ (BC) (Sallares et al. 2004). However, the first treatments for this disease only appeared in the 1600s and consisted of infusions made of barks from Cinchona trees found in the Peruvian Amazon (Achan et al. 2011). The main source of quinine (**5**) until the 1900s was also from Chinchona trees, first found and used by the Jesuits. Several expeditions to Peru to search for alternative sources of Cinchona seeds and plants were undertaken in the following years, occasionally with illegal smuggling abroad (Breedlove et al. 2015). Charles Ledger, with help from a local friend, managed to locate seeds of a Chinchona species from the Peruvian/Bolivian border whose bark contained up to 10% quinine (**5**), a significant improvement over other species (Gramiccia 1988). In 1865, these were sent to London; however, the British government showed little interest in them. They were eventually sold to the Dutch government who cultivated and improved the species in their colony Java (now Indonesia). This species, called *Chinchona ledgeriana* to honor Charles Ledger, was the basis for most of the world's supply of quinine (**5**) (Achan et al. 2011, Gramiccia 1988).

In the 1800s, Joseph Caventou and Pierre Pelletier, two French scientists, characterized the active principle of the plant infusions as quinine (**5**), which became a reference malaria treatment for centuries (Le Bras et al. 2003). Today, more than 400 yr after its pioneering use, quinine (**5**) is still an effective antimalarial, but large concentrations may cause severe side effects. Therefore, this compound is not recommended as a first choice for malaria treatment (WHO 2015).

During World War II, the Japanese had taken control of the Java region and thus the commerce of *C. ledgeriana* trees, which resulted in short supplies of quinine (**5**) worldwide and motivated the beginning of research programs that led to the first synthetic 4-aminoquinolines. Among them, CQ (**3**) was proven to be the least toxic and showed high efficacy against the fatal form of malaria caused by *P. falciparum.* This discovery opened new frontiers for the development of other synthetic 4-aminoquinoline compounds with antimalarial effect, e.g., amodiaquine (AQ, **6**) (Olliaro et al. 1996).

In 1946, hydroxychloroquine (HCQ, **7**) was synthesized as one of the first CQ (**3**) analogs by adding a hydroxyl group in the N-ethyl substituents of CQ (**3**). This chemical modification resulted in a less toxic compound when compared to its precursor without having a dramatic effect in its antimalarial activity. However, this compound is not able to overcome CQ (**3**) resistance, and therefore its use is limited in most parts of the world (Al-Bari 2015, Lim et al. 2009, Saenz et al. 2012). Due to its lower toxicity, HCQ (**7**) is nowadays still used in some countries, e.g., as chemoprophylaxis against malaria caused by *P. vivax* in the Republic of Korea's Army (Lim et al. 2009). Pyrimethamine (**8**), another synthetic drug derived from ethyl-pyrimidine, was simultaneously discovered and largely used later in African countries, usually administered with sulfonamides (Le Bras et al. 2003).

PQ (**2**), a synthetic 8-aminoquinoline resulting from the drug research programs during World War II, is still used to treat relapses caused by *P. vivax* and *P. ovale*. In spite of the limited knowledge of the liver stage of *Plasmodium* infection, malariologists recognized the importance to overcome the observed phenomenon of relapse in *P. vivax* malaria by using antimalarials with an effect on the dormant stages of the parasite (Elderfield et al. 1955). PQ (**2**) also played an important role in preventing reintroduction of endemic malaria to North America by targeting the *P. vivax* liver dormant stages in soldiers returning from World War II (Baird 2015, Ducharme et al. 1996). After decades counting only on this compound, a new 8-aminoquinoline analog of PQ (**2**) was recently developed: single-dose tafenoquine (**13**) kills liver stages (Campo et al. 2015, Commons et al. 2017). In July 2018, GSK and Medicines for Malaria Venture (MMV) announced that "*the FDA has approved, under Priority Review, single-dose Krintafel (tafenoquine, 13) for the radical cure (prevention of relapse) of P. vivax malaria in patients aged 16 yr and older who are receiving appropriate antimalarial therapy for acute P. vivax infection*". The importance of finding alternatives to PQ (**2**) is that this compound can cause severe side effects in patients with genetic G6PD variants leading to deficiency of the enzyme G6PD (Baird 2015). Tafenoquine (**13**) may also cause severe hemolysis in individuals with G6PD deficiency (Dow et al. 2014, Kitchakarn et al. 2017).

Treatments based on the quinoline compound mefloquine (MQ, **9**) and the sesquiterpene lactone ART (**4**) were developed years later post-World War II (Figure 4) (Frenette et al. 2007). An ACT based on these two compounds has been recommended for most cases of malaria in recent years. While treatments based on the combination of MQ (**9**) and ART (**4**) are still effective, resistance cases have also started to appear (Ashley et al. 2014, Satimai et al. 2012).

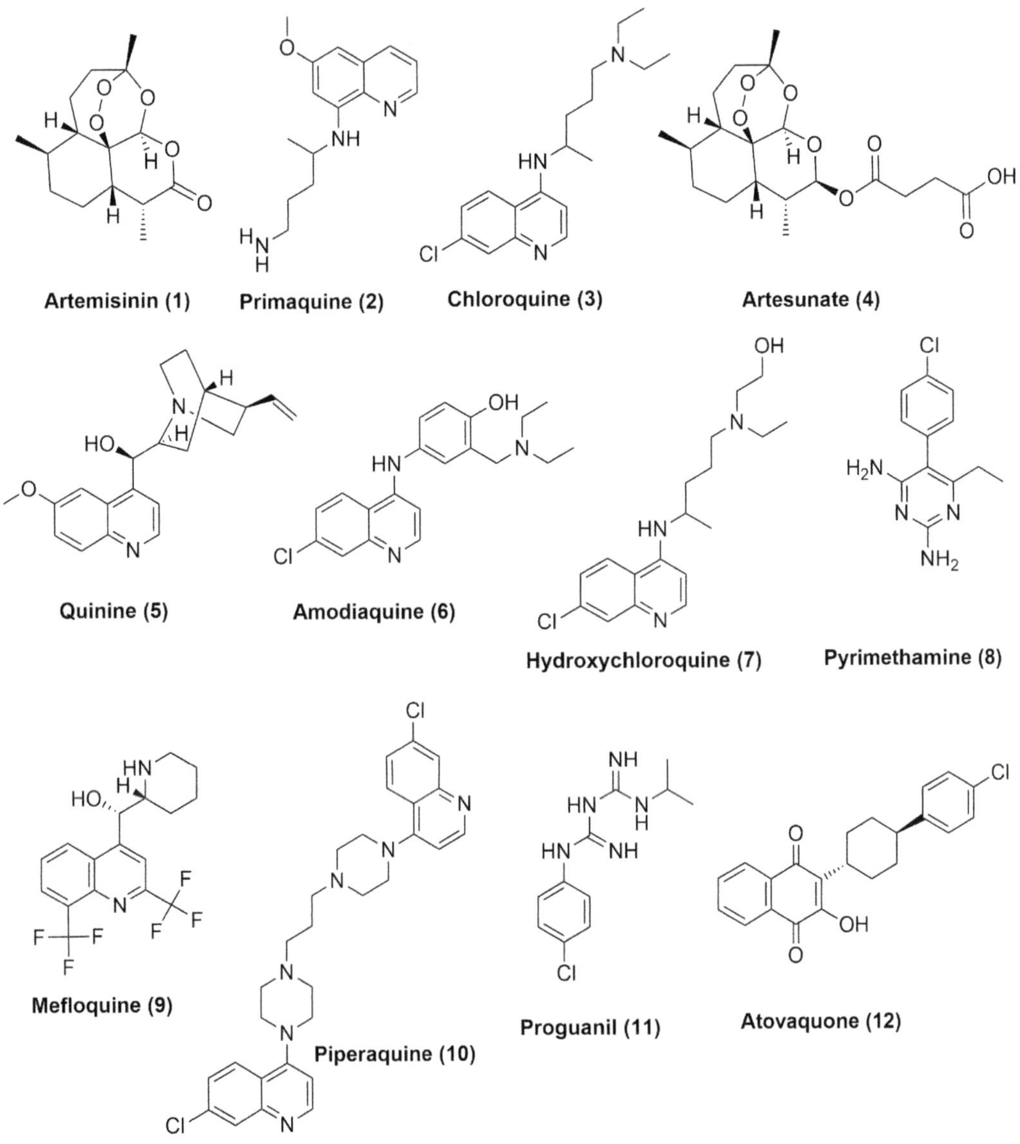

Figure 4. Antimalarials currently in therapy.

Aiming to overcome this resistance, and also in the search for less toxic and more active compounds, a considerable number of on-going medicinal chemistry projects around the world is looking for molecules inspired on modifications of the quinoline structure on novel pathways able to fight the defense mechanisms developed by different species of *Plasmodium*; the majority of them are in research phase (Aguiar et al. 2012a, Saenz et al. 2012). Additional compounds were identified and developed (Figure 5), which have progressed from pre-clinical to clinical trials in recent years, including ferroquine (FQ, **15**) (Biot et al. 2011), MMV048 (**18**) (Paquet et al. 2017), SJ733 (**14**) (Jiménez-Díaz et al. 2014c), KAE609 (**16**) (White et al. 2014), and DSM265 (**17**) (Phillips et al. 2015).

FQ (**15**, on the right), a compound that consisted of the addition of a ferrocene unit to the structure of CQ (**3**), is one of the most recent cases of successful chemical modifications on quinolones, highlighting the potential of chemical structure modifications as powerful approaches to overcome parasite drug resistance

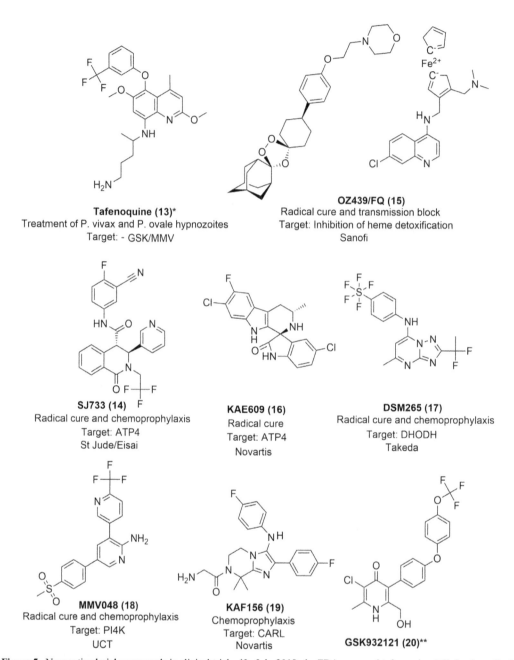

Figure 5. New antimalarial compounds in clinical trials. *In July 2018, the FDA approved tafenoquine (**13**) for the radical cure of *P. vivax* malaria in patients aged 16 yr and older who are receiving appropriate antimalarial therapy for acute *P. vivax* infection. **GSK932121 (**20**) has showed cardiotoxicity in phase-1 clinical trials (section 6.1).

(Wani et al. 2015). *In vitro* studies have suggested that ferrocene-containing compounds are active against both *P. falciparum* sensitive and resistant species and are advancing through clinical trials (McCarthy et al. 2016). FQ (**15**) is proposed to interact with haematin, it inhibits hemozoin (HZ) formation and is remarkably effective against CQ (**3**)-resistant *P. falciparum* (Christophe Biot et al. 2005).

MMV048 (**18**) is effective against resistant parasite strains across the entire parasite life cycle with the potential to cure and protect in a single dose. This medicine was the first new antimalarial to enter phase I studies in Africa (Paquet et al. 2017). The compound SJ733 (**14**) targets a *Plasmodium* cation-transporting ATPase, clearing parasites *in vivo* as quickly as ART (**4**) by specifically inducing eryptosis/senescence (Jiménez-Díaz et al. 2014a). The compound KAE609 (**16**) is a synthetic antimalarial drug belonging to the spiroindolone class that inhibits the *P. falciparum* Ca^{2+}-ATPase (*Pf*ATP4). KAE609 (**16**) kills blood stages of *P. falciparum in vitro* at low nanomolar concentrations, including late-stage gametocytes, and thus possesses transmission-blocking activity potential (van Pelt-Koops et al. 2012). A phase I study has shown KAE609 (**16**) to be well tolerated in healthy volunteers at doses up to 150 mg daily and to have favorable pharmacokinetic properties (Leong et al. 2014). Furthermore, a phase II trial revealed the potent and fast activity of KAE609 (**16**) against both *P. falciparum* and *P. vivax* malaria, with a short mean parasite clearance time of 12 hr and a parasite half-life clearance of ~ 0.9 hr. Importantly, KAE609 (**16**) was highly effective for the treatment of patients infected with *P. falciparum* strains bearing mutations in the K13 gene (White et al. 2014). The *DSM265* (**17**) compound is an experimental antimalarial that selectively inhibits the parasite dihydroorotate dehydrogenase (DHODH). *DSM265* (**17**) shows *in vitro* activity against liver and blood stages of *P. falciparum* (Phillips et al. 2015).

In addition to drugs in clinical evaluation, different structures and chemical classes are in pre-clinical phase for the treatment of malaria (Charman et al. 2011, Jiménez-Díaz et al. 2014b, Kuhen et al. 2014). MMV has assembled a total of 400 active antimalarial compounds called the Malaria Box, containing 200 drug-like and 200 probe-like compounds toward development of new, affordable and easily accessible antimalarial drugs for endemic regions. These compounds are being widely evaluated by the scientific community, and diverse chemical classes with different mechanisms of action have already been identified, such as triazolopyrimidine, trioxane, dihydroisoquinolone, aminopyridine, quinoline-4-carboxamide, imidazolopiperazine, triaminopyrimidine, and 2,4-diaminopyrimidine (Baragana et al. 2015, Hameed et al. 2015, Younis et al. 2012).

Search for New Antimalarials Inspired from Medicinal Plants

Inspired by the success of quinine (**5**), the search for new antimalarial from natural sources has been an interesting area of research for many decades (Kato et al. 2016, Kaur et al. 2010). The chemistry of natural products is still considered a promising approach, with some compounds showing antimalarial activity in research development stages (Aguiar et al. 2012b, Vennerstrom et al. 2004, Wells 2011). Although synthetic drugs are the current state-of-the-art treatments recommended by WHO, the use of medicinal plants against the disease is a common practice in sub-Saharan African countries and in the Brazilian Amazon, regions highly affected by malaria (Adebayo et al. 2012, Carvalho et al. 1991, Willcox et al. 2011). This frequent use of plants against the disease, mainly by local communities, continues to inspire chemists and biologists to isolate the compounds responsible for their activity, aiming to be used as lead molecules for further drug discovery (Bero et al. 2010, Carvalho et al. 1991).

In the western Brazilian Amazon, there is a wide use of one plant species of the *Rhamnaceae* family, *Ampelozizyphus amazonicus*, also known as "Indian Beer" (IB) or "Cerveja-de-Índio". The dried roots of IB are used as cold infusions by natives before leaving their homes, usually prior to their river bath, and is claimed to have protective effect against the disease. Nowadays, its use is largely spread among riverside populations and also among the Quilombola communities (Oliveira et al. 2015). Ethanolic extracts of the IB plant inhibit exo-erythrocytic development of *P. berghei* sporozoites *in vitro* and significantly delay the malaria pre-patent period in mice challenged with sporozoites, demonstrating its prophylactic effects, as claimed by the inhabitants of the Amazon region (Andrade-Neto et al. 2008). However, more studies are necessary to identify the compounds responsible for this *in vitro* activity, and we should be careful before assuming IB's prophylactic effect in humans.

Infusions of wood bark of *Aspidosperma nitidum* (*Apocynaceae*) are largely used to treat fever and malaria in the Brazilian Amazon, and the molecules responsible for this antimalarial activity are yet to be identified. Recent studies have shown antimalarial activity of the alkaloid-rich fractions from this species (Coutinho et al. 2013). Whether isolated compounds could be used as a basis for development of new alkaloid synthetic drugs has yet to be demonstrated.

Different species of the plant from the genus *Dodonaea*, present in Southern Africa, Arabia, Australia and New Zealand, have also been used to fight malaria. Some compounds from this plant (Figure 6), e.g., pinocembrin (**21**) and flavonol santin (**22**), have been isolated and showed pronounced antimalarial activities *in vivo* (Melaku et al. 2017).

The natural product lupinine (**23**), from *Lupinus luteus*, has inspired the synthesis of the molecular hybrid quinolizidine compound AM1 (**24**), with nanomolar inhibitory activity against CQ (**3**)-sensitive and resistant *P. falciparum* strains *in vitro*. This compound also presented high potency *ex vivo* against *P. vivax* field isolates, with high *in vivo* oral efficacy in both *P. berghei* and *P. yoelii* in experimentally infected mice and IC_{50} values comparable or better than those of CQ (**3**) (Basilico et al. 2017).

Most parts of the tree *Azadirachta indica A. Juss*, popularly known as "Neem tree", commonly found in India, are believed to present medicinal properties (Biswas et al. 2002). Epoxyazadiradione (**25**), a substance isolated from this plant, was further chemically modified and its analogs showed potent antiplasmodial activity against CQ (**3**)-sensitive and resistant parasites, at low nanomolar dose (Ashok Yadav et al. 2017).

A high throughput study (HTS), conducted by Zhang and co-workers on 16,177 fractions from 1,300 different plants, showed that several fractions from 35 plants had *in vitro* inhibitory activity against *P. falciparum*. In addition, triterpenoids α-betulinic acid (**26**) and β-betulinic acid (**27**) of *Eugenia rigida* were also isolated as potential lead molecules for further compound optimization (Zhang et al. 2016).

Plants provide prototype molecules and novel templates for drug development, especially for the treatment of malaria, but natural product drug discovery faces many challenges, e.g., presence of low

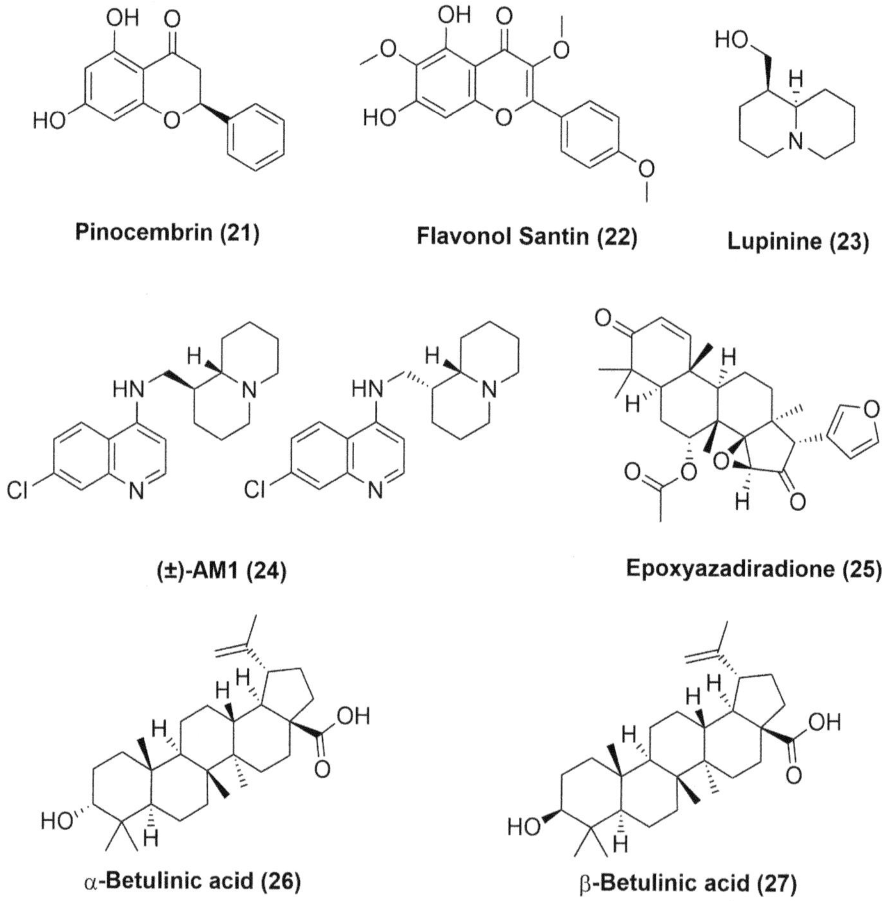

Pinocembrin (21) **Flavonol Santin (22)** **Lupinine (23)**

(±)-AM1 (24) **Epoxyazadiradione (25)**

α-Betulinic acid (26) **β-Betulinic acid (27)**

Figure 6. Chemistry of natural products in the search for new antimalarials.

quantities of an active constituent in crude extracts, interfering compounds present within extracts, and influence of multiple active or toxic compounds (Newman et al. 2012).

Mechanism of Action of Antimalarials

The current FDA approved antimalarial drugs act in many different processes involved in *Plasmodium* development, most of them against parasites inside the host RBC, where they degrade vast amounts of hemoglobin (Table 1). The aspartic proteases plasmepsins and cysteine proteases falcipains cleave haemoglobin into small fragments (Goldberg et al. 1991, Rosenthal et al. 1988). These fragments are then transported to the parasite cytosol for final degradation into amino acids utilized by the parasite in the early steps of the hemoglobin degradation pathway (Gluzman et al. 1994, Rosenthal et al. 1992). During hemoglobin degradation, toxic free heme (heme-Fe^{III}) is liberated and can generate an excessive amount of reactive oxygen species (ROS) (Goyal et al. 2012, Kumar et al. 2005). The malaria parasite has developed a unique mechanism to convert Fe^{III} into a less toxic heme adduct hemozoin (HZ), known as malarial pigment (Bendrat et al. 1995, Egan 2008). This process is facilitated by the action of heme detoxification proteins (HDP). Lipids as well as proteins have been suggested to catalyze HZ formation inside the food vacuole. Histidine-rich protein II was the first protein reported to be involved in HZ formation. The disruption of HZ formation, indispensable for the parasite survival, is an attractive target in killing the parasite. Antimalarials such as CQ (**3**), AQ (**6**), piperaquine (**10**) and MQ (**9**) seem to block the HZ formation, although additional targets may also be involved.

The cytotoxic effect of artemisinin (**1**) derivatives is mediated by free radicals followed by the alkylation of *P. falciparum* proteins. The active moiety of artemisinin (**1**) derivatives, a sesquiterpene lactone containing an endoperoxide bridge, is cleaved in the presence of ferrous iron, generating ROS such as hydroxyl radicals, superoxide anions, and carbon-centered free radicals (Asawamahasakda et al. 1994, Berman et al. 1997, Meshnick et al. 1993).

Although there is no consensus about the mechanism of action of artemisinin (**1**) derivatives, one of the most recent reports suggests that carbon-centered free radicals in the presence of catalytic quantities of Fe^{II} may inhibit *P. falciparum* sarco-endoplasmic reticulum Ca^{II}-ATPase (SERCA), a protein located outside the food vacuole, encoded by the *Pf*ATP6 gene (Eckstein-Ludwig et al. 2003, Shandilya et al. 2013). Deregulation of this protein's activity is proposed to correlate with the rapid swelling of endoplasmic reticulum in the parasites following exposure to artemisinin (**1**) (Eckstein-Ludwig et al. 2003). Other molecular targets for artemisinin (**1**) derivatives have been proposed, mainly involved in the glycolysis and hemoglobin digestion pathways, two important sources of energy and amino acid supply (Ismail et al. 2016, Wang et al. 2015).

Table 1. Current antimalarial drugs, target parasite stage and associated genetic marker.

Chemical class	Antimalarial	Targeted parasite stage	Drug resistance marker
Sesquiterpene lactone endoperoxides	artesunate, artemisinin, artemether, dihydroartemisinin	All stages	*Pf*Kelch 13
4-aminoquinolines	chloroquine, amodiaquine, piperaquine, pyronaridine, naphthoquine	Asexual blood stage	*Pf*crt, *Pf*mdr1, *Pf*plm2, *Pv*mdr1
Amino alcohols	quinine, mefloquine, lumefantrine, halofantrine	Asexual blood stage	*Pf*crt, *Pf*mdr1, *Pv*mdr1
Antifolates	pyrimethamine, sulfadoxine, proguanil	Asexual blood stage and liver schizont	*Pf*dhfr, *Pf*dhps, *Pv*dhfr, *Pv*dhps
Naphtoquinone	atovaquone	Asexual blood stage and liver schizonts	*Pf*cyb
Antibiotics	clindamycin, doxycycline, tetracycline	Asexual blood stage	Apicoplast target

Antimalarial Drug Resistance

Quinine (**5**) resistance was reported since the early 1900s, first in Brazil and later in Southeast Asia. It is usually correlated with polymorphisms in membrane transporters (Cui et al. 2015, da Silva et al. 2014, Pukrittayakamee et al. 1994). Membrane transporters are known to confer resistance in both cancer cells and parasites that cause infectious diseases, mostly by increasing efflux of medicines to the outside of cells (Cui et al. 2015). CQ (**3**) resistance, initially observed in Colombia and at the Cambodia-Thailand border in the 1950s, is widely spread nowadays (Wellems et al. 2001). Although the mechanisms by which parasites become resistant to CQ (**3**) are still not well understood and may involve multiple polymorphisms, in the early 2000s, the *Pf*crt gene, encoding a digestive vacuole transmembrane protein, was identified as an important cause of CQ (**3**) resistance (Ecker et al. 2012, Fidock et al. 2000). Other transporters like *Pf*mdr1 have been associated with MQ (**9**) resistance in Southeast Asia, as well as with AQ (**6**), and CQ (**3**) inefficacy (Duraisingh et al. 2005, Eyase et al. 2013, Price et al. 2004).

The folate metabolic pathway is a target for pyrimethamine (**8**) and proguanil (**11**). Mutations in genes encoding for enzymes in this pathway, e.g., dihydrofolate reductase (DHFR) and dihydropteroate synthase (DHPS), are associated with resistance to these antimalarials (Hyde 2005).

The naphthoquinone compound, atovaquone (AV, **12**), also presents a different mechanism of action than the quinoline derivatives. This inhibitor of electron transport is believed to target quinone-binding sites of cytochrome b, and mutations on the cytochrome b gene (*Pf*cytb) may affect the efficacy of AV (Cui et al. 2015).

ART (**4**) derivatives are believed to have a unique mechanism of resistance, which may not depend on the heme polymerization pathway. ART (**4**) is currently recommended for malaria treatment through ACT but has also become ineffective in some areas in Southeast Asia, China and Africa (Lu et al. 2017, Zaw et al. 2017). Recent cases of artemisinin (**1**) resistance have been associated with mutations in the gene encoding K13, underscoring the need to search for new compounds acting on different stages of the parasite life cycle, possibly through a multi-target approach. More recently, Mukherjee and co-workers analyzed sixty-eight parasites isolates from Cambodia and showed that other yet unidentified mutations may contribute to this mechanism of resistance developed by the parasite (Mukherjee et al. 2017).

The increasing resistance to CQ (**3**), and more recently to artemisinin (**1**), has motivated the development of more efficient ways of tracking resistance in different parts of the world. The malaria genomic epidemiology network (MalariaGEN), created in 2005, has as one of its goals to share data combining the power of large-scale genomic techniques to clinical and epidemiological assays, which would allow an efficient tracking of polymorphisms related to the use of current approved malaria treatments (Malaria Genomic Epidemiology 2008). A large database of Single Nucleotide Polymorphisms (SNPs), evidencing more than three million variants in 7,000 samples, has already been collected as part of the "*P. falciparum* community project" since 2010. The "worldwide antimalarial resistance network" (WWARN) is another platform that has increased significantly the power of identifying incoming resistance (Sibley et al. 2007). WWARN allows the identification of biomarkers related to antimalarial drug inefficacy, and how they connect with data of drug susceptibility and pharmacokinetic studies; it made possible to develop a model that estimates the prevalence of K13 mutations related to artemisinin resistance to reach values as high as 10% in some areas of Myanmar.

While most resistance cases described in this section are focused on *P. falciparum*, resistance has also been reported for *P. vivax* infections. However, it has been harder to track the latter since efficacy of treatment is usually confounded by malaria relapse from the dormant liver stages, urging for public policies aiming to improve methods for monitoring *P. vivax* drug resistance (Price et al. 2014).

Novel Methods for Screening for Potential Antimalarials

Phenotypic screening

A rational approach for finding new antimalarials has recently become more plausible based on the knowledge of potential targets. Phenotypic screening approaches have also shown to be efficient to find potential candidates for fighting malaria, e.g., searching compounds that may act on different stages of the parasite life cycle (Hovlid et al. 2016). In contrast to knowing the targets associated with the mechanism of action of these compounds, these HTS methods look for changes in the phenotype observed in cells under exposure to different drug concentrations. The Genome Wide Association Study (GWAS) has been extensively used for targeting discovery and chemical validation in malaria parasites (Luth et al. 2018).

A recent case of success was reported for the spiroindolone KAE609 (**16**), an inhibitor of the *Pf*ATP4 enzyme discovered after a phenotypic HTS that is advancing to late stages of clinical trials (Rottmann et al. 2010). The knowledge of the mechanism of action of KAE609 (**16**) has now opened new frontiers for using target-based screening approaches. In these assays, lead compounds are identified according to their potential of inhibiting a specific protein function, instead of looking for phenotype changes in cells.

After identifying promising candidates undergoing clinical trials with their respective target, it becomes easier for the design of more effective drugs by performing chemical structural changes empowered by *in silico* techniques, e.g., small molecule docking and molecular dynamics. These *in silico* techniques have not yet been successfully used to bring an antimalarial drug from early to late clinical phases. The recent increase on the knowledge of important protein targets for the parasite life cycle is about to change this scenario in the next 5 yr. Other examples of compounds with known targets in clinical trials for malaria treatment are MMV048 (**18**), an inhibitor of the *Pf*PI4K enzyme, and DSM265 (**17**), targeting *Pf*DHODH. Pre-clinical drug discovery programs have already identified the *in vitro* and *in vivo* antimalarial potential of antifungal compounds selected by docking studies (Penna-Coutinho et al. 2011). A considerable number of studies have focused on the pre-clinical computational design of potential antimalarials targeting proteins important for the parasite survival in different stages of its development, e.g., the pre-mRNA processing factor *Pf*CPSF3 (Sonoiki et al. 2017), the dihydrofolate reductase (Rastelli et al. 2003) and the parasite's mitochondrial bc1 complex (da Cruz et al. 2012). Capper and co-workers, however, highlight that careful modeling approaches are necessary before advancing with designed inhibitors to clinical trials. They found that 4(1H)-pyridone GSK932121 (**20**), a potential inhibitor of cytochrome bc1 that went through clinical trials phase 1, was initially designed and optimized by targeting the binding site Q_o of the protein. Further crystallization studies discovered another binding site for GSK932121, known as Q_i. This misunderstanding of the binding mode of GSK932121 may have resulted in an unpredictable cardiotoxicity, and led to its failure in the early stages of clinical trials (Capper et al. 2015).

Methods for in vitro, ex vivo and in vivo antimalarial drug efficacy testing

The human malaria parasite displays a complex life cycle, which is intermediate between two hosts, a female *Anopheles* mosquito and humans. Effective antimalarials against the whole parasite life cycle are urgently needed and many techniques are applied to this end. It was the *in vitro P. falciparum* cultivation described only in 1978, with further advances regarding parasite biology, material science, and technology, that soon allowed *in vitro* assays to screen antimalarial drugs against erythrocytic stages (Trager et al. 1978). The first such assay was described by Rieckmann and co-workers in 1978, a microtechnique based on schizonts maturation used to evaluate the CQ (**3**) *in vitro* sensitivity from two different *P. falciparum* strains obtained during infection of *Aotus* monkeys (Rieckmann et al. 1978). This microtechnique method is still used for screening compounds against *P. vivax* and *P. falciparum* in *ex vivo* isolates (Renapurkar et al. 1989, Russell et al. 2003). It requires basic cell culture items but is labor intensive and does not permit to screen large set of compounds simultaneously. In 1979, Desjardins and colleagues developed a rapid, semiautomated microdilution method for measuring the activity of potential drugs against cultured *P. falciparum* blood parasites using a radiolabeled nucleic acid precursor, H^3-hypoxanthine, as the indicator of antimalarial activity (Desjardins et al. 1979). This method was extensively used and adopted for drug screening in the US Army Antimalarial Drug Development Program at the Walter Reed Army Institute of Research (Washington, DC, United States), among others. The radioactive substances were soon replaced by other techniques due to the stringent regulations regarding handling and disposal of radioactive material, plus the compulsive use of highly expensive instruments such as liquid scintillation counters. Thus, the enzyme-linked immunosorbent assays (ELISA) became an option for drug test, thanks to monoclonal antibodies specific for the parasite enzyme lactate dehydrogenase (*Pf*LDH) or a parasite histidine-rich protein (HRPII) (Druilhe et al. 2001, Noedl et al. 2002). Although the assessment of parasite growth is effective in both tests, they are expensive and depend on the availability of monoclonal antibodies. Furthermore, they are ELISA susceptible to experimental variation.

Fluorescence-based techniques with fast automatic quantification of parasite growth after staining with fluorescent DNA intercalating dyes such as SYBR Green I, YOYO-1, and Pico Green are now widely used. A study carried out by Smilkstein and co-workers demonstrated that IC_{50} values were the same with SYBR Green I as those obtained with the radioisotope, [^{3}H] ethanolamine incorporation (Smilkstein et al. 2004).

HTS is also a useful technique based on miniaturized assays to screen thousands to millions of compounds from chemical libraries to find lead compounds with phenotypic importance. These assays have been widely used to identify new classes of hit compounds active against *P. falciparum* asexual or sexual stages. This approach is advantageous given that currently only a few clinically validated drug targets are available (Avery et al. 2014, Gamo et al. 2010). In addition, the technique increases the potential for the discovery of new chemotypes acting against new antimalarial targets (Delves et al. 2013, Guiguemde et al. 2010, Plouffe et al. 2008).

Several methods are applied to discover new transmission blocking approaches, such as targeting the *P. falciparum* stage V gametocytes, responsible for parasite transmission, aiming to discover drugs with gametocytocidal activity, e.g., PQ (**2**) and its derivatives, or MEFAS, a new compound in pre-clinical stages derived from MQ (**9**) and ART (**4**) (Aguiar et al. 2017, de Pilla Varotti et al. 2008, Penna-Coutinho et al. 2016). The 'gold-standard' laboratory assay for measuring transmission blocking is a membrane-feeding assay (SMFA). It embraces the complex cell biology of the parasite, the complex interactions of the parasites with the mosquito midgut microflora and the immune system of the mosquito. Unfortunately, it remains a very-low-throughput assay and prohibitively expensive for any HTS (Aguiar et al. 2017, Churcher et al. 2012, Miura et al. 2013).

The number of compounds identified against hypnozoites is limited, due to the difficulty of developing techniques to work with this stage of the parasite. An assay was described by Dembélé and co-workers using persistent nondividing uninucleate hepatic forms of *P. cynomolgi* in *in vitro*-cultured primary hepatocytes from the natural host *M. fascicularis*. However, this is a difficult model that depends on the availability of monkeys, and therefore limits the search for compounds with anti-relapse activity (Dembele et al. 2014).

Conclusion

The current pipeline of FDA approved drugs for malaria is based on combination therapies involving artemisinin (**1**) derivatives. Recent cases of resistance to artemisinin (**1**) are reported in Southeast Asia, China and Africa and urge for the search of new effective antimalarials, possibly targeting multiple stages of the parasite life cycle. Compounds advancing clinical trials with novel mechanisms of action, e.g., KAE609 (**16**) and DSM265 (**17**), have the potential of increasing the number of antimalarial compounds. In addition, new alternatives to PQ (**2**) such as tafenoquine (**13**) are extremely important for targeting dormant stages of *P. vivax* in the liver. State-of-the-art approaches for identifying antimalarial candidates usually consist of a combination of different techniques, e.g., phenotypic HTS, target-based screening, *in silico* design, *in vitro* enzyme-based and fluorescent dyes for parasite detection, as well as "gold-standard" methods for measuring transmission blocking potential such as SMFA. Platforms for tracking resistance, e.g., WWARN and MalariaGen, bring new perspectives in identifying resistance mechanisms developed by the parasite. Together, these techniques show state-of-the-art approaches for overcoming resistance and empowering the portfolio of promising antimalarials with high efficacy against all forms of *Plasmodium* infections.

References

Achan, J., A.O. Talisuna, A. Erhart, A. Yeka, J.K. Tibenderana, F.N. Baliraine et al. 2011. Quinine, an old anti-malarial drug in a modern world: role in the treatment of malaria. Malar. J. 10(144): 1–12.

Adebayo, J.O. and A.U. Krettli. 2011. Potential antimalarials from Nigerian plants: a review. J. Ethnopharmacol. 133(2): 289–302.

Adebayo, J.O., A.E. Santana and A.U. Krettli. 2012. Evaluation of the antiplasmodial and cytotoxicity potentials of husk fiber extracts from Cocos nucifera, a medicinal plant used in Nigeria to treat human malaria. Hum. Exp. Toxicol. 31(3): 244–9. doi: 10.1177/0960327111424298. Epub 2012 Jan 12.

Aguiar, A.C., M. Santos Rde, F.J. Figueiredo, W.A. Cortopassi, A.S. Pimentel, T.C. Franca et al. 2012a. Antimalarial activity and mechanisms of action of two novel 4-aminoquinolines against chloroquine-resistant parasites. PLoS One. 7(5): e37259.

Aguiar, A.C., E.M. Rocha, N.B. Souza, T.C. Franca and A.U. Krettli. 2012b. New approaches in antimalarial drug discovery and development: a review. Mem. Inst. Oswaldo Cruz. 107(7): 831–845.

Aguiar, A.C., F.J. Figueiredo, P.D. Neuenfeldt, T.H. Katsuragawa, B.B. Drawanz, W. Cunico et al. 2017. Primaquine-thiazolidinones block malaria transmission and development of the liver exoerythrocytic forms. Malar. J. 16(1): 110.

Al-Bari, M.A. 2015. Chloroquine analogues in drug discovery: new directions of uses, mechanisms of actions and toxic manifestations from malaria to multifarious diseases. J. Antimicrob. Chemother. 70(6): 1608–1621.

Aly, A.S., A.M. Vaughan and S.H. Kappe. 2009. Malaria parasite development in the mosquito and infection of the mammalian host. Annu. Rev. Microbiol. 63: 195–221.

Amino, R., D. Giovannini, S. Thiberge, P. Gueirard, B. Boisson, J.-F. Dubremetz et al. 2008. Host cell traversal is important for progression of the malaria parasite through the dermis to the liver. Cell Host & Microbe. 3(2): 88–96.

Andrade-Neto, V.F., M.G.L. Brandão, F. Nogueira, V.E. Rosário and A.U. Krettli. 2008. Ampelozyziphus amazonicus Ducke (Rhamnaceae), a medicinal plant used to prevent malaria in the Amazon Region, hampers the development of Plasmodium berghei sporozoites. Int. J. Parasitol. 38(13): 1505–1511.

Asawamahasakda, W., I. Ittarat, Y.M. Pu, H. Ziffer and S.R. Meshnick. 1994. Reaction of antimalarial endoperoxides with specific parasite proteins. Antimicrob. Agents Chemother. 38(8): 1854–1858.

Ashley, E.A., M. Dhorda, R.M. Fairhurst, C. Amaratunga, P. Lim, S. Suon et al. 2014. Spread of artemisinin resistance in Plasmodium falciparum malaria. N. Engl. J. Med. 371(5): 411–423.

Ashok Yadav, P., C. Pavan Kumar, B. Siva, K. Suresh Babu, A.D. Allanki, P.S. Sijwali et al. 2017. Synthesis and evaluation of anti-plasmodial and cytotoxic activities of epoxyazadiradione derivatives. Eur. J. Med. Chem. 134: 242–257.

Avery, V.M., S. Bashyam, J.N. Burrows, S. Duffy, G. Papadatos, S. Puthukkuti et al. 2014. Screening and hit evaluation of a chemical library against blood-stage Plasmodium falciparum. Malar. J. 13: 190.

Baird, K. 2015. Origins and implications of neglect of G6PD deficiency and primaquine toxicity in Plasmodium vivax malaria. Pathog Glob. Health. 109(3): 93–106.

Baker, D.A. 2010. Malaria gametocytogenesis. Mol. Biochem. Parasitol. 172(2): 57–65.

Baragana, B., I. Hallyburton, M.C. Lee, N.R. Norcross, R. Grimaldi, T.D. Otto et al. 2015. A novel multiple-stage antimalarial agent that inhibits protein synthesis. Nature. 522(7556): 315–320.

Barber, B.E., T. William, M.J. Grigg, J. Menon, S. Auburn, J. Marfurt et al. 2013. A prospective comparative study of knowlesi, falciparum, and vivax malaria in Sabah, Malaysia: high proportion with severe disease from Plasmodium knowlesi and Plasmodium vivax but no mortality with early referral and artesunate therapy. Clin. Infect. Dis. 56(3): 383–397.

Basilico, N., S. Parapini, A. Sparatore, S. Romeo, P. Misiano, L. Vivas et al. 2017. In vivo and in vitro activities and ADME-Tox profile of a Quinolizidine-Modified 4-Aminoquinoline: A potent Anti-P. falciparum and Anti-P. vivax Blood-stage antimalarial. Molecules. 22(12).

Bendrat, K., B.J. Berger and A. Cerami. 1995. Haem polymerization in malaria. Nature. 378 (6553): 138–139.

Berman, P.A. and P.A. Adams. 1997. Artemisinin enhances heme-catalysed oxidation of lipid membranes. Free Radic. Biol. Med. 22(7): 1283–1288.

Bero, J., M. Frédérich and J. Quetin-Leclercq. 2010. Antimalarial compounds isolated from plants used in traditional medicine. J. Pharm. Pharmacol. 61(11): 1401–1433.

Biot, C., D. Taramelli, I. Forfar-Bares, L.A. Maciejewski, M. Boyce, G. Nowogrocki et al. 2005. Insights into the mechanism of action of ferroquine relationship between physicochemical properties and antiplasmodial activity. Mol. Pharm. 2(3): 185–193.

Biot, C., F. Nosten, L. Fraisse, D. Ter-Minassian, J. Khalife and D. Dive. 2011. The antimalarial ferroquine: from bench to clinic. Parasite. 18(3): 207–214.

Biswas, K., I. Chattopadhyay, R.K. Banerjee and U. Bandyopadhyay. 2002. Biological activities and medicinal properties of neem (Azadirachta indica). Curr. Sci. 82(11): 1336–1345.

Breedlove, B. and P.M. Arguin. 2015. Portrait of the coveted cinchona. Emerg. Infect. Dis. 21(7): 1280–1281.

Campo, B., O. Vandal, D.L. Wesche and J.N. Burrows. 2015. Killing the hypnozoite—drug discovery approaches to prevent relapse in *Plasmodium vivax*. Pathog. Glob. Health. 109(3): 107–122.

Capper, M.J., P.M. O'Neill, N. Fisher, R.W. Strange, D. Moss, S.A. Ward et al. 2015. Antimalarial 4(1H)-pyridones bind to the Qi site of cytochrome bc1. Proc. Natl. Acad. Sci. USA. 112(3): 755–760.

Carvalho, L.H., M.G. Brandao, D. Santos-Filho, J.L. Lopes and A.U. Krettli. 1991. Antimalarial activity of crude extracts from Brazilian plants studied *in vivo* in *Plasmodium berghei*-infected mice and *in vitro* against *Plasmodium falciparum* in culture. Braz. J. Med. Biol. Res. 24(11): 1113–1123.

Charman, S.A., S. Arbe-Barnes, I.C. Bathurst, R. Brun, M. Campbell, W.N. Charman et al. 2011. Synthetic ozonide drug candidate OZ439 offers new hope for a single-dose cure of uncomplicated malaria. Proc. Natl. Acad. Sci. USA. 108(11): 4400.

Churcher, T.S., A.M. Blagborough, M. Delves, C. Ramakrishnan, M.C. Kapulu, A.R. Williams et al. 2012. Measuring the blockade of malaria transmission—an analysis of the Standard Membrane Feeding Assay. Int. J. Parasitol. 42(11): 1037–1044.

Commons, R.J., K. Thriemer, G. Humphreys, I. Suay, C.H. Sibley, P.J. Guerin et al. 2017. The vivax surveyor: Online mapping database for *Plasmodium vivax* clinical trials. Int. J. Parasitol. Drugs Drug Resist. 7(2): 181–190.

Coutinho, J.P., A.C. Aguiar, P.A. dos Santos, J.C. Lima, M.G. Rocha, C.L. Zani et al. 2013. Aspidosperma (Apocynaceae) plant cytotoxicity and activity towards malaria parasites. Part I: Aspidosperma nitidum (Benth) used as a remedy to treat fever and malaria in the Amazon. Mem. Inst. Oswaldo Cruz. 108(8): 974–982.

Cui, L., S. Mharakurwa, D. Ndiaye, P.K. Rathod and P.J. Rosenthal. 2015. Antimalarial drug resistance: Literature review and activities and findings of the ICEMR network. Am. J. Trop. Med. Hyg. 93(3 Suppl): 57–68.

da Cruz, F.P., C. Martin, K. Buchholz, M.J. Lafuente-Monasterio, T. Rodrigues, B. Sönnichsen et al. 2012. Drug screen targeted at *Plasmodium* liver stages identifies a potent multistage antimalarial drug. J. Infect. Dis. 205(8): 1278–1286.

da Silva, A.F.C. and J.L. Benchimol. 2014. Malaria and quinine resistance: A medical and scientific issue between Brazil and Germany (1907–19). Medical History. 58(1): 1–26.

de Pilla Varotti, F., A.C. Botelho, A.A. Andrade, R.C. de Paula, E.M. Fagundes, A. Valverde et al. 2008. Synthesis, antimalarial activity, and intracellular targets of MEFAS, a new hybrid compound derived from mefloquine and artesunate. Antimicrob. Agents Chemother. 52(11): 3868–3874.

Delves, M.J., A. Ruecker, U. Straschil, J. Lelièvre, S. Marques, M.J. López-Barragán et al. 2013. Male and female *Plasmodium falciparum* mature gametocytes show different responses to antimalarial drugs. Antimicrob. Agents Chemother. 57(7): 3268–3274.

Dembele, L., J.F. Franetich, A. Lorthiois, A. Gego, A.M. Zeeman, C.H. Kocken et al. 2014. Persistence and activation of malaria hypnozoites in long-term primary hepatocyte cultures. Nat. Med. 20(3): 307–312.

Desjardins, R.E., C.J. Canfield, J.D. Haynes and J.D. Chulay. 1979. Quantitative assessment of antimalarial activity *in vitro* by a semiautomated microdilution technique. Antimicrob. Agents Chemother. 16(6): 710–718.

Dondorp, A.M., F. Nosten, P. Yi, D. Das, A.P. Phyo, J. Tarning et al. 2009. Artemisinin resistance in *Plasmodium falciparum* malaria. N. Engl. J. Med. 361(5): 455–467.

Dow, G.S., W.F. McCarthy, M. Reid, B. Smith, D. Tang and G.D. Shanks. 2014. A retrospective analysis of the protective efficacy of tafenoquine and mefloquine as prophylactic anti-malarials in non-immune individuals during deployment to a malaria-endemic area. Malar. J. 13(1): 49.

Druilhe, P., A. Moreno, C. Blanc, P.H. Brasseur and P. Jacquier. 2001. A colorimetric *in vitro* drug sensitivity assay for *Plasmodium falciparum* based on a highly sensitive double-site lactate dehydrogenase antigen-capture enzyme-linked immunosorbent assay. Am. J. Trop. Med. Hyg. 64(5-6): 233–241.

Ducharme, J. and R. Farinotti. 1996. Clinical pharmacokinetics and metabolism of chloroquine. Clin. Pharmacokinet. 31(4): 257–274.

Duraisingh, M.T. and A.F. Cowman. 2005. Contribution of the pfmdr1 gene to antimalarial drug-resistance. Acta Trop. 94(3): 181–190.

Ecker, A., A.M. Lehane, J. Clain and D.A. Fidock. 2012. PfCRT and its role in antimalarial drug resistance. Trends Parasitol. 28(11): 504–514.

Eckstein-Ludwig, U., R.J. Webb, I.D. Van Goethem, J.M. East, A.G. Lee, M. Kimura et al. 2003. Artemisinins target the SERCA of *Plasmodium falciparum*. Nature. 424(6951): 957–961.

Egan, T.J. 2008. Recent advances in understanding the mechanism of hemozoin (malaria pigment) formation. J. Inorg. Biochem. 102(5): 1288–1299.

Elderfield, R.C., H.E. Mertel, R.T. Mitch, I.M. Wempen and E. Werble. 1955. Synthesis of primaquine and certain of its analogs 1. J. Am. Chem. Soc. 77(18): 4816–4819.

Elizalde-Torrent, A., F. Val, I.C.C. Azevedo, W.M. Monteiro, L.C.L. Ferreira, C. Fernandez-Becerra et al. 2018. Sudden spleen rupture in a *Plasmodium vivax*-infected patient undergoing malaria treatment. Malar. J. 17(1): 79.

Eyase, F.L., H.M. Akala, L. Ingasia, A. Cheruiyot, A. Omondi, C. Okudo et al. 2013. The role of Pfmdr1 and Pfcrt in changing chloroquine, amodiaquine, mefloquine and lumefantrine susceptibility in western-Kenya P. falciparum samples during 2008–2011. PLoS One. 8(5): e64299.

Fidock, D.A., T. Nomura, A.K. Talley, R.A. Cooper, S.M. Dzekunov, M.T. Ferdig et al. 2000. Mutations in the *P. falciparum* digestive vacuole transmembrane protein PfCRT and evidence for their role in chloroquine resistance. Mol. Cell. 6(4): 861–871.

Frenal, K., J.F. Dubremetz, M. Lebrun and D. Soldati-Favre. 2017. Gliding motility powers invasion and egress in Apicomplexa. Nat. Rev. Microbiol. 15(11): 645–660.

Frenette, P.S. and G.F. Atweh. 2007. Sickle cell disease: old discoveries, new concepts, and future promise. J. Clin. Invest. 117(4): 850–858.

Gamo, F.J., L.M. Sanz, J. Vidal, C. de Cozar, E. Alvarez, J.L. Lavandera et al. 2010. Thousands of chemical starting points for antimalarial lead identification. Nature. 465(7296): 305–310.

Gerald, N., B. Mahajan and S. Kumar. 2011. Mitosis in the human malaria parasite *Plasmodium falciparum*. Eukaryot Cell. 10(4): 474–482.

Gluzman, I.Y., S.E. Francis, A. Oksman, C.E. Smith, K.L. Duffin and D.E. Goldberg. 1994. Order and specificity of the *Plasmodium falciparum* hemoglobin degradation pathway. J. Clin. Inv. 93(4): 1602–1608.

Goldberg, D.E., A.F. Slater, R. Beavis, B. Chait, A. Cerami and G.B. Henderson. 1991. Hemoglobin degradation in the human malaria pathogen *Plasmodium falciparum*: a catabolic pathway initiated by a specific aspartic protease. J. Exp. Med. 173(4): 961.

Goyal, M., A. Alam and U. Bandyopadhyay. 2012. Redox regulation in malaria: Current concepts and pharmacotherapeutic implications. Curr. Med. Chem. 19(10): 1475–1503.

Gramiccia, G. 1988. The life of Charles Ledger (1818–1905): Alpacas and Quinine. Basingstoke: Macmillan Press.

Guiguemde, W.A., A.A. Shelat, D. Bouck, S. Duffy, G.J. Crowther, P.H. Davis et al. 2010. Chemical genetics of *Plasmodium falciparum*. Nature. 465(7296): 311–315.

Hameed, P.S., S. Solapure, V. Patil, P.P. Henrich, P.A. Magistrado, S. Bharath et al. 2015. Triaminopyrimidine is a fast-killing and long-acting antimalarial clinical candidate. Nat. Commun. 6: 6715.

Han, Y.S., J. Thompson, F.C. Kafatos and C. Barillas-Mury. 2000. Molecular interactions between Anopheles stephensi midgut cells and *Plasmodium berghei*: the time bomb theory of ookinete invasion of mosquitoes. The EMBO Journal. 19(22): 6030.

Hovlid, M.L. and E.A. Winzeler. 2016. Phenotypic screens in antimalarial drug discovery. Trends Parasitol. 32(9): 697–707.

Hyde, J.E. 2005. Exploring the folate pathway in *Plasmodium falciparum*. Acta Trop. 94(3): 191–206.

Ismail, H.M., V. Barton, M. Phanchana, S. Charoensutthivarakul, M.H.L. Wong, J. Hemingway et al. 2016. Artemisinin activity-based probes identify multiple molecular targets within the asexual stage of the malaria parasites *Plasmodium falciparum* 3D7. Proc. Natl. Acad. Sci. USA. 113(8): 2080–2085.

Jiménez-Díaz, M.B., D. Ebert, Y. Salinas, A. Pradhan, A.M. Lehane, M.-E. Myrand-Lapierre et al. 2014a. (+)-SJ733, a clinical candidate for malaria that acts through ATP4 to induce rapid host-mediated clearance of & lt;em> *Plasmodium* </em>. Proc. Nat. Acad. Sci. 111(50): E5455.

Jiménez-Díaz, M.B., D. Ebert, Y. Salinas, A. Pradhan, A.M. Lehane, M.-E. Myrand-Lapierre et al. 2014b. (+)-SJ733, a clinical candidate for malaria that acts through ATP4 to induce rapid host-mediated clearance of *Plasmodium*. Proc. Natl. Acad. Sci. USA. 111(50): E5455.

Jiménez-Díaz, M.B., D. Ebert, Y. Salinas, A. Pradhan, A.M. Lehane, M.-E. Myrand-Lapierre et al. 2014c. (+)-SJ733, a clinical candidate for malaria that acts through ATP4 to induce rapid host-mediated clearance of *Plasmodium*. Proc. Natl. Acad. Sci. USA. 111(50): E5455–E5462.

Kato, N., E. Comer, T. Sakata-Kato, A. Sharma, M. Sharma, M. Maetani et al. 2016. Diversity-oriented synthesis yields novel multistage antimalarial inhibitors. Nature. 538(7625): 344–349.

Kaur, K., M. Jain, R.P. Reddy and R. Jain. 2010. Quinolines and structurally related heterocycles as antimalarials. Eur. J. Med. Chem. 45(8): 3245–3264.

Kitchakarn, S., D. Lek, S. Thol, C. Hok, A. Saejeng, R. Huy et al. 2017. Implementation of G6PD testing and primaquine for P. vivax radical cure: Operational perspectives from Thailand and Cambodia. WHO South East Asia J. Public Health. 6(2): 60–68.

Kuhen, K.L., A.K. Chatterjee, M. Rottmann, K. Gagaring, R. Borboa, J. Buenviaje et al. 2014. KAF156 is an antimalarial clinical candidate with potential for use in prophylaxis, treatment, and prevention of disease transmission. Antimicrob. Agents Chemother. 58(9): 5060–5067.

Kumar, S. and U. Bandyopadhyay. 2005. Free heme toxicity and its detoxification systems in human. Toxicol. Lett. 157(3): 175–188.

Le Bras, J. and R. Durand. 2003. The mechanisms of resistance to antimalarial drugs in *Plasmodium falciparum*. Fundam. Clin. Pharmacol. 17(2): 147–153.

Leong, F.J., R. Li, J.P. Jain, G. Lefevre, B. Magnusson, T.T. Diagana et al. 2014. A first-in-human randomized, double-blind, placebo-controlled, single- and multiple-ascending oral dose study of novel antimalarial Spiroindolone KAE609 (Cipargamin) to assess its safety, tolerability, and pharmacokinetics in healthy adult volunteers. Antimicrob. Agents Chemother. 58(10): 6209–6214.

Lim, H.S., J.S. Im, J.Y. Cho, K.S. Bae, T.A. Klein, J.S. Yeom et al. 2009. Pharmacokinetics of hydroxychloroquine and its clinical implications in chemoprophylaxis against malaria caused by *Plasmodium vivax*. Antimicrob. Agents Chemother. 53(4): 1468–1475.

Lu, F., R. Culleton, M. Zhang, A. Ramaprasad, L. von Seidlein, H. Zhou et al. 2017. Emergence of indigenous artemisinin-resistant *Plasmodium falciparum* in Africa. N. Engl. J. Med. 376(10): 991–993.

Luth, M.R., P. Gupta, S. Ottilie and E.A. Winzeler. 2018. Using *in vitro* evolution and whole genome analysis to discover next generation targets for antimalarial drug discovery. ACS Infectious Diseases. 4(3): 301–314.

Malaria Genomic Epidemiology, N. 2008. A global network for investigating the genomic epidemiology of malaria. Nature. 456(7223): 732–737.

McCarthy, J.S., T. Ruckle, E. Djeriou, C. Cantalloube, D. Ter-Minassian, M. Baker et al. 2016. A Phase II pilot trial to evaluate safety and efficacy of ferroquine against early *Plasmodium falciparum* in an induced blood-stage malaria infection study. Malar. J. 15: 469.

Melaku, Y., T. Worku, Y. Tadesse, Y. Mekonnen, J. Schmidt, N. Arnold et al. 2017. Antiplasmodial compounds from leaves of Dodonaea angustifolia. Curr. Bioact. Compd. 13(3): 268–273.

Meshnick, S.R., Y.Z. Yang, V. Lima, F. Kuypers, S. Kamchonwongpaisan and Y. Yuthavong. 1993. Iron-dependent free radical generation from the antimalarial agent artemisinin (qinghaosu). Antimicrob. Agents Chemother. 37(5): 1108–1114.

Miller, L.H., S.J. Mason, D.F. Clyde and M.H. McGinniss. 1976. The resistance factor to *Plasmodium vivax* in blacks. The Duffy-blood-group genotype, FyFy. N. Engl. J. Med. 295(6): 302–304.

Miller, L.H., D.I. Baruch, K. Marsh and O.K. Doumbo. 2002. The pathogenic basis of malaria. Nature. 415(6872): 673–679.

Miura, K., B. Deng, G. Tullo, A. Diouf, S.E. Moretz, E. Locke et al. 2013. Qualification of standard membrane-feeding assay with *Plasmodium falciparum* malaria and potential improvements for future assays. PLoS One. 8(3): e57909.

Mol, C.D., K.B. Lim, V. Sridhar, H. Zou, E.Y. Chien, B.C. Sang et al. 2003. Structure of a c-kit product complex reveals the basis for kinase transactivation. J. Biol. Chem. 278(34): 31461–31464.

Mota, M.M., G. Pradel, J.P. Vanderberg, J.C.R. Hafalla, U. Frevert, R.S. Nussenzweig et al. 2001. Migration of *Plasmodium* sporozoites through cells before infection. Science. 291(5501): 141.

Mukherjee, A., S. Bopp, P. Magistrado, W. Wong, R. Daniels, A. Demas et al. 2017. Artemisinin resistance without pfkelch13 mutations in *Plasmodium falciparum* isolates from Cambodia. Malar. J. 16: 195.

Newman, D.J. and G.M. Cragg. 2012. Natural products as sources of new drugs over the 30 years from 1981 to 2010. J. Nat. Prod. 75(3): 311–335.

Noedl, H., C. Wongsrichanalai, R.S. Miller, K.S. Myint, S. Looareesuwan, Y. Sukthana et al. 2002. *Plasmodium falciparum*: effect of anti-malarial drugs on the production and secretion characteristics of histidine-rich protein II. Exp. Parasitol. 102(3-4): 157–163.

Noedl, H., D. Socheat and W. Satimai. 2009. Artemisinin-resistant malaria in Asia. N. Engl. J. Med. 361(5): 540–541.

Oliveira, D.R., A.U. Krettli, A.C.C. Aguiar, G.G. Leitao, M.N. Vieira, K.S. Martins et al. 2015. Ethnopharmacological evaluation of medicinal plants used against malaria by quilombola communities from Oriximina, Brazil. J. Ethnopharmacol. 173: 424–434.

Olliaro, P., C. Nevill, J. LeBras, P. Ringwald, P. Mussano, P. Garner et al. 1996. Systematic review of amodiaquine treatment in uncomplicated malaria. Lancet. 348(9036): 1196–1201.

Paquet, T., C. Le Manach, D.G. Cabrera, Y. Younis, P.P. Henrich, T.S. Abraham et al. 2017. Antimalarial efficacy of MMV390048, an inhibitor of *Plasmodium* phosphatidylinositol 4-kinase. Sci. Transl. Med. 9(387): eaad9735.

Penna-Coutinho, J., W.A. Cortopassi, A.A. Oliveira, T.C. Franca and A.U. Krettli. 2011. Antimalarial activity of potential inhibitors of *Plasmodium falciparum* lactate dehydrogenase enzyme selected by docking studies. PLoS One. 6(7): e21237.

Penna-Coutinho, J., M.J. Almela, C. Miguel-Blanco, E. Herreros, P.M. Sa, N. Boechat et al. 2016. Transmission-blocking potential of MEFAS, a hybrid compound derived from artesunate and mefloquine. Antimicrob. Agents Chemother. 60(5): 3145–3147.

Peters, A.L. and C.J. Van Noorden. 2009. Glucose-6-phosphate dehydrogenase deficiency and malaria: cytochemical detection of heterozygous G6PD deficiency in women. J. Histochem. Cytochem. 57(11): 1003–1011.

Phillips, M.A., J. Lotharius, K. Marsh, J. White, A. Dayan, K.L. White et al. 2015. A long-duration dihydroorotate dehydrogenase inhibitor (DSM265) for prevention and treatment of malaria. Sci. Transl. Med. 7(296): 296ra111.

Plouffe, D., A. Brinker, C. McNamara, K. Henson, N. Kato, K. Kuhen et al. 2008. *In silico* activity profiling reveals the mechanism of action of antimalarials discovered in a high-throughput screen. Proc. Natl. Acad. Sci. USA. 105(26): 9059–9064.

Price, R.N., A.C. Uhlemann, A. Brockman, R. McGready, E. Ashley, L. Phaipun et al. 2004. Mefloquine resistance in *Plasmodium falciparum* and increased pfmdr1 gene copy number. Lancet. 364(9432): 438–447.

Price, R.N., L. von Seidlein, N. Valecha, F. Nosten, J.K. Baird and N.J. White. 2014. Global extent of chloroquine-resistant *Plasmodium vivax*: a systematic review and meta-analysis. Lancet Infect. Dis. 14(10): 982–991.

Pukrittayakamee, S., W. Supanaranond, S. Looareesuwan, S. Vanijanonta and N.J. White. 1994. Quinine in severe falciparum malaria: evidence of declining efficacy in Thailand. Trans. R Soc. Trop. Med. Hyg. 88(3): 324–327.

Rastelli, G., S. Pacchioni, W. Sirawaraporn, R. Sirawaraporn, M.D. Parenti and A.M. Ferrari. 2003. Docking and database screening reveal new classes of *Plasmodium falciparum* dihydrofolate reductase inhibitors. J. Med. Chem. 46(14): 2834–2845.

Renapurkar, D.M., V.R. Pradhan, N.K. Sutar, R.A. Deshmukh, C.H. Pandit and S.N. Marathe. 1989. Micro test for assaying sensitivity of *Plasmodium vivax in vitro*. Chemotherapy. 35(3): 160–163.

Rieckmann, K.H., G.H. Campbell, L.J. Sax and J.E. Mrema. 1978. Drug sensitivity of *Plasmodium falciparum*. An *in-vitro* microtechnique. Lancet. 1(8054): 22–23.

Rosenthal, P.J., J.H. McKerrow, M. Aikawa, H. Nagasawa and J.H. Leech. 1988. A malarial cysteine proteinase is necessary for hemoglobin degradation by *Plasmodium falciparum*. J. Clin. Inv. 82(5): 1560–1566.

Rosenthal, P.J. and R.G. Nelson. 1992. Isolation and characterization of a cysteine proteinase gene of *Plasmodium falciparum*. Mol. Biochem. Parasitol. 51(1): 143–152.

Rottmann, M., C. McNamara, B.K. Yeung, M.C. Lee, B. Zou, B. Russell et al. 2010. Spiroindolones, a potent compound class for the treatment of malaria. Science. 329(5996): 1175–1180.

Russell, B.M., R. Udomsangpetch, K.H. Rieckmann, B.M. Kotecka, R.E. Coleman and J. Sattabongkot. 2003. Simple *in vitro* assay for determining the sensitivity of *Plasmodium vivax* isolates from fresh human blood to antimalarials in areas where *P. vivax* is endemic. Antimicrob. Agents Chemother. 47(1): 170–173.

Saenz, F.E., T. Mutka, K. Udenze, A.M. Oduola and D.E. Kyle. 2012. Novel 4-aminoquinoline analogs highly active against the blood and sexual stages of *Plasmodium in vivo* and *in vitro*. Antimicrob. Agents Chemother. 56(9): 4685–4692.

Saharan, S., U. Kohli, R. Lodha, A. Sharma and A. Bagga. 2009. Thrombotic microangiopathy associated with *Plasmodium vivax* malaria. Pediatr. Nephrol. 24(3): 623–624.

Sallares, R., A. Bouwman and C. Anderung. 2004. The spread of malaria to Southern Europe in antiquity: new approaches to old problems. Med. Hist. 48(3): 311–328.

Satimai, W., P. Sudathip, S. Vijaykadga, A. Khamsiriwatchara, S. Sawang, T. Potithavoranan et al. 2012. Artemisinin resistance containment project in Thailand. II: Responses to mefloquine-artesunate combination therapy among falciparum malaria patients in provinces bordering Cambodia. Malar. J. 11: 300.

Shandilya, A., S. Chacko, B. Jayaram and I. Ghosh. 2013. A plausible mechanism for the antimalarial activity of artemisinin: A computational approach. Sci. Rep. 3: 2513.

Sibley, C.H., K.I. Barnes and C.V. Plowe. 2007. The rationale and plan for creating a World Antimalarial Resistance Network (WARN). Malar. J. 6: 118.

Smilkstein, M., N. Sriwilaijaroen, J.X. Kelly, P. Wilairat and M. Riscoe. 2004. Simple and inexpensive fluorescence-based technique for high-throughput antimalarial drug screening. Antimicrob. Agents Chemother. 48(5): 1803–1806.

Sonoiki, E., C.L. Ng, M.C. Lee, D. Guo, Y.K. Zhang, Y. Zhou et al. 2017. A potent antimalarial benzoxaborole targets a *Plasmodium falciparum* cleavage and polyadenylation specificity factor homologue. Nat. Commun. 8: 14574.

Sturm, A., R. Amino, C. van de Sand, T. Regen, S. Retzlaff, A. Rennenberg et al. 2006. Manipulation of host hepatocytes by the malaria parasite for delivery into liver sinusoids. Science. 313(5791): 1287.

Sultan, A.A. 1999. Molecular mechanisms of malaria sporozoite motility and invasion of host cells. Int. Microbiol. 2(3): 155–160.

Tavares, J., P. Formaglio, S. Thiberge, E. Mordelet, N. Van Rooijen, A. Medvinsky et al. 2013. Role of host cell traversal by the malaria sporozoite during liver infection. J. Exp. Med. 210(5): 905–915.

Trager, W. and J.B. Jenson. 1978. Cultivation of malarial parasites. Nature. 273(5664): 621–622.

van Pelt-Koops, J.C., H.E. Pett, W. Graumans, M. van der Vegte-Bolmer, G.J. van Gemert, M. Rottmann et al. 2012. The spiroindolone drug candidate NITD609 potently inhibits gametocytogenesis and blocks *Plasmodium falciparum* transmission to anopheles mosquito vector. Antimicrob. Agents Chemother. 56(7): 3544–3548.

Vennerstrom, J.L., S. Arbe-Barnes, R. Brun, S.A. Charman, F.C. Chiu, J. Chollet et al. 2004. Identification of an antimalarial synthetic trioxolane drug development candidate. Nature. 430(7002): 900–904.

Vinetz, J.M. 2005. *Plasmodium* ookinete invasion of the mosquito midgut. Curr. Top. Microbiol. Immunol. 295: 357–382.

Wang, J., C.J. Zhang, W.N. Chia, C.C. Loh, Z. Li, Y.M. Lee et al. 2015. Haem-activated promiscuous targeting of artemisinin in *Plasmodium falciparum*. Nat. Commun. 6: 10111.

Wani, W.A., E. Jameel, U. Baig, S. Mumtazuddin and L.T. Hun. 2015. Ferroquine and its derivatives: new generation of antimalarial agents. Eur. J. Med. Chem. 101: 534–551.

Wassmer, S.C. and G.E. Grau. 2017. Severe malaria: what's new on the pathogenesis front? Int. J. Parasitol. 47(2-3): 145–152.

Weiss, G.E., P.R. Gilson, T. Taechalertpaisarn, W.H. Tham, N.W. de Jong, K.L. Harvey et al. 2015. Revealing the sequence and resulting cellular morphology of receptor-ligand interactions during *Plasmodium falciparum* invasion of erythrocytes. PLoS Pathog. 11(2): e1004670.

Wellems, T.E. and C.V. Plowe. 2001. Chloroquine-resistant malaria. J. Infect. Dis. 184(6): 770–776.

Wells, T.N.C. 2011. Natural products as starting points for future anti-malarial therapies: going back to our roots? Malaria Journal. 10(Suppl 1): S3–S3.

White, N.J., S. Pukrittayakamee, A.P. Phyo, R. Rueangweerayut, F. Nosten, P. Jittamala et al. 2014. Spiroindolone KAE609 for falciparum and vivax malaria. N. Engl. J. Med. 371(5): 403–410.

WHO. 2015. Guidelines for the Treatment of Malaria. Geneva.

WHO. 2018. Overview of malaria treatment, available in http://www.who.int/malaria/areas/treatment/overview/en/, acessed in 26 April 2018.

Willcox, M., F. Benoit-Vical, D. Fowler, G. Bourdy, G. Burford, S. Giani et al. 2011. Do ethnobotanical and laboratory data predict clinical safety and efficacy of anti-malarial plants? Malar. J. 10 Suppl 1: S7.

Woodrow, C.J. and N.J. White. 2017. The clinical impact of artemisinin resistance in Southeast Asia and the potential for future spread. FEMS Microbiol. Rev. 41(1): 34–48.

Younis, Y., F. Douelle, T.-S. Feng, D.G. Cabrera, C.L. Manach, A.T. Nchinda et al. 2012. 3,5-Diaryl-2-aminopyridines as a novel class of orally active antimalarials demonstrating single dose cure in mice and clinical candidate potential. J. Med. Chem. 55(7): 3479–3487.

Zaw, M.T., N.A. Emran and Z. Lin. 2018. Updates on k13 mutant alleles for artemisinin resistance in *Plasmodium falciparum*. J. Microbiol. Immunol. Infect. 51: 159–165.

Zhang, J., J.J. Bowling, D. Smithson, J. Clark, M.R. Jacob, S.I. Khan et al. 2016. Diversity-oriented natural product platform identifies plant constituents targeting *Plasmodium falciparum*. Malar. J. 15(1): 270.

Chapter **10**

Hits and Lead Discovery in the Identification of New Drugs against the Trypanosomatidic Infections

Theodora Calogeropoulou,[1,]* George E. Magoulas,[1] Ina Pöhner,[2] Joanna Panecka-Hofman,[3,2,9] Pasquale Linciano,[4] Stefania Ferrari,[4] Nuno Santarem,[5] Mª Dolores Jiménez-Antón,[5] Ana Isabel Olías-Molero,[5] José María Alunda,[6] Anabela Cordeiro da Silva,[7,5] Rebecca C. Wade[2,8,9] and Maria Paola Costi[4,]*

Introduction

The Neglected Tropical Diseases (NTDs) are a group of 17 pathologies, recognized by the World Health Organization (WHO), which are endemic in 149 countries in tropical and sub-tropical areas of the globe, and affect more than one billion people overall (Feasey et al. 2010). The pathologies are all caused by microparasites or macroparasites. Among the diseases provoked by microparasites, three result from infections with kinetoplastidae, a group of flagellated protozoa transmitted by insect vectors: Chagas disease, Human African Trypanosomiasis (HAT) and leishmaniasis. The focus of the present chapter is on the identification of new drugs for the treatment of trypanosomatidic infections such as Chagas disease, caused by *T. cruzi*, and Human African Trypanosomiasis, caused by *T. brucei* (Filardy et al. 2018).

[1] Institute of Chemical Biology, National Hellenic Research Foundation, Athens, Greece.
[2] Molecular and Cellular Modeling Group, Heidelberg Institute for Theoretical Studies (HITS), Heidelberg, Germany.
[3] Faculty of Physics, University of Warsaw, Warsaw, Poland.
[4] Dipartimento di Scienze della Vita, University of Modena and Reggio Emilia, Via Campi 103, 41125 Modena, Italy.
[5] Instituto de Investigação e Inovação em Saúde, Universidade do Porto, and Parasite Disease Group, Instituto de Biologia Molecular e Celular, Universidade do Porto, Porto, Portugal.
[6] Department of Animal Health, Faculty of Veterinary Medicine, Universidad Complutense de Madrid, Madrid, Spain.
[7] Departamento de Ciências Biológicas, Faculdade de Farmácia da Universidade do Porto, Porto, Portugal.
[8] Center for Molecular Biology (ZMBH), DKFZ-ZMBH Alliance, Heidelberg University, Heidelberg, Germany.
[9] Interdisciplinary Center for Scientific Computing (IWR), Heidelberg University, Heidelberg, Germany.
* Corresponding authors: tcalog@eie.gr; costimp@unimore.it

Chagas Disease

Chagas disease, also referred to as American Trypanosomiasis, represents a serious medical and socioeconomic burden for over 21 countries of Latin America. More than 8 million people worldwide are estimated to be infected by *T. cruzi* and more than 10,000 deaths per year are reported. Recently, a reduction in incidence and prevalence of the infection has been observed, but on the other hand, a spread of the disease to previously unaffected regions as a consequence of massive migration fluxes, congenital transmission, and blood and organ donations has been reported, making Chagas disease a world health issue (Figure 1) (Pérez-Molina and Molina 2018).

The disease usually evolves from an acute to a chronic phase. The acute phase arises just after the infection and can last from a few weeks to several months and is characterized by non-specific signs (i.e., fever, swelling of skin and mucosa). Thereafter, the disease enters an asymptomatic chronic stage and only 20–30% of the infected people manifest lethal complications after several years (Bern et al. 2011). The treatment of both the acute and chronic stages of Chagas disease is based on chemotherapy. For almost 50 years, benznidazole and nifurtimox (Figure 2) were the two first-line drugs for the treatment of Chagas disease (Rodriques Coura and de Castro 2002). Unfortunately, their efficacy is limited, and more frequently the side effects that the two drugs elicit during the treatment of the chronic stage induce the patients to quit the therapy. Nifurtimox treatment is discontinued in up to 75% of all cases, and benznidazole, which is better tolerated, is discontinued in 9 to 29% of the cases. Besides chemotherapy, serological cure is recommended for acute congenital Chagas during the first year of life, and for chronically infected children under 14 years (Pérez-Molina and Molina 2018).

Human African Trypanosomiasis (HAT)

Human African Trypanosomiasis (HAT), also known as sleeping sickness, is caused by the bloodstream form of the two protozoan parasites *Trypanosoma brucei gambiense* and *Trypanosoma brucei rhodesiense* (Büscher et al. 2017). The sleeping sickness is mainly spread in the poorest rural areas of sub-Saharan Africa,

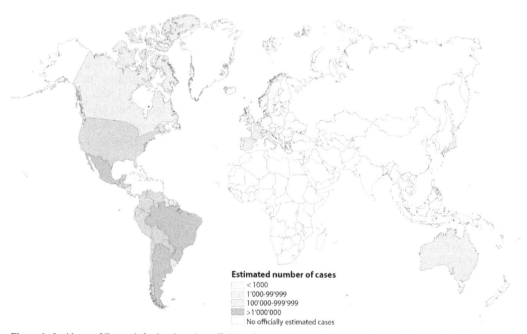

Figure 1. Incidence of *T. cruzi* infection, based on official estimates and status of vector transmission. Adapted from WHO 2010.

Color version at the end of the book

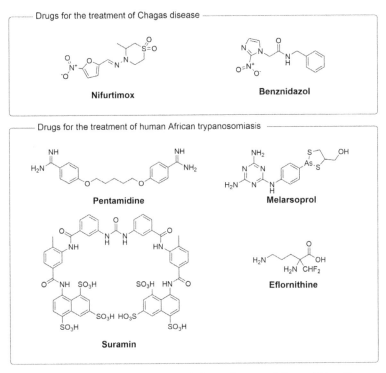

Figure 2. Drugs currently in use for the treatment of Chagas disease and Human African Trypanosomiasis.

where the habitat is suitable for the survival of the tsetse fly, the vector responsible for the transmission of the parasite. In particular, *T. b. gambiense* is widespread in Central and Western Africa and causes over 98% of chronic HAT, whereas *T. b. rhodensiense* only infects humans occasionally and is mainly spread in Southern and Eastern Africa (Figure 3). Starting from 2009, and for the first time in thirty years, mostly due to WHO launched programs of surveillance and treatment, less than 10.000 new cases per year of HAT were registered in 2009. This represents a drop of 76% with respect to the 300,000 cases observed in 1995. This trend suggests that a complete eradication of HAT by 2020 is possible (WHO 2017). However, the number of cases registered by the WHO covers only the visible part of HAT incidence, whereas around 70 million people living in sub-Saharan Africa are exposed to *T. brucei* infection (Simarro et al. 2012).

HAT can occur in an acute or chronic form. The acute form of the disease appears within few weeks of the initial injection of the trypomastigote form of the parasite into the host by the tsetse fly. It is characterized by non-specific flu-like symptoms including fever, headache and joint pain. Thereafter, similar to Chagas disease, the infection can remain quiescent for a long time period and re-emerge several years later (chronic form). The second stage starts when the parasite migrates across the blood-brain barrier into the central nervous system, resulting in neurological symptoms such as confusion, depleted coordination and sensory disturbances, and disruption of the normal sleeping cycle (from which the name sleeping sickness was derived). Ultimately, progressive mental deterioration leads to coma and death (Kennedy 2013). Other *Trypanosoma* species (e.g., *T. vivax*, *T. congolense*) are etiological agents of a variety of wasting diseases affecting domestic livestock, which collectively go by the name of Animal African Trypanosomiasis (AAT or Nagana). Nagana causes significant damage to cattle farming with 3 million heads lost each year, contributing to significant economical damage in countries with already fragile economic structures. Moreover, domestic animals can represent a reservoir for both *T. b. gambiense* and *T. b. rhodesiense*, exposing humans to a possible infection (Njiokou et al. 2010). Therefore, fighting both HAT and AAT in the one health approach (Okello et al. 2014) is the only way to the complete eradication of this pathology (Giordani et al. 2016). The

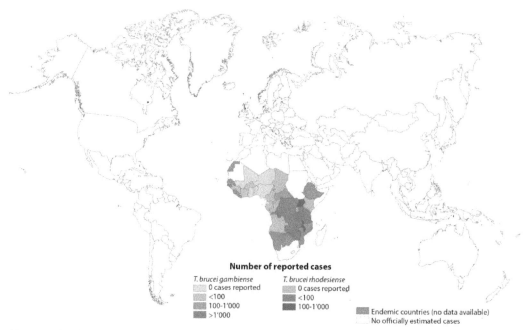

Figure 3. Distribution of Human African Trypanosomiasis (*T. b. gambiense* in green and *T. b. rhodesiense* in blue) worldwide. Adapted from WHO 2017.

Color version at the end of the book

treatment of HAT, diversified depending on the stage of infection, is only based on chemotherapy (Cullen and Mocerino 2017). Nowadays, only four drugs and one drug combination are employed in therapy (Figure 2). Pentamidine is currently the first-line option for treating the initial stage of HAT (Sands et al. 1985), whereas suramin is employed as a second choice or for the primary treatment of *T. b. rhodesiense* infection, for which it is more effective than pentamidine. However, both drugs suffer from important limitations: they are administered parenterally, require a healthcare professional, are ineffective in stage two and, more importantly, have adverse side effects that are often responsible for the suspension of the treatment. Melarsoprol, eflornithine and nifurtimox, instead, are the only drugs actually effective in the second stage of HAT (Eperon et al. 2014). Melarsoprol was the first drug to be developed for HAT; it has been medically used since 1949 and it has the great advantage of being effective against both *T. b. gambiense* and *T. b. rhodesiense* infections. However, it derives from arsenic, which is the reason for its undesirable effects, including fatal encephalopathy (Fairlamb and Horn 2018).

Eflornithine is the only recent drug approved for HAT in 2000. It is a less toxic alternative to melarsoprol, even though it is completely ineffective against *T. b. rhodesiense*. The main drawback of eflornithine is the complex regimen of intravenous infusions 4-times per day for 14 days of treatment (Chappuis et al. 2005). Today eflornithine is rarely used alone but is normally prescribed in combination with nifurtimox. Nifurtimox alone is less effective against *T. brucei* than *T. cruzi*, but in combination with eflornithine, the efficacy of the treatment is comparable to that of eflornithine alone, but with considerably fewer side-effects than the monotherapy. In addition, the regimen of eflornithine in combination with nifurtimox is more manageable, furthermore permitting an oral administration of the two drugs (Priotto et al. 2009).

HAT and Chagas Disease: Social Impact and Intervention

Although 1.4 billion people is exposed to the risk of NTDs, these pathologies remain neglected at several levels. At the local level, they are usually not mentioned by affected people, who are afraid of bias and marginalisation by the community. These pathologies barely spread outside the tropical area of origin therefore, they do not represent an immediate risk for the 'occidental' countries that tend to be disinterested. However, the price to be paid for this choice is high: the NTDs have an elevated impact on the life of every single person, family and community, drastically decreasing the quality of life, reducing productivity and contributing to a cycle of increased poverty in already economically fragile countries (Weiss 2008). Notwithstanding the social and economic burden, research and development on these illnesses is limited. For example, among all the 1,393 new drugs approved between 1975 and 1999, only 13 (0.9%) were targeted for NTDs, and only four of those were developed by pharmaceutical companies. The other nine were discovered as a result of veterinary and military research (Trouiller et al. 2002). Therefore, in order to encourage the research and development of new drugs that could be more effective, safe and economically sustainable, and to overcome the lack of interest of the major pharmaceutical companies in this health issue, associations between public and private institutions (PPP, public-private partnership) were recently initiated (Liese et al. 2010). These include the European Commission (Pierce et al. 2017) and other government agencies, private foundations and pharmaceutical multinationals such as the Drugs for Neglected Diseases Initiative (DNDi) (Chatelain and Ioset 2011) and the Medicines for Malaria Venture (MMV 2018). These PPPs coordinate the basic research conducted by universities and public health organizations with the experience and technology of the chemical and technological pharmaceutical industries to develop new drug candidates. The DNDi, along with partners including the Bill & Melinda Gates Foundation (WA, USA), Sanofi (Paris, France) and Médecins Sans Frontières (Geneva, Switzerland) are attempting to address the deficiency in accessible treatments and currently have two oral candidates in clinical trials. Acoziborole (SCYX-7158) emerged as a safe and promising candidate in late 2009 for the treatment of the second stage of HAT (Eperon et al. 2014). After successful preclinical trials, the drug entered clinical development in 2012. In 2016, acoziborole entered into a Phase II/III clinical trial, which is expected to be completed by April 2020 (Jacobs et al. 2011). Fexinidazole is currently the most advanced oral drug candidate being developed for first stage and early second stage HAT (Eperon et al. 2014). A pivotal Phase II/III trial was completed in 2016, although two additional 'plug-in' trials are currently ongoing to assess the efficacy of the drug in special population groups not examined in the initial cohort. In addition, DNDi is also running a Phase III trial examining the effectiveness of fexinidazole in patients treated on both an out-patient basis and in a clinical hospital setting—depending on status. These trials are going to be completed by March 2020 (Mesu et al. 2018). Besides acoziborole and fexinidazole, which are two successful examples of new drugs identified for the treatment of trypanosomatidic infections, new candidates continuously enter the drug discovery pipeline.

Drug Discovery Approaches

Usually, drug discovery for NTDs is carried out using classical ligand-based approaches, target-based approaches and phenotypic screening. Ligand-based approaches, which are discussed later in the chapter, are typically focused on the development of new compounds on the basis of already known active compounds, natural compounds or marketed drugs. Chemical structure modifications are then applied on the basis of classical medicinal chemistry strategies (Wermuth et al. 2015). Target-based approaches involve screening a library of compounds against a protein target and then optimizing the compounds for potency against the enzyme, selectivity, cellular activity, and pharmacokinetic properties. However, there are relatively few validated drug targets for trypanosomiatidic infections (Frearson et al. 2007). Targets of major interest in the field of drug discovery are reported in Gilbert et al. (2013) and, in this chapter, we focus on targets relevant for ergosterol biosynthesis, folate metabolism, phosphodiesterases, cysteine proteases and trypanothione metabolism. On the other hand, phenotypic screening has the advantage of identifying compounds that are active against the whole cell, meaning issues such as cell uptake and cell efflux have already been addressed (Haasen et al. 2017). There has been a major emphasis on phenotypic approaches to drug discovery for neglected diseases and a number of notable successes have been reported, like the above mentioned fexinidazole and acoziborole (Eperon et al. 2014). Nonetheless, a balanced portfolio of carefully selected ligand- and target-based approaches together with phenotypic approaches is probably the best strategy for drug discovery for NTDs. This must be complemented by studies in animal models, which are reviewed in the final section of this chapter.

Synthetic compounds active against Trypanosoma cruzi *and* Trypanosoma brucei

Over the years, numerous papers have been published aiming at new, more effective and safe drugs against trypanosomatidic infections. In the context of this chapter, the synthesis and structure-activity relationship (SAR) studies of the most important compound classes with promising antitrypanosomal activity are described, covering related literature from 2010 to present.

Quinoline derivatives

A series of ten 2-alkylaminomethylquinoline derivatives were synthesized (Muscia et al. 2011) and tested against different developmental stages of *T. cruzi* (epimastigotes, trypomastigotes and amastigotes).

The antiparasitic activity *in vitro* against epimastigotes of five compounds (IC_{50} = 3.4–11.8 μM vs 5.8 μM for benznidazole) led to the further evaluation against trypomastigotes and amastigotes. Compound **1** was the most active against trypomastigotes with IC_{50} = 3.1 μM, with cytotoxic activity against COS-7 line slightly better than the reference drug (CC_{50} = 770.9 μM vs 706 μM for benznidazole) (Figure 4). Furthermore, compound **1** showed good selectivity for both trypomastigotes and amastigotes with selectivity index (SI) of 248.7 and 60.2, respectively.

Reid et al. (2011) described the synthesis of derivatives of *N*-benzyl-1,2-dihydroquinolin-6-ols (Figure 5) and their evaluation against *T. b. rhodesiense* STIB900. The authors proceeded with an extensive SAR study in order to decipher the effect of the substituents on the biological activity. These studies are summarized in Figure 6. The most active compounds *in vitro* were **2**, **3**, **4** and **5** with IC_{50} values 0.012 ± 0.001, 0.011 ± 0.001, 0.013 ± 0.004 and 0.014 ± 0.004 μM, respectively. These compounds were selected for *in vivo* evaluation and were administered to mice infected with *T. b. rhodesiense* STIB900. Compound **2** suppressed parasitemia but a relapse occurred after 12.75 days after injection. Conversely, the ester prodrug **3** and the hydrochloride salts **4** and **5** resulted in cure even though at higher dosages (4 days × 50 mg/kg ip) than the reference drugs diminazene (4 days × 10 mg/kg ip) and pentamidine (4 days × 5 mg/kg ip).

Hiltensperger et al. (2012) described the synthesis of a library of quinolone-type compounds bearing a benzamide function at position 3 and an amine heterocycle at position 7 for SAR purposes (Figure 7). These compounds were tested against *T. b. brucei* and *T. b. rhodesiense.*

In the context of the SAR studies, synthetic intermediates were tested as well. It is apparent that the amidation at position 3 is essential for activity but only for benzylamide and not for phenylamide derivatives, indicating the necessity for flexibility at position 3. In addition, the presence of cyclic and acyclic amines at position 7 enhances the activity. The most potent compound proved to be compound **6**, which exhibited promising *in vitro* activity against *T. brucei* (IC_{50} = 47 nM) and *T. b. rhodesiense* (IC_{50} = 9 nM) combined with low cytotoxicity against macrophages J774.1. Hence, compound **6** was chosen for *in vivo* evaluation in a murine model of HAT. A preliminary formulation for oral administration was developed but was unsuccessful against *T. b. rhodesiense* (STIB900) infected NMRI mice.

Upadhayaya et al. (2013) described the synthesis of a series of compounds based on quinolines and indenoquinolines with variable side chains. From this library, five compounds (Figure 8) showed higher activity than benznidazole and nifurtimox (IC_{50} = 0.25–0.65 μM) against *T. cruzi* and *T. brucei.*

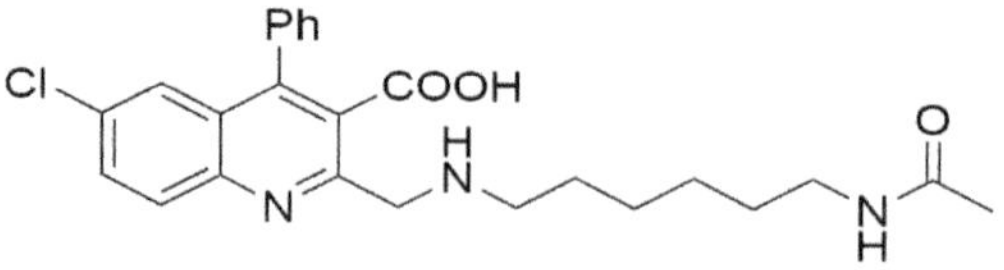

1

Figure 4. Structure of the 2-alkylaminomethylquinoline derivative **1**.

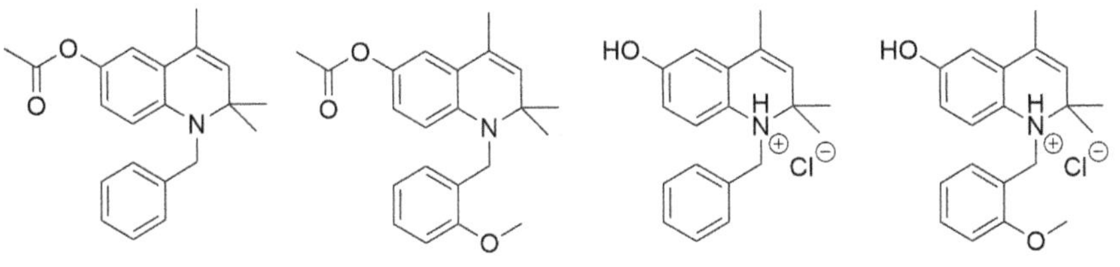

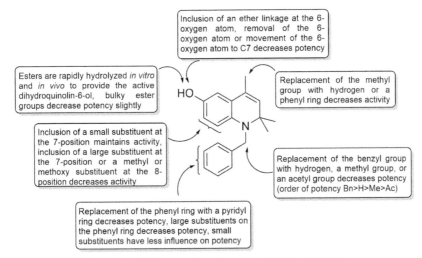

Figure 5. Structures of most active *N*-benzyl-1,2-dihydroquinolin-6-ols **2–5**.

Inclusion of an ether linkage at the 6-oxygen atom, removal of the 6-oxygen atom or movement of the 6-oxygen atom to C7 decreases potency

Esters are rapidly hydrolyzed *in vitro* and *in vivo* to provide the active dihydroquinolin-6-ol, bulky ester groups decrease potency slightly

Replacement of the methyl group with hydrogen or a phenyl ring decreases activity

Inclusion of a small substituent at the 7-position maintains activity, inclusion of a large substituent at the 7-position or a methyl or methoxy substituent at the 8-position decreases activity

Replacement of the benzyl group with hydrogen, a methyl group, or an acetyl group decreases potency (order of potency Bn>H>Me>Ac)

Replacement of the phenyl ring with a pyridyl ring decreases potency, large substituents on the phenyl ring decreases potency, small substituents have less influence on potency

Figure 6. Activity map of tested compounds (Reid et al. 2011).

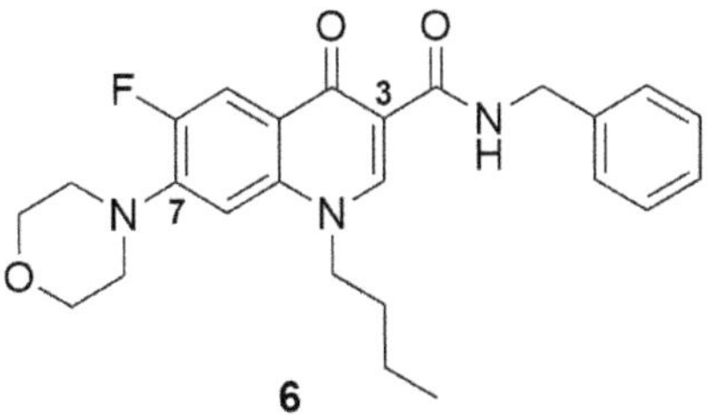

Figure 7. Structure of the most potent compound **6**.

A series of new 3-nitrotriazole and 2-nitrotriazole-linked quinolines and quinazolines were synthesized and their antitrypanosomal activity was tested (Papadopoulou et al. 2017). Even though almost all compounds showed activity against *T. cruzi* and *T. b. rhodesiense*, only two chloroquinoline derivatives (**12** and **13**, Figure 9) exhibited satisfactory selectivity indices.

Particularly, compound **12** which bears a nitroimidazole moiety showed IC_{50} values of 1.29 and 1.11 µM against *T. b. rhodesiense* and *T. cruzi*, respectively, while compound **13**, which bears a nitrotriazole moiety, showed IC_{50} values of 0.038 and 0.574 µM, respectively. Especially compound **13** exhibited an excellent SI against *T. b. rhodesiense* (SI = 1937).

Diamines and polyamines

Caminos et al. (2012) described the synthesis of 25 *N,N'*-disubstituted diamines through reductive amination of free aliphatic amines with various substituted benzaldehydes. This library was screened for antiparasitic

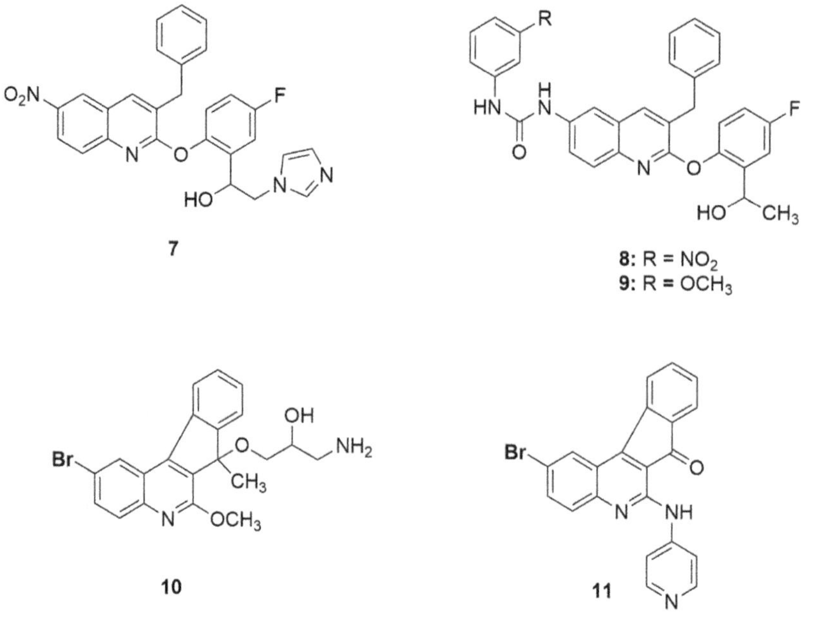

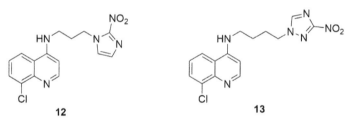

Figure 8. Structures of quinoline (**7–9**) and indenoquinoline (**10**, **11**) derivatives.

Figure 9. Structures of the most potent chloroquinolines **12** and **13**.

activity *in vitro* against *T. brucei* and *T. cruzi*. In terms of SAR studies, the length of the aliphatic chain between the two amino functions was studied, as well as the substitution of the benzyl moiety attached to the amines. The most promising compounds were **14** and **15** that bear a benzyloxy substitution at position 4, and an aliphatic chain with 3 or 4 carbons (Figure 10). These compounds exhibit medium activity against *T. cruzi* (IC_{50} = 0.78 and 0.76 μM, respectively); however, they are significantly more active against *T. brucei* (IC_{50} = 0.062 and 0.097 μM, respectively) with higher selectivity indices (SI = 97 and 60, respectively).

Sánchez-Moreno et al. (2012) published the synthesis of four pyrazole-containing macrocyclic and macrobicyclic polyamines and their *in vitro* and *in vivo* evaluation as potential antichagasic agents. Two of these compounds, **16** and **17** (Figure 11), were the most active from the compounds tested in *T. cruzi* epimastigote, axenic amastigote and intracellular amastigote forms. In addition, they proved to be more active than the reference drug benznidazole. More specifically, compound **16** showed an IC_{50} = 1.3 ± 0.1 μM and compound **17** showed an IC_{50} = 1.3 ± 0.3 μM (versus benznidazole IC_{50} = 15.9 ± 1.1 μM) against the epimastigote form. Concerning the axenic epimastigote form, the IC_{50} values for compounds **16** and **17** were 7.2 ± 2.2 μM and 8.8 ± 1.8 μM, respectively (benznidazole IC_{50} = 15.9 ± 1.1 μM). Finally, the IC_{50} values for compounds **16** and **17** were 6.2 ± 0.8 μM and 6.5 ± 1.6 μM, respectively, against the intracellular amastigote form, while for benznidazole, it was 23.3 ± 4.6 μM. Regarding the cytotoxicity evaluation against Vero cells, compounds **16** and **17** were substantially less toxic than the reference drug (IC_{50} = 149.1 and 178.5 μM, respectively, against 13.6 μM for benznidazole).

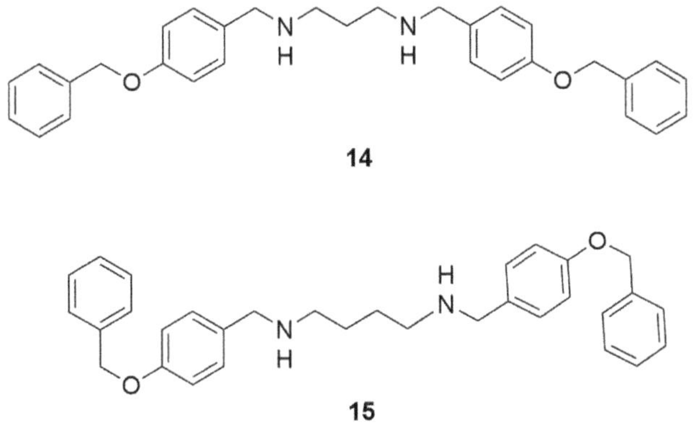

14

15

Figure 10. Structures of the most potent diamines **14** and **15**.

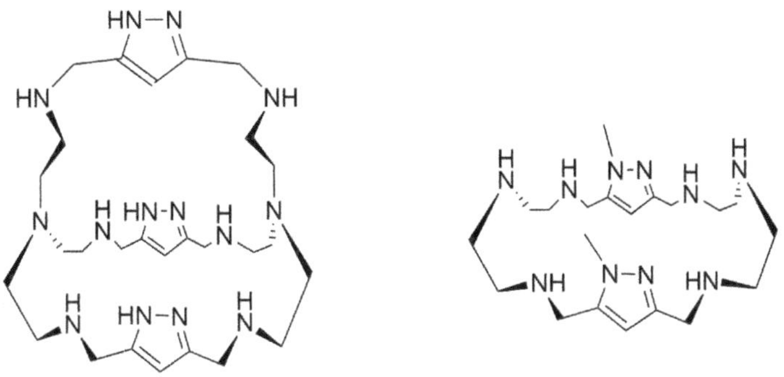

16   **17**

Figure 11. Structures of macrobicyclic and macrocyclic pyrazole-containing polyamines **16** and **17**.

Prompted by the *in vitro* results, these compounds were tested *in vivo* against female BALB/c mice and they proved to be more active than benznidazole in both the acute and chronic phase animal models (Sánchez-Moreno et al. 2012).

Acridones

A small library of acridones was synthesized and their antiparasitic activity was tested (Montalvo-Quirós et al. 2015). The most active compounds are depicted in Figure 12. Acridones **18–20** showed excellent activity against *T. b. rhodesiense* (IC$_{50}$ = 0.069, 0.007 and 0.062 µM, respectively), accompanied by very good selectivity (SI > 2000). The *N*-methylation of these compounds to the corresponding acridones **21–23** did not alter the activity of **22** and **23** but increased the activity of **21** 10-fold (IC$_{50}$ = 0.007 µM).

Compounds **18–20** were chosen for preliminary *in vivo* evaluation in the *T. b. rhodesiense* mouse model. Compound **19** confirmed its activity since three out of four mice were cured, with mean day of relapse over fifty days.

Thiohydantoins

During a high throughput screening for potential inhibitors of *T. brucei in vitro*, Buchynskyy et al. (2017a) discovered the substituted 2-thiohydantoin **24** (EC$_{50}$ = 346 nM) as a potential hit compound. An extensive SAR study, which comprised changes to each of the phenyl moieties in terms of lipophilicity, site of substitution, electron donating and electron withdrawing groups and the combination of them, led to two new compounds **25** and **26** (Figure 13). These compounds showed excellent *T. brucei* activity

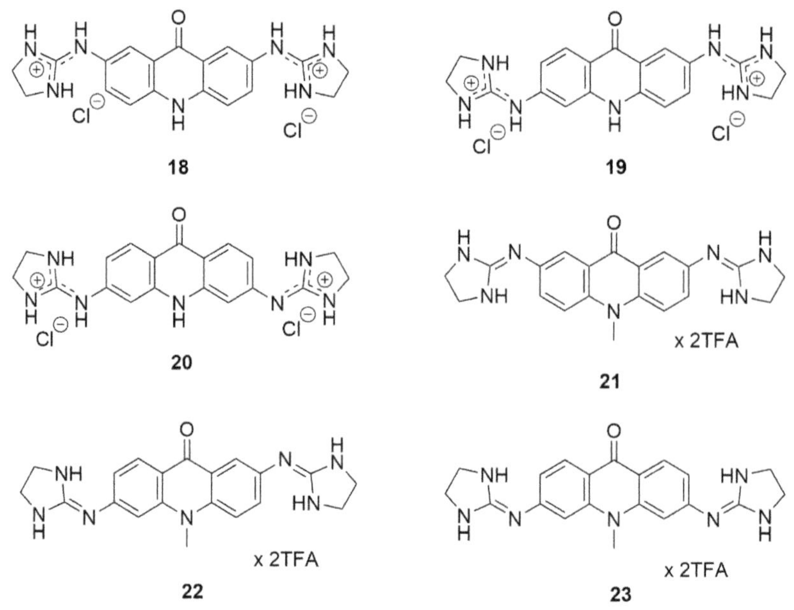

Figure 12. Acridones **18–23** with activity against *T. b. rhodesiense.*

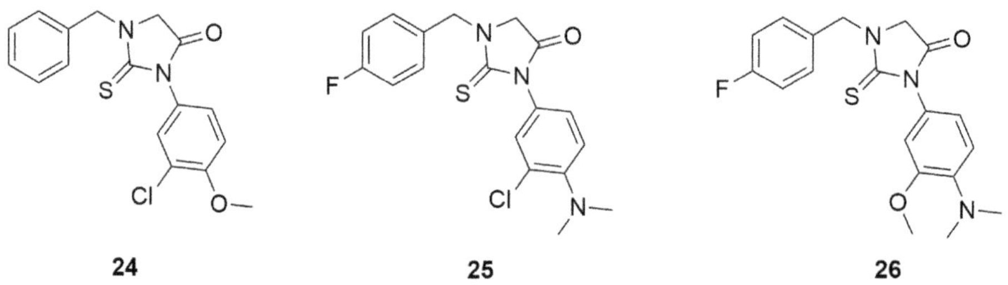

Figure 13. Hit compound **24** and lead compounds **25** and **26**.

in vitro (EC_{50} = 3 nM for **25** and EC_{50} = 2 nM for **26**). For this reason, they were also tested *in vivo* in the acute phase model of HAT. Both compounds cured all treated mice as no parasitemia was detected for 60 days after infection.

Quinones, quinoxalines and quinazolines

In recent years, naphthoquinone has drawn much attention as a scaffold with potential antitrypanosomatidic activity. Carneiro et al. (2012) reported the synthesis of new oxirane derivatives using naphthoquinones as starting materials. Even though most of the synthesized compounds proved more active than the reference drug benznidazole (IC_{50} = 11.5 μM, CC_{50} = 48 μM) against epimastigote forms of *T. cruzi*, only compound **27** (Figure 14) exhibited comparable cytotoxicity (IC_{50} = 0.09 μM, CC_{50} = 44 μM).

Khraiwesh et al. (2012) synthesized eleven new imido-substituted 1,4-naphthoquinones which were tested against *T. cruzi* epimastigotes. Interestingly, all compounds showed better activity (IC_{50} = 0.7–6.1 μM) than the reference drug nifurtimox (IC_{50} = 10.67 μM, SI = 10.86) but only four of them, compounds **28–31** (Figure 15), exhibited a higher selectivity index (SI = 31.83–275.3).

Samant and Chakaingesu (2013) synthesized a series of mono- and disubstituted naphthoquinones and all compounds were tested against *T. b. rhodesiense*. The most promising compounds are depicted in Figure 16. The monosubstituted compounds **33** and **34** were more active (IC_{50} = 0.07 ± 0.01 μM and 0.05 ± 0.01 μM, respectively) than the disubstituted one (**32**) (IC_{50} = 0.09 ± 0.01 μM). In addition,

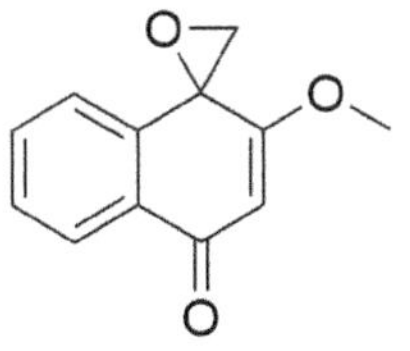

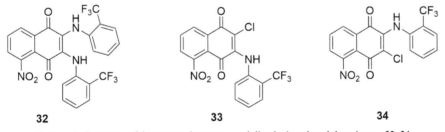

27

Figure 14. Structure of the most active oxirane derivative **27**.

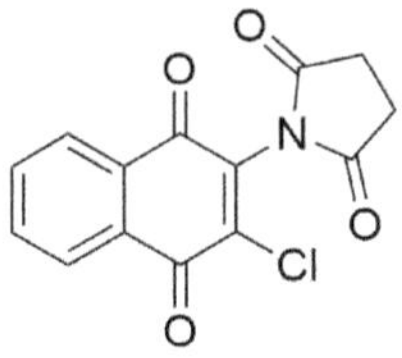

28
IC$_{50}$ = 2.77 µM, SI = 60.25

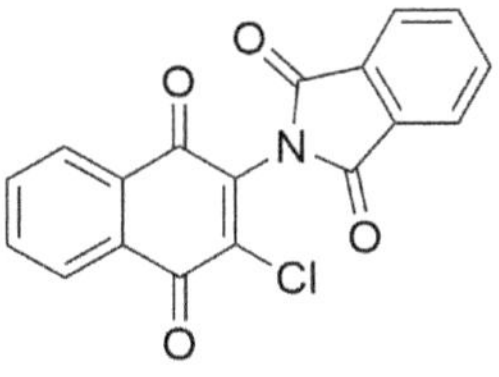

29
IC$_{50}$ = 4.83 µM, SI = 53.97

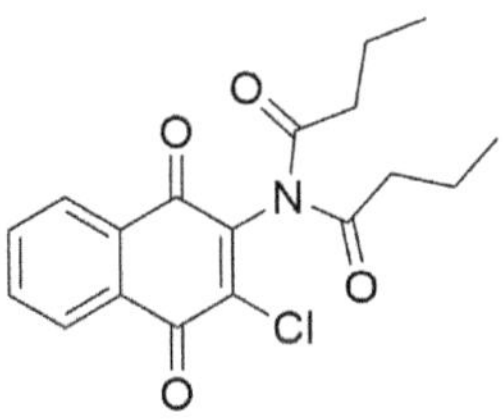

30
IC$_{50}$ = 0.70 µM, SI = 31.83

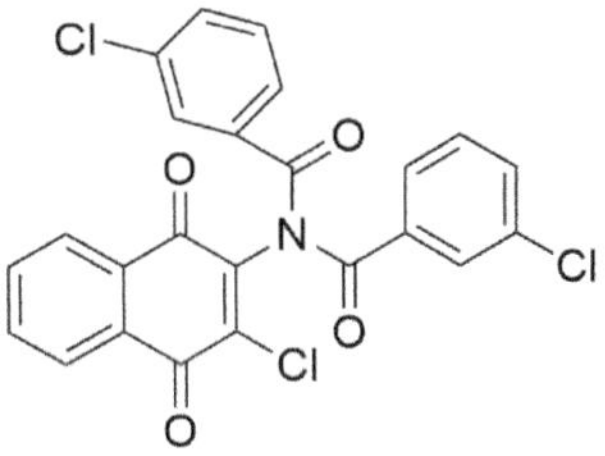

31
IC$_{50}$ = 2.23 µM, SI = 275.3

Figure 15. Structures of the most active imido-substituted 1,4-naphthoquinones **28–31**.

32

33

34

Figure 16. Structures of the most active mono- and di-substituted naphthoquinones **32–34**.

these three compounds (**32–34**) were the least cytotoxic from this library, with CC$_{50}$ = 88 ± 5 µM, CC$_{50}$ = 75 ± 5 µM and CC$_{50}$ = 95 ± 5 µM, respectively, when tested against L-6 rat skeletal myoblast cells.

A new library of aryloxy-quinone derivatives was synthesized by Vásquez et al. (2015). Interestingly, almost all new compounds were more active against *T. cruzi* Y strain epimastigotes and less toxic against J774 cells than the reference drug nifurtimox (IC$_{50}$ = 7.00 ± 0.3 µM, SI = 40). Thus, the combination of activity and selectivity led to four potential hits (Figure 17). Compound **35** was the most active (IC$_{50}$ = 0.02 ± 0.01 µM, SI = 625) followed by compounds **36–38** with IC$_{50}$ values 0.05 ± 0.02 µM, 0.04 ± 0.02 µM and 0.09 ± 0.04 µM, respectively.

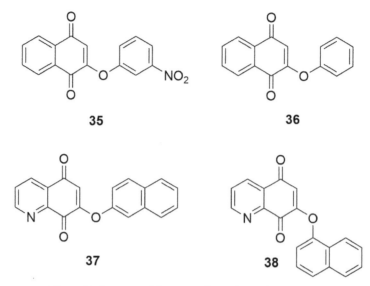

Figure 17. Structures of the most active aryloxy-quinones **35–38**.

In the last decade, quinoxaline derivatives have been characterised as potential anti-trypanosoma agents (Ancizu et al. 2009). Numerous compounds have been synthesized and evaluated and thus, some structural requirements have been established against trypanosomatids *in vitro*. These comprise the existence of the *N*-oxide moiety and the insertion of electron withdrawing groups on the quinoxaline ring.

Benitez et al. (2011) synthesized an extensive library of quinoxalines *N,N'*-dioxides as potential anti-*T. cruzi* agents. Initially, the evaluation of these compounds was carried out *in vitro* against the epimastigote form of the Talahuen 2 strain of *T. cruzi* by calculating the percentage of growth inhibition (PGI). The most active compounds were **39–47** (Figure 18). In addition, the IC_{50} concentrations were assessed with the most active compounds being **39** (IC_{50} = 0.4 µM), **40** (IC_{50} = 0.7 µM) and **42** (IC_{50} = 0.39 µM). Active compounds were also tested against two other *T. cruzi* strains, namely, colombiana and Y strains. In particular, the most potent compounds, **40** and **42,** were tested *in vivo* in murine models of acute Chagas' disease against the bloodstream trypomastigote form of CL Brener clone, showing a very interesting biological profile.

The aforementioned structural prerequisites concerning quinoxalines were confirmed by Torres et al. (2013). Eighteen new quinoxaline *N,N'*-dioxides were synthesized and evaluated against the epimastigote form of the Talahuen 2 strain of *T. cruzi*. 14 out of 18 compounds showed PGI values of 100% while the most active compounds were **48–53** (Figure 19) with IC_{50} values varying from 0.4–2.6 µM. Compound **52** was the most active compound (IC_{50} = 0.4 µM).

Patel et al. (2013), motivated by the activity of the cancer drug lapatinib against *T. brucei*, performed an extensive SAR study, in which 4-anilinoquinazoline **55** (NEU-617) emerged as the most potent, orally bioavailable inhibitor of trypanosome replication (Figure 20). All compounds were tested against cultures of *T. brucei brucei* Lister 427. Compound **55** (EC_{50} = 0.042 µM) was more active than lapatinib (EC_{50} = 1.54 µM) and it was even more selective against HepG2 cells (> 20 µM versus 6.2 µM for lapatinib).

In an effort to further optimize **55** (NEU-617) as antiparasitic lead compound, Devine et al. (2015) proceeded with the synthesis of new derivatives involving several replacements on the quinazoline scaffold. Even though **55** was superior against *T. brucei* compared to the new derivatives, several hits were discovered against other protozoal species, i.e. *T. cruzi, Leishmania major* and *Plasmodium falciparum*. Thus, compound **56** was found to be the most active compound against intracellular amastigotes of *T. cruzi* (EC_{50} = 0.09 µM) and compound **57** the most potent from the new library against *T. brucei* (EC_{50} = 0.21 µM) (Figure 21).

39 **40** **41**

42 **43** **44**

45 **46** **47**

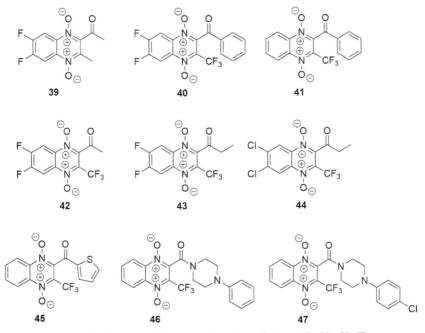

Figure 18. Structures of the most active quinoxaline *N,N'*-dioxides **39–47**.

48 **49** **50**

51 **52** **53**

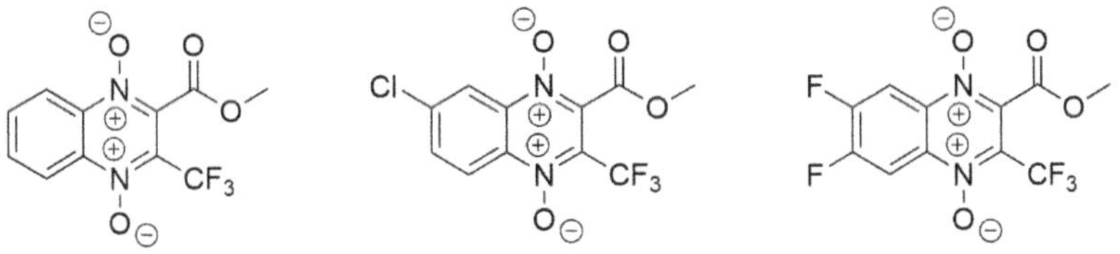

Figure 19. Structures of the most active quinoxaline *N,N'*-dioxides **48–53**.

54 **55 (NEU-617)**

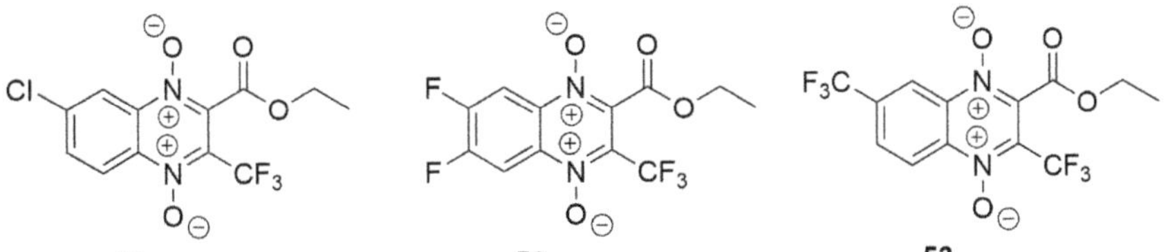

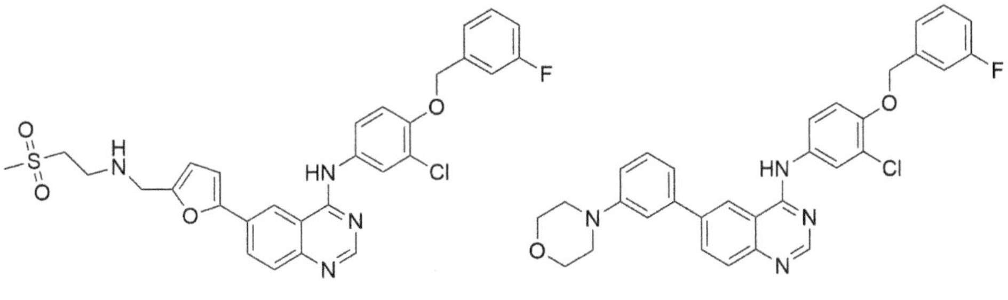

Figure 20. Structures of lapatinib (**54**) and the most potent inhibitor **55**.

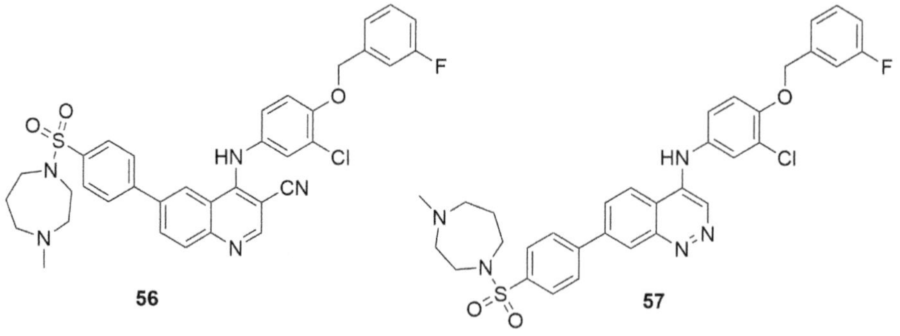

Figure 21. Structures of the most potent inhibitors **56** and **57**.

Benzamide derivatives

As a continuation of their previous findings, Hwang et al. (2010 and 2013a) reported their optimization efforts for chloronitrobenzamides (CNBs). Compound **58** was found to be active against *T. b. brucei* (EC$_{50}$ = 0.92 μM) which led to a new SAR study. Numerous compounds were synthesized and tested and finally compounds **59–61** were the most potent against *T. b. brucei* (EC$_{50}$ = 0.006, 0.027 and 0.041 μM, respectively) (Figure 22).

In addition, **59–61** were tested against *T. b. rhodesiense* and *T. b. gambiense* and they showed activity against *T. b. rhodesiense* (EC$_{50}$ = 0.013, 0.007 and 0.011 μM, respectively) as well as against *T. b. gambiense* (EC$_{50}$ = 0.036, 0.002 and 0.001 μM, respectively). However, these compounds exhibited poor to modest solubility, an issue that should be addressed in their further development.

In an effort to reduce complexity and molecular weight and at the same time to improve the pharmacological properties of CNBs, Hwang et al. (2013b) synthesized a new library of compounds by replacing the chloronitrobenzamide moiety. Even though most of the compounds were inactive, one potential lead (compound **62**, Figure 23) was found which bears the 4-chloropyridine carboxamide moiety. This compound showed good activity against *T. b. brucei* (EC$_{50}$ = 0.12 μM) and excellent activity against *T. b. rhodesiense* (EC$_{50}$ = 0.018 μM) and *T. b. gambiense* (EC$_{50}$ = 0.038 μM).

Pyridyl benzamides were further explored as potential anti-trypanosomatidic agents (Ferrins et al. 2014). An extensive SAR study was conducted based on hit compound **63** (IC$_{50}$ = 3.03 μM). A large library was synthesized and tested against *T. b. brucei*, *T. b. rhodesiense* and *T. cruzi*. Compounds **64–68** (Figure 24) showed activity with IC$_{50}$ values ranging between 0.41–1.1 μM against *T. b. brucei* and 0.045–0.64 μM against *T. b. rhodesiense*, with the most active compound being **65** (IC$_{50}$ = 0.045 μM). However, all compounds were inactive against *T. cruzi*. These compounds with low molecular weight have favorable properties for further optimization and have a very good prediction for CNS penetration which is essential for treating second stage HAT.

In the context of a high throughput screening campaign of 87000 compounds against *T. b. brucei*, Rahmani et al. (2015) identified a new class of potential trypanocides, pyrazine carboxamides. This screening delivered a starting hit, compound **69** (EC$_{50}$ = 0.49 μM), and subsequent SAR studies were conducted concerning structural changes around the core. Several compounds showed very good activity against *T. b. brucei* and *T. b. rhodesiense* but the most active compounds were **70** with EC$_{50}$ values of 0.035 and 0.024 μM against *T. b. brucei* and *T. b. rhodesiense*, respectively and compound **71** with EC$_{50}$ values 0.025 and 0.038 μM, respectively (Figure 25). It is worth mentioning that this class of compounds showed very low cytotoxicity and was selective for *T. brucei*, since no significant activity was observed against *T. cruzi*.

Cleghorn et al. (2015) conducted a phenotypic screening of compounds against *T. b. brucei* followed by a mammalian cell counterscreen (MRC-5 cells) to exclude nonselective compounds. This work led to indoline-2-carboxamide **72** (Figure 26) which showed good activity (EC$_{50}$ = 27 nM) and selectivity over mammalian cells (> 1600 fold). With compound **72** in hand, SAR studies were realized in terms of core modifications and the effect of stereochemistry on the chiral center. These studies led to the discovery of

58

59

60

61

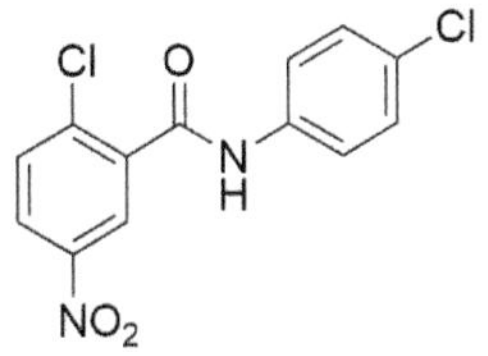

Figure 22. Structures of hit compound **58** and the most potent CNBs **59–61**.

62

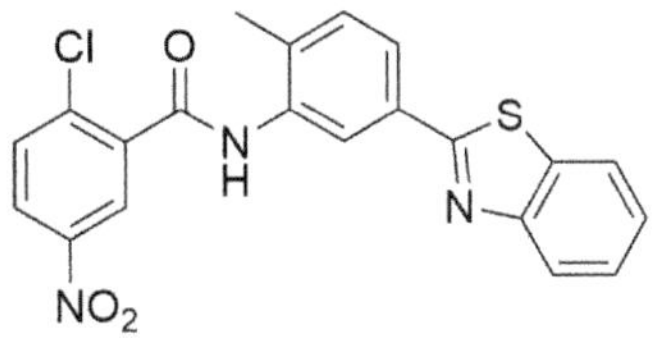

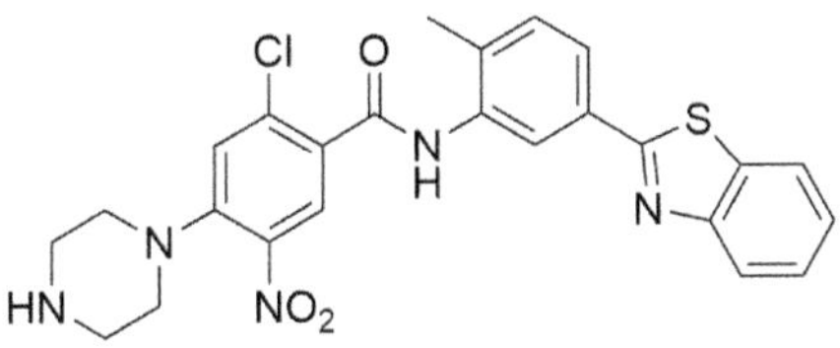

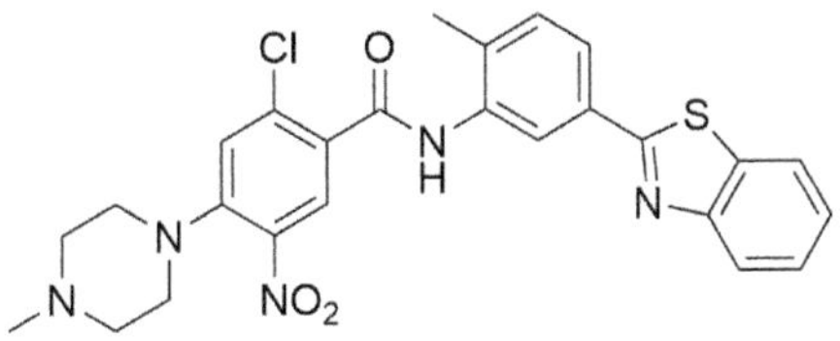

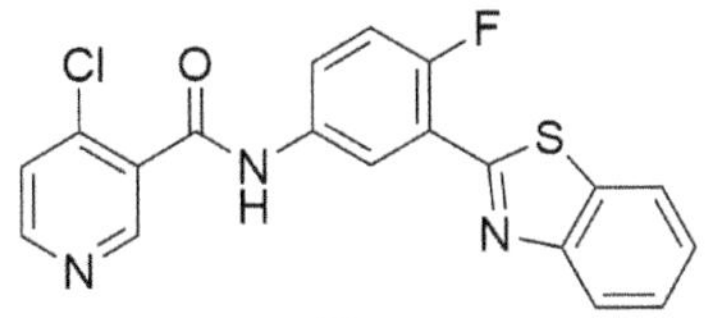

Figure 23. Structure of lead compound **62**.

63

64

65

66

67

68

Figure 24. Structures of hit compound **63** and lead pyridyl benzamides **64–68**.

69

70

71

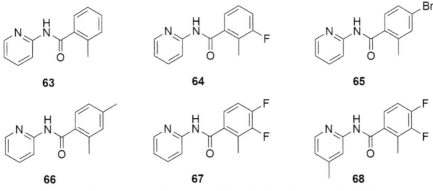

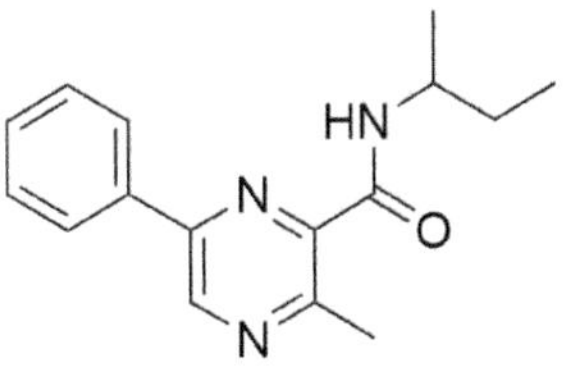

Figure 25. Structures of hit compound **69** and lead compounds **70** and **71**.

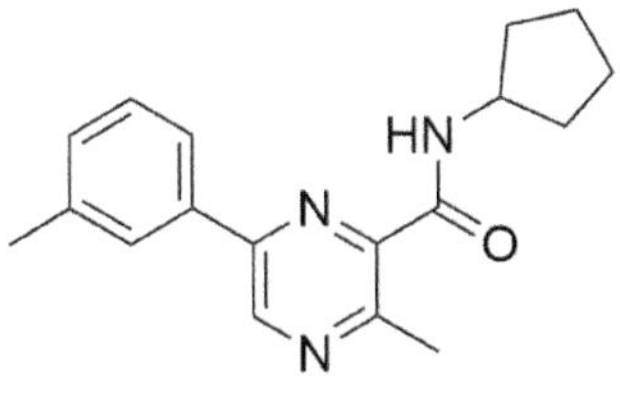

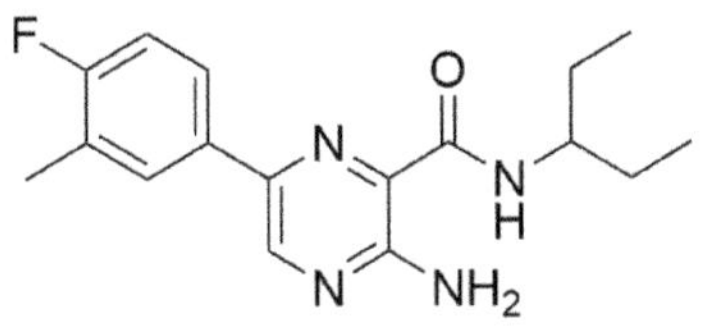

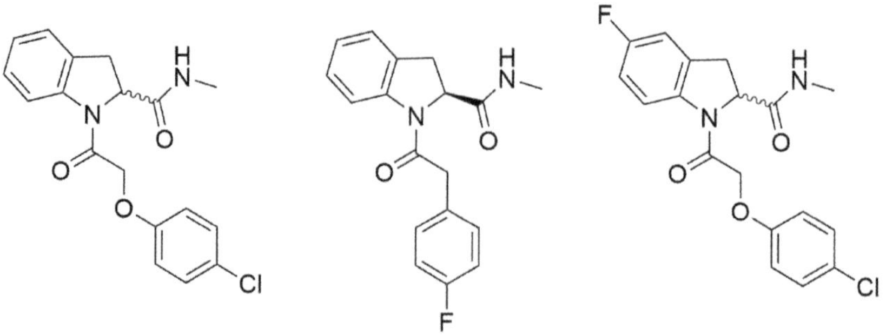

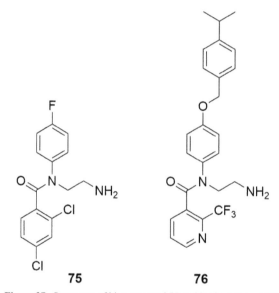

Figure 26. Structures of potent indoline-2-carboxamides **72–74**.

Figure 27. Structures of hit compound **75** and lead compound **76**.

two new compounds, **73** and **74** (racemic), with lower activity against *T. b. brucei* (EC$_{50}$ = 60 and 80 nM, respectively) but with improved metabolic stability and enhanced *in vivo* exposure. These compounds exhibited excellent pharmacokinetic properties, and resulted in a full cure in a HAT stage 1 mouse model, but unfortunately only a partial cure in stage 2.

Buchynskyy et al. (2017b) identified *N*-(2-aminoethyl)-*N*-phenyl benzamides as an interesting class of compounds with potential antiparasitic activity against *T. brucei*. Compound **75** (Figure 27) was selected as a hit compound for its activity (EC$_{50}$ = 1.21 µM) against *T. b. brucei*, its selectivity over mammalian cells (> 30 fold) and its drug-like features, including low molecular weight, clogP, H-bond donors and acceptors. The outcome of SAR studies was the discovery of some new lead compounds with EC$_{50}$ values ranging from 0.001–0.031 µM, with compound **76** being the most potent derivative (EC$_{50}$ = 0.001 µM against *T. b. brucei* and 0.002 µM against *T. b. rhodesiense*). However, in murine efficacy models of HAT infection, the compounds showed only partial cures or suppression.

Chalcones

Chalcones form another class of compounds with broad spectrum pharmacological activities. Recently, Borsari et al. (2017) reported the synthesis of a library of 13 2-hydroxy-chalcones bearing methoxy groups.

All the synthesized compounds were tested against the bloodstream form of *T. brucei* and the intracellular stage of *T. cruzi* at 10 μM. Compounds **77–79** (Figure 28) were the most potent against *T. brucei* with EC_{50} values 1.3 ± 0.02, 2.1 ± 0 and 2.1 ± 0.4 μM, respectively and with selectivity index > 12.

Bhambra et al. (2017) synthesized a small library of pyridylchalcones which were tested against *T. b. rhodesiense*. Even though none of these compounds showed better activity than the reference drugs pentamidine or melarsoprol, three compounds (**80–82**) can be considered as potential leads with IC_{50} values 0.29, 0.40 and 0.41 μM, respectively (Figure 29).

Hydroxamic acid derivatives

Fytas et al. (2011) discovered acetohydroxamic acids as a new class of compounds with potential antitrypanocidal activity. The synthesis of these compounds was realized through the attachment of an acetohydroxamic acid moiety to the imidic nitrogen of 2,6-diketopiperazines. A SAR study revealed that compounds **83** (S-enantiomer), **84** (R-enantiomer) and **85** (racemic mixture of **83** and **84**) (Figure 30) showed low nanomolar activity against the bloodstream-form of *T. brucei* with IC_{50} values 6.8 ± 1.4, 9.1 ± 0.2 and 17± 1 nM, respectively, while compound **83**, along with compounds **86** and **87**, displayed significant activity against *T. cruzi* with IC_{50} values 0.21 ± 0.04, 5.51 ± 0.68 and 3.62 ± 0.31 μM, respectively. Overall, compound **83** proved to be the most active compound against both species. In addition, these compounds showed very good selectivity indices. The fact that replacement of the hydroxamic acid moiety led to compounds with decreased activity makes this group a requisite for trypanocidal activity. A small library of hydroxamic acid derivatives, which inhibit human histone deacetylases, was synthesized and tested against cultured bloodstream form *T. brucei* (Kelly et al. 2012). Most of these compounds exhibited very good activity in the submicromolar range. Specifically, the most promising compounds were **88–90** (Figure 31) with IC_{50} values 0.034 ± 0.002, 0.064 ± 0.005 and 0.086 ± 0.009 μM, respectively.

Thiazole derivatives

Zelisko et al. (2012) described the synthesis and biological evaluation of a series of 6,6,7-trisubstituted thiopyrano[2,3-*d*][1,3] thiazoles. Interestingly, one compound, **91** (Figure 32), inhibited *T. b. brucei* and *T. b. gambiense* with IC_{50} values of 0.26 and 0.42 μM, respectively; thus, it can be considered as a potential lead for further optimization.

Cardoso et al. (2014) reported the ultrasound-assisted synthesis and the anti-*T. cruzi* activity of twenty four 2-(pyridine-2-yl)-1,3-thiazoles. The majority of this class of compounds demonstrated higher activity than the reference drug benznidazole, with compounds **92** and **93** (Figure 33) being the most potent with IC_{50} values of 1.2 μM each against *T. cruzi* trypomastigotes. In addition, this class of compounds showed no cytotoxicity against HepG2 cells.

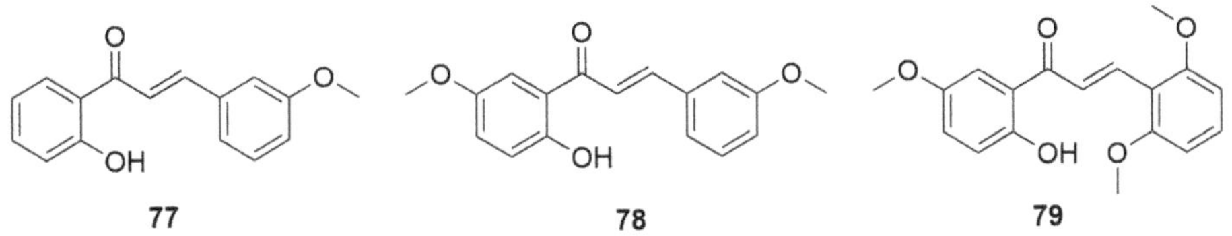

Figure 28. Structures of the most potent methoxylated 2-hydroxychalcones **77–79**.

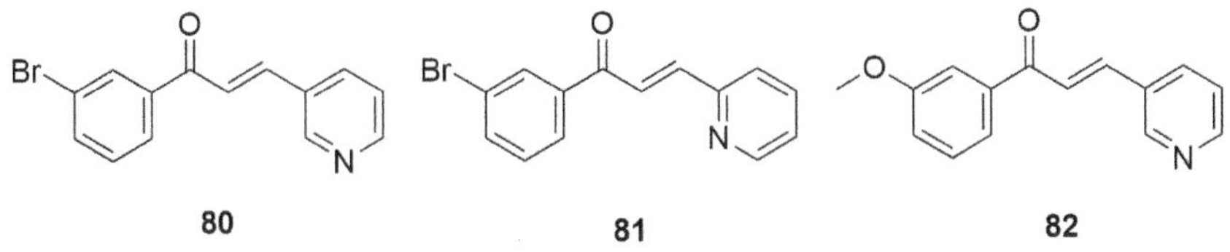

Figure 29. Structures of most potent pyridylchalcones **80–82**.

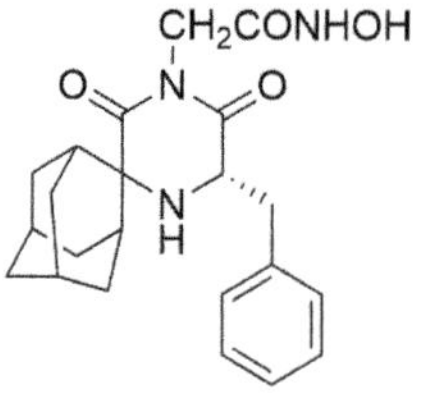

83

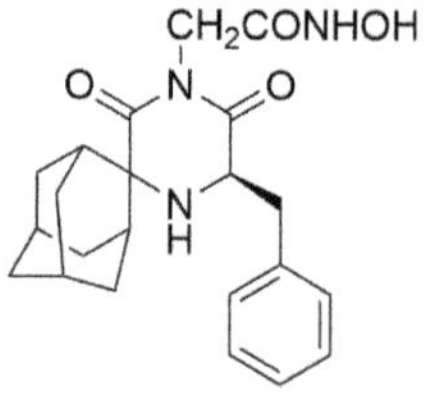

84

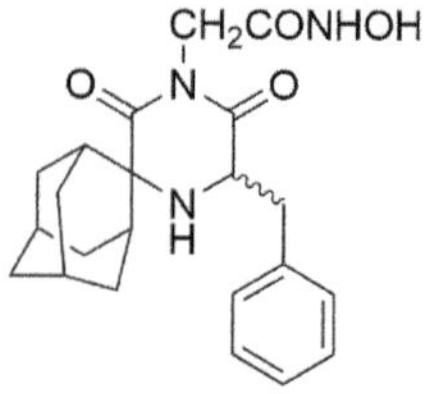

85

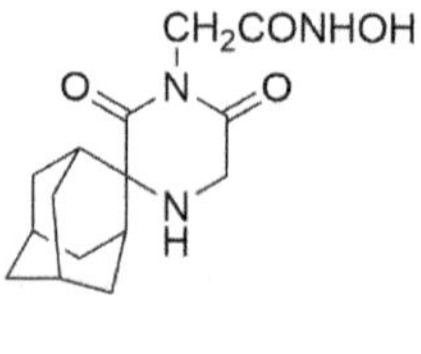

86

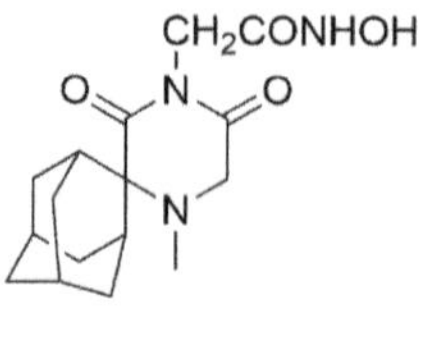

87

Figure 30. Structures of hydroxamic acids **83–87**.

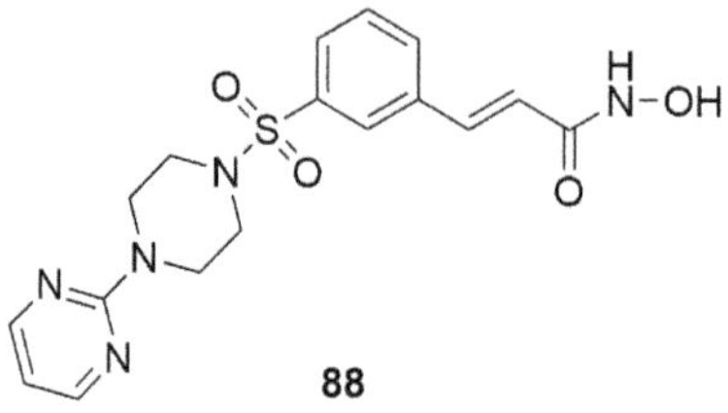

88

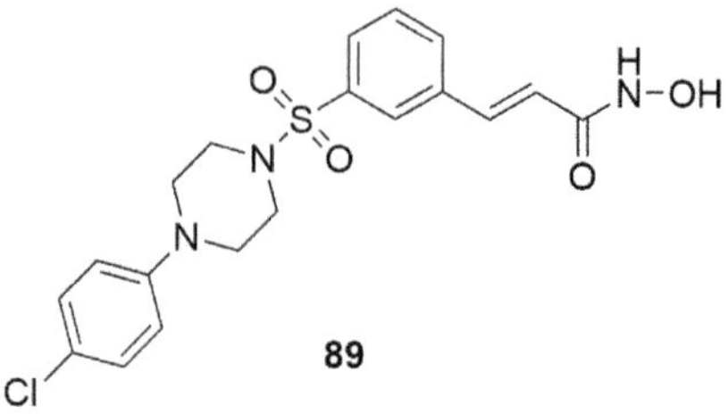

89

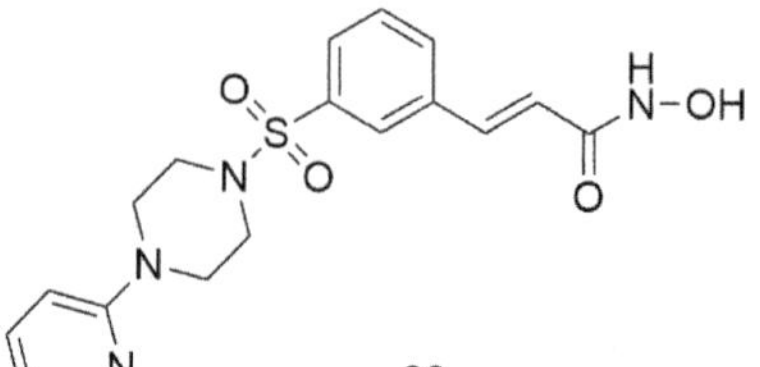

90

Figure 31. Structures of the most active hydroxamic acids **88–90**.

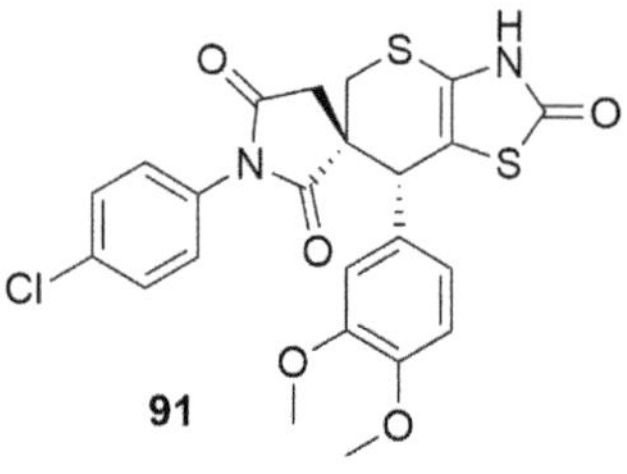

91

Figure 32. Structure of potential lead **91**.

Russell et al. (2016) published their work on hit to lead optimization of compound **94** (Figure 34), which emerged as a hit compound through high-throughput screening, exhibiting activity for *T. b. brucei*, *T. b. rhodesiense* and *T. cruzi*, (IC_{50} = 0.80, 1.5 and 2.3 μM, respectively) and favorable physicochemical properties. An extensive SAR study was conducted towards the discovery of new

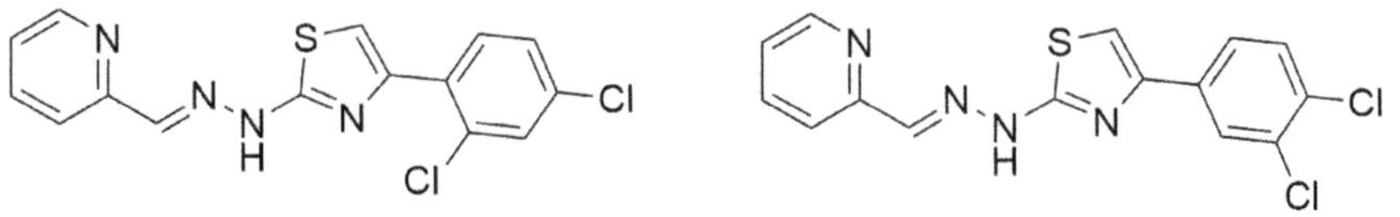

Figure 33. Structures of most potent thiazole derivatives **92** and **93**.

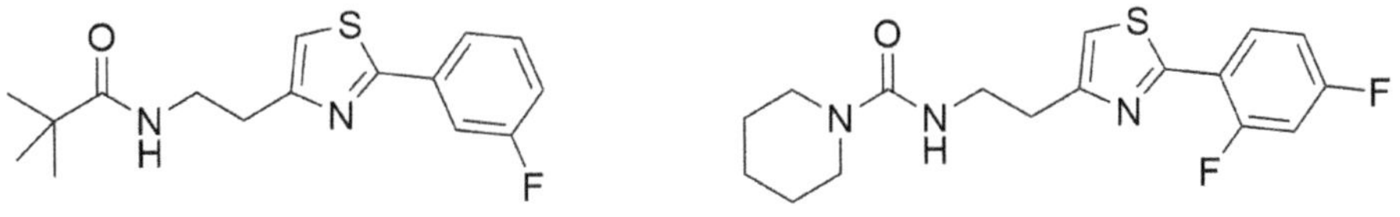

Figure 34. Structures of hit compound **94** and lead compound **95**.

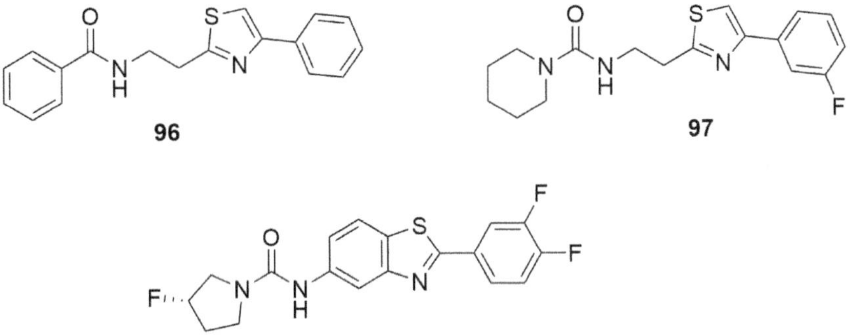

Figure 35. Structures of hit compound **96** and lead compounds **97** and **98**.

leads. Indeed, 2-(fluorophenyl)thiazole **95** was found to exhibit excellent activity against *T. b. brucei* (IC_{50} = 0.024 ± 0.003 µM, SI = 433) and *T. cruzi* (IC_{50} = 0.020 ± 0.01 µM, SI > 3162). Compound **95** was tested *in vivo* in mice infected with the trypomastigote form of *T. cruzi* Brazil strain. The compound showed encouraging results but, unfortunately, it was rapidly metabolized.

In a phenotypic high-throughput screening of 700,000 compounds, compound **96** (Figure 35) was identified, among others, as a potential anti-*T.b. rhodesiense* (IC_{50} = 0.632 µM, SI = 162). Patrick et al. (2016, 2017) with two back-to-back papers reported the efforts towards the optimization of the hit compound **96**. A SAR study was conducted by focusing on changes on both phenyl rings of compound **96**. Therefore, 72 new derivatives were synthesized and tested against *T. b. rhodesiense* STIB900 and L6 rat myoblast cells for cytotoxicity *in vitro*. Forty-four compounds were more active than **96** and eight of them showed IC_{50} values below 100 nM. The most potent compound was **97** (IC_{50} = 9 nM, SI > 18,000) but, unfortunately, the *in vivo* test showed that it was unable to cure infected mice. Even though the administration of **97** caused reduction of parasitemia, relapses occurred. This was attributed to poor metabolic stability. Prompted by these results, a second paper described a new SAR study of 65 additional compounds with modifications in other sites on hit **96** with the intention of maintaining the same activity and improving the metabolic stability. This led to compound **98** which was less active than **97** (IC_{50} = 35 nM) but with enhanced metabolic stability and brain penetration. Oral dosing of **98** cured five out of five mice in both acute and chronic murine models of HAT.

Many thiazole derivatives were synthesized and evaluated for their antiparasitic activity during the last year by several research groups. Compound **99** (Filho et al. 2017) showed activity against the trypomastigote form of *T. cruzi* (IC_{50} = 0.37 µM), compound **100** (Thompson et al. 2017) with IC_{50} = 0.055 µM against

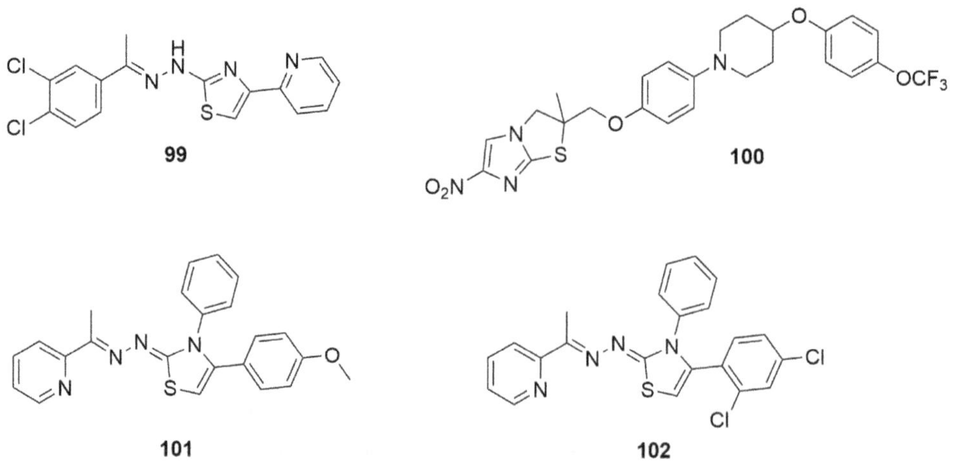

Figure 36. Structures of potential hits **99–102**.

T. cruzi, and compounds **101** and **102** (Silva et al. 2017b) with IC_{50} values 1.2 and 1.6 μM, respectively against the trypomastigote form of *T. cruzi* (Figure 36).

Thiophene derivatives

Bhambra et al. (2016) reported the synthesis of a small library of 2,6-disubstituted-4,5,7-trifluorobenzothiophenes. Compounds **103** and **104** (Figure 37) demonstrated attractive antitrypanosomal activity against *T. b. rhodesiense* with IC_{50} values 0.60 and 0.53 μM, respectively, and no toxicity to mammalian cells. It is apparent that the activity of these compounds can be attributed to the existence of the benzimidazole moiety since its replacement resulted in loss of activity.

Indole derivatives

Vega et al. (2012) prepared a series of nitro-indazolin-3-ones which were tested *in vitro* against epimastigote forms of *T. cruzi*. Compounds **105–107** (Figure 38) showed trypanocidal activity with IC_{50} = 0.93, 2.39, 1.17 μM, respectively and low toxicity. The authors found structural similarities with other known antiprotozoan drugs during their search, and therefore they introduced a new scaffold for further research and optimization.

Tapia et al. (2014) synthesized a series of indole-4,9-diones and their activity was evaluated against the epimastigote form of *T. cruzi*, Y strain. All new compounds showed better activity and selectivity compared to the reference drug nifurtimox. Interestingly, compound **108** (Figure 38) demonstrated nanomolar inhibitory activity (IC_{50} = 20 nM), and a high selectivity index (SI = 625).

Imidazole derivatives

A high-throughput screening of 303,286 compounds revealed a class of imidazole-based inhibitors (**109–111**, Figure 39) that can inhibit infection of mammalian host cells by *T. cruzi* trypomastigotes (Bettiol et al. 2009). In an effort to further optimize the activity, cytotoxicity and bioavailability, new inhibitors of *T. cruzi* CYP51 were synthesized (Andriani et al. 2013) with ring-constrained structures. The most promising inhibitors were **112** (EC_{50} = 72 nM) and **113** (EC_{50} = 80 nM).

The SAR study revealed that the substitution of the phenyl ring with lipophilic groups is essential. The absence of these groups was accompanied by loss of potency. In addition, replacement of the imidazole moiety by other nitrogen heterocycles, such as pyrazole or triazole, resulted in loss of activity. Hence, the presence of an imidazole ring is required for *T. cruzi* CYP51 binding.

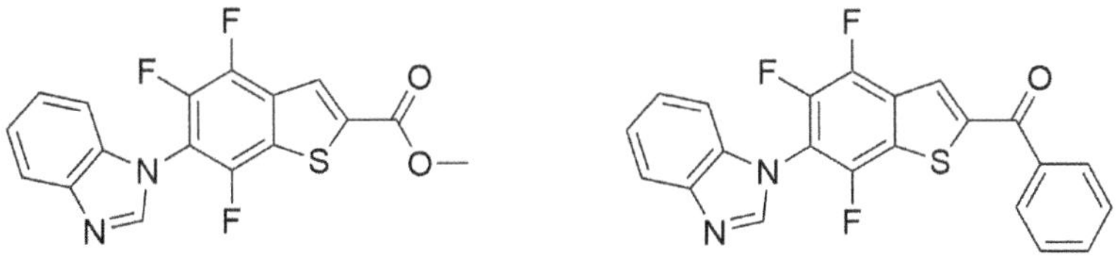

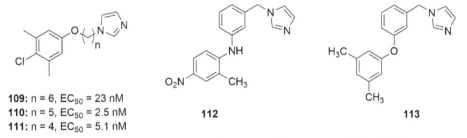

103 **104**

Figure 37. Structures of potential hits **103** and **104**.

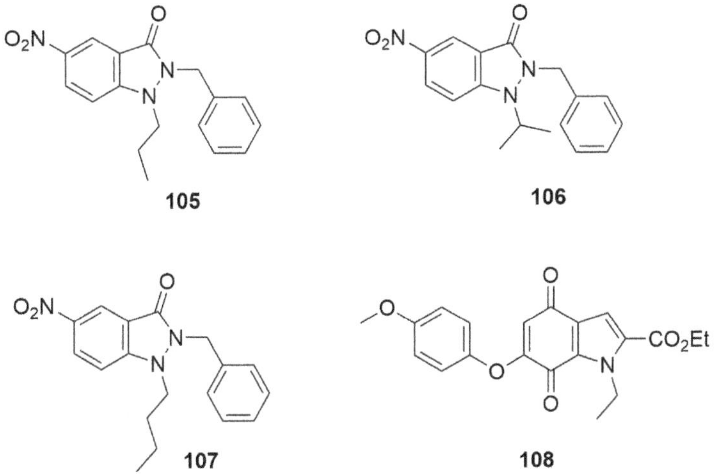

105 **106**

107 **108**

Figure 38. Structures of indole derivatives with potential trypanocidal activity.

109: n = 6, EC$_{50}$ = 23 nM
110: n = 5, EC$_{50}$ = 2.5 nM
111: n = 4, EC$_{50}$ = 5.1 nM

112 **113**

Figure 39. Structures of hit compounds **109–111** and lead compounds **112** and **113**.

More compounds bearing an imidazole ring have been synthesized and tested against the drug-targetable enzyme CYP51 due to structural similarities with its inhibitors. In particular, compounds **114–116** (Figure 40), even in their racemic form, showed activity against *T. cruzi* Talahuen C2C4 amastigote stage (Friggeri et al. 2013) with IC$_{50}$ values 14, 5 and 36 nM, respectively. The authors wanted to further explore the activity of the single enantiomers which led to the conclusion that *S*-enantiomers were more active than the corresponding *R*-enantiomers. Compound (*S*)-**114** showed IC$_{50}$ = 3.8 nM vs 193 nM of (*R*)-**114**, (*S*)-**115** showed IC$_{50}$ = 1.8 nM while (*R*)-**115** showed IC$_{50}$ =112 nM and (*S*)-**116** showed IC$_{50}$ = 23.6 nM vs 97.2 nM of (*R*)-**116**.

Suryadevara et al. (2013) described the synthesis of seventy-five dialkylimidazole-imidazole based inhibitors of CYP51. Interestingly, most of the compounds showed remarkable nanomolar activity against *T. cruzi* amastigotes. The most promising compounds and their EC values are depicted in Figure 41.

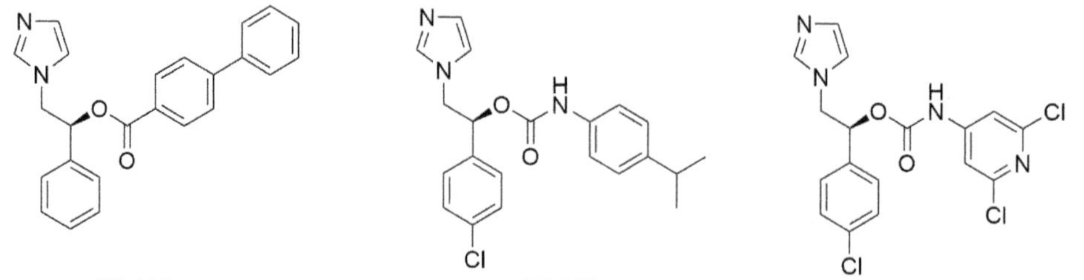

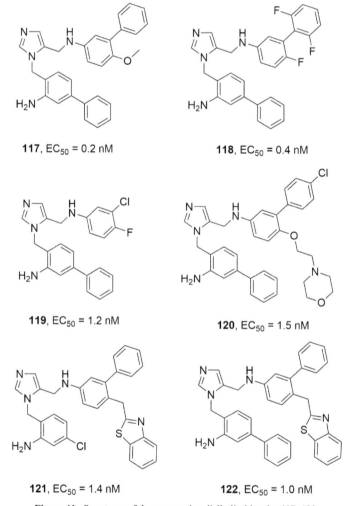

Figure 40. Structures of active compounds **114–116**.

117, EC$_{50}$ = 0.2 nM

118, EC$_{50}$ = 0.4 nM

119, EC$_{50}$ = 1.2 nM

120, EC$_{50}$ = 1.5 nM

121, EC$_{50}$ = 1.4 nM

122, EC$_{50}$ = 1.0 nM

Figure 41. Structures of the most active dialkylimidazoles **117–122**.

Computational and experimental structure-based drug design strategies against Trypanosoma cruzi *and* Trypanosoma brucei

In the above section, we presented a large number of synthetic compounds that have been optimized for their anti-trypanosomal properties; however, this was often done without taking specific molecular targets into account. Target-oriented methods provide an alternative strategy or can present an interesting complement to optimization based solely on anti-parasitic properties. In this section, we review some of the recent literature on structure-based drug design (SBDD) efforts to tackle trypanosomatidic infections by targeting specific metabolic pathways or enzymes that have been extensively explored in target-guided drug discovery approaches during the past years, namely, CYP51, folate pathway proteins, phosphodiesterases, cysteine proteases or enzymes of the trypanothione metabolism. In the discovery of new hits and lead optimization, experimental methods and computational techniques are widely used together to facilitate the process of compound library design and iterative improvement in the context of known (or predicted) biomolecular targets. We describe approaches to SBDD for key targets, as well as techniques for tackling typical challenges in SBDD, such as selectivity, off-target binding and deciphering the mechanism-of-action (MoA) of a drug. We conclude the section with a brief summary of the methods typically employed in anti-trypanosomatidic drug discovery, their potential applications and limitations.

Lanosterol 14α-demethylase (CYP51)

A particularly prominent example of a widely considered anti-trypanosomatid drug target is an enzyme involved in the ergosterol biosynthesis route, namely the lanosterol 14α-demethylase (or CYP51). CYP51s, which belong to the family of cytochrome P450s, are highly conserved heme-containing proteins involved in the production of plasma membrane building blocks and regulatory molecules (Lepesheva and Waterman 2004, 2007). Azole-based CYP51 inhibitors are known anti-fungal agents (Lass-Flörl 2011, Denning and Bromley 2015) and the trypanosomal ergosterol biosynthesis resembles that of fungi, making the repurposing of anti-fungal compounds a well-explored design strategy (Buckner and Urbina 2012). Furthermore, crystallographic complexes of TbCYP51 and TcCYP51 with anti-fungal compounds, such as fluconazole **123** and posaconazole **124** (Figure 42, Chen et al. 2010), paved the way for further optimization of azole-based and chemically distinct CYP51 inhibitors for trypanosomatidic infections. As another example, Hoekstra et al. (2015) reported the crystallographic complex of a 1-tetrazole-based anti-fungal clinical drug candidate with TcCYP51, providing an additional target-based starting point for future optimization of the compound as an anti-*T. cruzi* agent.

Hargrove et al. (2013) used X-ray crystallography to determine the binding modes of the promising pyridine-based drug candidates **125** and **126** (Figure 43) for Chagas disease. These compounds were found to be the first non-azole compounds showing as potent inhibition of TcCYP51 as posaconazole **124**. Importantly, the structural data show that the coordination bonds between the pyridine heterocycles of **125** and **126** and the ferric heme iron of TcCYP51 are longer than in the case of azoles. The authors highlight that this may allow higher selectivity between the trypanosomal enzyme and the human variant.

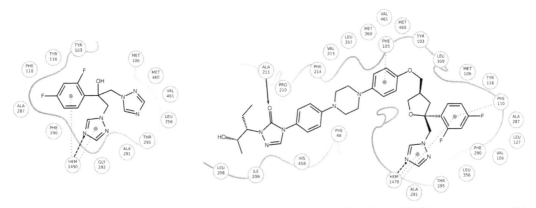

Figure 42. Interaction diagrams of the anti-fungal compounds fluconazole **123** (left) in TcCYP51 and posaconazole **124** (right) in TbCYP51. The diagrams are based on the crystallographic complexes with PDB-ID 2wuz and 2x2n (Chen et al. 2010), respectively. Pocket-lining residues and the pocket shape are shown. Black dashed lines indicate coordination bonds between the ferric heme iron and a nitrogen atom of the ligand, gray dotted lines indicate π-π interactions and black arrows indicate hydrogen-bonding interactions.

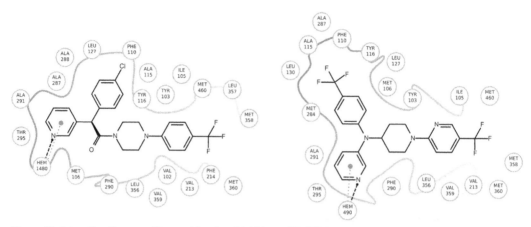

Figure 43. Interaction diagrams of two pyridine-based inhibitors of TcCYP51, **125** and **126**. The diagrams are based on the crystallographic complexes with PDB-ID 3zg2 and 3zg3 (Hargrove et al. 2013), respectively. Pocket-lining residues and the pocket shape are shown. Black dashed lines indicate coordination bonds between the ferric heme iron and a nitrogen atom of the ligand and gray dotted lines indicate π-π interactions.

Due to the weaker coordinating interaction, the other non-bonded interactions between the protein and the ligand, which differ between the targets, become more important determinants for compound binding affinities. However, as can be seen in Figure 43, the interaction of compounds **125** and **126** with TcCYP51 is mainly mediated by hydrophobic contacts.

The development of the aforementioned imidazole-based *T. cruzi* CYP51 inhibitors **112** and **113** (see Figure 39) by Andriani et al. (2013) as well as compounds **114–116** (Figure 40) by Friggeri et al. (2013) was similarly supported by crystallographic data (directly by structure determination or indirectly by docking studies to existing crystal structures). In a follow-up study, Friggeri et al. (2014) further optimized imidazole-based inhibitors and demonstrated their ability to bind to CYP51 in two different regions: either in the substrate-binding site close to the heme group or in the substrate access channel (compare binding mode of **127** in Figure 44).

Another example of a particularly successful SBDD approach is the drug candidate (R)-N-(1-(3,4'-difluorobiphenyl-4-yl)-2-(1H-imidazol-1-yl)ethyl)-4-(5-phenyl-1,3,4-oxadiazol-2-yl)benzamide (**128**, Figure 45) developed by Lepesheva et al. (2015). Based on **127**, which cured both acute and chronic Chagas disease in experimental models, and the existing structural knowledge for CYP51 (Lepesheva et al. 2010, Villalta et al. 2013), **128** was designed as a highly specific inhibitor of the trypanosomal enzyme by introducing additional aromatic interactions between the protein and the ligand in the depth of the CYP51 binding cavity (see Figures 44 and 45). Compound **128** displayed an improved anti-parasitic activity (EC$_{50}$ against *T. cruzi* amastigotes from infected cardiomyocytes 0.8 nM for **128** vs. 1.3 nM for **127**), cures experimental Chagas disease with 100% efficiency, is orally bioavailable and has low off-target activity as well as favorable pharmacokinetics.

Not only crystallography but also docking studies were employed in the design of CYP51 inhibitors. More recently, docking of imidazoles (De Vita et al. 2016) and pyrazolo[3,4-e][1,4]thiazepin-based inhibitors (Ferreira de Almeida Fuiza et al. 2018) against TcCYP51 crystal structures identified this enzyme as a potential target, which rationalized the observed anti-*T. cruzi* activities of the compounds.

An interesting complement to the efforts guided solely by static crystal structures are molecular dynamics (MD) simulations, performed by Yu et al. (2015, 2016), used to study ligand egress routes in *T. brucei* CYP51 in comparison with human CYP51. These studies highlight differences in the dynamics and composition of the ligand tunnel between the trypanosomal and human CYP51, which could be exploited in future anti-parasitic drug design efforts to enhance selectivity.

Gunatilleke et al. (2012) combined target-based high-throughput screening (HTS) with a screen against *T. cruzi*-infected skeletal myoblast cells to yield compounds with a known molecular target and activity against the parasite. Further, they used bioinformatics approaches to demonstrate similarities between

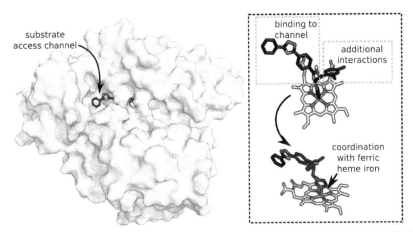

Figure 44. Compound **127** binding to TcCYP51 (see also Figure 45, based on PDB-ID 3gw9; Lepesheva et al. 2010), occupying the substrate access channel and coordinating with the ferric heme iron. The protein is shown as a semi-transparent surface with the ligand with black carbons and the heme group in white sticks. The channel opening towards the surface is marked. On the right side, the protein was removed for clarity. One part of the ligand binds to the channel, while a second portion forms additional interactions in the depth of the pocket. The top view was rotated by approx. 45° to show the coordination between the ligand and the ferric heme iron in the lower panel.

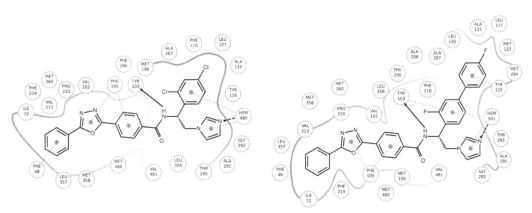

Figure 45. Interaction diagrams of two inhibitors of TbCYP51, **127** and its optimized derivative **128**. The diagrams are based on the crystallographic complexes with PDB-ID 3gw9 and 4g7g (Lepesheva et al. 2010, 2015), respectively. Pocket-lining residues and the pocket shape are shown. Black dashed lines indicate coordination bonds between the ferric heme iron and a nitrogen atom of the ligand, gray dotted lines with filled circles indicate π-π interactions, and black arrows show hydrogen-bonding interactions.

compounds preferentially bound by CYP51 and compounds bound by several other cytochrome P450 enzymes and an unrelated glutaminyl-peptide cyclotransferase. Inhibitors of these enzymes can hence serve as a potential pool of lead compounds.

It is not uncommon that large libraries of potential hit compounds are screened *in silico* against crystallographic databases of enzymatic targets. A drawback of such screens is that many studies lack experimental validation of their results. Nevertheless, *in silico* studies exploring, for example, potential targets of phytochemicals may provide some first insight when a target is not known or may be used to propose possible hits for a desired target. For example, compounds isolated from Nigerian medicinal plants have been studied by Setzer and Ogungbe (2012). Using *in silico* methods, they found potential inhibitors of, amongst others, TbCYP51 and two enzymes of the parasitic folate pathway: pteridine reductase 1 (PTR1) and dihydrofolate reductase (DHFR).

Further details on the current structural knowledge about CYP51 in trypanosomatids and the design of inhibitory compounds can be found in the recent review by Lepesheva et al. (2018).

Folate metabolism

Targeting the kinetoplastid folate pathway, unlike the corresponding malarial (Hawser et al. 2006) and bacterial (Yuthavong et al. 2005) pathways, requires not only the inhibition of dihydrofolate reductase (DHFR), but also of pteridine reductase 1 (PTR1) (Bello et al. 1994, Sienkiewicz et al. 2010). The latter enzyme is mainly responsible for the reduction of pterins, but can be upregulated when DHFR is inhibited and serve as a bypass for folate reduction to provide necessary educts for DNA synthesis and thus ensure parasite survival (Dawson et al. 2006, Vickers and Beverley 2011). In *T. brucei*, PTR1 was validated as a potential drug target by gene knockout and RNA interference experiments (Ong et al. 2011, Sienkiewicz et al. 2010). Herein, we mostly focus on inhibitor design for PTR1 from *T. cruzi* and *T. brucei*. Multiple drug design approaches have been used to target PTR1, starting from optimization of the substrate scaffold, through virtual screening (VS), to fragment-based drug design (FBDD).

An example of a classical substrate-like compound is methotrexate **129** (MTX), which is a subnanomolar inhibitor of DHFR, and an approved anti-cancer drug (Zuccotto et al. 1999, Shuvalov et al. 2017). However, it has also been shown to inhibit PTR1 at the submicromolar level (Dawson et al. 2006, Cavazzuti et al. 2008). Notably, the substrate, MTX and most other inhibitors of PTR1 occupy the main binding site in a π-sandwich between the nicotinamide of the NADPH/NADP$^+$ cofactor and a phenylalanine residue (Figure 46). MTX adopts a similar binding mode to folate **130**, but with a flipped orientation of the pteridine ring (Figure 46).

The aforementioned binding modes of folate and MTX were starting points in the study by Tulloch et al. (2010), who selected 3 scaffolds—pteridine, pyrrolopyrimidine and pyrimidine—for inhibitor design and optimization against *T. brucei* PTR1 (TbPTR1). Five pyrrolopyrimidine-based inhibitors were identified and crystallized in TbPTR1. Among those, **131** and **132** (Figure 47) with K_i values against TbPTR1 of 0.36 μM and 0.40 μM, respectively, were found to attain modest ED_{50} values against the *T. brucei* bloodstream form (BSF): 274 ± 7.5 μM and 123 ± 3.3 μM, respectively. **132** was also found to show a synergistic effect when combined with MTX. Later, Khalaf et al. (2014) used a similar approach for the development of 61 additional pyrrolopyrimidines, of which 23 were crystallized in TbPTR1, greatly expanding the structural data available for this enzyme. Two of the crystallized compounds, **133** and **134** (Figure 48), had TbPTR1 K_i^{app} values of 0.23 μM and 0.14 μM, respectively, and were found to have *T. brucei* BSF IC_{50} values of 3.20 μM and 0.25 μM, respectively, in Creek's minimal medium. However, these derivatives showed substantial toxicity in *in vivo* mouse models and thus were not suitable for further development.

VS approaches were used to identify novel non-pteridine scaffolds, including the 2-aminothiadiazole core and flavonoids as potential binders of the PTR1 substrate pocket (Ferrari et al. 2011, Borsari et al. 2016). Recently, a library of 2-aminothiadiazole-based TbPTR1 inhibitors has been developed (Linciano et al. 2017). X-ray crystallography and docking simulations confirmed the classical binding mode for these series (cf. Figure 46), with the amino moiety of the scaffold core interacting with a serine residue close to the active site, cofactor ribose and phosphates (Figure 49). Two thiadiazole-2,5-diamines **136** and **137** (Figure 49) reached TbPTR1 IC_{50} values of 16.0 μM and 25.0 μM, respectively. Despite being unable to inhibit the *T. brucei* BSF as single agents, both PTR1 inhibitors potentiated the EC_{50} of MTX by 4.1 and 2-fold, respectively.

Another class of hits against PTR1 is flavonoids, identified by computational and experimental screening of a natural products library (Borsari et al. 2016), with flavonols showing the most promising inhibitory effect on TbPTR1. A combination of crystallographic experiments and computational docking was then employed to explore the multiple possible binding modes and deduce a structure-activity relationship (SAR) for a set of synthetic flavonols. In a follow-up project, the same methods allowed in-depth characterization of the determinants of the activities of several flavonols and the corresponding flavanones (Di Pisa et al. 2017).

In another VS study, Dube et al. (2014) used a combination of docking and pharmacophore modeling to screen the ZINC database for putative inhibitors of TbPTR1 and predict their activities. The VS of fragments against TbPTR1 performed by Mpamhanga et al. (2009) identified 2-aminobenzothiazole and 2-aminobenzimidazole, binding in the substrate pocket, as promising cores that were further used for inhibitor development. Notably, the crystallographic studies revealed that some of the synthesized

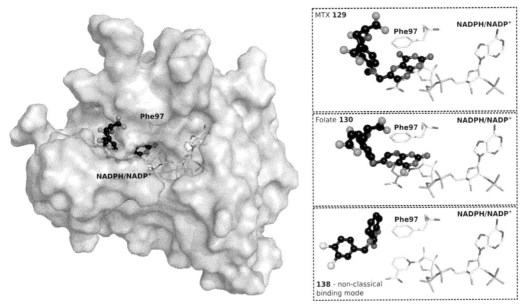

Figure 46. Illustration of compounds binding in the π-sandwich between Phe97 and the nicotinamide of the NADPH/NADP⁺ cofactor of TbPTR1 or in alternative modes adjacent to the active site. On the left, a monomer of the homotetrameric enzyme is shown as a semi-transparent surface representation with bound MTX **129** in dark ball-and-stick representation, and the cofactor and Phe97 in white sticks. In the right-hand panel, the same representation is used, omitting the protein apart from Phe 97. The complex with MTX **129** is based on PDB-ID 2c7v (Dawson et al. 2006), with folate **130**—on PDB-ID 3bmc (Tulloch et al. 2010) and with **138**, illustrating the non-classical binding mode outside the π-sandwich—on PDB-ID 3gn2 (Mpamhanga et al. 2009).

Color version at the end of the book

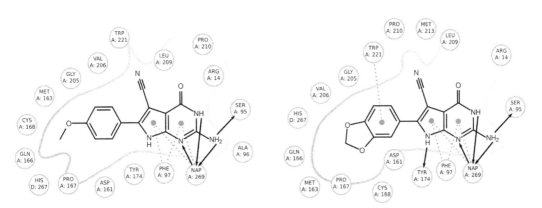

Figure 47. Interaction diagrams of two pyrrolopyrimidine-based inhibitors of TbPTR1, **131** and **132**. The diagrams are based on the crystallographic complexes with PDB-ID 3jqe and 3jq9 (Tulloch et al. 2010), respectively. Pocket-lining residues and the pocket shape are shown. Gray dotted lines indicate π-π interactions and black arrows show hydrogen-bonding interactions. NAP denotes NADP(H).

compounds with a 2-aminobenzimidazole scaffold adopted a non-classical binding mode in the TbPTR1-specific subsite adjacent to the primary substrate binding site (Mpamhanga et al. 2009; Figure 46, compound **138**). Compounds **138** and **139** (Figure 50) reached K_i^{app} of 0.4 μM and 0.007 μM, respectively, against TbPTR1. Despite its nanomolar on-target potency, **139** displayed an EC_{50} against *T. brucei* of only 10 μM. Spinks et al. (2011) further attempted to optimize the series of 2-aminobenzimidazoles to

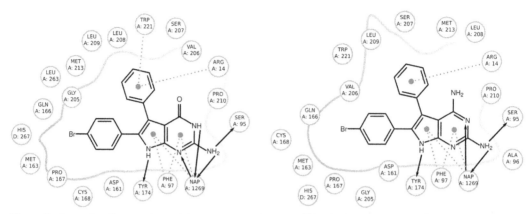

Figure 48. Interaction diagrams of two additional pyrrolopyrimidine-based inhibitors of TbPTR1, **133** and **134**. The diagrams are based on the crystallographic complexes with PDB-ID 4cmi and 4cmj (Khalaf et al. 2014), respectively. Pocket-lining residues and the pocket shape are shown. Gray dotted lines indicate π-π interactions and black arrows show hydrogen-bonding interactions. NAP denotes NADP(H).

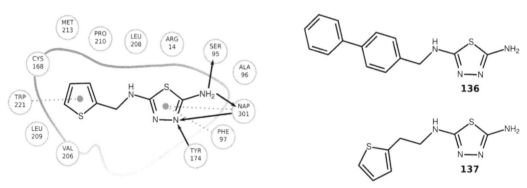

Figure 49. Interaction diagrams of a 2,5-diamino-1,3,4-thiadiazole inhibitor of TbPTR1, **135**, and structures of its derivatives **136** and **137**. Compounds **136** and **137** were predicted to show a similar binding mode in TbPTR1 by docking studies (Linciano et al. 2017). The interaction diagram is based on the crystallographic complex with PDB-ID 5izc. Pocket-lining residues and the pocket shape are shown. Gray dotted lines indicate π-π interactions and black arrows show hydrogen-bonding interactions. NAP denotes NADP(H).

target the alternative subsite, but anti-parasite activities did not improve, with the lowest EC_{50} value being 6.7 μM.

The non-classical binding mode of the amino-benzimidazole series discussed above inspired computational FBDD studies to combine a scaffold with a classical binding mode and an alternative subpocket-targeting scaffold. In principle, computational methods exist that may help in finding the best molecular fragment binding to the subsite. However, in the case of the TbPTR1 alternative subsite exploited by Mpamhanga et al. (2009) and Spinks et al. (2011), this was challenging due to the presence of halogen substituents in the most potent compounds. Many state-of-the-art force fields used in molecular docking suffer from short-comings in the representation of halogens (Wilcken et al. 2013). Thus, using the 2-aminobenzimidazole series by Mpamhanga et al. (2009) and Spinks et al. (2011), Jedwabny et al. (2017) demonstrated the application of a computationally efficient quantum-mechanics-based model for predicting binding affinities of fragments in the TbPTR1 binding site, which could be used to overcome these issues.

The majority of compounds have been developed to target TbPTR1 (or *L. major* PTR1). Although a crystal structure of a close homolog of TcPTR1, TcPTR2, was solved (Schormann et al. 2005), most drug design efforts did not consider the *T. cruzi* enzyme variants. Mendoza-Martínez et al. (2015) designed some quinazoline derivatives and used docking studies to support TcPTR2 and TcDHFR as reasonable potential targets. The compounds were evaluated against bloodstream trypomastigotes of two strains of

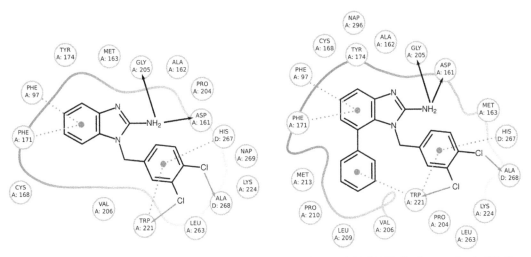

Figure 50. Interaction diagrams of two 2-aminobenzimidazole-based inhibitors of TbPTR1 binding in a non-classical binding mode, **138** and **139** (cf. also Figure 46). The diagrams are based on the crystallographic complexes with PDB-ID 3gn2 and 2wd8 (Mpamhanga et al. 2009), respectively. Pocket-lining residues and the pocket shape are shown. Gray dotted lines indicate π-π interactions, black arrows show hydrogen-bonding interactions and gray arrows indicate halogen-bonds NAP denotes NADP(H).

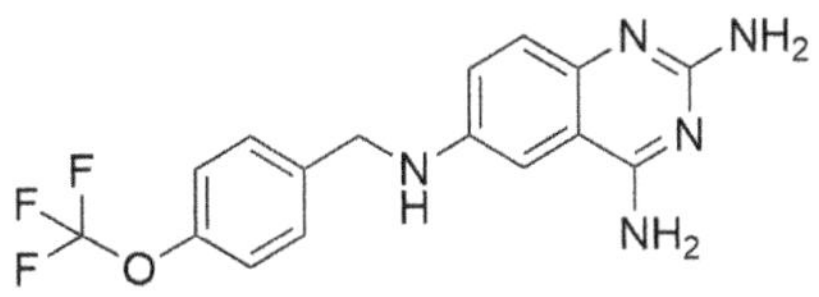

Figure 51. Structures of the quinazoline derivatives **140–142** that putatively target TcPTR2/TcDHFR.

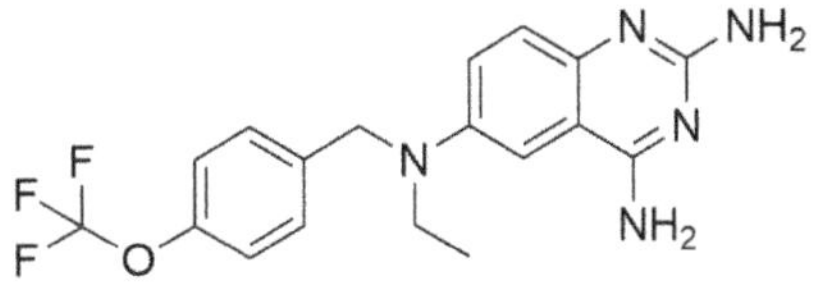

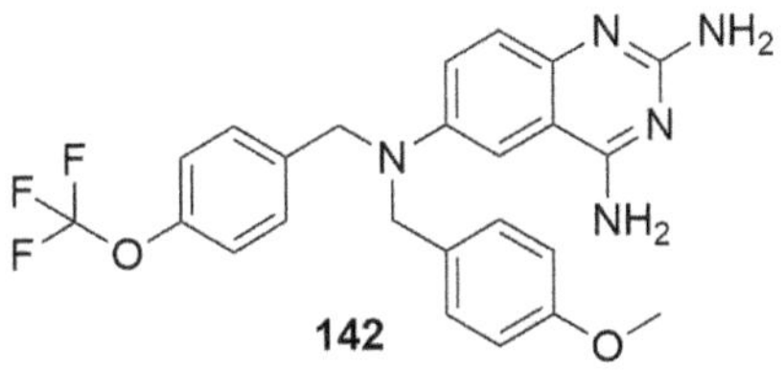

T. cruzi (NINOA and INC-5 strain) and compounds **140–142** (Figure 51) were found to be particularly interesting, since they showed a better activity profile than the reference drugs, nifurtimox and benznidazole.

Otherwise, for *T. cruzi*, mainly DHFR was considered in drug design efforts: Schormann et al. (2008) used 3D-QSAR models to guide the design of inhibitors selective for TcDHFR over human DHFR (hDHFR). In a subsequent study, guided by crystallography and docking experiments, they attempted to exploit amino acid differences between the pocket entrance regions of hDHFR and TcDHFR, including a substitution of Phe31 to Met49. A series of 2,4-diaminoquinazoline derivatives, similar to trimetrexate, with varying flexible groups in the tail, some of which were predicted to bind near Met49 of TcDHFR, had 7–8 14 times better K_i against TcDHFR than hDHFR (Schormann et al. 2010).

The above discussed study of Mendoza-Martínez et al. (2015) is an example of a dual inhibition approach, which is particularly important for targeting the trypanosomatid folate pathway. Ideally, this requires targeting both PTR1 and parasitic DHFR, while avoiding inhibitor binding to hDHFR, which is quite similar to the parasitic homologue. To address this issue, Panecka-Hofman et al. (2017) applied a variety of techniques (such as computational analysis of crystallographic structures, homology modeling and binding site mapping) for sequence and structural comparison of the folate pathway on- and off-targets. Ligand-target interactions, binding site properties and target conformational variability were computationally compared to yield guidelines for the design and optimization of selective inhibitors of the trypanosomatidic folate pathway. In an extension of this study, the conformational variability of the TcDHFR and hDHFR binding sites was analyzed with the TRAPP (TRAnsient Pockets in Proteins) web server based on the available crystallographic data (Stank et al. 2017). A transiently appearing subpocket was identified in the vicinity of Met49, which corresponds to Phe31 in hDHFR. The ProSAT+ tool integrated in TRAPP also identified position 31 as a known site of hDHFR mutation that alters binding of the MTX inhibitor **129**.

The majority of drug design efforts for the kinetoplastid folate pathway have so far focused on PTR1/PTR2 and DHFR. A few other folate pathway enzymes, such as the N^5,N^{10}-methylenetetrahydrofolate dehydrogenase/cyclohydrolase (DHCH) of *T. brucei*, were considered in compound development. Eadsforth et al. (2015) designed inhibitors of TbDHCH using a combination of crystallographic and docking experiments starting from an inhibitor of bacterial and human DHCH.

Despite the extensive design and development efforts to obtain potent and selective inhibitors of PTR1 and DHFR, there is often limited transferability of on-target-based activity to an *in vitro* or even *in vivo* activity against *T. brucei* or *T. cruzi*. For a more detailed overview on the efforts made, possible reasons for this limitation and other potential targets to be considered in the future, the reader is referred to the recent review by Cullia et al. (2018).

Phosphodiesterases

More recently, a phosphodiesterase (PDE) of *T. brucei*, the PDEB1 isoform, has gained attention as a potential drug target for Human African Trypanosomiasis (HAT). Phosphodiesterases cleave phosphodiester bonds in cyclic nucleotides like cyclic AMP (cAMP), which is an important second messenger involved in regulation of signal transduction. An overview about cAMP signalling in trypanosomatids and differences between parasitic and human pathways that can be exploited for drug discovery can be found in the review by Tagoe et al. (2015). Herein, we focus on the recent efforts made to develop inhibitors of TbPDEB1.

Since inhibitors of human PDEs, like cilomilast, piclamilast, sildenafil and tadalafil were known, design efforts were often focused on repurposing these drugs and developing analogs thereof (Amata et al. 2014, Ochiana et al. 2012, Wang et al. 2012, Woodring et al. 2013), but with rather limited success. For example, Amata et al. (2014) found that cilomilast **143** (Figure 52) had an IC_{50} of 16.4 μM against TbPDEB1 and the best derivative **144** (Figure 52) resulted in an IC_{50} of 0.95 μM. However, the EC_{50} of **144** in a cellular assay against *T. brucei* was still only modest (26 μM vs. cilomilast **143** $EC_{50} > 50$ μM).

A virtual screening of the ZINC database was carried out by Jansen et al. (2013) to broaden the chemical space of the potential TbPDEB1 inhibitors. Molecular docking in conjunction with a score based on receptor-compound interaction fingerprints was used to filter suitable compounds. This way, six novel inhibitors of TbPDEB1 with IC_{50} values between 10 and 80 μM were identified.

In another study, Orrling et al. (2012) used homology modeling and docking studies to exploit a parasite-specific subpocket, the so-called P-pocket of TbPDEB1 (Figure 53), for the design of the improved catechol pyrazolinone-based inhibitors. The most potent inhibitor **145** (Figure 54) achieved an IC_{50} of 49 nM against TbPDEB1 and was able to inhibit parasite trypomastigote proliferation in *in vitro* studies: *T. brucei rhodesiense* with IC_{50} of 60 nM, *T. brucei brucei* with IC_{50} of 520 nM and *T. cruzi* with IC_{50} of 7.6 μM. However, compound **145** was an even more potent inhibitor of human PDE isoforms. Thus, this study highlights the potential of PDE inhibitors against trypanosomal infections, but also indicates that further optimization of the selectivity for the TbPDEB1 target is required.

The P-pocket of TbPDEB1 has been recently further exploited by Blaazer et al. (2018) in their development of selective 4a,5,8,8a-tetrahydrophthalazinone-based inhibitors. Guided by the crystallographic analysis of non-specific TbPDEB1 inhibitors and the analysis of flexibility patterns of a TbPDEB1-inhibitor complex observed by MD simulations, several compounds specifically targeting the P-pocket were developed. **146** and **147** (Figure 55) were overall the best, both showing K_i of 100 nM against TbPDEB1, 10- and 19-fold selectivity for the parasitic over the human enzyme, and had IC_{50}s of 5.5 μM and 6.7 μM, respectively, when tested against *T. brucei*.

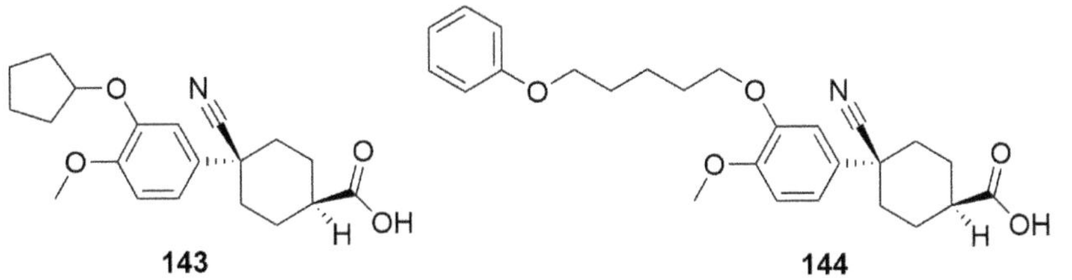

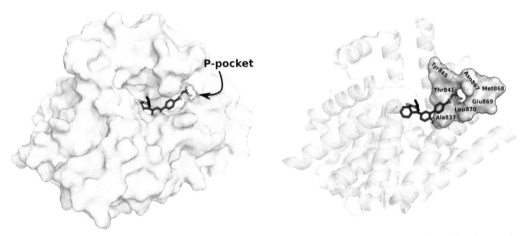

143
cilomast

144

Figure 52. Structures of the human PDE inhibitor cilomilast **143** and its derivative **144** optimized for TbPDEB1 targeting.

Figure 53. Compound **147** binding to TbPDEB1 (see also Figure 55, based on PDB-ID 5l8c) and targeting the parasite PDE-specific P-pocket. On the left, the protein is shown as a semi-transparent surface with the ligand in black sticks and the location of the P-pocket marked. On the right side, the protein is shown in the same orientation as cartoon and only the P-pocket residues are shown as a surface with residues labeled according to Blaazer et al. (2018).

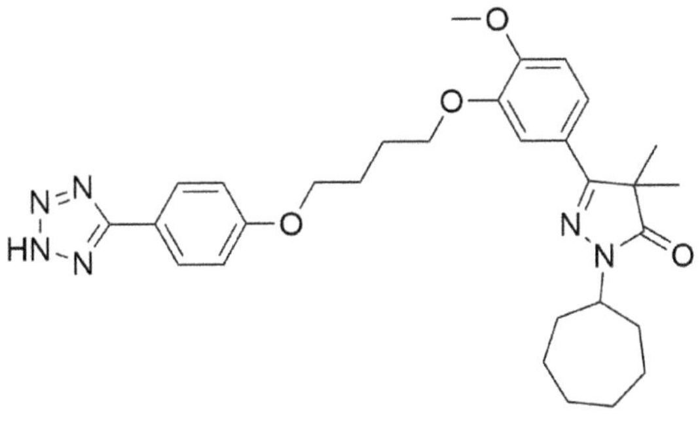

Figure 54. Structure of the P-pocket targeting TbPDEB1 inhibitor **145**.

Cysteine proteases

Two cysteine proteases structurally related to human cathepsin L, cruzain of *T. cruzi* and rhodesain of *T. brucei rhodesiense*, have been subject to drug development efforts, including many computational and mechanistic studies in the past years, which we review below. More details on inhibitor design against cysteine proteases in *Trypanosoma* can be found in the recent review by Ferreira and Andricopulo (2017).

Cruzain: Since cruzain is a protease, many inhibitors designed were based on peptides and typically bind covalently (see Figure 56). Database screening strategies led to non-peptide inhibitors of cruzain. Ferreira et al. (2010) illustrated for cruzain inhibitors how the combination of VS, HTS and prioritization

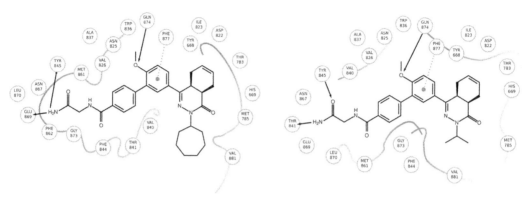

Figure 55. Interaction diagrams of the two P-pocket-targeting TbPDEB1 inhibitors, **146** and **147** (cf. Figure 53). The diagrams are based on the crystallographic complexes with PDB-ID 5g2b and 5l8c (Blaazer et al. 2018), respectively. Pocket-lining residues and the pocket shape are shown. Gray dotted lines indicate π-π interactions and black arrows show hydrogen-bonding interactions.

of molecular scaffolds can largely avoid false-positives. Wiggers et al. (2013) identified non-covalent cruzain inhibitors from the ZINC database. Further, Palos et al. (2017) performed VS of FDA-approved drugs against cruzain and confirmed the trypanocidal potential of four putative inhibitors *in vitro* and *in vivo*, which may thus represent starting scaffolds for further drug development.

Crystallography was also used for exploring compound binding modes, MoA, and for obtaining SARs. In the aforementioned VS study, Wiggers et al. (2013) used a molecular simplification approach to obtain a SAR for one of the compounds and found that the 2-acetamidothiophene-3-carboxamide scaffold was the critical component for the interactions with cruzain. Then, they confirmed the binding mode of this scaffold by crystallographic data, thus validating a potential new non-covalent, non-peptidic cruzain-binding scaffold. Avelar et al. (2015) characterized dipeptidyl nitriles as inhibitors of cruzain by extensive SAR studies and determining a crystallographic complex with compound **148** (Figures 56 and 57). Jones et al. (2015) synthesized and crystallized oxyguanidine analogs of existing cysteine protease inhibitors and were able to show that one of the compounds displays covalent (**149**, Figure 57) and the other non-covalent inhibition (**150**, Figure 57).

A variety of computational chemistry methods has been used to study cruzain interactions with inhibitors, to better understand their MoA, and to design new compounds. Hologram quantitative structure-activity relationship, comparative molecular field analysis and comparative molecular similarity index

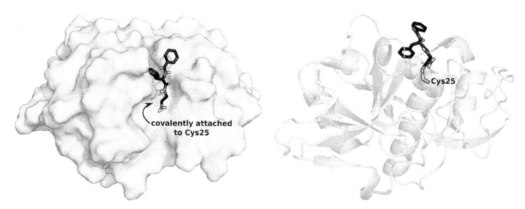

Figure 56. Example of a dipeptidyl nitrile ligand **148** covalently attached to the cysteine protease cruzain (see also Figure 57, based on PDB-ID 4qh6; Avelar et al. 2015). On the left, the protein is shown as a semi-transparent surface with the ligand in sticks with black carbons. On the right, the protein is shown in cartoon representation, rotated by about 90° and the site of the covalent attachment, Cys25, is labeled.

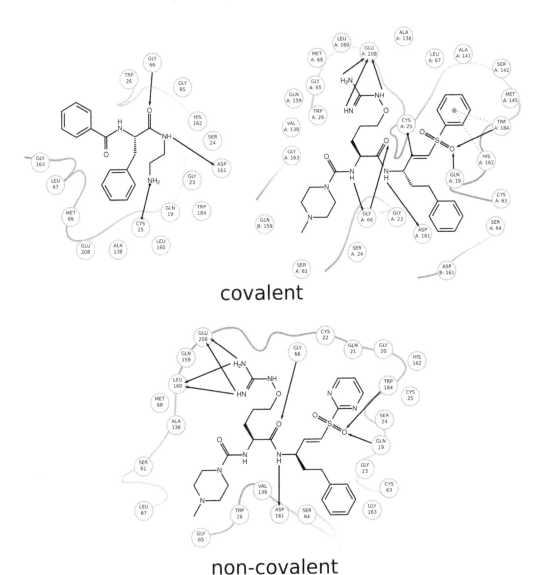

Figure 57. Interaction diagrams of cruzain inhibitors: the covalent dipeptidyl nitrile **148** (top left, see also Figure 56; Avelar et al. 2015) and oxyguanidine inhibitor **149** (top right; Jones et al. 2015) and the non-covalent oxyguanidine inhibitor **150** (bottom). The diagrams are based on the crystallographic complexes with PDB-ID 4qh6, 4pi3 and 4xui, respectively. Pocket-lining residues and the pocket shape are shown. Gray dotted lines indicate π-π interactions, black arrows show hydrogen-bonding interactions, and a black line ended with circles marks a covalent bond between ligand and protein.

analysis methods combined with docking simulations have been applied to a series of benzimidazole-based cruzain inhibitors by Pauli et al. (2017) to predict binding modes and activities. Silva et al. (2017) used docking studies and QSAR methods to study nitrile-containing cruzain inhibitors and predict their activities, leading to the proposal of new potential inhibitors. de Souza et al. (2017) used 2D- and 3D-QSAR methods to explore the interactions of oxadiazole-based compounds with different cruzain subsites. Elizondo-Jimenez et al. (2017) synthesized benzenesulfonyl and N-propionyl benzenesulfonyl hydrazone derivatives, evaluated their anti-*T. cruzi* activity and used docking studies to propose covalent binding to cruzain as the compounds' MoA. Silva-Júnior et al. (2016) synthesized several trypanocidal thiophen-2-iminothiazolidines and used molecular docking to demonstrate that the most active compound likely interacts simultaneously with two subsites of cruzain.

To gain more insight into cruzain dynamics and its interactions with inhibitors, MD simulations have been applied together with other molecular modelling techniques. Durrant et al. (2010) used sequence analysis and MD simulations to explore additional binding sites in cruzain. Hoelz et al. (2016) studied free and liganded cruzain dynamics at acidic pH, which corresponds to its environment in the cell. Very recently, Cianni et al. (2018) also used MD simulations to study the binding mode of reversible covalent inhibitors to the less frequently studied specific subsite S3 of cruzain. Finally, Martins et al. (2018) demonstrated a comprehensive computational approach including docking, MD, *ab initio* and MM/PBSA calculations for binding mode prediction and estimation of the contributions of specific amino acids to binding. Finally furthermore, more mechanistic approaches have been employed, for example by Arafet et al. (2015, 2017) who studied the MoA of peptidyl-epoxyketone- or peptidyl-halomethyl-ketone-based cruzain inhibitors with a QM/MM method.

Rhodesain: For rhodesain, several SBDD efforts were inspired by its structural similarity to human cathepsin. Triazine nitrile-based compounds were studied against rhodesain and extensive SAR analyses were performed to explore the binding preferences of the different subsites, supported by a crystallographic complex of the synthesized compounds with the structurally related human cathepsin L enzyme (Ehmke et al. 2013). Schirmeister et al. (2017) aimed at repurposing human cathepsin-targeting dipeptide nitriles for rhodesain and used covalent docking to support the development of a SAR. Later, Giroud et al. (2018) optimized a set of macrocyclic lactams, developed as human cathepsin L inhibitors, to target *T. brucei* rhodesain and elucidated their binding modes by crystallographic studies. The initial compound **151** (Figure 58) had a K_i of 11 nM against rhodesain, but also a K_i of 10 nM against human cathepsin L. One of the optimized, designed pyrazole derivatives **152** (Figure 58) was found to be about 11 times more effective as an inhibitor of rhodesain than human cathepsin L (K_i rhodesain 5.2 nM; K_i human cathepsin L 55.7 nM) and to be a potent inhibitor of *T. b. rhodesiense* with an IC_{50} of 0.6 nM.

Trypanothione metabolism

The redox metabolism of parasites like *T. brucei* relies, in contrast to humans, on the dithiol trypanothione **153** (N1,N8-bis(glutathionyl)spermidine; see Figure 59) being absent in humans and making enzymes involved in this pathway interesting as drug targets for trypanosomatidic diseases (Fairlamb and Cerami 1992, Leroux and Krauth-Siegel 2016). One of the best studied and genetically validated targets is trypanothione reductase (TrypR; see Figure 59), which is responsible for reducing trypanothione disulfide

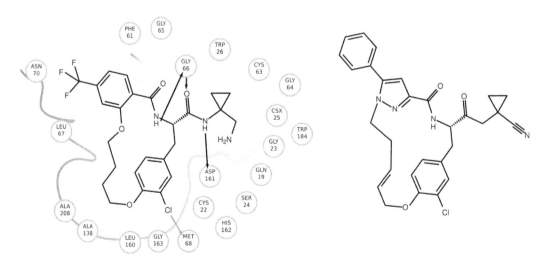

Figure 58. Interaction diagrams of a macrolactam inhibitor of rhodesain **151** (left) and structure of its derivative **152** (right). The interaction diagram is based on the crystallographic complex with PDB-ID 6ex8 (Giroud et al. 2018). Pocket-lining residues and the pocket shape are shown. Black arrows in the interaction diagram indicate hydrogen-bonding interactions and gray arrows indicate halogen-bonding interactions. CSX denotes a cysteine residue with an oxo-modification.

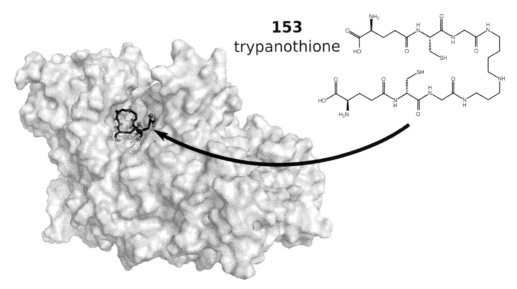

Figure 59. TrypR of *T. brucei* with trypanothione **153** bound at the interface between two chains (based on PDB-ID 2wow, chain A and B, ligand state A; Patterson et al. 2011). The protein is shown as a surface with trypanothione in black sticks.

(Fairlamb and Cerami 1992, Krieger et al. 2000). In humans, a similar reaction is performed by glutathione reductase, which, however, has an opposite net charge in the active site, facilitating the development of specific inhibitors (Faerman et al. 1996).

Structure-based modelling provided insights into the TrypR pocket regions that could be targeted in drug design approaches. For example, Patterson et al. (2011) designed 3,4-dihydroquinazoline-based inhibitors and solved several crystal structures of *T. brucei* TrypR. They observed conformational changes upon ligand binding, initiating the formation of a subpocket, which was exploited in further design and yielded compounds with improved TbTrypR and anti-trypanosomal activity: The initial hit compound **154** (Figure 60) had an IC$_{50}$ of 6.8 µM against TbTrypR and an EC$_{50}$ against *T. brucei* of 40 µM, while the best designed compound **155** (Figure 60) yielded a TbTrypR IC$_{50}$ of 0.23 µM and a *T. brucei* EC$_{50}$ of 0.73 µM.

In a later study, based on a series of peptide-based inhibitors, da Rocha Pita et al. (2012) developed receptor-dependent four-dimensional quantitative structure-activity relationship (RD-4D-QSAR) models (Pan et al. 2003) that allowed for identifying TrypR subsites that may be exploited in future inhibitor development.

Using a combined approach including mutation studies, docking simulations, and crystallography, Persch et al. (2014) developed analogs of 1-[1-(benzo[b]thien-2-yl)cyclohexyl]piperidine as inhibitors of *T. brucei* and *T. cruzi* TrypR, targeting the large substrate binding site (Figure 59). For example, compound **156** (Figure 61) displayed K$_i$ values of 4 ± 0.5 µM against TcTrypR and 12 ± 2 µM against TbTrypR, when assuming a competitive inhibition mechanism. The IC$_{50}$ against *T. cruzi* was 19.0 µM and against *T. brucei rhodesiense*—3.5 µM, with SI of 8 for L6 cells. However, there was some evidence that TrypR might not be the only target of the tested compounds. In a follow-up project (De Gasparo et al. 2018), again with the help of crystallographic studies, the cyclohexylpyrrolidine inhibitors were further optimized by retaining fragments that bind to the hydrophobic substrate binding site and by increasing the polarity of solvent-exposed moieties to improve aqueous solubility.

On the other hand, structure-based techniques helped in identifying TrypR as a potential target for some compounds active at the parasite level. This was the case for propyl/isopropyl quinoxaline-7-carboxylate 1,4-di-N-oxide-based compounds, active against *T. cruzi*, which were found to target TrypR by using docking simulations and enzymatic validation (Chaćon-Vargas et al. 2017). Arias et al. (2017) synthesized a set of nitrofuran derivatives, which demonstrated uncompetitive inhibition of TrypR in subsequent experiments. Docking studies indicated that the inhibitors may in fact be capable of binding to

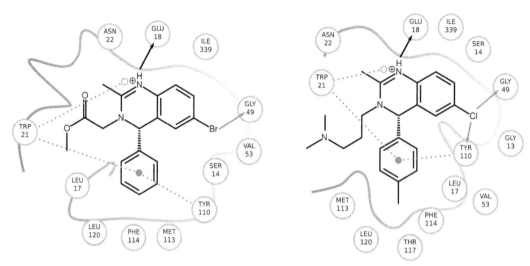

Figure 60. Interaction diagrams of two dihydroquinazoline-based inhibitors of TbTrypR, **154** and **155**. The diagrams are based on the crystallographic complexes with PDB-ID 2wp5 and 2wpf (Patterson et al. 2011), respectively. Pocket-lining residues and the pocket shape are shown. Gray dotted lines indicate π-π interactions and, with white circles, cation-π interactions, black arrows indicate hydrogen-bonding and, gray arrows indicate halogen-bonding interactions.

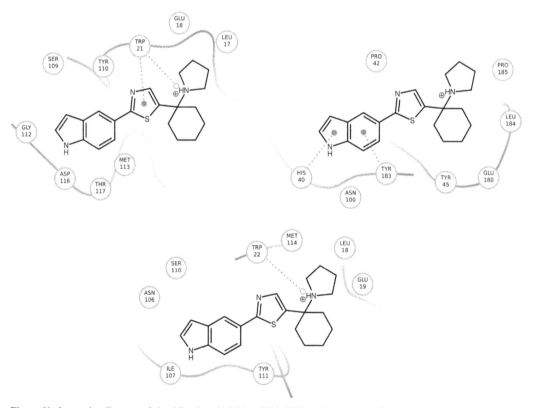

Figure 61. Interaction diagrams of piperidine-based inhibitor **156** in TbTrypR (top, two binding modes) and TcTrypR (bottom). The diagrams are based on the crystallographic complexes with PDB-ID 4nev and 4new (Persch et al. 2014), respectively. Pocket-lining residues and the pocket shape are shown. Gray dotted lines indicate π-π interactions and, with white circles, cation-π interactions.

the enzyme-substrate complex, thus explaining the observed behavior. Similar observations were previously made for mesoionic 1,3,4-thiadiazolium-2-aminide (Rodrigues et al. 2012), which was also found to dock to TrypR in the presence of the substrate molecule. Finally, natural products or natural product-derived compounds, such as alkaloids or neolignan derivatives were proposed as inhibitors of TcTrypR on the basis of *in silico* screening, docking studies, and 2D-QSAR analysis (Argüelles et al. 2016, Hartmann et al. 2017).

Other enzymes of the trypanothione pathway were also investigated as potential drug targets. A mathematical model of the *T. cruzi* trypanothione pathway was developed by Olin-Sandoval et al. (2012). The results demonstrated that a polypharmacology approach targeting γ-glutamylcysteine synthetase (γECS) and trypanothione synthetase (TrypS) as the enzymes that exert the highest control on the pathway fluxes may be more promising than targeting TrypR. TrypR was found to have less metabolic control and thus requires very high ligand binding affinities to shut the pathway down. Further, by the same approach, tryparedoxin was identified as a suitable potential drug target, since it shows low catalytic efficiency and exerts large metabolic control (González-Chávez et al. 2015).

In line with the above findings, Benítez et al. (2016) focused on identifying TrypS inhibitors, using target-based screening of a compound library. Furthermore, Vázquez et al. (2017) discovered buthionine sulfoximine as a dual inhibitor of γECS and TrypS, which was further confirmed by the docking and over-expression experiments.

For a more detailed review on the system and currently known inhibitors of both TrypR and TrypS, the reader is referred to Leroux and Krauth-Siegel (2016).

Perspectives and limitations of target-based drug discovery approaches

Many of the examples presented herein demonstrate that it is not always trivial to translate good activities against a specific biomolecular target into anti-parasitic activity. However, target-guided approaches, like crystallography and computational docking studies, provide important guidelines for scaffold optimization and aid the development of SARs. Further, off-target effects can be minimized by the same techniques and comparative studies of, for instance, sequences, structures and molecular interaction fields. Computational studies of target dynamics provide further hints for desirable flexibility profiles of designed molecules. Moreover, mechanistic insights are gained by studying drug-target interactions. Target-based methods are under continuous development and offer great potential for finding suitable starting points for medicinal chemistry programs and the design of specific, selective compounds with a well-defined MoA. The choice of the target and its impact on the pathway to be inhibited is often a critical bottleneck and mathematical models of trypanosomal metabolic pathways may shed light on which enzymes have most control over pathway fluxes and thus may present the most promising targets. In summary, while many interesting compounds have been developed by target-based design strategies, there are limitations to the approach which are best overcome by combining target-guided approaches with screening of the compounds' anti-parasitic properties early on in the drug discovery process.

In vivo murine models in trypanosomatidic infections

Murine models, due to their small size, availability of tools for genetic manipulation and immunological studies, are at the forefront of animal use in science (Vandamme 2015). Notwithstanding, the use of animals in scientific research has always been a socially polarizing subject even with the implementation of the three Rs (Replacement, Reduction and Refinement) proposed more than 60 years ago (Russell and Burch 1959). For an animal model to be considered, there must be similarities related to disease etiology, pathophysiology, symptomatology and also response to therapeutic or prophylactic agents. In this sense, animal models have contributed decisively to the understanding of pathophysiological processes associated with infection and disease and have also been instrumental in pre-clinical vaccine and drug development.

For HAT, the animal models are well established and have predictive value for drug development (Field et al. 2017). These models were further solidified using highly susceptible BALB/c mice and bioluminescent parasites that enable longitudinal evaluation of drug performance (McLatchie et al. 2013,

Burrell-Saward et al. 2015). Most models that exist are for stage 1 disease using the non-pathogenic *T. b. brucei* S427, although *T. b. rhodesiense* and to a lesser extent *T. b. gambiense* models also exist (Giroud et al. 2009, Muchiri et al. 2015, Field et al. 2017). Established models for stage 2 are also available using *T. b. brucei GVR35* that induces a slow progressing infection in invasion of the central nervous system (Jennings et al. 1983, Burrell-Saward et al. 2015). For Chagas disease, the situation is quite different, as the translatability of the existing mice models to human disease is not linear as demonstrated by the posaconazole failure (Francisco et al. 2015, Molina et al. 2015). Many of the standardization issues that affect *Leishmania* mice models are also present in Chagas disease with completely different infection outcomes depending on the parasite strain, stage, inoculum and inoculation route affecting treatment susceptibility (Chatelain and Konar 2015). Like in HAT, there are distinct animal models proposed for acute and chronic stages of the disease. The models for the acute stage are more common in drug development, which normally use high doses of parasites and are expected to be fatal after one month (Romanha et al. 2010). These models are typically used to demonstrate lack of efficacy of compounds and are considered not to be appropriate for lead development (Chatelain and Konar 2015). Chronic models also exist, requiring several months to be established with disease outcome being highly dependent on the strains used (Marinho et al. 2004, Marinho et al. 2009). Therefore, these chronic models are considered time consuming and are expensive for drug development, requiring in-depth studies of the tissue tropism of the used strains (Chatelain and Konar 2015). A known technical limitation of the Chagas models was, for a long time, the detection of infection. This was problematic as these parasites are often absent from blood, requiring extensive examination of distinct tissues (Field et al. 2017). Nonetheless, this difficulty has been somewhat minimized with the use of bioluminescent parasites that, in conjunction with immunosuppressive treatments with cyclophosphamide, enable a better assessment of cure (Lewis et al. 2015). Consequently, there is the notion that the existing mice models for Chagas disease have a limited predictive value for drug development, increasing the need to improve the available mice models for Chagas (Chatelain and Konar 2015, Field et al. 2017).

Hamsters can be infected with several *Trypanosoma* sp and this species has been considered the most satisfactory and economic animal for maintenance of *T. b. gambiense* infection for experimental studies in laboratories (Lee and Pan 1980). However, as a rule, the use of hamsters as experimental models for HAT has been considerably less relevant compared to mice models (Pink et al. 2005). In the case of *T. cruzi* infections, hamster is considered a valuable model for Chagas disease studies in both acute and chronic phases of the infection (Ramirez et al. 1994), since they reproduce a range of different outcomes of the disease in humans (Bilate et al. 2008).

Ultimately, no perfect animal models exist but they have been essential to advance our knowledge of pathogenic mechanisms involved in these diseases and also to develop successful control approaches through vaccine and drug development.

Conclusion and Perspectives

In the present chapter, we have highlighted key medicinal chemistry approaches to identifying and assessing new hits and optimizing leads for tackling Chagas disease and HAT. The drug discovery approaches to the identification of new drugs for Chagas disease and HAT take advantage of the scope for collaborative work by different stakeholders, including academic research scientists, national and international organizations and governmental initiatives as well as private research centers and pharmaceutical companies. More financial support for the early stages of research and development is needed. Unfortunately, many research programs start and develop early hits and leads but then fall prematurely into the "valley of death" of unused early and late candidate compounds. A major effort devoted to further developing the most valuable compounds identified should be a core part of future research programs.

Acknowledgements

The Authors acknowledge the European Union's Seventh Framework Programme for research, technological development and demonstration under grant agreement n° 603240 (NMTrypI—New Medicines for

Trypanosomatidic Infections). http://www.nmtrypi.eu/. JPH acknowledges support from the Polish National Science Centre (grant no. 2016/21/D/NZ1/02806) and the BIOMS program at the Interdisciplinary Center for Scientific Computing IWR, University of Heidelberg. IP, RCW and JPH gratefully acknowledge the support of the Klaus Tschira Foundation.

Abbreviations

AAT	Animal African Trypanosomiasis
BSF	bloodstream form
cAMP	cyclic AMP
CNB	chloronitrobenzamide
DHCH	N^5,N^{10}-methylenetetrahydrofolate dehydrogenase/cyclohydrolase
DHFR	dihydrofolate reductase
DNDi	Drugs for Neglected Diseases initiative
FBDD	fragment-based drug design
γECS	γ-glutamylcysteine synthetase
HTS	high-throughput screening
HAT	Human African Trypanosomiasis
MoA	mechanism-of-action
MTX	methotrexate
MD	molecular dynamics
NTDs	neglected tropical diseases
PDE	phosphodiesterase
PGI	percentage of growth inhibition
PTR1	pteridine reductase 1
QSAR	quantitative structure activity relationship
SAR	structure-activity-relationship
SBDD	structure-based drug design
SI	selectivity index
TbPTR1	*Trypanosoma brucei* pteridine reductase 1
TrypR	trypanothione reductase
TrypS	trypanothione synthetase
VS	virtual screening
WHO	World Health Organization

References

Amata, E., N.D. Bland, C.T. Hoyt, L. Settimo, R.K. Campbell and M.P. Pollastri. 2014. Repurposing human PDE4 inhibitors for neglected tropical diseases: design, synthesis and evaluation of cilomilast analogues as *Trypanosoma brucei* PDEB1 inhibitors. Bioorg. Med. Chem. Lett. 24: 4084–4089.

Ancizu, S., E. Moreno, E. Torres, A. Burguete, S. Pérez-Silanes, D. Benítez et al. 2009. Heterocyclic-2-carboxylic acid (3-Cyano-1,4-di-N-oxidequinoxalin-2-yl)amide derivatives as hits for the development of neglected disease drugs. Molecules. 14: 2256–2272.

Andriani, G., E. Amata, J. Beatty, Z. Clements, B.J. Coffey, G. Courtemanche et al. 2013. Antitrypanosomal lead discovery: identification of a ligand-efficient inhibitor of *Trypanosoma cruzi* CYP51 and parasite growth. J. Med. Chem. 56(6): 2556–2567.

Arafet, K., S. Ferrer and V. Moliner. 2015. First quantum mechanics/molecular mechanics studies of the inhibition mechanism of cruzain by peptidyl halomethyl ketones. Biochemistry. 54: 3381–3391.

Arafet, K., S. Ferrer, F.V. González and V. Moliner. 2017. Quantum mechanics/molecular mechanics studies of the mechanism of cysteine protease inhibition by peptidyl-2,3-epoxyketones. Phys. Chem. Chem. Phys. 19: 12740–12748.

Argüelles, A.J., G.A. Cordell and H. Maruenda. 2016. Molecular docking and binding mode analysis of plant alkaloids as *in vitro* and *in silico* inhibitors of trypanothione reductase from *Trypanosoma cruzi*. Nat. Prod. Commun. 11: 57–62.

Arias, D.G., F.E. Herrera, A.S. Garay, D. Rodrigues, P.S. Forastieri, L.E. Luna et al. 2017. Rational design of nitrofuran derivatives: Synthesis and valuation as inhibitors of *Trypanosoma cruzi* trypanothione reductase. Eur. J. Med. Chem. 25: 1088–1097.

Avelar, L.A.A., C.D. Camilo, S. de Albuquerde, W.B. Fernandes, C. Gonçalez, P.W. Kenny et al. 2015. Molecular design, synthesis and trypanocidal activity of dipeptidyl nitriles as cruzain inhibitors. PLoS Negl. Trop. Dis. 9: e0003916.

Bello, A.R., B. Nare, D. Freedman, L. Hardy and S.M. Beverley. 1994. PTR1: A reductase mediating salvage of oxidized pteridines and methotrexate resistance in the protozoan parasite *Leishmania major*. Proc. Natl. Acad. Sci. USA. 91: 11442–11446.

Benítez, D., M. Cabrera, P. Hernandez, L. Boiani, M.L. Lavaggi, R. Di Maio et al. 2011. 3-Trifluoromethylquinoxaline N,N'-Dioxides as anti-trypanosomatid agents. Identification of optimal anti-*T. cruzi* agents and mechanism of action studies. J. Med. Chem. 54: 3624–3636.

Benítez, D., A. Medeiros, L. Fiestas, E.A. Panozzo-Zenere, F. Maiwald, K.C. Prousis et al. 2016. Identification of novel chemical scaffolds inhibiting trypanothione synthetase from pathogenic trypanosomatids. PLoS Negl. Trop. Dis. 10: e0004617.

Bern, C., S. Kjos, M.J. Yabsley and S.P. Montgomery. 20101 Trypanosoma cruzi and Chagas' disease in the United States. Clin. Microbiol. Rev. 24(4): 655–81.

Bettiol, E., M. Samanovic, A.S. Murkin, J. Raper, F. Buckner and A. Rodriguez. 2009. Identification of three classes of heteroaromatic compounds with activity against intracellular *Trypanosoma cruzi* by chemical library screening. PLoS Neglected Trop. Dis. 3: e384.

Bhambra, A.S., M. Edgar, M.R.J. Elsegood, Y. Li, G.W. Weaver, R.R.J. Arroo et al. 2016. Design, synthesis and antitrypanosomal activities of 2,6-disubstituted-4,5,7-trifluorobenzothiophenes. Eur. J. Med. Chem. 108: 347–353.

Bhambra, A.S., K.C. Ruparelia, H.L. Tan, D. Tasdemir, H. Burrell-Saward, V. Yardley et al. 2017. Synthesis and antitrypanosomal activities of novel pyridylchalcones. Eur. J. Med. Chem. 128: 213–218.

Blaazer, A.R., A.K. Singh, E. de Heuvel, E. Edink, K.M. Orrling, J.J.N. Veerman et al. 2018. Targeting a subpocket in *Trypanosoma brucei* phosphodiesterase B1 (*Tbr*PDEB1) enables the structure-based discovery of selective inhibitors with trypanocidal activity. J. Med. Chem. 61: 3870–3888.

Borsari, C., R. Luciani, C. Pozzi, I. Poehner, S. Henrich, M. Trande et al. 2016. Profiling of flavonol derivatives for the development of antitrypanosomatidic drugs. J. Med. Chem. 59: 7598–7616.

Buckner, F.S. and J.A. Urbina. 2012. Recent developments in sterol 14-demethylase inhibitors for chagas disease. Int. J. Parasitol. Drugs. Drug. Resist. 2: 236–242.

Buchynskyy, A., J.R. Gillespie, Z.M. Herbst, R.M. Ranade, F.S. Buckner and M.H. Gelb. 2017a. 1-Benzyl-3-aryl-2-thiohydantoin derivatives as new anti-*Trypanosoma brucei* agents: SAR and *in-vivo* efficacy. ACS Med. Chem. Lett. 8: 886–891.

Buchynskyy, A., J.R. Gillespie, M.A. Hulverson, J. McQueen, S.A. Creason, R.M. Ranade et al. 2017b. Discovery of N-(2-aminoethyl)-N-benzyloxyphenyl benzamides: New potent *Trypanosoma brucei* inhibitors. Bioorg. Med. Chem. 25: 1571–1584.

Burrell-Saward, H., J. Rodgers, B. Bradley, S.L. Croft and T.H. Ward. 2015. A sensitive and reproducible *in vivo* imaging mouse model for evaluation of drugs against late-stage human African trypanosomiasis. J. Antimicrob. Chemother. 70(2): 510–7.

Büscher, P., G. Cecchi, V. Jamonneau and G. Priotto. 2017. Human African trypanosomiasis. Lancet. 390: 2397–2409.

Calvet, C.M., D.F. Viera, J.Y. Choi, D. Kellar, M.D. Cameron, J.L. Siqueira-Neto et al. 2014. 4-Aminopyridyl-based CYP51 inhibitors as anti-*Trypanosoma cruzi* drug leads with improved pharmacokinetic profile and *in vivo* potency. J. Med. Chem. 57(16): 6989–7005.

Caminos, A.P., E.A. Panozzo-Zenere, S.R. Wilkinson, B.L. Tekwani and G.R. Labadie. 2012. Synthesis and antikinetoplastid activity of a series of N,N'-substituted diamines. Bioorg. Med. Chem. Lett. 22: 1712–1715.

Cardoso, M.V.O., L.R.P. Siqueira, E.B. Silva, L.B. Costa, M.Z. Hernandes, M.M. Rabello et al. 2014. 2-Pyridyl thiazoles as novel anti-*Trypanosoma cruzi* agents: Structural design, synthesis and pharmacological evaluation. Eur. J. Med. Chem. 86: 48–59.

Carneiro, P.F., S.B. do Nascimento, A.V. Pinto, M. do Carmo, F.R. Pinto, G.C. Lechuga et al. 2012. New oxirane derivatives of 1,4-naphthoquinones and their evaluation against *T. cruzi* epimastigote forms. Bioorg. Med. Chem. 20: 4995–5000.

Cavazzuti, A., G. Paglietti, W.N. Hunter, F. Gamarro, S. Piras, M. Loriga et al. 2008. Discovery of potent pteridine reductase inhibitors to guide antiparasite drug development. Proc. Natl. Acad. Sci. USA. 105(5): 1448–1453.

Chacón-Vargas, K.F., B. Nogueda-Torres, L.E. Sánchez-Torres, E. Suarez-Contreras, J.C. Villalobos-Rocha, Y. Torres-Martinez et al. 2017. Trypanocidal activity of quinoxaline 1,4 Di-N-oxide derivatives as trypanothione reductase inhibitors. Molecules. 22: E220.

Chappuis, F., N. Udayraj, K. Stietenroth, A. Meussen and P.A. Bovier. 2005. Eflornithine is safer than melarsoprol for the treatment of second-stage *Trypanosoma brucei* gambiense human African trypanosomiasis. Clin. Infect. Dis. 41: 748–51.

Chatelain, E. and J.-R. Ioset. 2011. Drug discovery and development for neglected diseases: the DNDi model. Drug Des. Devel. Ther. Dove Medical Press. 5: 175–181.

Chen, C.-K., S.S.F. Leung, C. Guilbert, M.P. Jacobson, J.H. McKerrow and L.M. Podust. 2010. Structural characterization of CYP51 from *Trypanosoma cruzi* and *Trypanosoma brucei* bound to the antifungal drugs posaconazole and fluconazole. PLoS Negl. Trop. Dis. 4(4): e651.

Choi, J.Y., C.M. Calvet, S.S. Gunatilleke, C. Ruiz, M.D. Cameron, J.H. McKerrow et al. 2013. Rational development of 4-aminopyridyl-based inhibitors targeting *Trypanosoma cruzi* CYP51 as anti-chagas agents. J. Med. Chem. 56(19): 7651–7668.

Cianni, L., G. Sartori, F. Rosini, D. De Vita, G. Pires, B.R. Lopes et al. 2018. Leveraging the cruzain S3 subsite to increase affinity for reversible covalent inhibitors. Bioorg. Chem. 79: 285–292.

Cleghorn, L.A.T., S. Albrecht, L. Stojanovski, F.R.J. Simeons, S. Norval, R. Kime et al. 2015. Discovery of indoline-2-carboxamide derivatives as a new class of brain-penetrant inhibitors of *Trypanosoma brucei*. J. Med. Chem. 58: 7695–7706.

Cullen, D.R. and M. Mocerino. 2017. A brief review of drug discovery research for human African trypanosomiasis. Curr. Med. Chem. 24(7): 701–17.

Cullia, G., L. Tamborini, P. Conti, C. De Micheli and A. Pinto. 2018. Folates in *Trypanosoma brucei*: Achievements and opportunities. ChemMedChem. 13(20): 2150–2158.

da Rocha Pita, S.S., M.G.A. Albuquerque, C.R. Rodrigues, H.C. Castro and A.J. Hopfinger. 2012. Receptor-dependent 4D-QSAR analysis of peptidemimetic inhibitors of *Trypanosoma cruzi* trypanothione reductase with receptor-based alignment. Chem. Biol. Drug. Des. 79: 740–748.

Dawson, A., F. Gibellini, N. Sienkiewicz, L.B. Tulloch, P.K. Fyfe, K. McLuskey et al. 2006. Structure and reactivity of *Trypanosoma brucei* pteridine reductase: inhibition by the archetypal antifolate methotrexate. Mol. Microbiol. 61(6): 1457–1468.

De Gasparo, R., E. Brodbeck-Persch, S. Bryson, N.B. Hentzen, M. Kaiser, E.F. Pai et al. 2018. Biological evaluation and X-ray co-crystal structures of Cyclohexylpyrrolidine ligands for trypanothione reductase, an enzyme from the redox metabolism of trypanosoma. ChemMedChem. 3: 957–967.

de Souza, A.S., M.T. de Oliveira and A.D. Andricopulo. 2017. Development of a pharmacophore for cruzain using oxadiazoles as virtual molecular probes: quantitative structure-activity relationship studies. J. Comput. Aided Mol. Des. 31: 801–816.

De Vita, D., F. Moraca, C. Zamperini, F. Pandolfi, R. Di Santo, A. Matheeussen et al. 2016. *In vitro* screening of 2-(1H-imidazol-1-yl)-1-phenylethanol derivatives as antiprotozoal agents and docking studies on *Trypanosoma cruzi* CYP51. Eur. J. Med. Chem. 113: 28–33.

Denning, D.W. and M.J. Bromley. 2015. Infectious disease. How to bolster the antifungal pipeline. Science. 347(6229): 1414–1416.

Devine, W., J.L. Woodring, U. Swaminathan, E. Amata, G. Patel, J. Erath et al. 2015. Protozoan parasite growth inhibitors discovered by cross-screening yield potent scaffolds for lead discovery. J. Med. Chem. 58: 5522–5537.

Di Pisa, F., G. Landi, L. Dello Iacono, C. Pozzi, C. Borsari, S. Ferrari et al. 2017. Chroman-4-One derivatives targeting pteridine reductase 1 and showing anti-parasitic activity. Molecules. 22(3): 426.

Doerig, C. 2004. Protein kinases as targets for anti-parasitic chemotherapy. Biochim. Biophys. Acta: Proteins Proteomics. 1697: 155–168.

Dube, D., S. Sharma, T.P. Singh and P. Kaur. 2014. Pharmacophore mapping, *In Silico* screening and molecular docking to identify selective *Trypanosoma brucei* pteridine reductase inhibitors. Mol. Inform. 33(2): 124–134.

Durrant, J.D., H. Keränen, B.A. Wilson and J.A. McCammon. 2010. Computational identification of uncharacterized cruzain binding sites. PLoS Negl. Trop. Dis. 4: e676.

Eadsforth, T.C., A. Pinto, R. Luciani, L. Tamborini, G. Cullia, C. De Micheli et al. 2015. Characterization of 2,4-Diamino-6-oxo-1,6-dihydropyrimidin-5-yl Ureido based inhibitors of *Trypanosoma brucei* fold and testing for antiparasitic activity. J. Med. Chem. 58: 7938–7948.

Ehmke, V., E. Winkler, D.W. Banner, W. Haap, W.B. Schweizer, M. Rottmann et al. 2013. Optimization of triazine nitriles as rhodesain inhibitors: structure-activity relationships, bioisosteric imidazopyridine nitriles, and X-ray crystal structure analysis with human cathepsin L. ChemMedChem. 8: 967–975.

Elizondo-Jimenez, S., A. Moreno-Herrera, R. Reyes-Olivares, E. Dorantes-Gonzalez, B. Nogueda-Torres, E.A.G. de Oliveira et al. 2017. Synthesis, biological evaluation and molecular docking of new benzenesulfonylhydrazone as potential anti-*Trypanosoma cruzi* agents. Med. Chem. 13: 149–158.

Eperon, G., M. Balasegaram, J. Potet, C. Mowbray, O. Valverde and F. Chappuis. 2014. Treatment options for second-stage gambiense human African trypanosomiasis. Expert. Rev. Anti. Infect. Ther. England. 12: 1407–1417.

Faerman, C.H., S.N. Savvides, C. Strickland, M.A. Breidenbach, J.A. Ponasik, B. Ganem et al. 1996. Charge is the major discriminating factor for glutathione reductase versus trypanothione reductase inhibitors. Bioorg. Med. Chem. 4: 1247–1253.

Fairlamb, A.H. and A. Cerami. 1992. Metabolism and functions of trypanothione in the Kinetoplastida. Annu. Rev. Microbiol. 46: 695–729.

Fairlamb, A.H. and D. Horn. 2018. Melarsoprol resistance in African trypanosomiasis. Trends Parasitol. 34: 481–492.

Feasey, N., M. Wansbrough-Jones, D.C.W. Mabey and A.W. Solomon. 2010. Neglected tropical diseases. Br. Med. Bull. England. 93: 179–200.

Ferrari, S., F. Morandi, D. Motiejunas, E. Nerini, S. Henrich, R. Luciani et al. 2011. Virtual screening identification of nonfolate compounds, including a CNS drug, as antiparasitic agents inhibiting pteridine reductase. J. Med. Chem. 54: 211–221.

Ferreira, L.G. and A.D. Andricopulo. 2017. Targeting cysteine proteases in trypanosomatid disease drug discovery. Pharmacol. Ther. 180: 49–61.

Ferreira, R.S., A. Simeonov, A. Jadhav, O. Eidam, B.T. Mott, M.J. Keiser et al. 2010. Complementarity between a docking and a high-throughput screen in discovering new cruzain inhibitors. J. Med. Chem. 53: 4891–4905.

Ferreira de Almeida Fuiza, L., R.B. Peres, M.R. Simões-Silva, P.B. da Silva, D. da Gama Jaen Batista, C. da Silva et al. 2018. Identification of Pyrazolo[3,4-e][1,4]thiazepin based CYP51 inhibitors as potential Chagas disease therapeutic alternative: *In vitro* and *in vivo* evaluation, binding mode prediction and SAR exploration. Eur. J. Med. Chem. 149: 257–268.

Ferrins, L., M. Gazdik, R. Rahmani, S. Varghese, M.L. Sykes, A.J. Jones et al. 2014. Pyridyl benzamides as a novel class of potent inhibitors for the kinetoplastid *Trypanosoma brucei*. J. Med. Chem. 57: 6393–6402.

Field, M.C., D. Horn, A.H. Fairlamb, M.A. Ferguson, D.W. Gray, K.D. Read et al. 2017. Anti-trypanosomatid drug discovery: an ongoing challenge and a continuing need. Nat. Rev. Microbiol. 15(4): 217–31.

Filardy, A.A., K. Guimaraes-Pinto, M.P. Nunes, K. Zukeram, L. Fliess L. Pereira et al. 2018. Human kinetoplastid protozoan infections: Where Are We Going Next? Front Immunol. Switzerland. 9: 1493.

Filho, G.B.O., M.V.O. Cardoso, J.W.P. Espíndola, D.A.O. Silva, R.S. Ferreira, P.L. Coelho et al. 2017. Structural design, synthesis and pharmacological evaluation of thiazoles against *Trypanosoma cruzi*. Eur. J. Med. Chem. 141: 346–361.

Francisco, A.F., M.D. Lewis, S. Jayawardhana, M.C. Taylor, E. Chatelain and J.M. Kelly. 2015. Limited ability of posaconazole to cure both acute and chronic *Trypanosoma cruzi* infections revealed by highly sensitive *in vivo* imaging. Antimicrob. Agents. Chemother. 59(8): 4653–61.

Frearson, J.A., P.G. Wyatt, I.H. Gilbert and A.H. Fairlamb. 2007. Target assessment for antiparasitic drug discovery. Trends Parasitol. 23: 589–595.

Friggeri, L., L. Scipione, R. Costi, M. Kaiser, F. Moraca, C. Zamperini et al. 2013. New promising compounds with *in vitro* nanomolar activity against *Trypanosoma cruzi*. ACS Med. Chem. Lett. 4(6): 538–541.

Friggeri, L., T.Y. Hargrove, G. Rachakonda, A.D. Williams, Z. Wawrzak, R. Di Santo et al. 2014. Structural basis for rational design of inhibitors targeting *Trypanosoma cruzi* sterol 14α-demethylase: two regions of the enzyme molecule potentiate its inhibition. J. Med. Chem. 57(15): 6704–6717.

Fytas, C., G. Zoidis, N. Tzoutzas, M.C. Taylor, G. Fytas and J.M. Kelly. 2011. Novel lipophilic acetohydroxamic acid derivatives based on conformationally constrained spiro carbocyclic 2,6-diketopiperazine scaffolds with potent trypanocidal activity. J. Med. Chem. 54: 5250–5254.

Gilbert, I.H. 2013. Drug discovery for neglected diseases: molecular target-based and phenotypic approaches: Miniperspectives series on phenotypic screening for antiinfective targets. J. Med. Chem. American Chemical Society. 56: 7719–7726.

Giordani, F., L.J. Morrison, T.G. Rowan, H.P. De Koning and M.P. Barrett. 2016. The animal trypanosomiasis and their chemotherapy: a review. Parasitology. 143: 1862–1889.

Giroud, C., F. Ottones, V. Coustou, D. Dacheux, N. Biteau, B. Miezan et al. 2009. Murine models for *Trypanosoma brucei gambiense* disease progression—from silent to chronic infections and early brain tropism. PLoS Negl. Trop. Dis. 3(9): e509.

Giroud, M., U. Dietzel, L. Anselm, D. Banner, A. Kuglstatter, J. Benz et al. 2018. Repurposing a library of human cathepsin L ligands: Identification of macrocyclic lactams as potent rhodesain and *Trypanosoma brucei* inhibitors. J. Med. Chem. 61: 3350–3369.

González-Chávez, Z., V. Olin-Sandoval, J.S. Rodíguez-Zavala, R. Moreno-Sánchez and E. Saavedra. 2015. Metabolic control analysis of the *Trypanosoma cruzi* peroxide detoxification pathway identifies tryparedoxin as a suitable drug target. Biochim. Biophys. Acta. 1850: 263–273.

Guedes, P.M.M., G.K Silva, F.R.S. Gutierrez and J.S. Silva. 2011. Current status of Chagas disease chemotherapy. Expert. Rev. Anti Infect. Ther. 9: 609–620.

Gunatilleke, S.S., C.M. Calvet, J.B. Johnston, C.-K. Chen, G. Erenburg, J. Gut et al. 2012. Diverse inhibitor chemotypes targeting *Trypanosoma cruzi* CYP51. PLoS Negl. Trop. Dis. 6(7): e1736.

Haasen, D., U. Schopfer, C. Antczak, C. Guy, F. Fuchs and P. Selzer. 2017. How phenotypic screening influenced drug discovery: Lessons from five years of practice. Assay Drug Dev Technol. United States. 15: 239–246.

Hargrove, T.Y., Z. Wawrzak, P.W. Alexander, J.H. Chaplin, M. Keenan, S.A. Charman et al. 2013. Complexes of *Trypanosoma cruzi* sterol 14α-demethylase (CYP51) with two pyridine-based drug candidates for Chagas disease: structural basis for pathogen selectivity. J. Biol. Chem. 288(44): 31602–31615.

Hartmann, A.P., M.R. de Carvalho, L.S.C. Bernandes, M.H. de Moraes, E.B. de Melo, C.D. Lopes et al. 2017. Synthesis and 2D-QSAR studies of neolignan-based diaryl-tetrahydrofuran and -furan analogues with remarkable activity against *Trypanosoma cruzi* and assessment of the trypanothione reductase activity. Eur. J. Med. Chem. 140: 187–199.

Hawser, S., S. Lociuro and K. Islam. 2006. Dihydrofolate reductase inhibitors as antibacterial agents. Biochem. Pharmacol. 71(7): 941–948.

Hiltensperger, G., N.G. Jones, S. Niedermeier, A. Stich, M. Kaiser, J. Jung et al. 2012. Synthesis and structure-activity relationships of new quinolone-type molecules against *Trypanosoma brucei*. J. Med. Chem. 55: 2538–2548.

Hoekstra, W. J., T.Y. Hargrove, Z. Wawrzak, D. da Gama Jaen Batista, C.F. da Silva, A.S.G. Nefertiti et al. 2015. Clinical candidate VT-1161's antiparasitic effect *in vitro*, activity in a murine model of chagas disease, and structural characterization in complex with the target enzyme CYP51 from *Trypanosoma cruzi*. Antimicrob. Agents Chemother. 60(2): 1058–1066.

Hoelz, L.V.B., V.F. Leal, C.R. Rodrigues, P.G. Pascutti, M.G. Albuquerque, E.M.F. Muri et al. 2016. Molecular dynamics simulations of the free and inhibitor-bound cruzain systems in aqueous solvent: insights on the inhibition mechanism in acidic pH. J. Biomol. Struct. Dyn. 34: 1969–1978.

Hwang, J.Y., D. Smithson, M. Connelly, J. Maier, F. Zhu and K.R. Guy. 2010. Discovery of halo-nitrobenzamides with potential application against human African trypanosomiasis. Bioorg. Med. Chem. Lett. 20: 149–152.

Hwang, J.Y., D. Smithson, F. Zhu, G. Holbrook, M.C. Connelly, M. Kaiser et al. 2013a. Optimization of Chloronitrobenzamides (CNBs) as therapeutic leads for Human African Trypanosomiasis (HAT). J. Med. Chem. 56: 2850–2860.

Hwang, J.Y., D.C. Smithson, G. Holbrook, F. Zhu, M.C. Connelly, M. Kaiser et al. 2013b. Optimization of the electrophile of chloronitrobenzamide leads active against *Trypanosoma brucei*. Bioorg. Med. Chem. Lett. 23: 4127–4131.

Jacobs, R.T., B. Nare, S.A. Wring, M.D. Orr, D. Chen, J.M. Sligar et al. 2011. SCYX-7158, an orally-active benzoxaborole for the treatment of stage 2 human African trypanosomiasis. PLoS Negl. Trop. Dis. 5(6): e1151.

Jansen, C., H. Wang, A.J. Kooistra, C. de Graaf, K. Orrling, H. Tenor et al. 2013. Discovery of novel *Trypanosoma brucei* phosphodiesterase B1 inhibitors by virtual screening against the unliganded *Tbr*PDEB1 crystal structure. J. Med. Chem. 56: 2087–2096.

Jedwabny, W., J. Panecka-Hofman, E. Dyguda-Kazimierowicz, R.C. Wade, W.A. Sokalski. 2017. Application of a simple quantum chemical approach to ligand fragment scoring for *Trypanosoma brucei* pteridine reductase 1 inhibition. J. Comput. Aided Mol. Des. 31(8): 715–728.

Jennings, F.W., G.M. Urquhart, P.K. Murray and B.M. Miller. 1983. Treatment with suramin and 2-substituted 5-nitroimidazoles of chronic murine *Trypanosoma brucei* infections with central nervous system involvement. Trans. R Soc. Trop. Med. Hyg. 77(5): 693–8.

Jones, B.D., A. Tochowicz, Y. Tang, M.D. Cameron, L.-I. McCall, K. Hirata et al. 2015. Synthesis and evaluation of oxyguanidine analogues of the cysteine protease inhibitor WRR-483 against Cruzain. ACS Med. Chem. Lett. 7: 77–82.

Jones, A.J. and V.M. Avery. 2015. Future treatment options for human African trypanosomiasis. Expert Rev. Anti Infect. Ther. 13: 1429–1432.

Kelly, J.M., M.C. Taylor, D. Horn, E. Loza, I. Kalvinsh and F. Björkling. 2012. Inhibitors of human histone deacetylase with potent activity against the African trypanosome *Trypanosoma brucei*. Bioorg. Med. Chem. Lett. 22: 1886–1890.

Kennedy, P.G.E. 2013. Clinical features, diagnosis, and treatment of human African trypanosomiasis (sleeping sickness). Lancet Neurol. Elsevier Ltd. 12: 186–194.

Khalaf, A.I., J.K. Huggan, C.J. Suckling, C.L. Gibson, K. Stewart, F. Giordani et al. 2014. Structure-based design and synthesis of antiparasitic pyrrolopyrimidines targeting pteridine reductase 1. J. Med. Chem. 57(15): 6479–6494.

Khraiwesh, M.H., C.M. Lee, Y. Brandy, E.S. Akinboye, S. Berhe, G. Gittens et al. 2012. Antitrypanosomal activities and cytotoxicity of some novel imidosubstituted 1,4-Naphthoquinone derivatives. Arch. Pharm. Res. 35: 27–33.

Krieger, S., W. Schwarz, M.R. Ariyanayagam, A.H. Fairlamb, R.L. Krauth-Siegel and C. Clayton. 2000. Trypanosomes lacking trypanothione reductase are avirulent and show increased sensitivity to oxidative stress. Mol. Microbiol. 35: 542–552.

Lass-Flörl, C. 2011. Triazole antifungal agents in invasive fungal infections: a comparative review. Drugs. 71(18): 2405–2419.

Lee, K.M. and P.C. Fan. 1980. Experimental transmission of *Trypanosoma gambiense* by syringe passage from albino-mouse to mice, rats, gerbil and hamster. Int. J. Zoonoses. 7(2): 142–149.

Lepesheva, G.I. and M.R. Waterman. 2004. CYP51—the omnipotent P450. Mol. Cell. Endocrinol. 215(1-2): 165–170.

Lepesheva, G.I. and M.R. Waterman. 2007. Sterol 14alpha-demethylase cytochrome P450 (CYP51), a P450 in all biological kingdoms. Biochim. Biophys. Acta. 1770(3): 467–477.

Lepesheva, G.I., H.-W. Park, T.Y. Hargrove, B. Vanhollebeke, Z. Wawrzak, J.M. Harp et al. 2010. Crystal structures of *Trypanosoma brucei* sterol 14alpha-demethylase and implications for selective treatment of human infections. J. Biol. Chem. 285: 1773–1780.

Lepesheva, G.I., T.Y. Hargrove, G. Rachakonda, Z. Wawrzak, S. Pomel, S. Cojean et al. 2015. VFV as a new effective CYP51 structure-derived drug candidate for chagas disease and visceral leishmaniasis. J. Infect. Dis. 212(9): 1439–1448.

Lepesheva, G.I., L. Friggeri and M.R. Waterman. 2018. CYP51 as drug targets for fungi and protozoan parasites: past, present and future. Parasitology. 1–17.

Leroux, A.E. and R.L. Krauth-Siegel. 2016. Thiol redox biology of trypanosomatids and potential targets for chemotherapy. Mol. Biochem. Parasitol. 206: 67–74.

Lewis, M.D., A.F. Francisco, M.C. Taylor and J.M. Kelly. 2015. A new experimental model for assessing drug efficacy against *Trypanosoma cruzi* infection based on highly sensitive *in vivo* imaging. J. Biomol. Screen. 20(1): 36–43.

Liese, B., M. Rosenberg and A. Schratz. 2010. Programmes, partnerships, and governance for elimination and control of neglected tropical diseases. Lancet. 375: 67–76.

Linciano, P., A. Dawson, I. Pöhner, D.M. Costa, M.S. Sá, A. Cordeiro-da-Silva et al. 2017. Exploiting the 2-Amino-1,3,4-thiadiazole scaffold to inhibit *Trypanosoma brucei* pteridine reductase in support of early-stage drug discovery. ACS Omega. 2: 5666–5683.

Marinho, C.R., D.Z. Bucci, M.L. Dagli, K.R. Bastos, M.G. Grisotto, L.R. Sardinha et al. 2004. Pathology affects different organs in two mouse strains chronically infected by a *Trypanosoma cruzi* clone: A model for genetic studies of Chagas' disease. Infect. Immun. 72(4): 2350–7.

Marinho, C.R., L.N. Nunez-Apaza, K.R. Bortoluci, A.L. Bombeiro, D.Z. Bucci, M.G. Grisotto et al. 2009. Infection by the Sylvio X10/4 clone of *Trypanosoma cruzi*: relevance of a low-virulence model of Chagas' disease. Microbes Infect. 11(13): 1037–45.

Martins, L.C., P.H.M. Torres, R.B. de Oliveira, P.G. Pascutti, E.A. Cino, R.S. Ferreira. 2018. Investigation of the binding mode of a novel cruzain inhibitor by docking, molecular dynamics, *ab initio* and MM/PBSA calculations. J. Comput. Aided Mol. Des. 32: 591–605.

McLatchie, A.P., H. Burrell-Saward, E. Myburgh, M.D. Lewis, T.H. Ward, J.C. Mottram et al. 2013. Highly sensitive *in vivo* imaging of *Trypanosoma brucei* expressing "red-shifted" luciferase. PLoS Negl. Trop. Dis. 7(11): e2571.

Mendoza-Martínez, C., J. Correa-Basurto, R. Nieto-Meneses, A. Márquez-Navarro, R. Aguilar-Suárez, M.D. Montero-Cortes et al. 2015. Design, synthesis and biological evaluation of quinazoline derivatives as anti-trypanosomatid and anti-plasmodial agents. Eur. J. Med. Chem. 96: 296–307.

Mesu, V.K.B.K., W.M. Kalonji, C. Bardonneau, O.V. Mordt, S. Blesson, F. Simon et al. 2018. Oral fexinidazole for late-stage African *Trypanosoma brucei* gambiense trypanosomiasis: a pivotal multicentre, randomised, non-inferiority trial. Lancet. 391(10116): 144–54.

MMV Medicines for Malaria Venture. 2018. Developing antimalarials to save lives. https://www.mmv.org/.

Molina, I., F. Salvador and A. Sanchez-Montalva. 2015. The use of posaconazole against Chagas disease. Curr. Opin. Infect. Dis. 28(5): 397–407.

Montalvo-Quirós, S., A. Taladriz-Sender, M. Kaiser and C. Dardonville. 2015. Antiprotozoal activity and DNA binding of dicationic acridones. J. Med. Chem. 58: 1940–1949.

Mpamhanga, C.P., D. Spinks, L.B. Tulloch, E.J. Shanks, D.A. Robinson, I.T. Collie et al. 2009. One scaffold, three binding modes: Novel and selective pteridine reductase 1 inhibitors derived from fragment hits discovered by virtual screening. J. Med. Chem. 52(14): 4454–4465.

Muchiri, M.W., K. Ndung'u, J.K. Kibugu, J.K. Thuita, P.K. Gitonga, G.N. Ngae et al. 2015. Comparative pathogenicity of *Trypanosoma brucei rhodesiense* strains in Swiss white mice and *Mastomys natalensis* rats. Acta Trop. 150: 23–8.

Muscia, G.C., S.I. Cazorla, F.M. Frank, G.L. Borosky, G.Y. Buldain, S.E. Asís et al. 2011. Synthesis, trypanocidal activity and molecular modeling studies of 2-alkylaminomethylquinoline derivatives. Eur. J. Med. Chem. 46: 3696–3703.

Njiokou, F., H. Nimpaye, G. Simo et al. 2010. Domestic animals as potential reservoir hosts of *Trypanosoma brucei* gambiense in sleeping sickness foci in Cameroon. Parasite. 17: 61–66.

Ochiana, S.O., A. Gustafson, N. Bland, C. Wang, M.J. Russo, R.K. Campbell et al. 2012. Synthesis and evaluation of human phosphodiesterases (PDE) 5 inhibitor analogs as trypanosomal PDE inhibitors. Part 2. Tadalafil analogs. Bioorg. Med. Chem. Lett. 22: 2582–2584.

Olin-Sandoval, V., Z. González-Chávez, M. Berzunza-Cruz, I. Martínez, R. Jasso-Chávez, I. Becker et al. 2012. Drug target validation of the trypanothione pathway enzymes through metabolic modelling. FEBS J. 279: 1811–1833.

Okello, A.L., K. Bardosh, J. Smith and S.C. Welburn. 2014. One health: Past successes and future challenges in three African contexts. PLoS Negl. Trop. Dis. 8: 1–7.

Ong, H.B., N. Sienkiewicz, S. Wyllie and A.H. Fairlamb. 2011. Dissecting the metabolic roles of pteridine reductase 1 in *Trypanosoma brucei* and *Leishmania major*. J. Biol. Chem. 286(12): 10429–10438.

Orrling, K.M., C.X.L. Jansen Jansen, V. Balmer, P. Bregy, A. Shanmugham, P. England et al. 2012. Catechol pyrazolinones as trypanocidals: fragment-based, synthesis, and pharmacological evaluation of nanomolar inhibitors of trypanosomal phosphodiesterase B1. J. Med. Chem. 55: 8745–8756.

Palos, I., E.E. Lara-Ramirez, J.C. Lopez-Cedillo, C. Garcia-Perez, M. Kashif, V. Bocanegra-Garcia et al. 2017. Repositioning FDA drugs as potential cruzain inhibitors from *Trypanosoma cruzi*: Virtual screening, *in vitro* and *in vivo* studies. Molecules. 22: E1015.

Pan, D., Y. Tseng and A.J. Hopfinger. 2003. Quantitative structure-based design: formalism and application of receptor-dependent RD-4D-QSAR analysis to a set of glucose analogue inhibitors of glycogen phosphorylase. J. Chem. Inf. Comput. Sci. 43: 1591–1607.

Panecka-Hofman, J., I. Pöhner, F. Spyrakis, T. Zeppelin, F. Di Pisa, L. Dello Iacono et al. 2017. Comparative mapping of on-targets and off-targets for the discovery of anti-trypanosomatid folate pathway inhibitors. Biochim. Biophys. Acta. 1861: 3215–3230.

Papadopoulou, M.V., W.D. Bloomer, H.S. Rosenzweig and M. Kaiser. 2017. The antitrypanosomal and antitubercular activity of some nitro(triazole/imidazole)-based aromatic amines. Eur. J. Med. Chem. 138: 1106–1113.

Patel, G., C.E. Karver, R. Behera, P.J. Guyett, C. Sullenberger, P. Edwards et al. 2013. Kinase scaffold repurposing for neglected disease drug discovery: Discovery of an efficacious, Lapatanib-derived lead compound for trypanosomiasis. J. Med. Chem. 56: 3820–3832.

Patrick, D.A., T. Wenzler, S. Yang, P.T. Weiser, M.Z. Wang, R. Brun et al. 2016. Synthesis of novel amide and urea derivatives of thiazol-2-ethylamines and their activity against *Trypanosoma brucei rhodesiense*. Bioorg. Med. Chem. 24: 2451–2465.

Patrick, D.A., J.R. Gillespie, J. McQueen, M.A. Hulverson, R.M. Ranade, S.A. Creason et al. 2017. Urea derivatives of 2-aryl-benzothiazol-5-amines: A new class of potential drugs for human African trypanosomiasis. J. Med. Chem. 60: 957–971.

Patterson, S., M.S. Alphey, D.C. Jones, E.J. Shanks, I.P. Street, J.A. Frearson et al. 2011. Dihydroquinazolines as a novel class of *Trypanosoma brucei* trypanothione reductase inhibitors: Discovery, synthesis, and characterization of their binding mode by protein crystallography. J. Med. Chem. 54: 6514–6530.

Pauli, I., L.G. Ferreira, M.L. de Souza, G. Oliva, R.S. Ferreira, M.A. Dessoy et al. 2017. Molecular modeling and structure-activity relationships for a series of benzimidazole derivatives as cruzain inhibitors. Future Med. Chem. 9: 641–657.

Pérez-Molina, J.A. and I. Molina. 2018. Chagas disease. Lancet. 391: 82–94.

Persch, E., S. Bryson, N.K. Todoroff, C. Eberle, J. Thelemann, N. Dirdjaja et al. 2014. Binding to large enzyme pockets: small-molecule inhibitors of trypanothione reductase. ChemMedChem. 9: 1880–1891.

Pierce, R.J., J. MacDougall, R. Leurs and M.P. Costi. 2017. The future of drug development for neglected tropical diseases: How the European commission can continue to make a difference. Trends Parasitol. Elsevier Ltd. 33: 581–583.

Price, H.P., M.R. Menon, C. Panethymitaki, D. Goulding, P.G. McKean and D.F. Smith. 2003. Myristoyl-CoA:protein N-myristoyl-transferase, an essential enzyme and potential drug target in kinetoplastid parasites. J. Biol. Chem. 278: 7206–7214.

Priotto, G., S. Kasparian, W. Mutombo, D. Ngouama, S. Ghorashian, U. Arnold et al. 2009. Nifurtimox-eflornithine combination therapy for second-stage African *Trypanosoma brucei gambiense* trypanosomiasis: a multicentre, randomised, phase III, non-inferiority trial. Lancet (London, England). England. 374: 56–64.

Rahmani, R., K. Ban, A.J. Jones, L. Ferrins, D. Ganame, M.L. Sykes et al. 2015. 6-Arylpyrazine-2-carboxamides: A new core for *Trypanosoma brucei* inhibitors. J. Med. Chem. 58: 6753–6765.

Reid, C.S., D.A. Patrick, S. He, J. Fotie, K. Premalatha, R.R. Tidwell et al. 2011. Synthesis and antitrypanosomal evaluation of derivatives of N-benzyl-1,2-dihydroquinolin-6-ols: Effect of core substitutions and salt formation. Bioorg. Med. Chem. 19: 513–523.

Rodriques Coura, J. and S.L. de Castro. 2002. A critical review on Chagas disease chemotherapy. Mem. Inst. Oswaldo Cruz. Brazil. 97: 3–24.

Rodrigues, R.F., D. Castro-Pinto, A. Echevarria, C.M. dos Reis, C.N. Del Cistia, C.M. Sant'Anna et al. 2012. Investigation of trypanothione reductase inhibitory activity by 1,3,4-thiadiazolium-2-aminide derivatives and molecular docking studies. Bioorg. Med. Chem. 20: 1760–1766.

Romanha, A.J., S.L. Castro, N. Soeiro Mde, J. Lannes-Vieira, I. Ribeiro, A. Talvani et al. 2010. *In vitro* and *in vivo* experimental models for drug screening and development for Chagas disease. Mem. Inst. Oswaldo Cruz. 105(2): 233–8.

Russell, S., R. Rahmani, A.J. Jones, H.L. Newson, K. Neilde, I. Cotillo et al. 2016. Hit-to-lead optimization of a novel class of potent, broad-spectrum trypanosomacides. J. Med. Chem. 59: 9686–9720.

Samant, B.S. and C. Chakaingesu. 2013. Novel naphthoquinone derivatives: Synthesis and activity against human African trypanosomiasis. Bioorg. Med. Chem. Lett. 23: 1420–1423.

Sánchez-Moreno, M., C. Marín, P. Navarro, L. Lamarque, E. García-España, C. Miranda et al. 2012. *In vitro* and *in vivo* trypanosomicidal activity of pyrazole-containing macrocyclic and macrobicyclic polyamines: Their action on acute and chronic phases of Chagas disease. J. Med. Chem. 55: 4231–4243.

Sands, M., M.A. Kron and R.B. Brown. 1985. Pentamidine: a review. Rev Infect Dis. United States. 7: 625–63.

Schirmeister, T., J. Schmitz, S. Jung, T. Schmenger, R.L. Krauth-Siegel and M. Gütschow. 2017. Evaluation of dipeptide nitriles as inhibitors of rhodesain, a major cysteine protease of *Trypanosoma brucei*. Bioorg. Med. Chem. Lett. 27: 45–50.

Schormann, N., B. Pal, O. Senkovich, M. Carson, A. Howard, C. Smith et al. 2005. Crystal structure of *Trypanosoma cruzi* pteridine reductase 2 in complex with a substrate and an inhibitor. J. Struct. Biol. 152: 64–75.

Schormann, N., O. Senkovich, K. Walker, D.L. Wright, A.C. Anderson, A. Rosowsky et al. 2008. Structure-based approach to pharmacophore identification, *in silico* screening, and three-dimensional quantitative structure-activity relationship studies for inhibitors of *Trypanosoma cruzi* dihydrofolate reductase function. Proteins. 73: 889–901.

Schormann, N., S.E. Velu, S. Murugesan, O. Senkovich, K. Walker, B.C. Chenna et al. 2010. Synthesis and characterization of potent inhibitors of *Trypanosoma cruzi* dihydrofolate reductase. Bioorg. Med. Chem. 18: 4056–4066.

Setzer, W.N. and I.V. Ogungbe. 2012. *In-silico* investigation of antitrypanosomal phytochemicals from Nigerian medicinal plants. PLoS Negl. Trop. Dis. 6(7): e1727.

Shuvalov, O., A. Petukhov, A. Daks, O. Fedorova, E. Vasileva, N.A. Barlev. 2017. One-carbon metabolism and nucleotide biosynthesis as attractive targets for anticancer therapy. Oncotarget. 8(14): 23955–23977.

Sienkiewicz, N., H.B. Ong and A.H. Fairlamb. 2010. *Trypanosoma brucei* pteridine reductase 1 is essential for survival *in vitro* and for virulence in mice. Mol. Microbiol. 77(3): 658–671.

Silva, D.G., J.R. Rocha, G.R. Sartori and C.A. Montanari. 2017a. Highly predictive hologram QSAR models of nitrile-containing cruzain inhibitors. J. Biomol. Struct. Dyn. 35: 3232–3249.

Silva, E.B., D.A.O. Silva, A.R. Oliveira, C.H.S. Mendes, T.A.R. dos Santos, A.C. da Silva et al. 2017b. Desing and synthesis of potent anti-*Trypanosoma cruzi* agents new thiazoles derivatives which induce apoptotic parasite death. Eur. J. Med. Chem. 130: 39–50.

Silva-Júnior, E.F., E.P.S. Silva, P.H.B. França, J.P.N. Silva, E.O. Barreto, E.B. Silva et al. 2016. Design, synthesis, molecular docking and biological evaluation of thiophen-2-iminothiazolidine derivatives for use against *Trypanosoma cruzi*. Bioorg. Med. Chem. 24: 4228–4240.

Simarro, P.P., G. Cecchi, J.R. Franco et al. 2012. Estimating and mapping the population at risk of sleeping sickness. PLoS Negl. Trop. Dis. 6: e1859

Spinks, D., H.B. Ong, C.P. Mpamhanga, E.J. Shanks, D.A. Robinson, I.T. Collie et al. 2011. Design, synthesis and biological evaluation of novel inhibitors of *Trypanosoma brucei* pteridine reductase 1. ChemMedChem. 6: 302–308.

Stank, A., D.B. Kohk, M. Horn, E. Sizikova, R. Neil, J. Panecka et al. 2017. TRAPP webserver: predicting protein binding site flexibility and detecting transient binding pockets. Nucleic Acids Res. 45: W325–W330.

Suryadevara, P.K., K.K. Racherla, S. Olepu, N.R. Norcross, H.B. Tatipaka, J.A. Arif et al. 2013. Dialkylimidazole inhibitors of *Trypanosoma cruzi* sterol 14α-demethylase as anti-Chagas disease agents. Bioorg. Med. Chem. Lett. 23: 6492–6499.

Tagoe, D.N.A., T.D. Kalejaiye and H.P. de Koning. 2015. The ever unfolding story of cAMP signaling in tryptrypanosoma: vive la difference! Front. Pharmacol. 6: 185.

Tapia, R.A., C.O. Salas, K. Vázquez, C. Espinosa-Bustos, J. Soto-Delgado, J. Varela et al. 2014. Synthesis and biological characterization of new aryloxyindole-4,9-diones as potent trypanosomicidal agents. Bioorg. Med. Chem. Lett. 24: 3919–3922.

Thompson, A.M., A. Blaser, B.D. Palmer, R.F. Anderson, S.S. Shinde, D. Launay et al. 2017. 6-Nitro-2,3-dihydroimidazo[2,1-b][1,3]thiazoles: Facile synthesis and comparative appraisal against tuberculosis and neglected tropical diseases. Bioorg. Med. Chem. Lett. 27: 2583–2589.

Torres, E., E. Moreno-Viguri, S. Galiano, G. Devarapally, P.W. Crawford, A. Azqueta et al. 2013. Novel quinoxaline 1,4-di-N-oxide derivatives as new potential antichagasic agents. Eur. J. Med. Chem. 66: 324–334.

Torrie, L.S., S. Wyllie, D. Spinks, S.L. Oza, S. Thompson, J.R. Harrison et al. 2009. Chemical validation of trypanothione synthetase. J. Biol. Chem. 284: 36137–36145.

Trouiller, P., E. Olliaro, J. Torreele, R. Orbinski and Laing, N. Ford. 2002. Drug development for neglected diseases: a deficient market and a public-health policy failure, Lancet (London, England). 359: 2188–94.

Tulloch, L.B., V.P. Martini, J. Iulek, J.K. Huggan, J.H. Lee, C.L. Gibson et al. 2010. Structure-based design of pteridine reductase inhibitors targeting African sleeping sickness and the leishmaniases. J. Med. Chem. 53(1): 221–229.

Upadhayaya, R.S., S.S. Dixit, A. Földesi and J. Chattopadhyaya. 2013. New antiprotozoal agents: Their synthesis and biological evaluations. Bioorg. Med. Chem. Lett. 23: 2750–2758.

Vázquez, C., M. Mejia-Tlachi, Z. González-Chávez, A. Silva, J.S. Rodríguez-Zavala, R. Moreno-Sánchez et al. 2017. Buthionine sulfoximine is a multitarget inhibitor of trypanothione synthesis in *Trypanosoma cruzi*. FEBS Lett. 591: 3881–3894.

Vázquez, K., C. Espinosa-Bustos, J. Soto-Delgado, R.A. Tapia, J. Varela, E. Birriel et al. 2015. New aryloxy-quinone derivatives as potential Anti-Chagasic agents: Synthesis, trypanosomicidal activity, electrochemical properties, pharmacophore elucidation and 3D-QSAR analysis. RSC Adv. 5: 65153–65166.

Vega, M.C., M. Rolón, A. Montero-Torres, C. Fonseca-Berzal, J.A. Escario, A. Gómez-Barrio et al. 2012. Synthesis, biological evaluation and chemometric analysis of indazole derivatives. 1,2-disubstituted 5-nitroindazolinones, new prototypes of antichagasic drug. Eur. J. Med. Chem. 58: 214–227.

Vickers, T.J. and S.M. Beverley. 2011. Folate metabolic pathways in Leishmania. Essays Biochem. 51: 63–80.

Viera, D.F., J.Y. Choi, C.M. Calvet, J.L. Siqueira-Neto, J.B. Johnston, D. Kellar et al. 2014a. Binding mode and potency of N-Indolyloxopyridinyl-4-aminopropanyl-based inhibitors targeting *Trypanosoma cruzi* CYP51. J. Med. Chem. 57(23): 10162–10175.

Viera, D.F., J.Y. Choi, W.R. Roush and L.M. Podust. 2014b. Expanding the binding envelope of CYP51 inhibitors targeting *Trypanosoma cruzi* with 4-aminopyridyl-based sulfonamide derivatives. ChemBioChem. 15(8): 1111–1120.

Villalta, F., M.C. Dobish, P.N. Nde, Y.Y. Kleshchenko, T.Y. Hargrove, C.A. Johnson et al. 2013. VNI cures acute and chronic experimental Chagas disease. J. Infect. Dis. 208(3): 504–511.

Wang, C., T.D. Ashton, A. Gustafson, N.D. Bland, S.O. Ochiana, R.K. Campbell et al. 2012. Synthesis and evaluation of human phosphodiesterases (PDE) 5 inhibitor analogs as trypanosomal PDE inhibitors. 1. Sildenafil analogs. Bioorg. Med. Chem. Lett. 22: 2579–2581.

Wermuth, C., D. Aldous, P. Raboisson and D. Rognan. 2015. The practice of medicinal chemistry. 4th edition.

WHO. 2010. Chagas disease: epidemiology. http://www.who.int/chagas/epidemiology/en/.

WHO. 2017. Human African trypanosomiasis: epidemiological situation. http://www.who.int/trypanosomiasis_african/country/en/.

Weiss, M.G. 2008. Stigma and the social burden of neglected tropical diseases. PLoS Negl. Trop. Dis. Public Library of Science. 2: e237.

Wiggers, H.J., J.R. Rocha, W.B. Fernandes, R. Sesti-Costa, Z.A. Carneiro, J. Cheleski et al. 2013. Non-peptidic cruzain inhibitors with trypanocidal activity discovered by virtual screening and *in vitro* assay. PLoS Negl. Trop. Dis. 7: e2370.

Wilcken, R., M.O. Zimmermann, A. Lange, A.C. Joerger and F.M. Boeckler. 2013. Principles and applications of halogen bonding in medicinal chemistry and chemical biology. J. Med. Chem. 56(4): 1363–1388.

Woodring, J.L., N.D. Bland, S.O. Ochiana, R.K. Campbell and M.P. Pollastri. 2013. Synthesis and assessment of catechol diether compounds as inhibitors of trypanosomal phosphodiesterase B1 (*Tbr*PDEB1). Bioorg. Med. Chem. Lett. 23: 5971–5974.

Yu, X., V. Cojocaru, G. Mustafa, O.M.H. Salo-Ahen, G.L. Lepesheva and R.C. Wade. 2015. Dynamics of CYP51: implications for function and inhibitor design. J. Mol. Recognit. 28(2): 59–73.

Yu, X., P. Nandekar, G. Mustafa, V. Cojocaru, G.L. Lepesheva and R.C. Wade. 2016. Ligand tunnels in *T. brucei* and human CYP51: Insights for parasite-specific drug design. Biochim. Biophys. Acta. 1860(1): 67–78.

Yuthavong, Y., J. Yuvaniyama, P. Chitnumsub, J. Vanichtanankul, S. Chusacultanachai, B. Tarnchompoo et al. 2005. Malarial (*Plasmodium falciparum*) dihydrofolate reductase-thymidylate synthase: structural basis for antifolate resistance and development of effective inhibitors. Parasitology. 130(3): 249–259.

Zelisko, N., D. Atamanyuk, O. Vasylenko, P. Grellier and R. Lesyk. 2012. Synthesis and antitrypanosomal activity of new 6,6,7-trisubstituted thiopyrano[2,3-d][1,3]thiazoles. Bioorg. Med. Chem. Lett. 22: 7071–7074.

Zuccotto, F., R. Brun, D. Gonzalez Pacanowska, L.M. Ruiz Perez and I.H. Gilbert. 1999. The structure-based design and synthesis of selective inhibitors of *Trypanosoma cruzi* dihydrofolate reductase. Bioorg. Med. Chem. Lett. 9: 1463–1468.

Chapter **11**

New Chemical Scaffolds to Selectively Target the Trypanothione Metabolism

Andrea Ilari* and Gianni Colotti*

Introduction

Leishmaniasis, Chagas disease and sleeping sickness are poverty-related diseases characterized by high morbidity deeply linked to malnutrition, complex humanitarian emergencies and environmental changes that affect vector biology. Leishmaniases and trypanosomiases-related disabilities impose a great social burden, especially for women, impair economic productivity and impede social development. Leishmaniasis is widespread in 22 countries in the New World and in 66 nations in the Old World and endemic regions have been spreading further over the last 10 yr with a sharp increase in the number of recorded cases. Two million new cases are estimated to occur annually, with an estimated 12 million people presently infected worldwide (World Health Organization 2016). Chagas disease affects about 8 million people in Latin America, of whom 30–40% either have or will develop cardiomyopathy, digestive megasyndromes, or both. Human African Trypanosomiasis (HAT), also known as sleeping sickness, leads to a debilitating and progressive neurological disease that includes sleep disorders, coma and death in all untreated individuals (Boelaert et al. 2010). This killer disease is endemic to several countries, putting millions of people at risk with around 12,000 people infected every year (Barrett et al. 2007, Barrett and Croft 2012). Despite these figures, the therapy of infectious diseases caused by protozoan parasites of the trypanosomatid family is a neglected area of research and drug development.

Treatment of these diseases is unsatisfactory in terms of safety and efficacy, which sharply contrasts with the therapeutic need in terms of people at risk, number of affected patients, and associated fatalities. This discrepancy is primarily due to the prevalence of these diseases in tropical and subtropical poor countries with little research capacities.

As a consequence, efficacious new drugs have not been developed, and available ones (Table 1) still comprise toxic arsenicals (melarsoprol, **1**) used to treat the second stage of the African trypanosomiasis, antimony-containing compounds (Glucantime, **2** and Pentostam, **3**) used against Leishmaniasis (Frezard et al. 2009, Haldar et al. 2011) and Nifurtimox (**4**), a 5-nitrofuran which came into medication use in 1965, against Chagas Disease. However, the number of drugs used against these diseases has been enriched by other compounds originally developed for different pathologies such as eflornithine (α-difluoromethylornithine,

Istituto di Biologia e Patologia Molecolari, Consiglio Nazionale delle Ricerche (IBPM-CNR), Dipartimento di Scienze Biochimiche, "Sapienza" Università di Roma., P.le A. Moro, 5, 00185 Rome, Italy.
* Corresponding authors: andrea.ilari@uniroma1.it; gianni.colotti@uniroma1.it

Table 1. Structures of drugs used against trypanosomatids. The table reports the number used in the paper, name and chemical structure of each compound.

Compound	Chemical structure	Target
1: Melarsoprol		Thiol-containing enzymes
2: Meglumine antimoniate (Glucantime)		TR and other thiol-containing enzymes
3: Sodium stibogluconate (Pentostam)		TR and other thiol-containing enzymes
4: Nifurtimox		Nucleic acids
5: α-difluoromethylornithine (DFMO)		Ornithine decarboxylase
6: Miltefosine		Interaction with lipids, inhibition of cytochrome c oxidase
7: Amphotericin B		Binding of ergosterol
8: Paromomycin		Binding of 16S ribosomal RNA: protein synthesis inhibition

or DFMO, **5**) and miltefosine (**6**) that originally were developed for cancer therapy, used against Sleeping Sickness and visceral leishmaniasis (VL), amphotericin B (AmB, **7**), a polyene antifungal drug now used against VL, and paromomycin (**8**), an antiprotozoal antibiotic used against VL (Chawla et al. 2011, Vincent et al. 2010, Freitas-Junior et al. 2012, Hotez et al. 2007, 2004, Rassi et al. 2010) (Table 1).

Different approaches have been used in order to shorten courses of therapy, reduce toxicities through lower dosage and diminish the selection of resistant mutations (Ouellette et al. 2004). For HAT, the only advances in treatment over the past two decades have been the introduction of an eflornithine/nifurtimox co-administration (Barrett and Croft 2012). For VL, the use of liposomes to deliver AmB directly to macrophage has drastically reduced the toxicity of this drug (Davidson et al. 1991, Moore and Lockwood 2010). The major goal of drug discovery in this neglected field is the development of lead compounds specifically targeting unique metabolic pathways of trypanosomatids, capitalizing on the sequencing of several species, including *L. major*, *L . donovani* and *L. infantum*, of *T. cruzi* CL Brener strain, *T. brucei gambiense* and *Crithidia fasciculata* genomes (Aslett et al. 2010, El-Sayed et al. 2005). Trypanosomatid parasites possess a unique thiol metabolism based on trypanothione, replacing many of the antioxidant functions of glutathione in mammals (Colotti et al. 2013a, Colotti and Ilari 2011, Ilari et al. 2015, 2017). Trypanothione, synthesized by trypanothione synthetase-amidase (TSA) and reduced by trypanothione reductase (TR), is used as a source of electrons by the tryparedoxin/tryparedoxin peroxidase system (TXN/TXNPx) to reduce the hydroperoxides produced by macrophages during infection (Figure 1) (Comini and Flohé 2013, Cunningham and Fairlamb 1995, Krauth-Siegel and Comini 2008). This detoxification pathway is not only unique to the parasites but is also essential for their survival in the human host; therefore, it constitutes a key relevant drug target (Frearson et al. 2007). The vital importance of the pathway was verified in *Trypanosoma brucei* by dsRNA technology and knock-out in other trypanosomatids, respectively, and is explained by its role in the parasite's antioxidant defense against Reactive Oxygen Species (ROS) produced by host macrophages during infection (Dumas et al. 1997, Krieger et al. 2000, Oza et al. 2005).

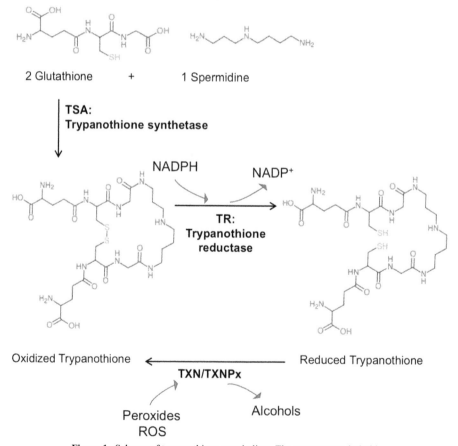

Figure 1. Scheme of trypanothione metabolism. The enzymes are in bold.

In the last 20 years, the structure of different enzymes of the trypanothione metabolic pathway has been solved and through structure-based drug design, many class of compounds have been identified as inhibitors of the pathways and consequently of the protozoan growth.

Trypanothione Synthesis: Glutathionylspermidine Synthetase (GspS) and Trypanothione Synthetase-amidase (TSA)

Trypanosomatids, which are exposed to high amounts of reactive oxygen species, produced by both host macrophage and the protozoa itself, use Trypanothione (T(SH)$_2$) (*N*1,*N*8-bis(glutathionyl)spermidine), a dithiol molecule synthesized starting from two glutathione molecules and one spermidine (Spd), as an efficient detoxification system. T(SH)$_2$ is more reactive than glutathione used by the human host, since the pKa of the cysteines coincides with the intracellular pH. A high T(SH)$_2$ concentration (1–2 mM) is always present in the parasite, meaning that high levels of inhibition of T(SH)$_2$ synthesis/ reduction has to be obtained in order to decrease parasite survival and virulence (Krauth-Siegel and Comini 2008).

T(SH)$_2$ is synthesized by means of two consecutive reactions. In the first reaction, the ATP-dependent addition of glutathione (GSH) to one of the amino groups of the polyamine spermidine (Spd), to form glutathionylspermidine (Gsp), takes place. This reaction can be catalyzed by Glutathionylspermidine synthetase (GspS) (present in some *Leishmania* species and in *T. cruzi*) and by the Trypanothione synthetase-amidase (TSA) (present in all trypanosomatids). In the second reaction, exclusively catalyzed by TSA, a second GSH is added to a terminal amino group of Gsp to form trypanothione (Figure 1) (Colotti and Ilari 2011, Krauth-Siegel and Comini 2008).

GspS and TSA proteins of *L. infantum*, with theoretical molecular weights of 81 and 74 kDa, are only 28.8% identical, but are predicted to conserve a similar fold. The gene for GspS is considered non-essential for *Leishmania* species, since it is poorly or not expressed in *L. infantum*, GspS overexpressing parasites are not permissive to TSA inactivation and a *gsps(–/–)* knockout line was viable and capable of replicating in both life cycle stages of the parasite, while TSA is essential for *Leishmania* parasites: elimination of both TSA alleles is not possible in *L. infantum* unless parasites were previously complemented with an episomal copy of the gene (Oza et al. 2005, Sousa et al. 2014, Torrie et al. 2009).

TSAs of trypanosomatids are very similar: TSA from *L. infantum* (*Li*TSA) shares 99.4, 95.2, 78.5, 61.1, and 58.9% identity with the TSAs from *L. donovani*, *L. major*, *C. fasciculata*, *T. brucei*, and *T. cruzi*, respectively (Table 2) (Sousa et al. 2014).

The X-ray crystal structure of TSA from *L. major* was solved at 2.3 Å resolution by Fyfe and colleagues (PDB code 2VOB) (Fyfe et al. 2008) and has furnished important information on protein function and have paved the way for structure-based rational drug design. The protein displays two distinct domains: an N-terminal amidase domain (residues 1-215 and 634-652), a papain-like cysteine protease domain with two α-helices and a β-barrel; and a C-terminal synthetase domain displaying an ATP-grasp family fold common to C:N ligases (216-633). The C-terminal synthetase domain, despite no obvious sequence homology (sequence identity 10%), belongs to the ATP-grasp superfamily and is structurally similar to the synthetase domain of GspS from *E. coli*, and to human glutathione synthetase (PDB code: 2HGS). The synthetase domain is composed of three subdomains (A, B and C) (Figure 2). Subdomain A comprises residues 216-393 and 595-633, subdomain B residues 394-511 and subdomain C, which creates one side of the ATP binding cleft, residues 512-595. The catalytic clefts accommodating the substrates are placed at the interface of the three subdomains and appear as a triangle-shaped gorge. The interface between the two subdomain A and C shapes the ATP binding site (S1). The GSH-binding cleft is formed mainly by subdomain B (S2), and the polyamine-binding site (spermidine and glutathionylspermidine) (S3) is a cleft between subdomains A and B. The knowledge of the structure allowed the modeling of substrates into each active site which provides insight into the specificity and reactivity of this unusual enzyme, able to catalyze four reactions by acting as a GspS, a trypanothione synthetase, a trypanothione amidase, and a glutathionylspermidine amidase (Figure 2).

Table 2. Alignment of the sequences of the most important proteins of the trypanothione metabolism in trypanosomatids and in *Homo sapiens*. The sequence identity percentages and the query cover (qc) with respect to *L. infantum* sequences are reported in the Table.

	L. major strain *Friedlin*	*L. donovani*	*T. brucei gambiense DAL972*	*T. cruzi* strain *CL Brener*	*Homo sapiens* (homologous proteins)
GspS	Not present	99% (qc 100%)	Not present	49% (qc 97%)	Not present
TSA	95% (qc 100%)	99% (qc 100%)	62% (qc 94%)	60% (qc 96%)	Not present
TR	96% (qc 100%)	99% (qc 100%)	67% (qc 100%)	67% (qc 99%)	Glutathione reductase: 35% (qc 95%)
TXN	86% (qc 100%)	100% (qc 100%)	60% (qc 97%)	60% (qc 99%)	Nucleoredoxin: 43% (qc 77%)
TXNPx	91% (qc 100%)	99% (qc 100%)	73% (qc 98%)	71% (qc 98%)	Peroxiredoxin-1: 60% (qc 100%)

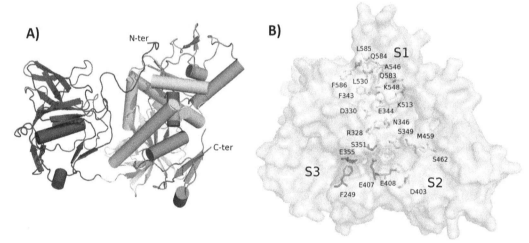

Figure 2. (A). TSA (TryS) overall fold. The amidase domain is colored blue (residues 1–215; 634–652). The synthetase domain is composed by three subdomains: A, residues 216–393 and 595–633, colored in green; B, residues 394–511, colored in magenta; C, residues 512–595, colored in red. (**B). The synthetase active site**. The protein surface is depicted as a *gray* semi-transparent van der Waals surface, except for ATP binding site (*yellow*) (S1), GSH binding site (*cyan*) (S2), spermidine binding site (magenta) (S3). The residues lining the three binding sites are indicated and depicted as sticks.

Color version at the end of the book

TSA as drug target

The importance of TSA activity for parasite viability has been demonstrated *in vitro* and *in vivo* for *T. brucei* and *L. infantum* by means of genetic and pharmacological approaches. TSA was demonstrated to be a good candidate to find new and more affordable drugs against neglected diseases caused by trypanosomatids since it is not present in the human host and is essential for the parasite survival (Sousa et al. 2014, Torrie et al. 2009). Moreover, it is encoded by a single copy gene (El-Sayed et al. 2005, Berriman et al. 2005, Ivens et al. 2005), has a known structure, provides metabolic control to the trypanothione pathway in *T. cruzi* (Olin-Sandoval et al. 2012) and kinetic information is available for several TSAs (Benitez et al. 2016).

Despite the high degree of homology, the TSAs of *Leishmania*, *T. cruzi* and *T. brucei* display different kinetic behavior, indicating the existence of structural differences between the three TSAs that change their affinity for the different substrates. In support of this observation, single amino acid substitutions in the homologue enzyme from *C. fasciculata* were reported to produce drastic changes in enzyme activity. For this reason, it is difficult to find a molecule targeting all *Leishmania*, *T. cruzi* and *T. brucei* through TSA inhibition (Oza et al. 2005).

Early studies of TSA inhibition

Before the resolution of TSA structure, rational inhibitor design was undertaken using GspS from *C. fasciculata* (*Cf*GspS) and *Escherichia coli* (*Ec*GspS) as test enzymes, or compounds isosteric with GSH or related transition state analogues as chemical scaffolds. Preliminary studies with GSH analogues identified the γ-glutamyl moiety as critical for molecular recognition. The addition of acidic groups to the L-γ-Glu-L-Leu dipeptide has brought to the synthesis of *Cf*GspS inhibitors of reasonable potency such as its phosphonic acid (Ki ~ 60 μM), the boronic acid (Ki ~ 81 μM) and the diaminopropionic acid derivatives (Ki ~ 7.2 μM) (Benitez et al. 2016). Derivatives mimicking the transition state, previously identified as potent inhibitors of *Ec*GspS, were proved to be equally active against recombinant *Cf*GspS. In particular, a Gsp-phosphinate derivative was found capable of inhibiting recombinant TSAs from *L. major*, *T. cruzi* and *T. brucei*, albeit with apparent Ki values 16–40-fold higher than that obtained for *Cf*GspS (Ki = 18.6 nM) (Oza et al. 2008). These compounds are the only ones able to target the three TSA, but unfortunately displayed null biological activity against pathogenic trypanosomatids at 100 μM concentration.

Identification of TSA inhibitors through high and medium throughput screenings

Chemical validation of TSA has been successfully carried out in recent years by Torrie et al. who developed an *in vitro* enzyme high throughput screening. They screened a library of 63,362 compounds, identifying three novel series of TSA inhibitors and designed lead compounds with nanomolar potency, which displayed mixed, uncompetitive, and allosteric-type inhibition with respect to spermidine, ATP, and glutathione (Torrie et al. 2009). Representatives of all three series were able to inhibit growth of *T. brucei in vitro*, and one of the lead compounds (DDD86243, **9**) (Table 3) decreased intracellular trypanothione levels to less than 10% and increased glutathione levels by 5-fold with respect to wild type.

Spinks et al., by using the same approach, identified six series of compounds able to inhibit *T. brucei* TSA (Spinks et al. 2012). The best compounds belong to the indazole series and were able to inhibit TSA with IC_{50} values below 100 nM but had micromolar potency in a trypanosome proliferation assay.

Other compounds were identified as TSA inhibitors: among the most intriguing ones were oxabicyclo[3.3.1]nonanones compounds, able to inhibit both TSA and TR of *Leishmania* (Saudagar et al. 2013).

Recent studies demonstrated that 5-substituted 3-chlorokenpaullone derivatives are potent inhibitors of *T. brucei* bloodstream forms (Orban et al. 2016) and that N,N'-bis(3,4-substituted-benzyl) diamine derivatives and an N5-substituted paullone (MOL2008, **10**) decreased the proliferation of *T. brucei* (EC_{50} in the nM range) and *L. infantum* promastigotes (EC_{50} = 12 μM) by inhibiting TSA (Benitez et al. 2016) (Table 3).

Recently, Benitez et al. screened a library composed of 144 compounds from 7 different families and several singletons against TSA from three major pathogen species of the trypanosomatid family (*Trypanosoma brucei*, *Trypanosoma cruzi* and *Leishmania infantum*) (Benitez et al. 2016). Only 4 compounds out of 15 active on at least one TSA, i.e., two BDA (N,N'-bis(3,4-substituted-benzyl) diamine derivatives) and two AI (4,5-dihydroazepino[4,5-b]indol-2(1H,3H,6H)-one derivatives, 4-azapaullones derivatives) compounds, were able to target multiple TSA: EAP1-47 [N1,N10-bis(4-isopropylbenzyl) decane-1,10-diamine] (**11**, Table 3), APC1-111 [N1,N8-bis(4-(benzyloxy)-3-methoxybenzyl)octane1,8-diamine], MOL2008 and FS-554. Among them, EAP1-47 is the only one able to halve the activity at 30 μM of all three TSA.

Table 3. Structures of some of the best inhibitors of the enzymes of the trypanothione pathway. The table reports the name and formula of the compounds, the chemical structure, the target, and the reference.

Compound	Chemical structure	Target enzyme	Reference
9: compound DDD86243		TSA	Torrie et al. 2009
10: (P),4,5-dihydroazepino[4,5-b]indol-2(1H,3H,6H)-one paullone derivative (compound MOL2008)		TSA	Benitez et al. 2016
11: EAP1-47: *N,N'*-bis(3,4-substituted-benzyl) diamine derivative		TSA	Benitez et al. 2016
12: Auranofin: Au¹⁺;(2S,3R,4S,5R,6R)-3,4,5-triacetyloxy-6-(acetyloxymethyl) oxane-2-thiolate;triethylphosphane		TR	Ilari et al. 2012
13: Lunarine: 22H-Benzofuro(3a,3-h)(1,5,10) triazacycloeicosine-3,14,22-trione, 4,5,6,7,8,9,10,11,12,13,20a,21,23,24-tetradecahydro-17,19-etheno		TR	Bond et al. 2009
14: 4-((1-(4-ethylphenyl)-2-methyl-5-(4-(methylthio)phenyl)-1H-pyrrol-3 yl) methyl) thio-morpholine		TR	Baiocco et al. 2013
15: RDS 777: 6-(Sec-butoxy)-2-((3-chlorophenyl)thio)pyrimidin-4-amine		TR	Saccoliti et al. 2017
16: (E)-1-(2-methoxy-4-((3-methylb-ut-2-en-1-yl)oxy)phenyl)-3-(4-nitro-phenyl)prop-2-en-1-one (chalcone compound 6)		TR	Ortalli et al. 2018

Table 3 contd. ...

...Table 3 contd.

Compound	Chemical structure	Target enzyme	Reference
17: N-{4-methoxy-3-[(4-ethoxyphenyl) sulfamoyl]phenyl}-5-nitrothiophene-2-carboxamide (compound A1/7 of the LeishBox)		TR	Ilari et al. 2018
18: 3-((((1-Benzyl-1H-tetrazol-5-yl) methyl)(1-adamantylmethyl)amino) methyl)-6,7-dimethoxyquinolin-2(1H)-one		TXNPx	Brindisi et al. 2015

Trypanothione Reductase (TR)

Trypanothione Reductase (TR) keeps trypanothione reduced in order to be used by the parasite to neutralize the ROS produced by the macrophage during the infection (Figure 3). Since the Leishmania protozoan live and multiply inside macrophages, this enzyme is essential for the parasite survival in amastigote stage during infection (Tovar et al. 1998, Dumas et al. 1997).

TR belongs to the family of FAD-dependent NAD(P)H ooxidoreductases, as GR, the human homologous enzyme and is quite similar to it in terms of sequence (about 40% identity), structure and mechanism of action. The crystal structures of the TR enzymes deposited in the PDB (*L. infantum*, *C. fasciculata* and *T. cruzi* TR) conserve the same three-dimensional structures (the sequence identity among TRs in trypanosomatids is rather high, ranging between 65 and 100%).

TR is a dimeric protein where each monomer is formed by three distinct domains: the FAD-binding domain (residues 1-160 and 289-360), the NADPH-binding domain (residues 161-289) and the interface domain (residues 361-488) (Baiocco et al. 2009a, b). The trypanothione binding pocket is quite large and is lined by hydrophobic and negatively charged residues differently from the human ortholog enzyme GR that possesses a substrate binding site smaller and is lined by positively charged residues (Bond et al. 1999, Zhang et al. 1996). This difference allows a selective targeting of TR enzyme.

The TR enzyme facilitates the transfer of two electrons from the NADPH cofactor to oxidized trypanothione (TS_2). Sequentially, NADPH binds to TR, its electrons are transferred to the FAD coenzyme; and finally, the $FADH_2$ reduces the Cys52–Cys57 disulfide bridge by formation of a transient charge transfer complex between the flavin and Cys57 thiolate. Upon entry of TS_2 in the active pocket of TR, Cys52 (deprotonated by the His461'-Glu466' pair) attacks nucleophilically the disulfide bridge of TS_2, forming with it a mixed disulfide bridge. The last step of the reaction implies a nucleophilic attack of Cys57 to Cys52 with the formation of the Cys52–Cys57 disulfide bridge and the release of reduced trypanothione molecule (Figure 3).

Soft Lewis acid metals as TR inhibitors

Pentavalent antimonials are prodrugs that become active upon reduction to trivalent antimony in the cell. Cunningham and Fairlamb demonstrated that antimonials interfere with the trypanothione metabolism by inhibiting the enzymatic activity of TR (Cunningham et al. 1995).

The antimonials are complexes of Sb(V) (Table 3), which have a low degree of toxicity. Once the complexes enter inside the macrophages, they are reduced by a reductase identified for the first time in Leishmania major, *Lm*ACR2 (Zhou et al. 2004), to Sb(III), which kills the protozoan.

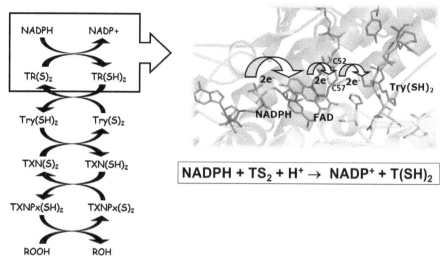

Figure 3. Trypanothione-dependent hydroperoxide reduction. Left Panel Electrons transfer from NADPH to the alkyl hydroperoxide and hydrogen peroxide. Two electrons pass through TR to trypanothione (Try(S)$_2$) which reduces tryparedoxin (TXN). The reduced tryparedoxin furnishes two electrons to the Tryparedoxin peroxidase to reduce alkyl hydroperoxides and hydrogen peroxide to alcohol and water, respectively. **Right Panel. Electron passage from NADPH to Try(S)$_2$.** Two electrons jump from NADPH to FAD and from FADH$_2$ to the two TR catalytic cysteines (Cys52 and Cys57). The two catalytic cysteines finally reduce trypanothione.

Baiocco et al. (2009a) demonstrated that TR is one of Sb(III) targets. Indeed, they solved the structure of reduced *Leishmania* TR in complex with NADPH and Sb(III), disclosing the molecular basis of the antimonial antileishmanial activity. As shown by the structural analysis, Sb(III) binds to the active residues of the catalytic pocket, namely Cys52, Cys57, His461' and Thr335, forming a stable complex. The described mechanism allows Sb(III) to inhibit the enzymatic activity of TR with high efficiency (Ki = 1.5 μM) (Figure 4).

In addition to antimonials, several metals, such as As(III), gold(I) and silver derivatives, are effective against *Leishmania* (Colotti et al. 2018). One of the target of these metals is the trypanothione reductase. Baiocco and coworkers have shown that As$_2$O$_3$ is able to inhibit TR of *L. infantum* in the micromolar range but with an inhibition constant one order of magnitude higher that antimonials (Ki = 14 ± 4 μM) (Baiocco et al. 2009a). The ability to bind the cysteines makes gold compounds able to inhibit TR with high efficiency. Auranofin (**12**, Table 3), used for decades against rheumatoid arthritis (Colotti et al. 2018), is also able to inhibit *L. infantum* TR. Indeed, auranofin is able to inactivate the enzyme with high efficiency (Ki = 0.15 ± 0.04 μM), thereby killing the parasite in the promastigote stage (IC$_{50}$ = 9.7 ± 1.0 μM). The low-resolution crystal structure of auranofin–TR complex allowed the comprehension of the molecular basis of this inhibition (Ilari et al. 2012). As expected, the gold ion was found to be tightly bound to the two catalytic cysteines (Cys52 and Cys57) in the active site of the enzyme, thereby hampering hydride transfer from the protein to trypanothione, while the thiosugar moiety of auranofin binds to the trypanothione binding site; thus auranofin inhibits TR through a dual mechanism (Figure 4B and 4C).

This finding paved the way to the study of the inhibition effects on TR activity of structurally different Au(I) and Au(III) compounds. Among the tested compounds, the most potent TR inhibitor is (Cl$_2$Au(III) (Pbi)Au(I)(PPh3)) (PF$_6$) (Pbi= 2-(2'-pyridyl)benzimidazole), which displays an apparent Ki value of 22 ± 11 nM, much lower than that of Sb(III) (1.5 μM). This compound is possibly the best candidate for further evaluation, since it also displays a low toxicity compared to other gold compounds (IC$_{50}$ = 0.6 μM, measured against human ovarian carcinoma cell line) (Colotti et al. 2013a).

Baiocco and coworkers have shown that silver is also able to inhibit with high efficiency TR (Baiocco et al. 2011). In particular, they showed that Ferritin-based encapsulated silver nanoparticles are effective against *L. infantum,* with an IC$_{50}$ against promastigote stage of 2.2 ± 0.3 μM and an IC$_{50}$ evaluated against

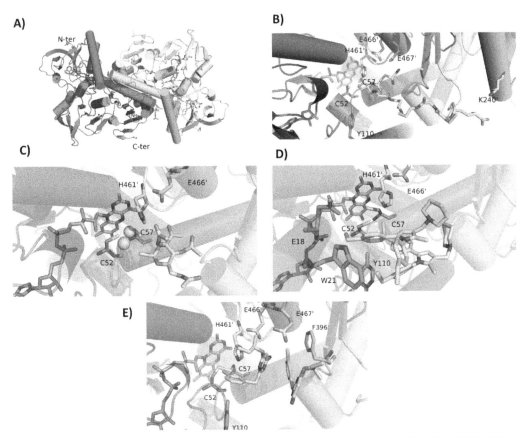

Figure 4. (A). TR overall fold (PDB code 4ADW). The two TR monomers are colored cyan and violet. The NADPH, FAD and trypanothione molecules are depicted as sticks. **(B).** Blow-up of TR-trypanothione complex catalytic cavity. The trypanothione molecule is depicted as sticks and colored green. The residues interacting with trypanothione are depicted as sticks. **(C).** Blow-up of the Auranofin-TR complex catalytic cavity (PDB code 2YAU). The 3,4,5-triacetyloxy-6-(acetyloxymethyl)oxane-2-thiol moiety is depicted as sticks and colored green, the gold ion is depicted as sphere and colored yellow, the chloride ion is depicted as sphere and colored green. The residues interacting with trypanothione are depicted as sticks. **(D).** Blow-up of the compound1-TR complex catalytic cavity (PDB code 4APN). The two compound 1 molecules present in the cavity are colored in green and lime green. All the residues interacting with the compound 1 molecules as well as the residues important for catalysis are indicated and depicted as sticks. **(E)** Blow-up of the RDS 777-TR complex catalytic cavity (PDB code 5EBK). The two RDS 777 molecules present in the cavity of TR monomer 1 are colored in green and lime green. All the residues interacting with the RDS 777 molecules as well as the residues important for catalysis are indicated and depicted as sticks.

Color version at the end of the book

amastigote in murine macrophages from Balb/c mice of 1.8 ± 0.2 µM. These values are lower than the IC_{50} of antimonial drugs in free and encapsulated forms, which range from 30 to 900 µM. The X-ray structure of the TR in complex with Ag shows that this metal as Sb(III) and Au(I) is able to bind the two catalytic cysteines (Cys52 and Cys57) and the His461', thereby inhibiting, with high efficiency, TR activity (the Ki calculated for Ag(0) and Ag(I) are 500 ± 200 nM and 50 ± 10 nM, respectively) (Baiocco et al. 2011).

Tricyclic trypanothione reductase (TR) inhibitors

Several tricyclic TR inhibitors have been identified (for a review, Kumar et al. 2014). Richardson et al. screened 1266 pharmacologically active compounds from the Sigma-Aldrich LOPAC1280 library

(Richardson et al. 2009). These compounds were screened against TR and live *T. brucei* parasites. Among all the compounds from the library, several tricyclic derivatives were shown to have a low degree of inhibition against the human GR ($IC_{50} > 100$ μM) and to be potent inhibitor of TR: clomipramine, $IC_{50} = 3.8$ μM; chlorpromazine $IC_{50} = 6.3$ μM; prochlorperazine $IC_{50} = 7.4$ μM; triflupromazine $IC_{50} = 7.5$ μM; mepacrine $IC_{50} = 133.8$ μM. Lunarine (**13**), composed of a spermidine chain with the terminal nitrogen atoms forming amide linkages with two α,β-unsaturated carboxylic acid functions disposed upon an unusual 3-oxohexahydrodibenzofuranyl tricyclic scaffold (Table 3), has been identified as a competitive, time-dependent inhibitor of TR (Bond et al. 1999). Hamilton et al. showed a possible mechanism for this inhibition, based on the covalent modification of a redox-active cysteine residue in the active site of TR by conjugate addition to one of the amide groups of lunarine (Hamilton et al. 2002). Hamilton et al. also studied benzofuranyl-based acyclic bis-polyamine analogues of lunarine (Hamilton et al. 2003). Other tricyclic compounds have been studied by Bonnet et al. (2000) who designed and synthesized a series of symmetrical substituted 1,4-bis(3-aminopropyl)piperazine derivatives and tested them for their inhibitory potency towards *T. cruzi* TR, their trypanocidal effects against both *T. cruzi* and *T. brucei* trypomastigote stage, and for their cytotoxicity towards human MRC-5 cells. The most potent TR inhibition was observed for polyphenyl derivatives indicated as 7 and 8 ($IC_{50} = 32$ μM and 28 μM, respectively); these two compounds showed 100% inhibition on *T. brucei* at concentrations of 6.3 and 3.1 μM, respectively (Bonnet et al. 2000).

In another study, Chibale et al. designed and synthesized 9,9-dimethylxanthene derivatives able to bind in the hydrophobic pocket involved in recognition of the spermidine moiety of trypanothione, and also introduced terminal tertiary amino groups into the compounds to impair their binding to the positively charged cavity of GR, the host off-target enzyme (Chibale et al. 2000). Only the compounds carrying two or three carbon methylene spacer between the tricyclic moiety and the secondary nitrogen atom display the ability to inhibit over 50% TR activity. However, they were not able to find a clear correlation between potency as inhibitors of TR and the *in vitro* antiparasitic activities. Girault et al. designed and optimized various bis(2-aminodiphenylsulfides) derivatives to find good inhibitors of *T. cruzi* TR (Girault et al. 2001). The results of the TR inhibition screening showed that the most potent tricyclic inhibitor possesses an $IC_{50} = 250$ nM. All the compounds were also tested *in vitro* against *T. cruzi* and *L. infantum* amastigotes and against *T. brucei* trypomastigotes.

Multitarget lead compounds

Chibale et al. (2003) showed that some compounds including mepacrine, promazine and clomipramine display the ability to both reverse the chloroquine resistance in Plasmodium and to inhibit TR. Based on this observation, they designed and developed a series of xanthene derivatives with intrinsic antimalarial activity, as potential TR inhibitor. Among all the derivatives of xanthenes, compound 16 showed the highest inhibitory activity (IC_{50} of 35.7 μM), conserving an antimalarial activity ($IC_{50} = 1.75$ μM). Chibale et al. also synthesized a series of sulfonamide and urea derivatives of quinacrine with varying methylene spacer lengths, tested for inhibition of TR and for activity *in vitro* against strains of the parasitic protozoa Trypanosoma, Leishmania and Plasmodium (Chibale et al. 2001, 2000). They succeeded in finding inhibitors with higher activity against TR with respect to quinacrine, with the best compound with an IC_{50} of 3.3 μM, 40 times better than that of quinacrine ($IC_{50} = 133$ μM). Their studies revealed that sulfonamide derivatives were more active than urea in inhibiting TR but this trend of activity did not correlate with the *in vitro* activities against *L. donovani*, *T. cruzi*, and *T. brucei*.

Recently, Uliassi et al. proposed for the first time the natural compound crassiflorone as a potential dual *Tb*GAPDH/*Tc*TR inhibitor and designed and synthesized novel synthetic crassiflorone derivatives. They found that among the tested compounds, only 19 displayed a balanced dual profile against the selected targets (% inhibition at 10 μM, *Tb*GAPDH = 64% and *Tc*TR = 65%). Despite their ability to inhibit TR, these compounds were not active against *T. cruzi* trypomastigote and *L. infantum* amastigote forms, whereas *T. brucei* bloodstream parasite was more susceptible to the compounds (Uliassi et al. 2017).

Polyamine analogs

Hamilton et al. (2003) prepared some benzofuranyl-based acyclic bis-polyamine analogues of lunarine. In their approach, they removed skew boat cyclohexanone moiety of lunarine leaving a planar bicyclic benzofuranyl scaffold. The acyclic bis-polyamine derivatives such as *N*1-glutathionylspermidine disulfide and the synthetic bis-dimethylaminopropyl- and bis-*N*-methylpiperazinyl amides of Ellman's reagent (DTNB), which are known TR substrates, were chosen for functionalization of a 3,5-disubstituted benzofuranyl template to give potential inhibitors. In their series of compounds, the bis-polyaminoacrylamide derivatives were shown to be competitive inhibitors (with respect to trypanothione) of TR, but only the bis-4-methyl-piperazin-1-yl-propylacrylamide derivative 3 displayed time-dependent activity.

Structure-based drug design

Structure-based studies pointed to the design of several organic compounds able to inhibit TR, such as acridines, 1,4-naphthoquinone derivatives and aniline-based diaryl sulfides. In *T. cruzi* TR, mepacrine forms a complex interacting with residues lining the trypanothione binding site important for substrate binding and positioning such as Glu18, Trp21 and Met113 (Jacoby et al. 1996).

The 3,4-dihydroquinazoline scaffold binds in a similar position in the trypanothione binding cavity of *T. brucei* TR interacting with residues Trp21, Tyr110, Met113, Phe114 (Patterson et al. 2011). Baiocco and coworkers have shown that the same residues are responsible for the binding of 4-((1-(4-ethylphenyl)-2-methyl-5-(4-(methylthio)phenyl)-1H-pyrrol-3-yl)methyl) thio-morpholine, a diaryl pyrrole compound (**14**, Table 3) that inhibits *L. infantum* TR in the micromolar range (Jacoby et al. 1996, Patterson et al. 2011, Baiocco et al. 2013). The indicated residues are conserved in the TR of *Leishmania*, *T. cruzi* and *T. brucei* and form a small hydrophobic pocket that can accommodate hydrophobic organic compounds and that could be used as preferred target to design TR lead compounds against all the three trypanosomatid diseases (Figure 4D).

Stump et al. have also shown the ability of diarylsulfide derivatives to bind *T. cruzi* TR and proposed a modeling-based binding mode for this class of compounds (Stump et al. 2008). In order to study the mechanism of inhibition exerted by these compounds and determine the binding mode of the diaryldisulfide derivatives, Saccoliti et al. solved the X-ray structure of *L. infantum* TR in its oxidized state in complex with RDS 777 (LiTR-777) at 3.5 Å resolution (Figure 4E). RDS 777 (**15**, Table 3) is able to inhibit the parasite growth (IC$_{50}$ = 29.4 ± 1.3 µM) by binding to the trypanothione binding site of TR with high efficiency (K$_i$ = 0.25 ± 0.18 µM). This compound binds the catalytic site engaging in hydrogen bonds the residues more involved in the catalysis, namely Cys57, Cys52, His461', Glu466' and Glu467' (Saccoliti et al. 2017).

Many successful studies have been carried out on TR, with the identification of several types of TR inhibitors, belonging to different classes and types of inhibition. Among the best ones, a worthy mention is of analogues of 1-[1-(benzo[b]thien-2-yl)cyclohexyl]piperidine (BTCP), nitroheterocyclic compounds, phenothiazine derivatives, 2-aminodiphenylsulfides, N-(3-phenylpropyl) substituted polyamines, polyamine-peptide conjugates, kukoamine A derivatives, and chalcone compounds (**16**) (Smith and Bradley 1999, Chitkul and Bradley 2000, Khan et al. 2000, Girault et al. 2001, Persch et al. 2014, Beig et al. 2015, Ortalli et al. 2018). Only a small number of TR-inhibiting compounds possess inhibition constants in the submicromolar range, possibly because the active site is large and with scarce features; in addition, most of these compounds have inadequate anti-parasitic activity. Importantly, studies on conditional TR knockout in *T. brucei* demonstrated that only the parasites with TR activity lower than 10% with respect to wild type are unable to grow and infect mice: due to the high amount of trypanothione, which may displace a competitive inhibitor with low affinity, TR should be inhibited at submicromolar range to prevent parasite growth (Krieger et al. 2000, Bernardes et al. 2013). A recent interesting study concerns the analysis of the 192 compounds identified in the GlaxoSmithKline HTS diversity set of 1.8 million compounds, and demonstrated to be effective by whole-cell phenotypic assays against *L. donovani* (Pena et al. 2015): recently, Ilari et al. characterized these inhibitors in *in vitro* assays on TR from *L. infantum* and human GR, thereby identifying 3 specific highly potent specific TR inhibitors and two partially selective TR inhibitors (Ilari et al. 2018). The most potent compound, i.e., N-(4-bromo-3-methylphenyl)-5-nitrothiophene-2-carboxamide (**17**), showed competition with respect to trypanothione binding, and is able to efficiently inhibit the growth of *L. donovani*, *T. cruzi* and *T. brucei*: the inhibition of TR, a validated target conserved in all trypanosomatids, may thus lead to the development of antikinetoplasmid drugs (Ilari et al. 2018, Pena et al. 2015).

The Trypanothione-dependent Redox Metabolism of *Leishmania*: Tryparedoxin (TXN), and Tryparedoxin-dependent Peroxidase (TXNPx)

Detoxification of peroxides in mammalian cells relies on catalase and on the glutathione peroxidase, which are absent in trypanosomatids. Trypanosomatids use the TXN/TXNPx redox couple to reduce the peroxides produced by macrophages during the infection by means of two reactions. In the first reaction, TXN in the reduced form binds oxidized TXNPx to reduce the intersubunit disulfide bridge between the two catalytic cysteines in the TXNPx dimer, with the formation of a mixed disulfide bridge between the N-terminal Cys40 of TXN and the resolving cysteine (Cr') of TXNPx, and the reduction of the peroxidatic cysteine (Cp). The TXN-TXNPx disulfide bond undergoes nucleophilic attack by the second Cys of TXN, to leave TXNPx Cr' as a thiol or a thiolate, while TXN returns to the oxidized form and is reduced again by $T(SH)_2$. In the second reaction, the reduced TXNPx reduces peroxides, and the Cp thiolate is oxidized to sulfenic acid, that can react again with the resolving cysteine Cr' from the other monomer, forming again an intermolecular disulfide bridge. TXNPx oxidation is associated with a conformational change from fully folded (FF) to locally unfolded (LU) conformation, essential for catalysis (Figure 5).

The crystal structures of cytosolic *L. major* TXN (*Lm*TXN) and of *L. major* TXNPx (*Lm*TXNPx) were solved by Fiorillo et al. (2012). *Lm*TXN is mostly monomeric, and its structure, similar to those of TXNs from *C. fasciculata* and from *T. brucei* (with about 60% identity with respect to LmTXN), is formed by a seven-stranded twisted β-sheet, surrounded by four α-helices and two short 3_{10}-helices. The active site (Trp39-Cys40-Pro41-Pro42-Cys43) is at the N-terminus of the α1-helix.

The asymmetric unit of *Lm*TXN crystal contains a possibly biologically relevant dimer showing extensive contacts between adjacent monomers, where dimerization occurs by a two-fold symmetry related domain-swapping of the two monomers that exchange their α0 helices.

*Lm*TXNPx is a toroidal decamer formed by 5 dimers that are the active physiological units of the enzyme (Figure 6). As in TXN and in other proteins of the thioredoxin superfamily, the fold of *Lm*TXNPx monomers consists of a seven-stranded twisted β-sheet, surrounded by four α-helices and two short 3_{10}-helices, with the peroxidatic cysteine Cys52 (Cp) located at the N-terminus of the α-helix (α1), in

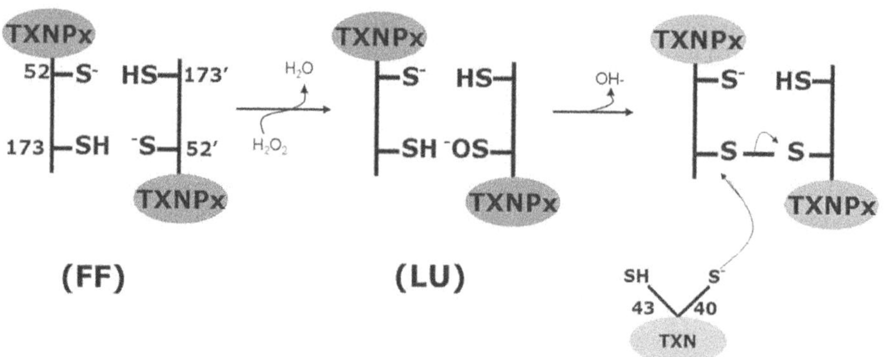

Figure 5. Mechanism of action of the TXN/TXNPx couple. The reduced TXNPx in fully folded conformation (FF) reduces hydrogen peroxide to water with the consequent oxidation of the peroxidatic cysteine (Cys52) to sulfenic acid. The oxidation of Cys52 induces a protein conformational change from the FF to the locally unfolded conformation (LU) which allows the formation of a disulfide bridge between the Cys52 and Cys173' (the resolving cysteine). The disulfide bridge is reduced by TXN.

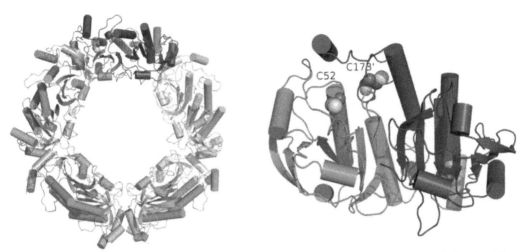

Figure 6. LmTXNPx structure (PDB code 3TUE). **Left:** Decameric assembly. The monomer A and B of a functional dimer are colored clear gray and dark gray, respectively. The two catalytic cysteines are represented as spheres. **Right:** Functional dimer. The two monomers A and B are colored clear grey and dark grey, respectively. The two catalytic cysteines are represented as spheres.

> **Color version at the end of the book**

a position similar to that of Cys43 in TXN, while the resolving cysteine (Cys173, Cr') and the whole C-terminal part of the protein are disordered and not visible in the structure of the protein in the reduced form (LU).

A redox-dependent structural switch occurs between FF and LU conformations during catalysis (Fiorillo et al. 2012, Brindisi et al. 2015), and conformational changes appear to take place only in the 43–53 loop containing the Cp and the C-terminal tail (residues 169–199) containing Cr', which in FF conformation is visible in the structure and folds in a long loop and a α-helix (Figure 6). In *Lm*TXNPx-FF, Cp is located in the α1-helix, in a narrow solvent-accessible pocket that constitutes the active site, while in *Lm*TXNPx-LU the helix partially unwinds and Cp becomes completely exposed to the solvent and available to be attacked by Cr' to form a disulfide bridge.

TXN and TXNPx inhibition

Fueller et al. recently used a high throughput screening approach with nearly 80,000 chemicals to identify inhibitors of TXN, taking advantage of the fact that parasite TXN has a WCPPC active site motif instead of the canonical WCGPC sequence in mammalian thioredoxins (Trx), and that with 16,000 Da, it is larger than human Trx (12,000 Da). They identified time-dependent, irreversible inhibitors of TXN-modifying Cys40, the first cysteine of its active site WCPPC motif. Although irreversible inhibitors are considered as non-ideal, the compounds inhibited the proliferation of *T. brucei* with good EC_{50} values, even below 1 μM (Fueller et al. 2012).

A series of compounds able to inhibit *Lm*TXNPx was identified by Brindisi et al. (2015), by high-throughput docking techniques (Brindisi et al. 2015). The analysis of the enzyme-inhibitor docked models, together with Surface Plasmon Resonance (SPR) experiments and activity assays, allowed Brindisi and coworkers to rationally design and synthesize a series of *N,N*-disubstituted 3-aminomethyl quinolones, that showed inhibitory potency against *Lm*TXNPx in the micromolar range; among these, compound 12, i.e., 3-((((1-Benzyl-1H-tetrazol-5-yl)methyl)(1-adamantylmethyl)amino)methyl)-6,7-dimethoxyquinolin-2(1H)-one, shows a 93% inhibition of TXNPx activity at 100 μM concentration, and a KD, measured by SPR technique, of 39 μM (**18**, Table 3). This study may pave the way to the discovery of a new class of antileishmanial drugs.

Conclusion

The search for new drugs against trypanosomatids appears to be slow. This is because little money is spent on these so called neglected diseases since they affect mainly poor and underdeveloped countries. However, recent efforts, based on classical and high-throughput approaches, are giving promising results, and an increasing number of protein targets, essential for the parasites and absent in the human host, is studied by several groups in the world. In addition, recent collaborations between academic researchers and pharmaceutical companies, which have data on millions of potential drug molecules, are starting to be possible positive factors for the search of new and more affordable drugs against leishmaniasis (Pena et al. 2015).

The enzymes of the trypanothione pathway are not present in human host and are essential for the parasite survival during the infection and for these reasons represent the most promising targets against the diseases caused by trypanosomatids. The structure-function relationships of trypanothione reductase of *L. infantum*, *T. cruzi* and *T. brucei* have been deeply studied and new scaffolds able to inhibit TR have been identified. However, at least 90% TR inactivation needs to be obtained by inhibitor compounds to kill the parasite avoiding the interference of the reduced trypanothione accumulation. Thus, to find new lead compounds targeting TR is quite difficult since effective molecules should have submicromolar inhibition activity as well as show very good selectivity over GR.

TSA is to date the most promising target: it is a low-abundance, essential enzyme in *Leishmania*, with no human homologs. The presence of druggable substrate binding pockets was demonstrated by the analysis of TSA crystal structure, and TSA inhibitors obtained from high-throughput studies have been demonstrated to be effective against *T. brucei*.

Of course, synergistic effects between inhibition of enzymes of the trypanothione pathway and of trypanothione itself can take place. Further, to overcome the problem of drug resistance and to make a therapy against trypanosomatids more effective, drug combinations may be used. Another possible option is represented from multi-targeted therapy involving single small molecules that can target multiple vital targets in parasites' metabolic pathways. In this respect, the research of Belluti and coworkers is of particular interest, who have recently developed a series of quinone–coumarin hybrids targeting both trypanosoma glyceraldehyde-3-phosphate dehydrogenase and TR (Belluti et al. 2014).

Acknowledgements

We acknowledge CNCCS CNR (National Collection of Chemical Compounds 2018), MIUR PRIN 20154JRJPP and FaReBio di qualità CNR to AI and GC.

References

Aslett, M., C. Aurrecoechea, M. Berriman, J. Brestelli, B.P. Brunk, M. Carrington et al. 2010. TriTrypDB: a functional genomic resource for the Trypanosomatidae. Nucleic Acids Res. 38(Database issue): D457–62.

Baiocco, P., G. Colotti, S. Franceschini and A. Ilari. 2009a. Molecular basis of antimony treatment in leishmaniasis. J. Med. Chem. 52(8): 2603–12.

Baiocco, P., S. Franceschini, A. Ilari and G. Colotti. 2009b. Trypanothione reductase from Leishmania infantum: cloning, expression, purification, crystallization and preliminary X-ray data analysis. Protein Pept. Lett. 16(2): 196–200.

Baiocco, P., A. Ilari, P. Ceci, S. Orsini, M. Gramiccia, T. Di Muccio et al. 2011. Inhibitory effect of silver nanoparticles on trypanothione reductase activity and Leishmania infantum proliferation. ACS Med. Chem. Lett. 2(3): 230–3.

Baiocco, P., G. Poce, S. Alfonso, M. Cocozza, G.G. Porretta, G. Colotti et al. 2013. Inhibition of Leishmania infantum trypanothione reductase by azole-based compounds: a comparative analysis with its physiological substrate by X-ray crystallography. ChemMedChem. 8(7): 1175–83.

Barrett, M.P., D.W. Boykin, R. Brun and R.R. Tidwell. 2007. Human African trypanosomiasis: pharmacological re-engagement with a neglected disease. Br. J. Pharmacol. 152(8): 1155–71.

Barrett, M.P. and S.L. Croft. 2012. Management of trypanosomiasis and leishmaniasis. Br. Med. Bull. 104: 175–96.

Beig, M., F. Oellien, L. Garoff, S. Noack, R.L. Krauth-Siegel and P.M. Selzer. 2015. Trypanothione reductase: a target protein for a combined *in vitro* and *in silico* screening approach. PLoS Negl. Trop. Dis. 9(6): e0003773.

Belluti, F., E. Uliassi, G. Veronesi, C. Bergamini, M. Kaiser, R. Brun et al. 2014. Toward the development of dual-targeted glyceraldehyde-3-phosphate dehydrogenase/trypanothione reductase inhibitors against Trypanosoma brucei and Trypanosoma cruzi. ChemMedChem. 9(2): 371–82.

Benitez, D., A. Medeiros, L. Fiestas, E.A. Panozzo-Zenere, F. Maiwald, K.C. Prousis et al. 2016. Identification of novel chemical scaffolds inhibiting trypanothione synthetase from pathogenic trypanosomatids. PLoS Negl. Trop. Dis. 10(4): e0004617.

Bernardes, L.S., C.L. Zani and I. Carvalho. 2013. Trypanosomatidae diseases: from the current therapy to the efficacious role of trypanothione reductase in drug discovery. Curr. Med. Chem. 20(21): 2673–96.

Berriman, M., E. Ghedin, C. Hertz-Fowler, G. Blandin, H. Renauld, D.C. Bartholomeu et al. 2005. The genome of the African trypanosome Trypanosoma brucei. Science. 309(5733): 416–22.

Boelaert, M., F. Meheus, J. Robays and P. Lutumba. 2010. Socio-economic aspects of neglected diseases: sleeping sickness and visceral leishmaniasis. Ann. Trop. Med. Parasitol. 104(7): 535–42.

Bond, C.S., Y. Zhang, M. Berriman, M.L. Cunningham, A.H. Fairlamb and W.N. Hunter. 1999. Crystal structure of Trypanosoma cruzi trypanothione reductase in complex with trypanothione, and the structure-based discovery of new natural product inhibitors. Structure. 7(1): 81–9.

Bonnet, B., D. Soullez, S. Girault, L. Maes, V. Landry, E. Davioud-Charvet et al. 2000. Trypanothione reductase inhibition/trypanocidal activity relationships in a 1,4-bis(3-aminopropyl)piperazine series. Bioorg. Med. Chem. 8(1): 95–103.

Brindisi, M., S. Brogi, N. Relitti, A. Vallone, S. Gemma, E. Novellino et al. 2015. Structure-based discovery of the first non-covalent inhibitors of Leishmania major tryparedoxin peroxidase by high throughput docking. Sci. Rep. 5: 9705.

Chawla, B., A. Jhingran, A. Panigrahi, K.D. Stuart and R. Madhubala. 2011. Paromomycin affects translation and vesicle-mediated trafficking as revealed by proteomics of paromomycin -susceptible -resistant Leishmania donovani. PLoS One. 6(10): e26660.

Chibale, K., M. Visser, V. Yardley, S.L. Croft and A.H. Fairlamb. 2000. Synthesis and evaluation of 9,9-dimethylxanthene tricyclics against trypanothione reductase, Trypanosoma brucei, Trypanosoma cruzi and Leishmania donovani. Bioorg. Med. Chem. Lett. 10(11): 1147–50.

Chibale, K., H. Haupt, H. Kendrick, V. Yardley, A. Saravanamuthu, A.H. Fairlamb et al. 2001. Antiprotozoal and cytotoxicity evaluation of sulfonamide and urea analogues of quinacrine. Bioorg. Med. Chem. Lett. 11(19): 2655–7.

Chibale, K., M. Visser, D.A. van Schalkwyk, A.H. Fairlamb, P.J. Smith and A. Saravanamuthu. 2003. Exploring the potential of xanthene derivatives as trypanothione reductase inhibitors and chloroquine potentiating agents. Tetrahedron. 59: 2289–96.

Chitkul, B., and M. Bradley. 2000. Optimising inhibitors of trypanothione reductase using solid-phase chemistry. Bioorg. Med. Chem. Lett. 10(20): 2367–9.

Colotti, G. and A. Ilari. 2011. Polyamine metabolism in Leishmania: from arginine to trypanothione. Amino Acids. 40(2): 269–85.

Colotti, G., P. Baiocco, A. Fiorillo, A. Boffi, E. Poser, F. Di Chiaro et al. 2013a. Structural insights into the enzymes of the trypanothione pathway: targets for antileishmaniasis drugs. Future Med. Chem. 5(15): 1861–75.

Colotti, G., A. Ilari, A. Fiorillo, P. Baiocco, M.A. Maiore, F. Scaletti et al. 2013b. Metal-based compounds as prospective antileishmanial agents: inhibition of trypanothione reductase by selected gold complexes. ChemMedChem. 8(10): 1634–7.

Colotti, G., A. Fiorillo and A. Ilari. 2018. Metal- and metalloid-containing drugs for the treatment of trypanosomatid diseases. Front Biosci. (Landmark Ed). 23: 954–966.

Comini, Marcelo A. and Leopold Flohé. 2013. Trypanothione-based redox metabolism of trypanosomatids. In *Trypanosomatid Diseases*: Wiley-VCH Verlag GmbH & Co. KGaA.

Cunningham, M.L. and A.H. Fairlamb. 1995. Trypanothione reductase from Leishmania donovani. Purification, characterisation and inhibition by trivalent antimonials. Eur. J. Biochem. 230(2): 460–8.

Davidson, R.N., S.L. Croft, A. Scott, M. Maini, A.H. Moody and A.D. Bryceson. 1991. Liposomal amphotericin B in drug-resistant visceral leishmaniasis. Lancet. 337(8749): 1061–2.

Dumas, C., M. Ouellette, J. Tovar, M.L. Cunningham, A.H. Fairlamb, S. Tamar et al. 1997. Disruption of the trypanothione reductase gene of Leishmania decreases its ability to survive oxidative stress in macrophages. EMBO J. 16(10): 2590–8.

El-Sayed, N.M., P.J. Myler, G. Blandin, M. Berriman, J. Crabtree, G. Aggarwal et al. 2005. Comparative genomics of trypanosomatid parasitic protozoa. Science. 309(5733): 404–9.

Fiorillo, A., G. Colotti, A. Boffi, P. Baiocco and A. Ilari. 2012. The crystal structures of the tryparedoxin-tryparedoxin peroxidase couple unveil the structural determinants of Leishmania detoxification pathway. PLoS Negl. Trop. Dis. 6(8): e1781.

Frearson, J.A., P.G. Wyatt, I.H. Gilbert and A.H. Fairlamb. 2007. Target assessment for antiparasitic drug discovery. Trends Parasitol. 23(12): 589–95.

Freitas-Junior, L.H., E. Chatelain, H.A. Kim and J.L. Siqueira-Neto. 2012. Visceral leishmaniasis treatment: What do we have, what do we need and how to deliver it? Int. J. Parasitol. Drugs Drug Resist. 2: 11–9.

Frezard, F., C. Demicheli and R.R. Ribeiro. 2009. Pentavalent antimonials: new perspectives for old drugs. Molecules. 14(7): 2317–36.

Fueller, F., B. Jehle, K. Putzker, J.D. Lewis and R.L. Krauth-Siegel. 2012. High throughput screening against the peroxidase cascade of African trypanosomes identifies antiparasitic compounds that inactivate tryparedoxin. J. Biol. Chem. 287(12): 8792–802.

Fyfe, P.K., S.L. Oza, A.H. Fairlamb and W.N. Hunter. 2008. Leishmania trypanothione synthetase-amidase structure reveals a basis for regulation of conflicting synthetic and hydrolytic activities. J. Biol. Chem. 283(25): 17672–80.

Girault, S., T.E. Davioud-Charvet, L. Maes, J.F. Dubremetz, M.A. Debreu, V. Landry et al. 2001. Potent and specific inhibitors of trypanothione reductase from Trypanosoma cruzi: bis(2-aminodiphenylsulfides) for fluorescent labeling studies. Bioorg. Med. Chem. 9(4): 837–46.

Haldar, A.K., P. Sen and S. Roy. 2011. Use of antimony in the treatment of leishmaniasis: current status and future directions. Mol. Biol. Int. 2011: 571242.

Hamilton, C.J., A.H. Fairlamb and I.M. Eggleston. 2002. Regiocontrolled synthesis of the macrocyclic polyamine alkaloid (±)-lunarine, a time-dependent inhibitor of trypanothione reductase. J. Chem. Soc. Perkin. 1(1): 1115–23.

Hamilton, C.J., A. Saravanamuthu, A.H. Fairlamb and I.M. Eggleston. 2003. Benzofuranyl 3,5-bis-polyamine derivatives as time-dependent inhibitors of trypanothione reductase. Bioorg. Med. Chem. 11(17): 3683–93.

Hotez, P.J., J.H. Remme, P. Buss, G. Alleyne, C. Morel and J.G. Breman. 2004. Combating tropical infectious diseases: Report of the disease control priorities in developing countries project. Clin. Infect. Dis. 38(6): 871–8.

Hotez, P.J., D.H. Molyneux, A. Fenwick, J. Kumaresan, S.E. Sachs, J.D. Sachs et al. 2007. Control of neglected tropical diseases. N. Engl. J. Med. 357(10): 1018–27.

Ilari, A., P. Baiocco, L. Messori, A. Fiorillo, A. Boffi, M. Gramiccia et al. 2012. A gold-containing drug against parasitic polyamine metabolism: the X-ray structure of trypanothione reductase from Leishmania infantum in complex with auranofin reveals a dual mechanism of enzyme inhibition. Amino Acids. 42(2-3): 803–11.

Ilari, A., A. Fiorillo, P. Baiocco, E. Poser, G. Angiulli and G. Colotti. 2015. Targeting polyamine metabolism for finding new drugs against leishmaniasis: a review. Mini. Rev. Med. Chem. 15(3): 243–52.

Ilari, A., A. Fiorillo, I. Genovese and G. Colotti. 2017. Polyamine-trypanothione pathway: an update. Future Med. Chem. 9(1): 61–77.

Ilari, A., I. Genovese, F. Fiorillo, T. Battista, I. De Ionna, A. Fiorillo et al. 2018. Toward a drug against all kinetoplastids: From leishbox to specific and potent trypanothione reductase inhibitors. Mol. Pharm.

Ivens, A.C., C.S. Peacock, E.A. Worthey, L. Murphy, G Aggarwal, M. Berriman et al. 2005. The genome of the kinetoplastid parasite, Leishmania major. Science. 309(5733): 436–42.

Jacoby, E.M., I. Schlichting, C.B. Lantwin, W. Kabsch and R.L. Krauth-Siegel. 1996. Crystal structure of the Trypanosoma cruzi trypanothione reductase.mepacrine complex. Proteins. 24(1): 73–80.

Khan, M.O., S.E. Austin, C. Chan, H. Yin, D. Marks, S.N. Vaghjani et al. 2000. Use of an additional hydrophobic binding site, the Z site, in the rational drug design of a new class of stronger trypanothione reductase inhibitor, quaternary alkylammonium phenothiazines. J. Med. Chem. 43(16): 3148–56.

Krauth-Siegel, R.L. and M.A. Comini. 2008. Redox control in trypanosomatids, parasitic protozoa with trypanothione-based thiol metabolism. Biochim. Biophys. Acta. 1780(11): 1236–48.

Krieger, S., W. Schwarz, M.R. Ariyanayagam, A.H. Fairlamb, R.L. Krauth-Siegel and C. Clayton. 2000. Trypanosomes lacking trypanothione reductase are avirulent and show increased sensitivity to oxidative stress. Mol. Microbiol. 35(3): 542–52.

Kumar, S., M.R. Ali and S. Bawa. 2014. Mini review on tricyclic compounds as an inhibitor of trypanothione reductase. J. Pharm. Bioallied. Sci. 6(4): 222–8.

Moore, E.M. and D.N. Lockwood. 2010. Treatment of visceral leishmaniasis. J. Glob. Infect. Dis. 2(2): 151–8.

Olin-Sandoval, V., Z. Gonzalez-Chavez, M. Berzunza-Cruz, I. Martinez, R. Jasso-Chavez, I. Becker et al. 2012. Drug target validation of the trypanothione pathway enzymes through metabolic modelling. FEBS J. 279(10): 1811–33.

Orban, O.C., R.S. Korn, D. Benitez, A. Medeiros, L. Preu, N. Loaec et al. 2016. 5-Substituted 3-chlorokenpaullone derivatives are potent inhibitors of Trypanosoma brucei bloodstream forms. Bioorg. Med. Chem. 24(16): 3790–800.

Ortalli, M., A. Ilari, G. Colotti, I. De Ionna, T. Battista, A. Bisi et al. 2018. Identification of chalcone-based antileishmanial agents targeting trypanothione reductase. Eur. J. Med. Chem. 152: 527–541.

Ouellette, M., J. Drummelsmith and B. Papadopoulou. 2004. Leishmaniasis: drugs in the clinic, resistance and new developments. Drug Resist Updat. 7(4-5): 257–66.

Oza, S.L., M.P. Shaw, S. Wyllie and A.H. Fairlamb. 2005. Trypanothione biosynthesis in Leishmania major. Mol. Biochem. Parasitol. 139(1): 107–16.

Oza, S.L., S. Chen, S. Wyllie, J.K. Coward and A.H. Fairlamb. 2008. ATP-dependent ligases in trypanothione biosynthesis—kinetics of catalysis and inhibition by phosphinic acid pseudopeptides. FEBS J. 275(21): 5408–21.

Patterson, S., M.S. Alphey, D.C. Jones, E.J. Shanks, I.P. Street, J.A. Frearson et al. 2011. Dihydroquinazolines as a novel class of Trypanosoma brucei trypanothione reductase inhibitors: discovery, synthesis, and characterization of their binding mode by protein crystallography. J. Med. Chem. 54(19): 6514–30.

Pena, I., M. Pilar Manzano, J. Cantizani, A. Kessler, J. Alonso-Padilla, A.I. Bardera et al. 2015. New compound sets identified from high throughput phenotypic screening against three kinetoplastid parasites: an open resource. Sci. Rep. 5: 8771.

Persch, E., S. Bryson, N.K. Todoroff, C. Eberle, J. Thelemann, N. Dirdjaja et al. 2014. Binding to large enzyme pockets: small-molecule inhibitors of trypanothione reductase. ChemMedChem. 9(8): 1880–91.

Rassi, A., Jr., A. Rassi and J.A. Marin-Neto. 2010. Chagas disease. Lancet. 375(9723): 1388–402.

Richardson, J.L., I.R. Nett, D.C. Jones, M.H. Abdille, I.H. Gilbert and A.H. Fairlamb. 2009. Improved tricyclic inhibitors of trypanothione reductase by screening and chemical synthesis. ChemMedChem. 4(8): 1333–40.

Saccoliti, F., G. Angiulli, G. Pupo, L. Pescatori, V.N. Madia, A. Messore et al. 2017. Inhibition of Leishmania infantum trypanothione reductase by diaryl sulfide derivatives. J. Enzyme Inhib. Med. Chem. 32(1): 304–310.

Saudagar, P., P. Saha, A.K. Saikia and V.K. Dubey. 2013. Molecular mechanism underlying antileishmanial effect of oxabicyclo[3.3.1]nonanones: inhibition of key redox enzymes of the pathogen. Eur. J. Pharm. Biopharm. 85(3 Pt A): 569–77.

Smith, H.K. and M. Bradley. 1999. Comparison of resin and solution screening methodologies in combinatorial chemistry and the identification of a 100 nM inhibitor of trypanothione reductase. J. Comb. Chem. 1(4): 326–32.

Sousa, A.F., A.G. Gomes-Alves, D. Benitez, M.A. Comini, L. Flohé, T. Jaeger et al. 2014. Genetic and chemical analyses reveal that trypanothione synthetase but not glutathionylspermidine synthetase is essential for Leishmania infantum. Free Radic. Biol. Med. 73: 229–38.

Spinks, D., L.S. Torrie, S. Thompson, J.R. Harrison, J.A. Frearson, K.D. Read et al. 2012. Design, synthesis and biological evaluation of Trypanosoma brucei trypanothione synthetase inhibitors. ChemMedChem. 7(1): 95–106.

Stump, B., C. Eberle, M. Kaiser, R. Brun, R.L. Krauth-Siegel and F. Diederich. 2008. Diaryl sulfide-based inhibitors of trypanothione reductase: inhibition potency, revised binding mode and antiprotozoal activities. Org. Biomol. Chem. 6(21): 3935–47.

Torrie, L.S., S. Wyllie, D. Spinks, S.L. Oza, S. Thompson, J.R. Harrison et al. 2009. Chemical validation of trypanothione synthetase: a potential drug target for human trypanosomiasis. J. Biol. Chem. 284(52): 36137–45.

Tovar, J., M.L. Cunningham, A.C. Smith, S.L. Croft and A.H. Fairlamb. 1998. Down-regulation of Leishmania donovani trypanothione reductase by heterologous expression of a trans-dominant mutant homologue: effect on parasite intracellular survival. Proc. Natl. Acad. Sci. USA. 95(9): 5311–6.

Trypanosomatid Diseases: Molecular Routes to Drug Discovery. Drug Discovery in Infectious Diseases. T. Jager, O. Koch, L. Flohe [eds.]. Series Editor Selzer PM, Wiley-Blackwell Ed. 2013.

Uliassi, E., G. Fiorani, R.L. Krauth-Siegel, C. Bergamini, R. Fato, G. Bianchini et al. 2017. Crassiflorone derivatives that inhibit Trypanosoma brucei glyceraldehyde-3-phosphate dehydrogenase (TbGAPDH) and Trypanosoma cruzi trypanothione reductase (TcTR) and display trypanocidal activity. Eur. J. Med. Chem. 141: 138–148.

Vincent, I.M., D. Creek, D.G. Watson, M.A. Kamleh, D.J. Woods, P.E. Wong et al. 2010. A molecular mechanism for eflornithine resistance in African trypanosomes. PLoS Pathog. 6(11): e1001204.

World Health Organization. 2016. Global Health Observatory Data—Leishmaniasis. Available at: http://www.who.int/gho/neglected_diseases/leishmaniasis/en/Global Health Observatory. 2016.

Zhang, Y., C.S. Bond, S. Bailey, M.L. Cunningham, A.H. Fairlamb and W.N. Hunter. 1996. The crystal structure of trypanothione reductase from the human pathogen Trypanosoma cruzi at 2.3 A resolution. Protein Sci. 5(1): 52–61.

Zhou, Y., N. Messier, M. Ouellette, B.P. Rosen and R. Mukhopadhyay. 2004. Leishmania major LmACR2 is a pentavalent antimony reductase that confers sensitivity to the drug pentostam. J. Biol. Chem. 279(36): 37445–51.

Chapter 12

The Renewal of Interest in Nitroaromatic Drugs

Towards New Anti-Kinetoplastid Agents

Nicolas Primas,[1,*] *Caroline Ducros,*[1] *Patrice Vanelle*[1,*]
and *Pierre Verhaeghe*[2]

Introduction

Currently, the World Health Organization (WHO) lists 20 Neglected Tropical Diseases (NTDs) affecting low-income populations from 149 countries. They are caused by a variety of pathogens such as viruses, bacteria, protozoa and helminths (Molyneux et al. 2017). These vector-borne parasites generate an economic and social burden in endemic areas, undermining the improvement of human health (Weiss 2008). Among these NTDs, kinetoplastid infections are estimated to put more than one billion people at risk (WHO 2015). Leishmaniases are infectious diseases caused by parasites of the *Leishmania* genus, transmitted to a mammal host (human, dog, monkey, rodent, etc.) by the bite of an infected female sandfly. Leishmaniases include several clinical forms such as visceral leishmaniasis (VL), fatal if untreated. It is due to the development of the intracellular amastigote form of the parasite, especially in the liver and spleen. The two main *Leishmania* species responsible for VL are *L. donovani* and *L. infantum* (Liévin-Le Moal and Loiseau 2016). Human African Trypanosomiasis (HAT) is an endemic vector-borne parasitic disease in sub-Saharan Africa. It is caused by a parasite called *Trypanosoma brucei* (*T. b.*) and transmitted by a tsetse fly (*Glossina* sp.) bite during a blood meal. Two different parasites are involved: *T. b. gambiense* responsible for chronic disease and *T. b. rhodesiense* responsible for acute disease. HAT first develops in a hemolymphatic stage, which can progress to a second nerve-affecting stage, causing serious meningo-encephalitis that can lead to death (Simarro et al. 2012, Franco et al. 2014, Büscher et al. 2017). Chagas disease (CD) or American Trypanosomiasis is caused by a parasite called *Trypanosoma cruzi* transmitted *via* the feces of the blood-sucking triatomine bug. CD evolves in two successive phases, an acute phase

[1] Aix-Marseille Univ, CNRS, Institut de Chimie Radicalaire, UMR 7273, Equipe Pharmaco-Chimie Radicalaire, Faculté de Pharmacie, 27 Boulevard Jean Moulin, 13385 Marseille cedex 05, France.
[2] CNRS, Université de Toulouse, UPR 8241, Laboratoire de chimie de coordination, 205 Route de Narbonne, 31077 Toulouse cedex 4, France.
* Corresponding authors: nicolas.primas@univ-amu.fr; patrice.vanelle@univ-amu.fr

with minor symptoms and a chronic phase with non-specific symptoms or clinical forms like cardiac, digestive or neurological. If untreated, this disease is fatal (Pérez-Molina and Molina 2018). Despite a considerable human burden, these diseases are called "neglected" mainly because the pharmaceutical industry has abandoned this research filed long ago for economic reasons (Willyard 2013). As a result, there are very few drugs available against kinetoplastid parasites and the marketed molecules display unacceptable side effects (arsenical encephalopathic for melarsoprol, kidney toxicity for amphotericin B, teratogenicity for miltefosine, etc). Furthermore, resistance to treatment has been increasing for many years, as noted with *L. donovani*: a 60% of resistance to antimony derivatives is found in India (Fairlamb 2003, García-Hernández et al. 2012, Copeland and Aronson 2015, Junior et al. 2017) (Table 1). Consequently, there is an urgent need for new, safe, effective, affordable and orally-active molecules to treat these lethal parasitic tropical neglected diseases.

Table 1. Data summary: kinetoplastid NTDs.

Species	Distribution	People at risk	Death/year	Treatments		New chemical entities in clinical trials
T. b. gambiense	West and Central Africa	61 million	Impossible to evaluate	*Stage 1* Fexinidazole Pentamidine	*Stage 2* Fexinidazole NECT	Acoziborole (SCYX-7158) (phase IIb/III)
T. b. rhodesiense	East and South Africa			*Stage 1* Suramine	*Stage 2* Melarsoprol	Fexinidazole
T. cruzi	South America	25 million	10,000	Benznidazole, Nifurtimox		Fexinidazole (Proof of Concept phase II)
L. donovani	South America, India, East Africa	616 million	20,000 to 30,000	Amphotericin B, Pentavalent antimony derivatives, Pentamidine, Miltefosine		DNDI-0690 (Phase I), DNDI-6148 (Phase I)
L. infantum						

First Nitroaromatic Drugs as Antiparasitic Agents

In the 1940s, nitroaromatic compounds showed their potential as chemotherapeutic agents. Many furans were synthesized as part of the search for new antibacterials. The particular ability of a nitro group in the 5th position of 2-substituted furans to confer antibacterial activity was clearly demonstrated (Dodd et al. 1944). The chemotherapeutic activity was displayed by a number of semicarbazone substituted nitrofurans. This work led to the nitrofuran antibacterial nitrofurazone (**1**) (Furacin®) (Main 1947, Dodd et al. 1950). The same drug also showed curative properties against experimental *T. b. gambiense* infections in mice (Packchanian 1955). The oral bioavailability of nitrofurazone (**1**) and its capacity to cross the blood-brain barrier (BBB) encouraged the first trials in patients infected by *T. b. gambiense* (Evens et al. 1957) or *T. b. rhodesiense* (Apted 1960). However, although these trials were mainly conducted in patients refractory to the other current treatments (pentamidine (**2**), suramin (**3**), melarsoprol (**4**), Figure 3), cure rates were variable and toxicities related to the nitrodrug appeared (Williamson 1962a, b), leading to the suspension of trials with nitrofurazone (**1**). However, its efficacy continued to be assessed on other NTDs: an animal model of Chagas disease (Packchanian 1957) and both cutaneous and visceral leishmaniases (Neal et al. 1988). Unfortunately, it showed a low level of *in vivo* efficacy and the evaluations were stopped.

Though nitrofurazone (**1**) did not find applications in the treatment of NTDs, its structure encouraged the industry to synthesize and test numerous nitro-containing heterocycles (Grunberg and Titsworth 1973). These studies led to the discovery of furaltadone (**5**) (Seneca et al. 1964), a nitrofuran derivative, metronidazole (**6**) (Furtado and Viegas 1967) and megazol (**7**) (Burden and Racette 1968), nitroimidazole derivatives, both with anti-trypanosomal activity. However, further development was also stopped due to neurotoxicity and low efficacy, except for megazol (**7**).

Fortunately, Bayer laboratory subsequently identified nifurtimox (**8**) (Lampit®), a nitrofuran derivative active against *T. cruzi*. It was introduced in 1965 for use in the treatment of acute CD in Latin America

(Ferreira 1967). However, due to gastrointestinal tract and central nervous system (CNS) side effects, the resistance of some *T. cruzi* strains and its genotoxicity, nifurtimox (**8**) use has now been discontinued in Brazil, Argentina, Chile, Uruguay and the USA (Rodriques Coura and de Castro 2002).

Several years later, in 1971, benznidazole (**9**) (Radanil®, Rochagan®), a 2-nitroimidazole, was introduced by Roche (Ferreira 1976) in the treatment of CD and is still in use. Although it was considered as better tolerated than nifurtimox (**8**), it still presents serious side-effects like dermatological reactions, agranulocytosis and neurotoxicity (Bern et al. 2007). Structure of nitroaromatic drugs are presented in Figure 1.

Nitroaromatics and toxicity issues

Toxicity concerns related to nitro-containing drugs emerged a long time ago (Strauss 1979), particularly due to the mutagenic potential of these compounds (McCann et al. 1975). Reduction of the nitro group was essential to observe the mutagenicity: in fact, the use of nitroreductase-deficient *Salmonella* in the bacterial reverse mutation assay (Ames test) abolished the mutagenicity of the niridazole (**10**) (Figure 2), a nitrothiazole (Blumer et al. 1980). However, these potential mutagenic issues prompted the pharmaceutical companies to preventively exclude the nitro group from drug-likeness predictor rules, to avoid drug development failures. Systematically excluded from screenings as "undesirable group", nitro-containing

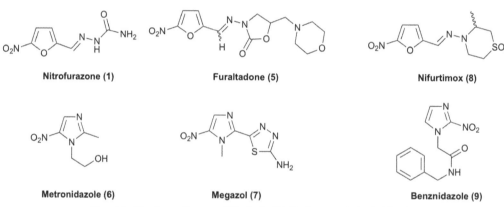

Nitrofurazone (1)   **Furaltadone (5)**   **Nifurtimox (8)**

Metronidazole (6)   **Megazol (7)**   **Benznidazole (9)**

Figure 1. Structures of some antikinetoplastid nitrofurans and nitroimidazoles.

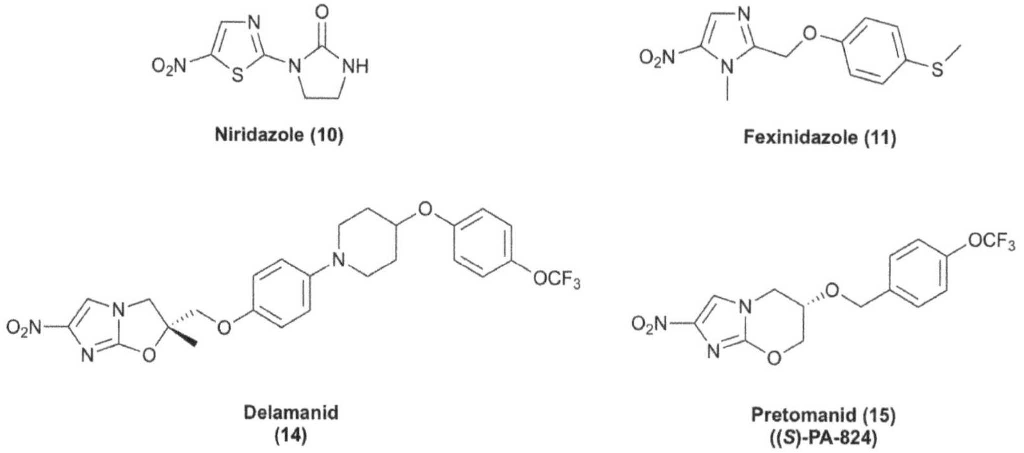

Niridazole (10)   **Fexinidazole (11)**

Delamanid   **Pretomanid (15)**
(14)   **((S)-PA-824)**

Figure 2. Structure of non-mutagenic nitroaromatics.

derivatives were therefore underdeveloped (Brenk et al. 2008, Shultz 2013). However, there have been several attempts to dissociate their anti-infective activity from their genotoxic character, considering that these molecules require to be bioactivated into genotoxic derivatives, to kill the parasite (Walsh et al. 1987, Crozet et al. 2009, Fersing et al. 2019). For fexinidazole (**11**) (see 5.1), nitroreductase-dependent mutagenic activity was observed in the Ames test. On the other hand, its genotoxicity was evaluated as negative by the micronucleus test (*in vitro* on human cells and *in vivo* in the rat), both for the parent molecule and for its two metabolites (sulfoxide (**12**) and sulfone (**13**), Figure 6) (Tweats et al. 2012). This result strongly suggests that the mutagenicity associated with nitroheterocycles is not an intrinsic parameter of this drug class and highlights the nitro reduction potential as a possible criterion for identifying the mutagenic properties during the nitrodrug development process (Hanaki et al. 2017). Moreover, 4-nitroimidazole-related molecules such as delamanid (**14**) (Deltyba®) and pretomanid (**15**) ((*S*)-PA-824), both antitubercular drug or drug-candidate, did not exhibit genotoxicity in the Ames test, suggesting the possibility of designing non-mutagenic anti-kinetoplastid nitroheterocycles (Stover et al. 2000, Matsumoto et al. 2006) (Figure 2).

Renewed Interest in Nitrodrugs

Nifurtimox—Eflornithine combination therapy and rediscovery of fexinidazole (11)

In 2001, a clinical trial compared three drug combination treatments for second-stage HAT due to *T. b. gambiense*: melarsoprol (**4**) with eflornithine (**16**), melarsoprol (**4**) with nifurtimox (**8**), and eflornithine (**16**) with nifurtimox (**8**) (Priotto et al. 2006). The existing anti-trypanosomal drugs were combined as a way of reducing the required dosages to avoid the related toxicities and the emergence of drug-resistance. Against all expectations, the trial was interrupted prematurely due to high drug-related mortality in the melarsoprol arms. Fortunately, Nifurtimox-Eflornithine Combination Therapy (NECT) demonstrated good tolerance and sufficient efficacy for further investigations to be performed. Cure rates with the NECT drug-combination (96.5%) were comparable with monotherapy using eflornithine (**16**), but with lower side-effects. Moreover, it allowed the dose and the duration of the eflornithine (**16**) infusion to be reduced (Priotto et al. 2009). The Drugs for Neglected Diseases Initiative (DNDi) successfully repositioned nifurtimox (**8**), originally designed as an antichagasic drug, and prompted the WHO in 2009 to add NECT to the Model Lists of Essential Medicines, as more than 60% of late-stage *T. b. gambiense* HAT could be treated using this combination. NECT represented a significant achievement, providing the first new drug regimen for HAT in nearly two decades. DNDi is a public-private partnership that focuses on drug discovery and clinical development. It has developed target product profiles (TPPs) and compound progression criteria for trypanosomatid diseases (Don and Ioset 2014). The ideal TPPs focus on new regimens that are active against all strains/subspecies, with good oral bioavailability, short treatment durations, improved safety to efficacy ratios and low cost. Alongside the NECT success, the potential of the old nitroimidazole megazol (**7**) was rediscovered in combination with suramin (**3**) and showed to be curative in a stage 2 HAT-infected mouse model (Enanga et al. 1998, Darsaud et al. 2004), although the study was stopped due to the genotoxicity of megazol (**7**) (Enanga et al. 2003). Drugs used in the combination therapy are shown in Figure 3.

Given the urgent need for new anti-trypanosomatid agents, the historical use of several nitrodugs in this field and the success of NECT, the DNDi sourced and screened more than 700 nitroaromatics. This screening led to a hit compound belonging to the 5-nitroimidazole series: fexinidazole (**11**). In fact, fexinidazole (**11**) was first described in 1978 by Hoechst (Winkelmann and Raether 1978) and its antiparasitic properties were known at the time: fexinidazole (**11**) was active *in vitro* and *in vivo* against *T. brucei* (Jennings and Urquhart 1983), *T. cruzi* and also trichomonads such as *Entamoeba histolytica* (Raether and Seidenath 1983). Although fexinidazole (**11**) was found to cure stage 2 HAT in a mouse model, development was stopped because the pharmaceutical industry was unwilling to explore nitrodrugs further owing to their possible toxicity.

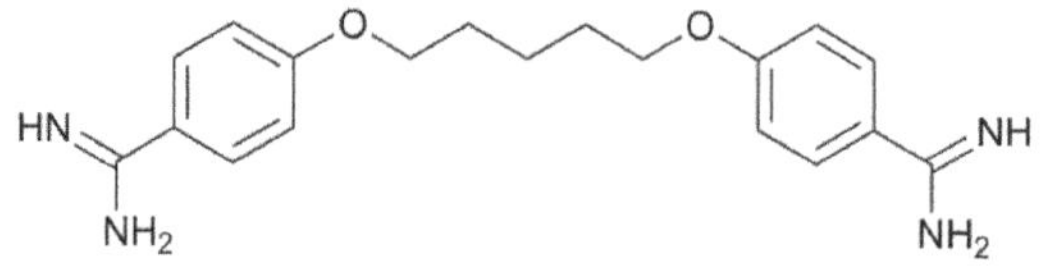

Pentamidine (2)

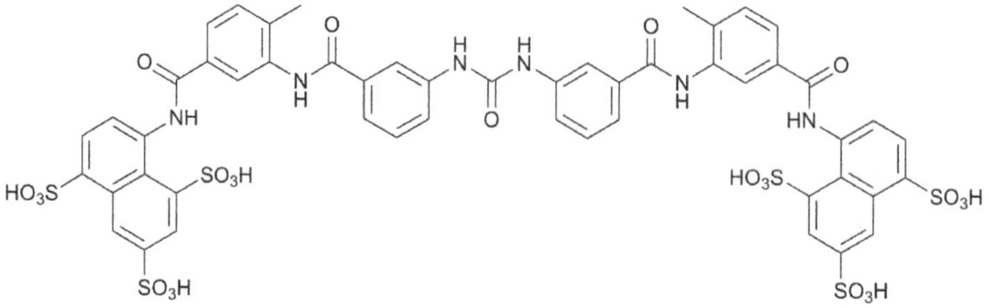

Suramin (3)

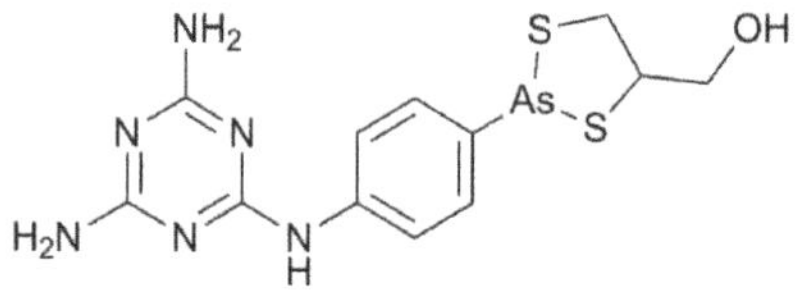

Melarsoprol (4) 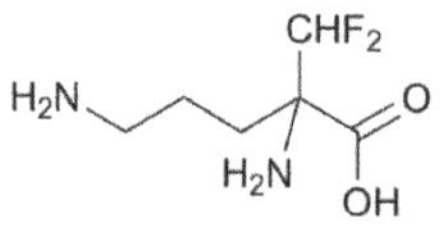   **Eflornithine (16)**

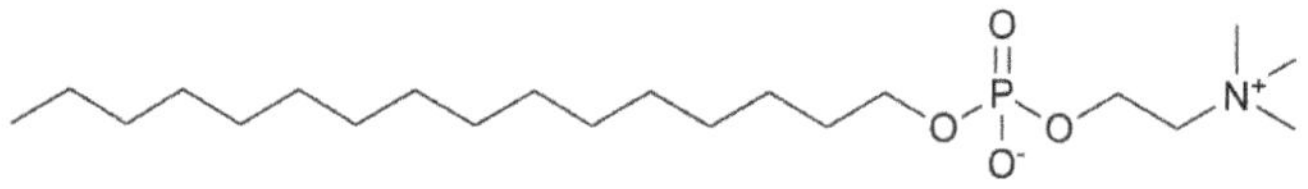

Miltefosine (19)

Figure 3. Structures of some non-nitrated antitrypanosomatid drugs.

Mechanism of action of nitroaromatic derivatives

Key role of the nitro group

Anti-infective nitroheterocycles act as prodrugs requiring the bioactivation of their nitro group before presenting antibacterial or antiparasitic properties (Blumer et al. 1980). While this nitro group is mandatory to the activity of this family of molecules, diverse substituents on the other positions of the heterocyclic ring may allow the modulation of their spectrum of activity and physicochemical parameters (Goldman 1982). The recognized mechanism of action for 5-nitroimidazoles first involves their penetration into the target cell by passive diffusion, followed by the reduction of the nitro group into Reactive oxygen species (ROS), including radical species (Race et al. 2005). Finally, the reaction of these reactive metabolites with cellular components such as DNA or proteins forms covalent adducts leading to the death of the infective agent (Azam et al. 2015). The reduction of nitroimidazole drugs by microorganisms is governed both by the reduction potential of the molecule and the number of electrons involved in the reduction (Edwards 1993, Spain 1995). In kinetoplastids, the enzymes catalyzing this type of reaction are called nitroreductases (NTR) (Fairlamb and Patterson 2018).

Nitroreductases (NTRs)

NTRs cover a family of proteins whose first members were discovered in eubacteria and were classified by sequence similarities (Bryant et al. 1981). These enzymes can catalyze the reduction of nitroaromatics by using flavin mononucleotide (FMN) or flavin adenine dinucleotide (FAD) as prosthetic groups, and nicotinamide adenine dinucleotide (NADH) or nicotinamide adenine dinucleotide phosphate (NADPH) as reducing agents (de Olivera 2010a). The biological function of NTR is currently poorly known: most likely, it serves as a response to oxidative stress (Roldán et al. 2008, de Olivera et al. 2010b).

To date, two types of NTRs have been characterized according to whether a single or two electrons are transferred:

- Type I NTR or NTR1, oxygen-insensitive, are frequently found in bacteria but are rare among eukaryotes (identified nevertheless in *Leishmania* and *Trypanosoma*). They catalyze the reduction of nitro groups by sequential two-electron reductions finally yielding primary amines (Figure 4). The nitroso and hydroxylamine intermediates can react with biomolecules to exert toxic and mutagenic effects (Whitmore and Varghese 1986, Koder et al. 2002).

- Type II NTR or NTR2, oxygen-dependent, catalyze the monoelectronic reduction of nitroaromatic derivatives, leading to a nitro radical anion. The instability of such species in the presence of oxygen can, by oxidation, generate the parent nitro molecule and a reactive superoxide anion. This so-called "futile" cycle causes oxidative stress by generating large quantities of superoxides (Figure 4). In the absence of oxygen, two nitro radical anions can react by a disproportionation reaction to afford one parent nitroaromatic molecule and a nitroso intermediate which could possibly react with a type I NTR (Peterson et al. 1979, Angermaier and Simon 1983).

To date, no structural data such as crystallography was available for kinetoplastid nitroreductase, which upset the rational drug design of new nitroaromatics.

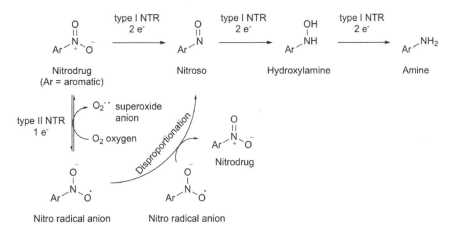

Figure 4. Reduction mechanisms of nitroaromatic compound by NTR of type I and type II (Patterson and Wyllie 2014).

Nitroreductase-catalyzed bioactivation of nifurtimox (8) and benznidazole (9)

With the DNDi reintroducing nitrodrugs to target NTDs, further mechanistic explorations were performed to identify toxic metabolites that could lead to the death of kinetoplastids. Mechanistic studies of the bioactivation of nifurtimox (**8**) showed that it was bioactivated by a type I NTR in *T. brucei* and *T. cruzi* (Wilkinson et al. 2008, Hall et al. 2011), and a similar observation was made with benznidazole (**9**) (Hall and Wilkinson 2012, Trochine et al. 2014).

The NTR1 bioactivation of nifurtimox (**8**) led to an unsaturated open-chain nitrile product (**17**) characterized by LC/MS (Figure 5). This metabolite was shown to inhibit both parasite and mammalian cell growth at equivalent concentrations, in marked contrast to the parent prodrug. The unsaturated open-

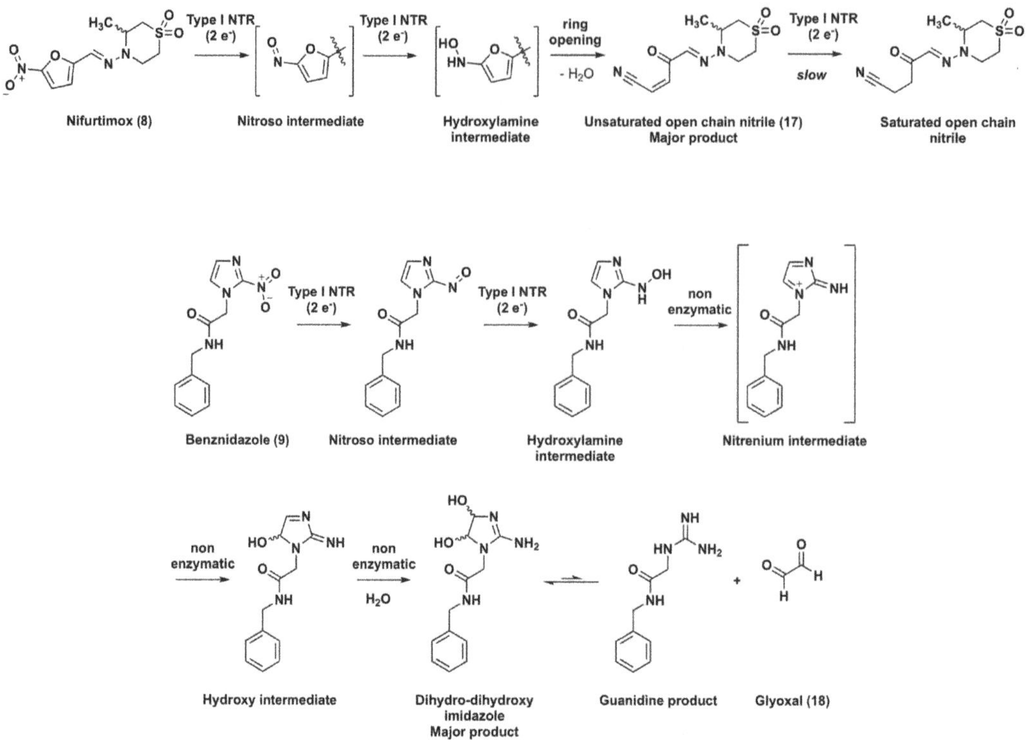

Figure 5. Bioactivation mechanism of nifurtimox (**8**) and benznidazole (**9**) by type I NTR (Patterson and Wyllie 2014).

chain nitrile derived from nifurtimox (**8**) had the potential to function as a Michael acceptor and could react non-specifically with a range of cellular components. This may explain the pleiotropic effects of nifurtimox on trypanosomes (Hall et al. 2011). It was initially thought that bioactivation of benznidazole (**9**) by NTR1 could give glyoxal (**18**) (Figure 5), a well-known toxic metabolite, postulated to contribute to the pleiotropic effects that benznidazole (**9**) induces in trypanosomes (Hall and Wilkinson 2012). However, the biotransformation of benznidazole (**9**) in *T. cruzi* was not directly investigated, but it was addressed in a metabolomic study in which low molecular weight adducts of glyoxal (**18**) were not detected. Finally, it was proposed that the covalent binding of benznidazole (**9**), both with low molecular weight thiols and with thiols-containing proteins, is a primary cause of the drug's activity against *T. cruzi* (Trochine et al. 2014).

Nitroaromatic derivatives under preclinical or clinical development

Fexinidazole (11)

The reassessment of the pharmacological and toxicological properties of fexinidazole (**11**), a result of the successful compound-mining efforts pursued by the DNDi in 2005, confirmed the excellent safety profile of the nitro-compound, with no genotoxicity to mammalian cells (Torreele et al. 2010). *In vivo*, fexinidazole is effective in curing both *T. b. rhodesiense* and *T. b. gambiense* acute models of infection at an oral dose of 100 mg/kg/day for 4 days. Most significantly, in a *T. b. brucei* infected mouse model of stage 2 HAT involving brain infection, 100% cure was obtained in groups of 5 mice receiving an oral dose of 100 mg/kg, twice per day for 5 days. As predicted by Winkelmann and Raether (Winkelmann and Raether 1978), fexinidazole (**11**) was extensively metabolized on the sulfur atom *in vivo* to give the corresponding sulfoxide (**12**) and the sulfone (**13**) metabolites (Figure 6), both of which display *in vitro* potency approximately equal to that of fexinidazole (**11**) itself (though *in vivo* efficacy of these metabolites was

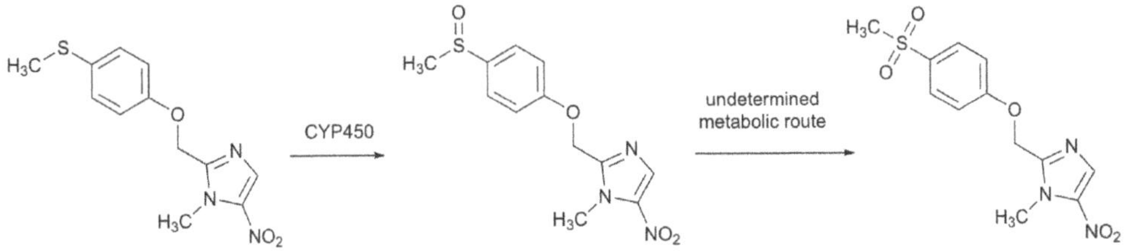

Fexinidazole (11)
IC$_{50}$ *T. b. gambiense* = 1,84 µM
IC$_{50}$ *T. b. rhodesiense* = 2,17 µM

Sulfoxide metabolite (12)
IC$_{50}$ *T. b. gambiense* = 0,91 µM
IC$_{50}$ *T. b. rhodesiense* = 1,44 µM

Sulfone metabolite (13)
IC$_{50}$ *T. b. gambiense* = 0,94 µM
IC$_{50}$ *T. b. rhodesiense* = 1,64 µM

Reference drug activities on *T. b. gambiense* : Melarsoprol = 0,005 µM ; Eflornithine = 1,67 µM ; Nifurtimox = 1,08 µM
Reference drug activities on *T. b. rhodesiense* : Melarsoprol = 0,007 µM ; Eflornithine = 3,80 µM ; Nifurtimox = 1,44 µM

Figure 6. Structures of fexinidazole (**11**) and its two active metabolites (**12–13**).

lower than that of the parent drug). This allows a lengthy combined exposure time over which antiparasitic activity can be exerted (Kaiser et al. 2011).

Fexinidazole (**11**), like other nitrodrugs, is a prodrug that requires activation by a nitroreductase (Wyllie et al. 2016a). A first *L. donovani* type 1 NTR (Ld)NTR1 was discovered and was found essential for parasite growth and replication, as it cannot be experimentally repressed (Voak et al. 2013). However, it was proved possible to generate a parasite strain overexpressing this (Ld)NTR1 in which a 15-fold increase in sensitivity to fexinidazole (**11**) was observed (Wyllie et al. 2012), confirming the direct involvement of (Ld)NTR1 in the activation of fexinidazole (Wyllie et al. 2013).

Phase II/III study results published in 2017 confirmed that fexinidazole (**11**) is safe and effective and presents significant advantages over NECT for HAT disease. In fact, it eliminates both the need for a lumbar puncture and systematic patient hospitalization (Mesu et al. 2018). Fexinidazole (**11**) received a positive scientific opinion by the European Medicines Agency's Committee in November 2018 and was registered in the Democratic Republic of Congo in December 2018. Fexinidazole is indicated as a 10-day once-a-day oral treatment for *T. b. gambiense* sleeping sickness that works both for two stages of the disease. A phase IIIb (clinical trial NCT03025789) study is currently underway, aiming to provide additional information on the efficacy and safety of fexinidazole and to assess its use under conditions as close as possible to real life, ideally allowing patients to take their medication at home, the results are expected by 2020 (Pollastri 2018). A new Phase II/III study is also being prepared in Malawi to assess fexinidazole (**11**) to treat HAT caused by *T. b. rhodesiense*, the other subspecies of the parasite that causes a more virulent strain of the disease. The study should start in mid-2019 (DNDi 2019a).

The DNDi also reassessed the potential of fexinidazole (**11**) to treat Chagas disease. New *in vivo* studies showed that fexinidazole (**11**) is effective in reducing parasitaemia and preventing mortality in a *T. cruzi* infected animal model, with identical cure rates to those obtained with benznidazole (**9**) (Bahia et al. 2012). Although active in the chronic phase of the infection, fexinidazole (**11**) and fexinidazole sulfone (**13**) are more effective than nifurtimox (**8**) and benznidazole (**9**) as curative treatments, particularly for acute stage infections (Franscico et al. 2016). Presenting a broad spectrum of activity on several genotypes of *T. cruzi* (Moares et al. 2014), metabolite fexinidazole sulfone (**13**) was found superior to benznidazole (**9**) or fexinidazole (**11**) itself in a mouse model of acute infection (Bahia et al. 2014). In view of these promising results, a first phase II Proof-of-Concept (PoC) study was initiated in 2014 in Bolivia. A total of 47 patients were included, but the study was interrupted due to safety and tolerability issues. Interim data efficacy and safety analysis suggested high efficacy rates for fexinidazole (**11**) and a decision was made to extend clinical study follow-up to 12 months. Analysis of key efficacy outcomes and safety demonstrated high efficacy at the lowest dose tested and for all treatment durations, with safety concerns around treatment with high doses tested for more than 14 days. In addition, acceptable safety and tolerability were found at low doses and short treatment durations. Taken together, these results suggest that further investigation of fexinidazole (**11**) for Chagas disease is warranted (DNDi 2018).

Given its efficacy against other trypanosomatid infections, the antileishmanial potential of fexinidazole (**11**) was evaluated *in vitro* and *in vivo* (Wyllie et al. 2012). The sulfoxide (**12**) and sulfone

(**13**) metabolites showed activity on intramacrophagic amastigote forms of *L. donovani*, while the parent molecule was inactive on this parasitic stage (Koniordou et al. 2017). With oral results comparable to those of miltefosine (**19**) (Figure 3) and pentamidine (**2**), fexinidazole (**11**) rapidly entered the Phase II PoC in 2013, to evaluate its safety and efficacy in humans as a potential treatment for VL. However, this study ended after 2 years, due to a lack of efficacy in this indication, with relapses observed (Zulfiqar et al. 2017). A fexinidazole (**11**)/miltefosine (**19**) combination was later envisaged by the DNDi but appears to have been on hold since 2016 (DNDi 2016).

Drug repositioning: bicyclic nitroimidazoles

Discovery of anti-TB activity

The first bicyclic nitroimidazole, a nitroimidazooxazole, that was reported to display *in vitro* and *in vivo* antitubercular activity was CGI-17341 (**20**) (Figure 7), discovered by Hindustan Ciba-Geigy in 1989 (Nagarajan et al. 1989, Ashtekar et al. 1993). However, it was found to be mutagenic in the Ames test, discouraging the company from carrying out further development and investigations in this series. In 2000, PathoGenesis (now Novartis) described a lead compound Pretomanid (**15**) ((*S*)-PA-824, Figure 7) from a series of over 300 nitroimidazopyrans (Stover et al. 2000, Denny and Palmer 2010). Pretomanid (**15**) showed excellent safety (not mutagenic) and bactericidal efficacy in phase II clinical trials on TB (Diacon et al. 2012). In 2006, Otsuka Pharmaceutical overcame the mutagenicity problem of the nitroimidazooxazole series by substituting the 2-position of the side chain with a heteroatom. This new series led to compound OPC-67683, now called Delamanid (**14**) (Deltyba®) (Figure 7), approved since 2014 for the treatment of adult pulmonary multidrug-resistant TB (MDR-TB) in combination therapies (Matsumoto et al. 2006, Gler et al. 2012, Gupta et al. 2016). Numerous analogs of bicyclic nitroimidazoles have been investigated in the wake of the success of Delamanid (**14**) (Mukherjee and Boshoff 2011).

Discovery of the anti-Visceral Leishmaniasis (VL) activity of pretomanid (**15**) and delamanid (**14**)

In the field of NTD drug discovery, the repurposing of drugs and clinical candidates offers a valuable alternative to *de novo* drug discovery, reducing research and development costs (Andrews et al. 2014). Given the potential activity of the antitubercular nitroimidazole (*S*)-PA-824 (**15**) (Pretomanid) (Figure 2) against *L. donovani* amastigotes (Jiricek et al. 2008), and the fact that both *M. tuberculosis* and *L. donovani* reside in macrophages *in vivo*, antitubercular agents should be an appropriate starting point in the search for VL treatments. Patterson et al. showed that (*S*)-PA-824 (**15**) is active against *L. donovani*

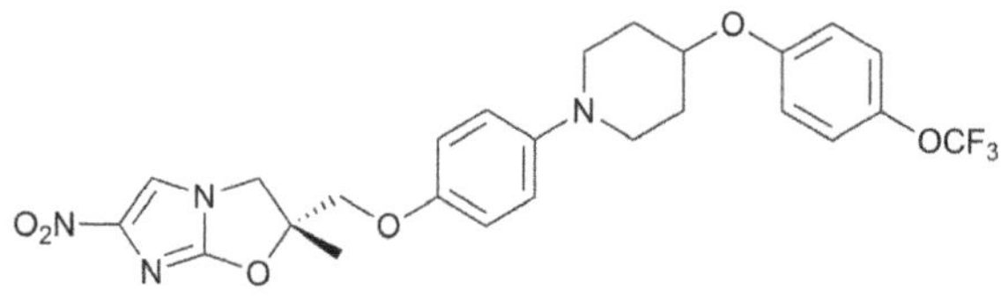

Delamanid (**14**)

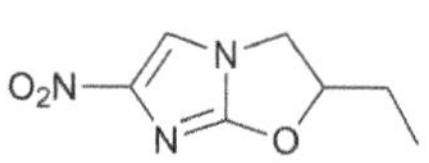

CGI-17341 (**20**) 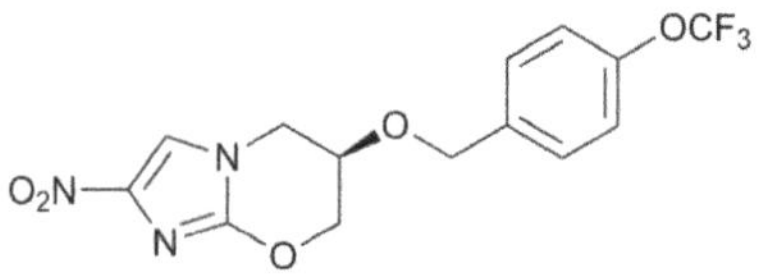   (*R*)-PA-824 (**21**)

Figure 7. Structures of nitro-containing bicyclic derivatives.

intracellular amastigotes at a potency comparable to that of fexinidazole sulfone (**13**) (EC$_{50}$ = 4.9 µM vs 5.3 µM) (Patterson et al. 2013). However, unlike the structure-activity relationships for *M. tuberculosis*, where the *S*-enantiomer of PA-824 is > 100-fold more active than the *R*-enantiomer, (*R*)-PA-824 (**21**) was found to be 5-fold more potent than the *S*-enantiomer in *L. donovani* (Figure 7). In a VL mouse model, at 100 mg.kg^{-1}, administered twice daily orally for 5 days, (*R*)-PA-824 (**21**) led to almost complete clearance of infection (Patterson et al. 2013). *In vitro* drug-combination studies indicate that fexinidazole (**11**) and (*R*)-PA-824 (**21**) are additive whereas (*S*)-PA-824 (**15**) and (*R*)-PA-824 (**21**) show mild antagonistic behavior. Moreover, *Leishmania* type I NTR cannot activate (*R*)-PA-824 (**21**), the nitro group remaining essential to the leishmanicidal activity. It was later demonstrated that the bicyclic PA-824 is activated in *Leishmania* by a novel type 2 nitroreductase (Wyllie et al. 2016b). As other more potent bicyclic nitroimidazoles were discovered concurrently, (*R*)-PA-824 (**21**) was not selected as preclinical agent in VL.

A similar study on the antitubercular bicyclic nitroimidazole delamanid (**14**) showed that it was a potent inhibitor of *L. donovani* both *in vitro* and *in vivo* (Patterson et al. 2016). Delamanid (**14**) (EC$_{50}$ = 0.087 µM) was found to be more active than the standard drug miltefosine (**19**) (EC$_{50}$ = 3.3 µM) and the active fexinidazole metabolite (**13**) (EC$_{50}$ = 5.3 µM) when assessed against intracellular *L. donovani* amastigotes. The (*S*)-enantiomer of delamanid was less potent, in line with its enantiomeric specificity in *M. tuberculosis* (Sasaki et al. 2006). Twice-daily oral dosing of delamanid (**14**) at 30 mg.kg^{-1} for 5 days resulted in sterile cures in a mouse model of VL. Despite this favorable *in vivo* activity called for preclinical evaluation, the recent identification of DNDI-VL-2098 (**22**) (Figure 8) as a preclinical candidate by the DNDi stopped the development of delamanid (**14**). It was recently showed that bicyclic nitroaromatics delamanid (**14**), DNDI-VL-2098 (**22**) and (*R*)-PA-824 (**21**) were activated by a type 2 nitroreductase (Wyllie et al. 2016b).

Bicyclic DNDi preclinical candidates

TB Alliance, a not-for-profit product development partnership dedicated to the discovery and development of new tuberculosis medicines, was granted access to a selected library of 72 antimycobacterial nitroimidazoles belonging to four chemical subclasses, under a contractual agreement with DNDi. These molecules belonging to the backup program for the clinical trial agent pretomanid were evaluated for their antileishmanial activity, leading to the identification of DNDI-VL-2098 (**22**) as a preclinical candidate for the oral treatment of VL (Mukkavilli et al. 2014, Gupta et al. 2015). DNDI-VL-2098 (**22**) is the *R*-enantiomer of the racemate DNDI-VL-2001 (**23**) (Figure 8), which possesses the same bicyclic moiety as delamanid (**14**) and was found more potent than the *S*-enantiomer. DNDI-VL-2098 (**22**) showed both good *in vitro* activity (IC$_{50}$ = 0.03 µM for the *L. donovani* DD8 strain, Table 2) and *in vivo* activity in mouse models, with an ED$_{90}$ value of 3.7 mg/kg. Together with its leishmanicidal activity, DNDI-VL-2098 (**22**) was also capable of inducing host-protective immune cells to suppress *Leishmania* parasites in hamsters. Unfortunately, testicular toxic effects were noted in the animal model and the development of the compound was stopped in 2015 (DNDi 2015, Charlton et al. 2018).

Fortunately, two new lead bicyclic nitroimidazoles, DNDI-0690 (**24**) and DNDI-8219 (**25**) (Figure 8 and Table 2), were selected as backup for the compound DNDI-VL-2098.

Following the discontinuation of DNDI-VL-2098 (**22**), Thompson et al. attempted to identify non-toxic backup compounds having an improved physicochemical and pharmacological profile. This new study also provided wider SAR conclusions for the nitroimidazooxazole class against TB and three kinetoplastid NTDs, together with a first *in vivo* appraisal of the best new leads for VL (Thompson et al. 2016). Several less lipophilic analogs displayed improved aqueous solubility, particularly at low pH, although stability toward liver microsomes was highly variable. Evaluated in a mouse model of acute *L. donovani* infection, one new nitroimidazooxazine derivative DNDI-0690 (**24**) (Figure 8), bearing a phenylpyridine side-chain, provided efficacy surpassing the original preclinical lead DNDI-VL-2098 (**22**). Nearly total parasite clearance was observed at 25 mg/kg for 5 days and 98% inhibition at 1.56 mg/kg (Thompson et al. 2016). Overall, the *R*-enantiomer of DNDI-0690 (**24**) displayed better pharmacokinetic parameters, leading to its selection as the preferred development candidate over the *S*-enantiomer. In terms of safety, DNDI-0690 (**24**) showed low inhibition of hERG (IC$_{50}$ > 30 µM), did not inhibit CYP3A4 (IC$_{50}$ > 100 µM), and was not mutagenic (Ames test). Interestingly, DNDI-0690 (**24**) belonging to the novel

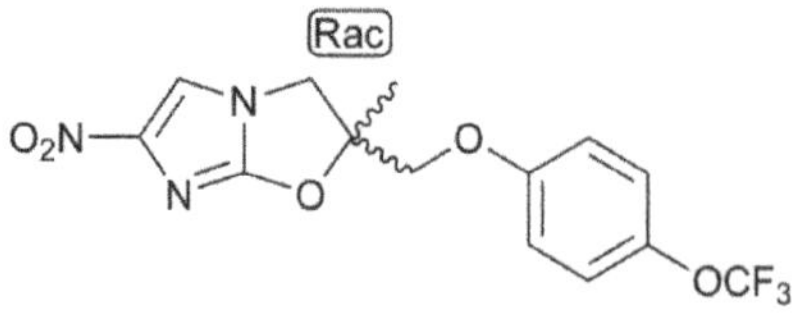

DNDI-VL-2001 (23)
racemate

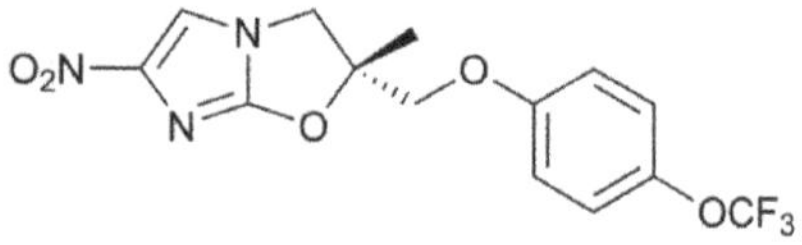

DNDI-VL-2098 (22)

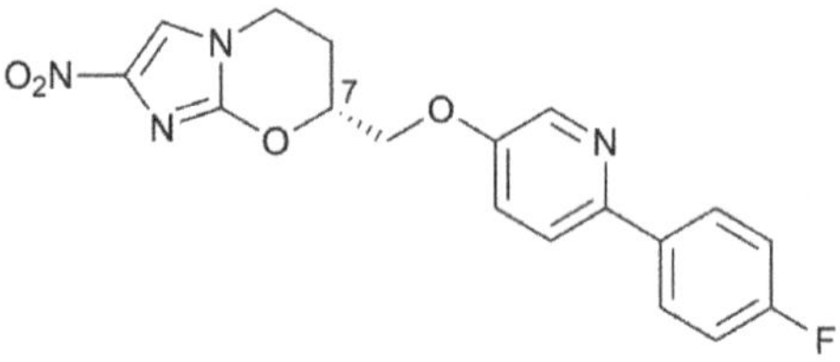

DNDI-0690 (24)

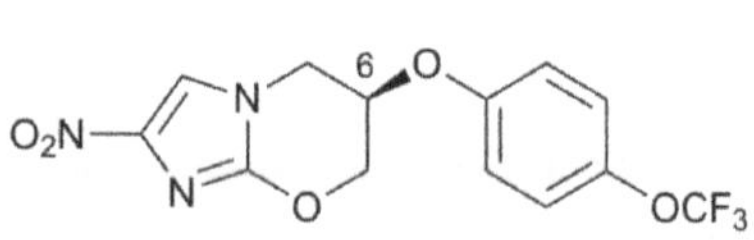

DNDI-8219 (25)

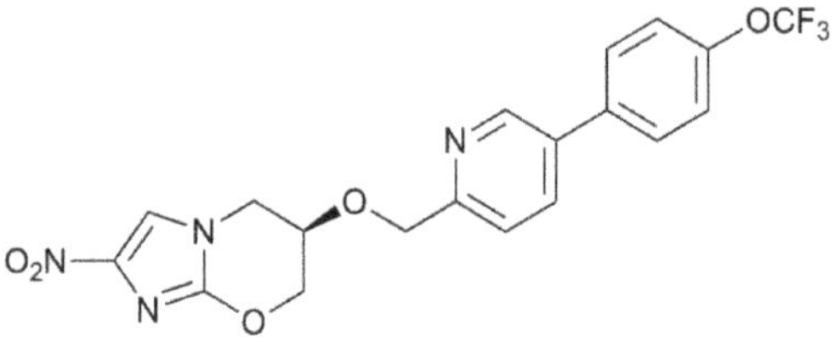

(26)
hERG inhibitor

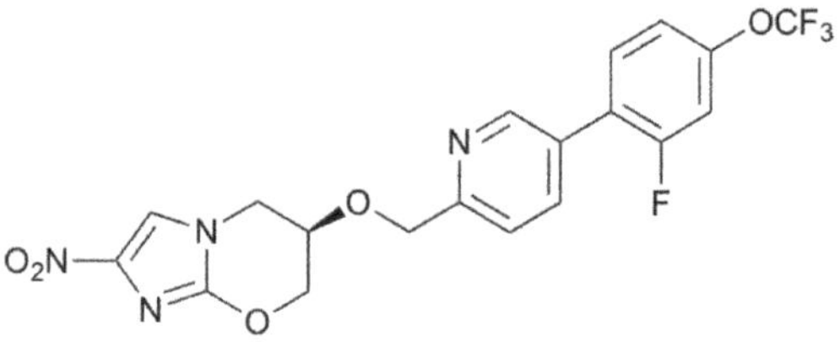

(27)
hERG inhibitor

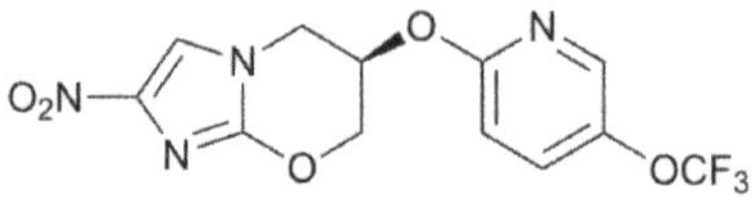

(28)
Ames positive

Figure 8. Structures of new antileishmanials leads DNDI-0690 (**24**) and DNDI-8219 (**25**) DNDI-VL-2001 (**23**), DNDI-VL-2098 (**22**) and related analogs (**22**, **23**, **26–28**).

Table 2. *In vitro* data on DNDi VL lead compounds.

	L. donovani	*L. infantum*	*T. cruzi*	*T. brucei*	MRC-5
DNDI-VL-2098 (22)	0.03	0.17	2.6	–	> 64
DNDI-0690 (24)	0.03	0.08	0.35	> 64	> 64
DNDI-8219 (25)	0.19	0.53	0.15	> 64	> 64

IC_{50} in μM values for inhibition of the growth of *L. donovani* and *L. infantum* (in mouse macrophages), *T. cruzi* (on MRC-5 cells), and *T. brucei*, or for cytotoxicity toward human lung fibroblasts (MRC-5 cells).

7-substituted 2-nitroimidazooxazine class showed good activity against both TB and Chagas disease, but not against HAT (Thompson et al. 2017).

DNDI-0690 (**24**) has now been selected and is in preclinical development. The first in human phase I study of safety, tolerability, and pharmacokinetics after single oral ascending doses of DNDI-0690 (**24**) was submitted to UK authorities in February 2019 (DNDi 2019b).

In order to secure backup derivatives against VL, a screening of a 900-compound pretomanid analog library was made, highlighting several hits with more suitable potency, solubility, and microsomal stability. These derivatives showed higher efficacy in a *L. donovani* mouse model of newly synthesized *R*-enantiomers with phenylpyridine-based side chains DNDI-0690 (**24**) at position 6 of the bicycle (Figure 8). Two new leads (**26**) and (**27**) displayed promising activity in the more stringent *L. infantum* hamster model but were unexpectedly found to be potent inhibitors of hERG. An extensive structure-activity relationship investigation highlighted two compounds, pyridine (**28**) and phenyl (**25**), with better solubility and pharmacokinetic properties along with an excellent oral efficacy in the same hamster model (> 97% parasite clearance at 25 mg/kg, twice daily) with minimal hERG inhibition. Additional profiling, however, showed that (**28**) was positive in the Ames test, preventing its further advancement. Finally, (**25**), now known as DNDI-8219 (Figure 8), was the favored VL backup candidate for DNDI-0690 (**24**) (Thompson et al. 2018). *In vitro* and *in vivo* data for these compounds are shown in Tables 2 and 3.

Table 3. Percentage reduction of amastigote burdens in liver, spleen and bone marrow after 5-day oral treatment with DNDi lead compounds in the early curative *L. infantum* model in the hamster (Van den Kerkhof et al. 2018).

Compounds	Dose	% reduction		
	mg/kg/day	Liver	Spleen	Bone marrow
Miltefosine (19)	40 SID	97.9	99.6	97.3
DNDI-VL-2098 (22)	50 SID	100	100	100
	25 SID	100	99.9	99.7
	12.5	99.0	98.7	94
DNDI-0690 (24)	12.5 BID	96.4	97.5	96.5
	6.25 BID	92.6	86.3	86.7
	12.5 SID	65.8	69.7	51.6
DNDI-8219 (25)	25 BID	98.4	99.2	97.0

Results are expressed as percentage reduction of amastigote burdens and are based on one experiment with five animals per group. Treatment was given once a day (SID) or twice a day (BID).

Other nitroaromatic derivatives under pre-clinical stage of development (screening, Hit-to-Lead)

The recent literature concerning anti-kinetoplastid nitroaromatics is surveyed below, covering the last ten years. The molecules are presented according to their biological activity: antichagasic derivatives, anti-*Trypanosoma brucei* derivatives (HAT) and antileishmanial derivatives, active only against the visceral form caused by *L. donovani* and *L. infantum*.

Antichagasic Nitrocompounds

5-Nitrofuran derivatives

The 5-nitrofuran series has been extensively studied over the past 50 years, but it still attracts a great interest in the field of medicinal chemistry.

Closely related analogs of nifuroxazide (**29**) (Figure 9), a 5-nitrofuran antibacterial marketed since 1966, were synthesized and tested against various strains of *T. cruzi*. Like nifurtimox (**8**) or nitrofurazone (**1**) (Figure 1), nifuroxazide (**29**) possesses a hydrazide moiety as a lateral chain. It should be pointed out

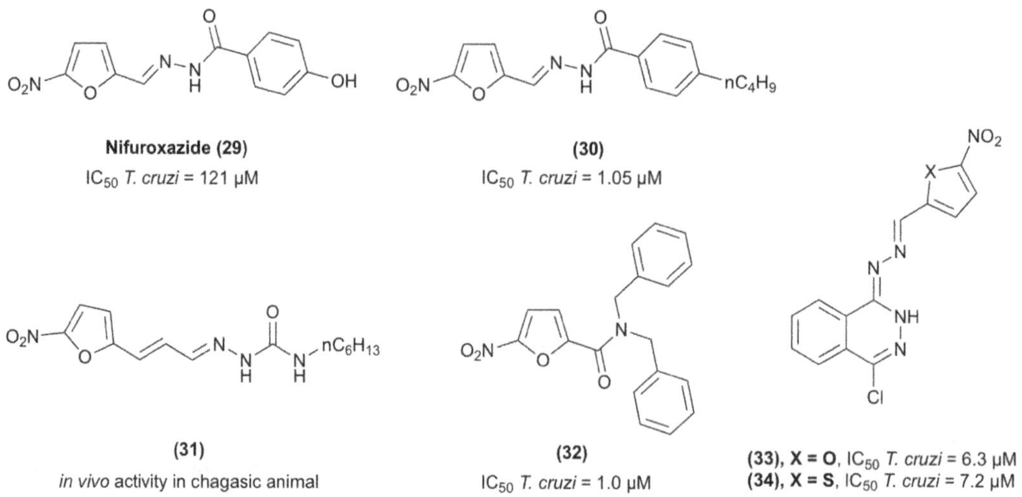

Figure 9. Structures of some antichagasic 5-nitrofurans.

that nifuroxazide (**29**) was almost inactive against *T. cruzi* compared to reference drugs (nifuroxazide (**29**) IC_{50} = 120.46 μM; benznidazole (**9**) IC_{50} = 22.69 μM and nifurtimox (**8**) IC_{50} = 3.78 μM).

Compound (**30**) (Figure 9) presented threefold higher *in vitro* activity than nifurtimox (**8**) against epimastigote forms of Y strain of *T. cruzi*. In the cytotoxicity assay, metronidazole (**6**) (Figure 1) presented an IC_{50} value of 28.05 μM (Selectivity index (SI) = cytotoxicity/activity ratio = 26.71) against J774 cells (Palace-Berl et al. 2013).

Replacement of the *n*-butylphenyl group by naphthalene led to very similar activity against three other *T. cruzi* strains (Silvio X10 cl1, Bug 2149 cl10 and Colombiana: IC_{50} values from 1.17 to 3.17 μM) (Palace-Berl et al. 2015). Similar activities were obtained when the aliphatic chain of (**6**) was increased to eight carbons (Palace-Berl et al. 2015). Cytotoxicity assays using human fibroblast cells demonstrated high selectivity indexes for these compounds.

However, the replacement of the 5-nitrofuran moiety by a 5-nitrothiophen led to a significant decrease in activity (Paula et al. 2009). Related (5-nitro-2-furyl)propene derivatives were also prepared and exhibited *in vivo* activity against *T. cruzi*. The semicarbazone (**31**) (Figure 9) was the most potent in the histopathological studies of Chagasic animals, where it showed greater efficacy in the presence of amastigotes and inflammatory infiltrates in heart and muscle than reference drug nifurtimox (**8**) (Cabrera et al. 2009).

Some derivatives of 5-nitro-2-furoic acid were designed by Arias et al. against *T. cruzi*. Among them, compound **32** (Figure 9) exhibited improved efficacy four-fold lower than that determined for nifurtimox (**8**), and a selectivity index of 70 in its toxicity against HeLa cells (Arias et al. 2017).

Other *N'*-[(5-nitrofuran-2-yl)methylene] substituted hydrazones were investigated, notably when the substituent was a phthalazine ring, leading to highly conjugated derivatives. The *in vitro* antitrypanosomal profile of these 5-nitroheteroarylphthalazine derivative (**33**) (Figure 9) was good, exhibiting low micromolar EC_{50} values against proliferative epimastigote of *T. cruzi* and minimal toxicity toward Vero cells. The replacement of the furan ring by a thiophene one (**34**) (Figure 9) led to similar biological profile. These derivatives (**33–34**) were more potent than the reference drug benznidazole (**9**) (EC_{50} = 30 μM) against the epimastigote stage of the parasite (Romero et al. 2017).

Nitrothiazoles

Also studied were other 5-membered heterocycles like the 5-nitrothiazoles. Nitazoxanide (**35**) (Figure 10), belonging to the thiazolide family (thiazole-amide), is a broad-spectrum antiparasitic molecule indicated for the treatment of infection by *Cryptosporidium parvum* and *Giardia lamblia* infections. In humans,

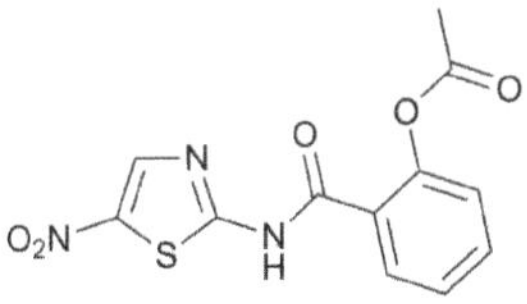

Nitazoxanide (35)

IC_{50} *T. cruzi epi* = 18.7 μM

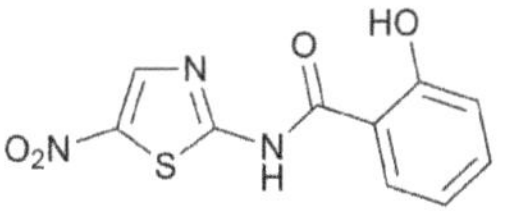

Tizoxanide (36)

IC_{50} *T. cruzi epi* = 17.5 μM

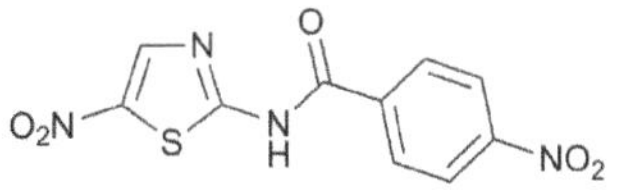

(37)

IC_{50} *T. cruzi epi* = 15.0 μM

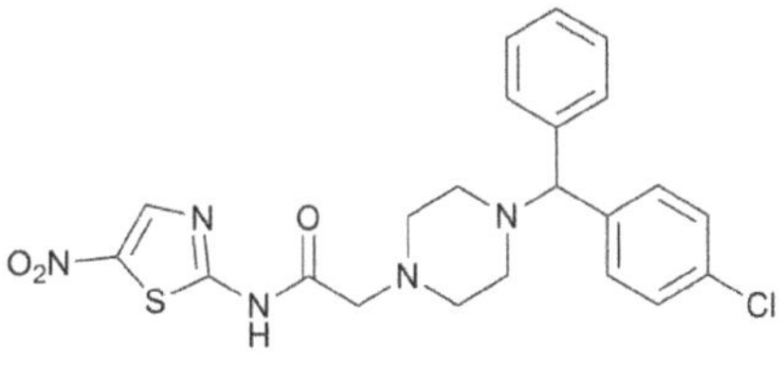

(38)

IC_{50} *T. cruzi ama* = 0.571 μM

Figure 10. Structures of some antichagasic 5-nitrothiazoles.

the salicylate moiety of nitazoxanide (**35**) is rapidly metabolized to tizoxanide (**36**) (Figure 10), which is as effective as the parent drug (Broekhuysen et al. 2000). Chan-Bacab et al. assessed the activity of both nitazoxanide (**35**) and its de-acetyl metabolite tizoxanide (**36**), as well as one other related compound (**37**) (Figure 10) (Chan-Bacab et al. 2009). These derivatives were twice active as benznidazole (**9**) against *T. cruzi* epimastigotes.

Other 5-nitrothiazoles were prepared by the Papadopoulou team and showed appreciable activity against the Tulahuen *T. cruzi* amastigote strain. It is noteworthy that there was an excellent correlation between antichagasic activity and lipophilicity. Piperazine amide (**38**) (Figure 10), bearing a diphenylmethylpiperazine moiety (the same as chlorcyclizine anti-H1 drug), with the highest clogP value (4.51) was the most active compound against *T. cruzi*, 3.86-fold more active than benznidazole (**9**). As (**38**) was not a good substrate for type I NTR, the mechanism of action of such derivatives was unclear (Papadopoulou et al. 2016a).

Nitrotriazole-based molecules

In collaboration with DNDi, the Papadopoulou team screened compounds that were originally designed as DNA-targeting anti-cancer agents (Papadopoulou and Bloomer 1993, Rosenzweig et al. 2005). These compounds belonging to the nitro(imidazole/triazole)-linked acridines were significantly and selectively active against *T. cruzi* amastigotes in infected L6 myoblasts, without showing toxicity for the host cells (L6 cells).Thus, compound (**39**) (Figure 11) administered at just 2 mg/kg/day for 50 days in a Chagas-infected mice model resulted in a rapid and persistent drop in peripheral parasite levels and a proportion of cures (20%). However, (**39**) was a topoisomerase I and II inhibitor and demonstrated toxicity at 15 mg/kg when administered i.p. for 30 days. These encouraging results prompted the development of less toxic and more efficacious 3-nitrotriazole-based amine compounds as trypanocidal agents.

In all, forty-two compounds were synthesized in 3-nitro-1,2,4-triazole and 2-nitroimidazole series, with various linkers bearing different heterocycles (Papadopoulou et al. 2011). Among them, eighteen in the 3-nitro-1,2,4-triazole series and only one in the 2-nitroimidazole series exhibited significant growth inhibiting *T. cruzi* amastigotes (0.04 < IC_{50} < 1.97 μM). Figure 11 summarizes the most potent derivatives (**40–42**) against Tulahuen *T. cruzi* amastigotes (up to 34-fold more active than benznidazole (**9**)). Selectivity indexes were determined by comparison with the cytotoxicity of the derivatives against L6 cells (Papadopoulou et al. 2011, 2017).

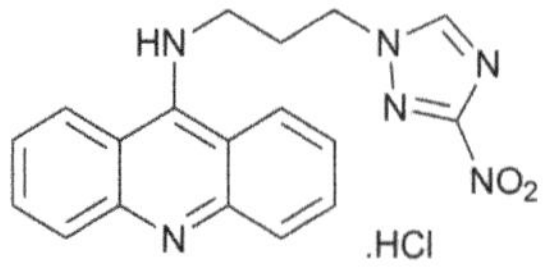

(39)
IC$_{50}$ *T. cruzi* ama = 0.14 µM, , SI = 146

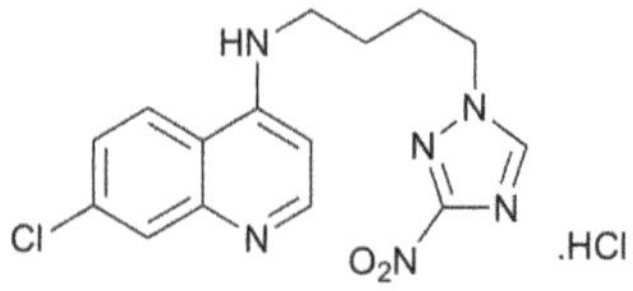

(40)
IC$_{50}$ *T. cruzi* ama = 0.14 µM, SI = 976

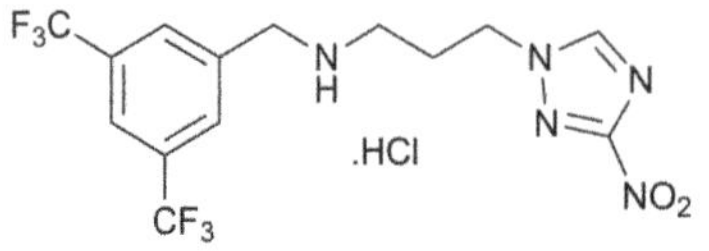

(41)
IC$_{50}$ *T. cruzi* ama = 0.17 µM, SI = 816

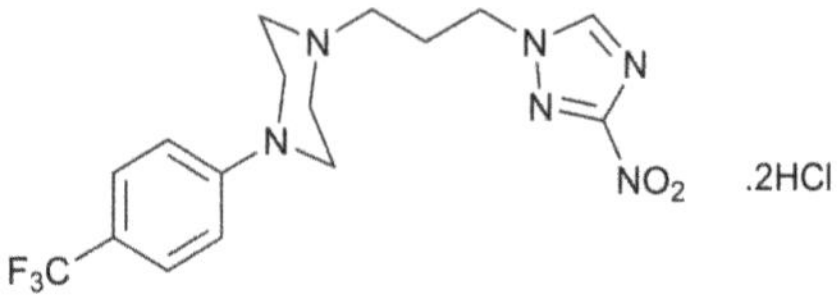

(42)
IC$_{50}$ *T. cruzi* ama = 0.04 µM, SI = 1320

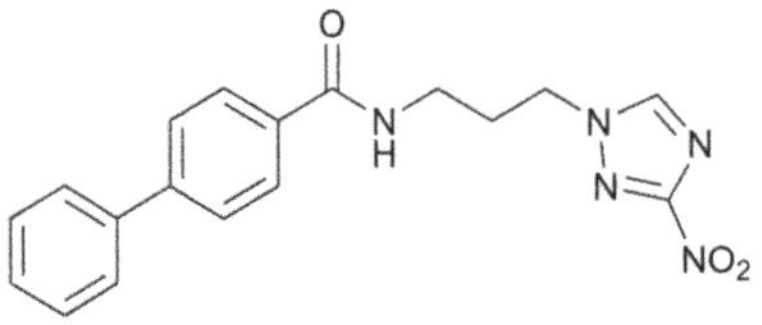

(43)
IC$_{50}$ *T. cruzi* ama = 43 nM, SI = 2782

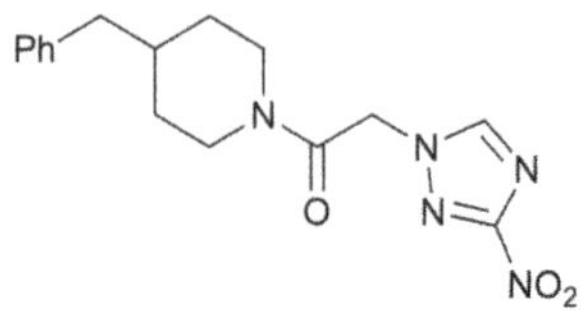

(44)
IC$_{50}$ *T. cruzi* ama = 307 nM, SI = 468

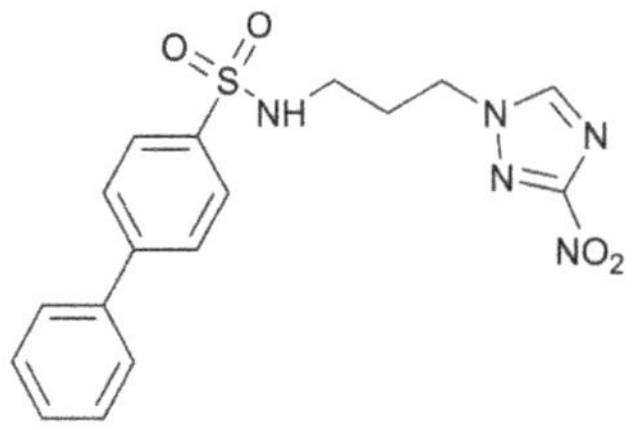

(45)
IC$_{50}$ *T. cruzi* ama = 28 nM, SI = 1764

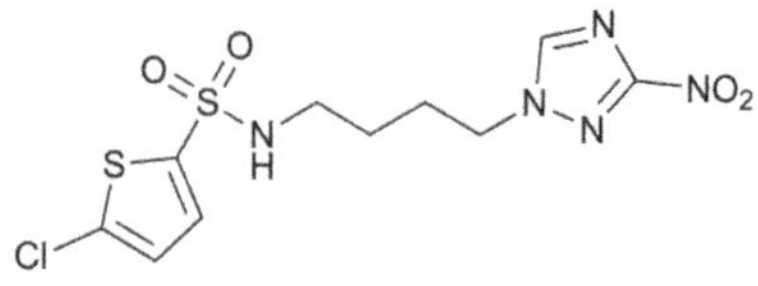

(46)
IC$_{50}$ *T. cruzi* ama = 462 nM, SI = 278

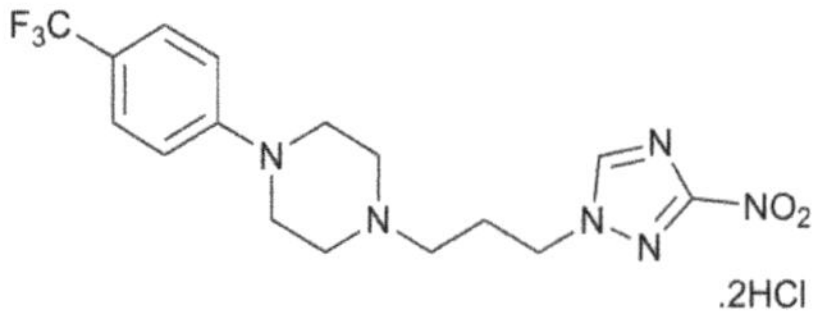

(47)
IC$_{50}$ *T. cruzi* ama = 40 nM, SI = 1320

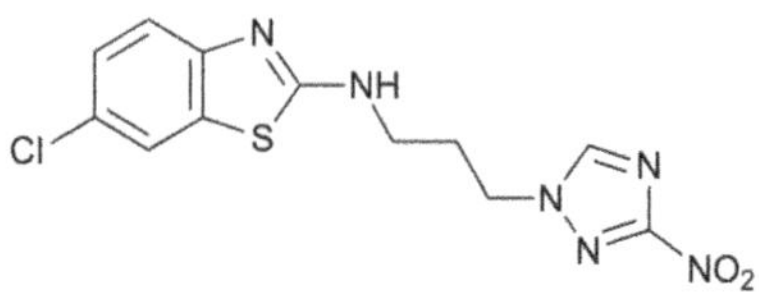

(48)
IC$_{50}$ *T. cruzi* ama = 59 nM, SI = 1725

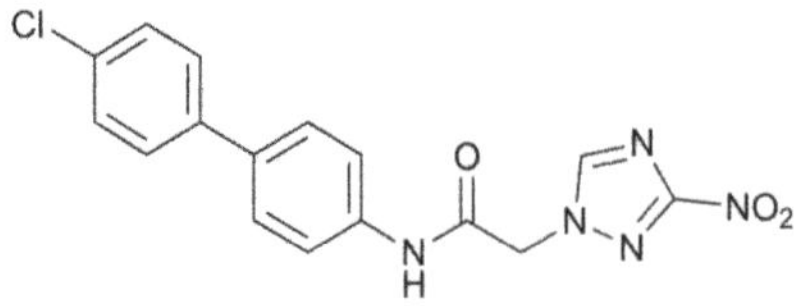

(49)
IC$_{50}$ *T. cruzi* ama = 45 nM, SI = 2797

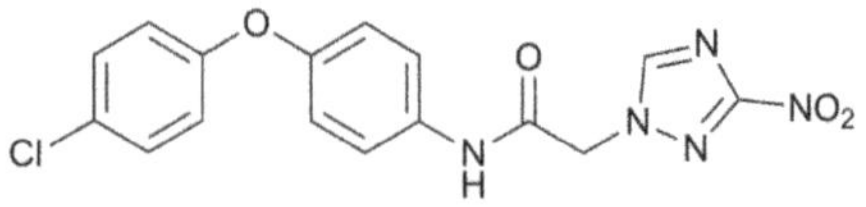

(50)
IC$_{50}$ *T. cruzi* ama = 8 nM, SI = 3615

Figure 11. Structure of 3-nitrotriazole-based derivatives.

Encouraged by the fact that the 3-nitrotriazole-based amine series was found negative for mutagenicity in the Ames test, investigations were expanded to the classes of 3-nitro-1*H*-1,2,4-triazole-based amides (**43–44**) and sulfonamides (**45–46**) (Figure 11) with thirty-six new molecules (Papadopoulou et al. 2012, 2014).

The most potent 3-nitro-1,2,4-triazole-based sulfonamide (**45**) (Figure 11) was 54-fold more active than benznidazole (**9**) against Tulahuen *T. cruzi* amastigotes. It was also demonstrated that these families of derivatives were bioactivated by NTR and were not inhibitors of trypanothione reductase (Papadopoulou et al. 2012).

The *in vivo* antichagasic activity of the compounds was assessed *via* a fast luminescence assay in which mice were infected with transgenic parasites that express luciferase. Animals were treated with each candidate compound for 5–10 days and were imaged. Compounds (**43**) and (**46**) (Figure 11) demonstrated greater activity than benznidazole (**9**) at 15 mg/kg/day, with no detectable parasite signal after 10 days of treatment (Papadopoulou et al. 2013a, 2014). Other more potent *in vitro* derivatives failed to cure the animals due to poor drug-like properties such as poor metabolic stability or poor permeability (Caco-2 model).

Other 3-nitro-1,2,4-triazole-based compounds were also studied in piperazine (**47**) and benzothiazole (**48**) series (Figure 11). Some of them (**47–48**) showed very potent *in vitro* activity against *T. cruzi* amastigotes compared to benznidazole (**9**) but failed *in vivo* to totally cure infected mice (Papadopoulou et al. 2013b, 2015c).

Some of the 3-nitrotriazole-based amides (**49–50**) (Figure 11) with a linear rigid core were synthesized as dual-acting antichagasic agents. These compounds are excellent substrates of type I nitroreductase (NTR) located in the mitochondrion of trypanosomatids, and also act as inhibitors of the sterol 14α-demethylase (*T. cruzi* CYP51) enzyme. Such dual-acting derivatives could introduce a new generation of antitrypanosomal drugs (Papadopoulou et al. 2015a, b, 2016b). Evaluation of compounds (**49**) and (**50**) for *in vivo* antichagasic activity in an acute *T. cruzi*-infected murine model at 13 mg/kg/day administered i.p. showed that parasites were reduced to undetectable levels after only 5 days of treatment.

5-Nitroindazole derivatives

Other nitroheterocycles investigated for their antichagasic activity include indazole-based derivatives. A series of 3-alkoxy-1-alkyl-5-nitro-1*H*-indazoles were evaluated against the CL-Brener clone of *T. cruzi* epimastigotes, affording moderately active derivatives (**51**) (Figure 12) (Rodríguez et al. 2009a, b). Closely related analogs in 5-nitroindazolin-3-one series showed interesting sub-micromolar activity for the compound (**52**) (Vega et al. 2012, Fonseca-Berzal et al. 2016a). Varying the 1-alkyl chain led to a marked improvement in the anti-*Trypanosoma cruzi* activity, which became as potent as the reference drug benznidazole (**9**). SAR analysis suggests that electron-donating groups at position 1 of the indazolinone ring are associated with improved antichagasic activity. Compound (**53**), although only moderately active on the epimastigote form, was very efficacious against amastigotes from CL-Brener as well as Tulahuen and Y strains of *T. cruzi* ($IC_{50} = 0.22$, 0.81 and 0.60 μM, respectively), and showed low cytotoxicity against fibroblasts and cardiac cells (Fonseca-Berzal et al. 2016b). The SAR analysis suggests that electron-

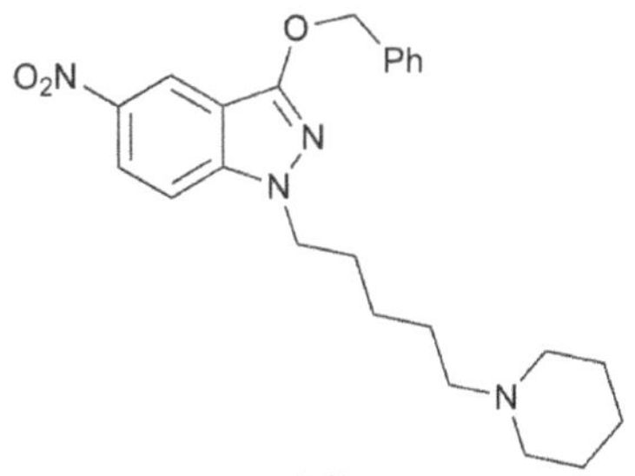

(51)
IC_{50} *T. cruzi* epi = 6.6 μM

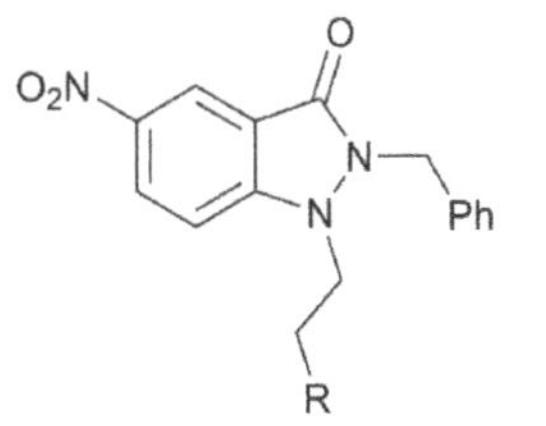

(52), R= -Me, IC_{50} *T. cruzi* epi = 0.93 μM
(53), R= -OH, IC_{50} *T. cruzi* epi = 1.58 μM
(54), R= -CH$_2$NH$_2$, IC_{50} *T. cruzi* epi = 0.24 μM

Figure 12. Structures and *in vitro* activities of 5-nitroindazole derivatives against epimastigote *T. cruzi*.

donating groups at position 1 of the indazolinone ring are associated with improved antichagasic activity. When the water-soluble amino group was introduced (**54**), there was a great improvement of the activity on the epimastigote form of the parasite and the activity on the amastigote form was also very potent (IC_{50} = 0.25 μM). In addition, (**54**) was active against other *T. cruzi* strains without cytotoxicity on fibroblastic or cardiac cells (Aran et al. 2018). Structure of compounds (**51–53**) is shown in Figure 12.

Metal complexes

Some earlier studies showed that metal complexes could have valuable antichagasic activity (Navarro et al. 2000), but such ruthenium complexes were plagued by low water solubility.

Amine-containing ruthenium complex *trans*-[Ru(Benznidazole)(NH$_3$)$_4$SO$_2$](CF$_3$SO$_3$)$_2$ (**55**) (Figure 13) is more hydrosoluble and more active ($IC_{50try/1\ h}$ = 79 μM) than free benznidazole (**9**) ($IC_{50try/1\ h}$ > 1 mM). This complex also exhibits low acute toxicity *in vitro* on macrophages and *in vivo* (400 μmol/kg < LD_{50} < 600 μmol/kg). In murine acute models of Chagas disease, (**55**) was more active than benznidazole (**9**) even when only one dose was administered. Moreover, (**55**), at a thousand-fold smaller concentration than the considered optimal dose for benznidazole (**9**), proved to be sufficient to protect all infected mice, eliminating the amastigotes in hearts and skeletal muscles (Nogueira Silva et al. 2008).

Other metal complexes of antichagasic drugs were synthesized and assessed for their biological properties. Nifurtimox-based cyrhetrenyl complex (**56**) (centered on rhenium metal, Figure 13) was active on both epimastigote and trypomastigote forms of *T. cruzi* (IC_{50} = 12.7 and 0.4 μM respectively, nifurtimox (**8**) IC_{50} = 17.2 and 17.2 μM). It was observed that (**56**) increased intracellular radical oxygen species (ROS) (Arancibia et al. 2011, Echeverría et al. 2016).

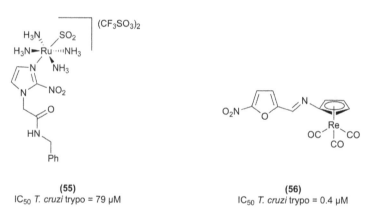

(55)
IC_{50} *T. cruzi* trypo = 79 μM

(56)
IC_{50} *T. cruzi* trypo = 0.4 μM

Figure 13. Structure of metal-based complexes (**55**) and (**56**).

Other nitroaromatics

Phthalazine derivatives containing imidazole rings showed remarkable anti-*T. cruzi* activity in an immunodeficient-mouse model of infection (Sánchez-Moreno et al. 2012). The introduction of a nitro group on such derivatives led to the 8-nitrosubstituted compound (**57**) (Figure 14) which was more active *in vitro* against *T. cruzi* and less toxic against Vero cells than the reference drug benznidazole (**9**). The SI value was 47-fold better for (**57**) than the reference drug in amastigote forms. It also remarkably reduced the infectivity rate in Vero cells and decreased the reactivation of parasitemia in immunodeficient mice (Olmo et al. 2015).

Aziridinyl dinitrobenzamide CB1954 (**58**) (Tetrazicar) (Figure 14) is a weak monofunctional alkylating agent originally synthesized at the Chester Beatty Laboratories in the late 1960s (Khan and Ross 1969). It was studied as an anticancer prodrug which could form DNA-DNA interstrand crosslinks upon enzymatic activation, generating a bifunctional agent (Knox et al. 2003). The anti-*T. brucei* activity

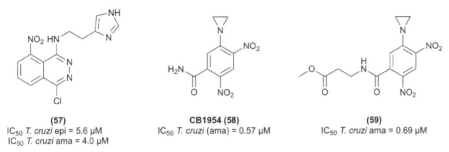

(57)
IC$_{50}$ *T. cruzi* epi = 5.6 µM
IC$_{50}$ *T. cruzi* ama = 4.0 µM

CB1954 (58)
IC$_{50}$ *T. cruzi* (ama) = 0.57 µM

(59)
IC$_{50}$ *T. cruzi* ama = 0.69 µM

Figure 14. Structure and *in vitro* anti-*T. cruzi* activity of some nitroaromatics.

of CB1954 (**58**) was identified in a phenotypic screening by the Fairlamb team (Sokolova et al. 2010). Derivatives of CB1954 were screened against *T. cruzi* amastigote parasites and submicromal activities were obtained without toxicity against Vero cells, leading to therapeutic indexes of > 900-fold against *T. cruzi* amastigotes (**59**) (Bot et al. 2010).

Anti-*Trypanosoma brucei* Nitroaromatics

5-Nitrofuran derivatives

Analogs of 5-nitrofurans were also widely studied for their action against *T. brucei*. Nitro heterocycles like melarsoprol (**4**) were coupled with a melamine moiety with the aim of selectively delivering these compounds to parasites. Indeed, *T. brucei* lacks the ability to synthesize the nutrients important to survival: the P2 transporter mediates the uptake of motifs such as melamine (Carter and Fairlamb 1993).

Some derivatives had similar *in vitro* trypanocidal activities to melarsoprol (**4**) against the bloodstream form (BSF or trypomastigote) of the parasite, with 50% growth-inhibiting concentrations in the submicromolar range. Selected compounds were also evaluated *in vivo* in rodent models infected with *T. brucei brucei* and *T. brucei rhodesiense*. Compound (**60**) (Figure 15) was able to cure mice infected with *T. b. brucei* at a dose of 20 mg/kg for 4 days. It was also tested with the more stringent *T. b. rhodesiense* model STIB 900 using the same treatment schedule, but it cured only one in four infected animals, with a mean survival of 35 days compared to eight days for untreated controls (Baliani et al. 2005, 2009).

In a study assessing aldehyde dehydrogenase (ALDH) 2 as a putative target responsible for the toxicity of 5-nitrofurans, a 5-nitro-2-furancarboxylamide (**61**) was identified with promising anti-*T. brucei* activity 77-fold more potent than nifurtimox (**8**) (Zhou et al. 2012).

A pharmacomodulation study was realized on the basis of the 5-nitro-2-furancarboxylamide scaffold. Finally, a nanomolar active derivative (**62**) (Figure 15) was obtained against the bloodstream-form *T. b. brucei*, three orders of magnitude more potent than nifurtimox (**8**) with a selectivity index > 8000 on HeLa cells. 5-Nitrofuran (**62**) showed the same degree of activity against *T. b. rhodesiense*. Very interestingly, cross-resistance studies showed that the 5-nitro-2-furancarboxylamide analogs displayed low levels of resistance to nifurtimox-resistant cells and vice versa (Zhou et al. 2013). Unfortunately, there were no further studies on derivative (**62**) fully exploring the potential of such a compound (mutagenic potential, blood-brain barrier permeability, metabolic stability and *in vivo* data on animal model).

Wilkinson et al. (2008) studied some derivatives of nitrofurazone against bloodstream-form *T. b. brucei* (Bot et al. 2013). Best compound (**63**) (Figure 15) was about ten-fold more potent than nifurtimox (**8**) with SI > 100 on Vero cells. These derivatives were bioactivated by type I TbNTR, and led to open-chain unsaturated nitrile metabolites like nifurtimox (**8**) (Figure 5).

5-Nitrothiazole derivatives

Some 5-nitrothiazoles were also investigated for their anti-*T. brucei* activity, with only moderate activity against the bloodstream-form of *T. brucei*. The bioactivation of these 5-nitrothiazoles was assessed,

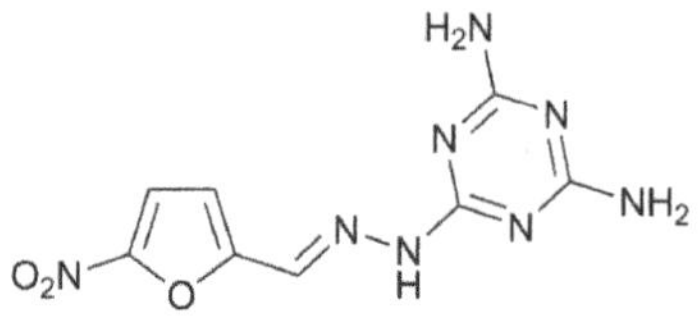

(60)
IC$_{50}$ *T. b. b.* BSF = 0.23 µM
IC$_{50}$ *T. b. r.* BSF = 0.025 µM

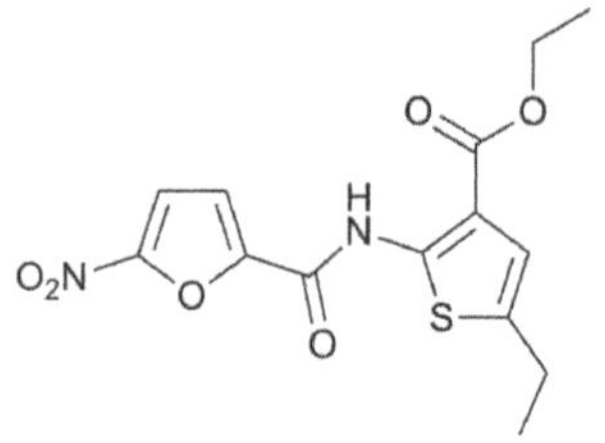

(61)
IC$_{50}$ *T. b. b.* BSF = 31.3 nM, SI > 640

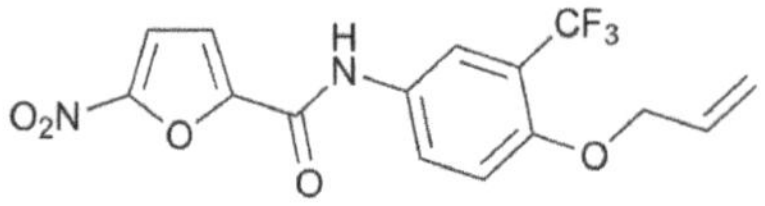

(62)
IC$_{50}$ *T. b. b.* BSF = 2.4 nM, SI > 8330
IC$_{50}$ *T. b. r.* BSF = 2.9 nM

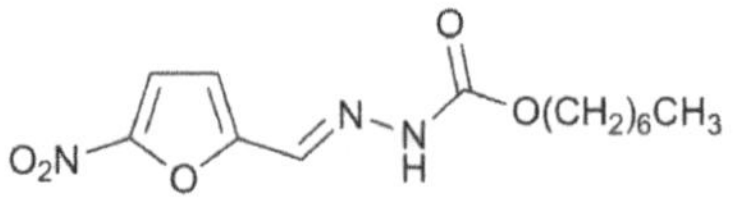

(63)
IC$_{50}$ *T. b. b.* BSF = 120 nM, SI = 116

Figure 15. Structure and *in vitro* anti-*T. brucei* activities 5-nitrofuran derivatives.

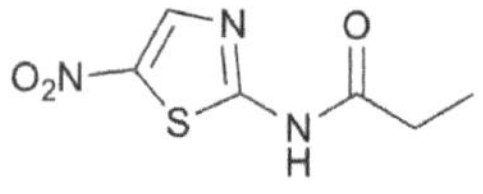

(64)
IC$_{50}$ *T. b. b.* BSF = 3.67 µM

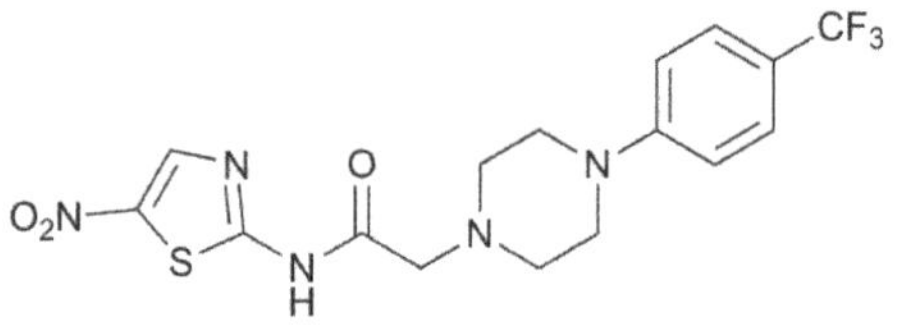

(65)
IC$_{50}$ *T. b. b.* BSF = 1.02 µM

Figure 16. Structures and anti-HAT activities of 5-nitrothiazole derivatives.

showing the implication of type I TbNTR for compound (**64**) (Figure 16) whereas, curiously, (**65**) was not activated by TbNTR. Although micromolar activity was obtained against *T. b. brucei*, the activity against *T. b. rhodesiense* dropped about one-fold (O'Shea et al. 2016, Papadopoulou et al. 2016a).

3-Nitro-1,2,4-triazole-based derivatives

Nitrotriazole derivatives were extensively investigated as antichagasic compounds. It should be pointed out that some compounds exhibiting the best antichagasic activity (**40**) (Figure 11) also displayed submicromolar activity against bloodstream-form *T. b. brucei* and *T. b. rhodesiense* (Papadopoulou et al. 2011). Activation by NTR played a role in the anti-parasitic activity, since BSF *T. b. brucei* trypomastigotes with elevated TbNTR levels were hypersensitive to tested compounds. Sulfonamide derivative (**66**) (Figure 17) was slightly less active against *T. b. rhodesiense*, whereas 3-nitro-1,2,4-triazole-based amide (**67**) was as potent as (**40**) (Papadopoulou et al. 2012, 2014). More recently, by merely switching the chlorine atom from position 7 of quinoline (**40**) to position 8, the activity of the resulting analog (**68**) was strongly improved against BSF *T. b. rhodesiense* (Papadopoulou et al. 2017).

Other antichagasic 3-nitro-1,2,4-triazole-based piperazine and benzothiazole derivatives are the compound (**48**) (Figure 11) with IC$_{50}$ *T. b. b.* BSF = 0.231 µM, SI = 180 and the compound (**69**) (Figure 17) which showed moderate *in vitro* activity against BSF *T. b. rhodesiense* (Papadopoulou et al. 2013b).

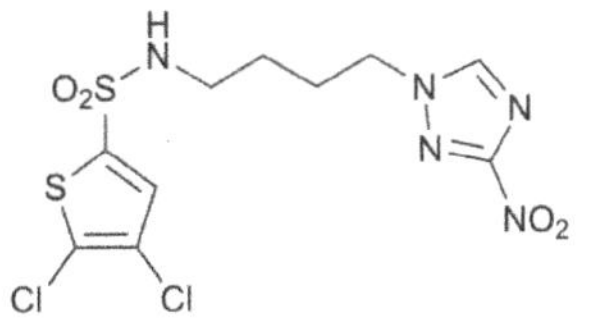

(66)
IC$_{50}$ *T.b.r.* BSF = 0.218 µM, SI = 447

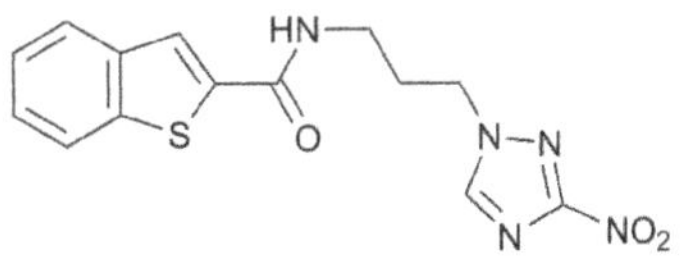

(67)
IC$_{50}$ *T.b.r.* BSF = 0.187 µM, SI = 665

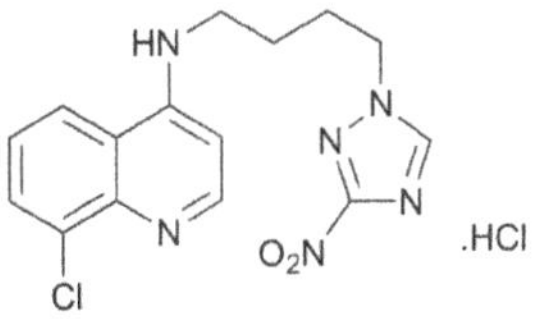

(68)
IC$_{50}$ *T.b.r.* BSF = 0.038 µM, SI = 1937

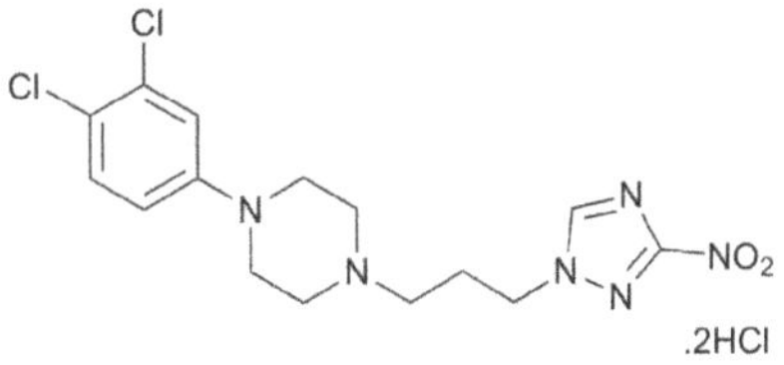

(69)
IC$_{50}$ *T.b.r.* BSF = 0.204 µM, SI = 500

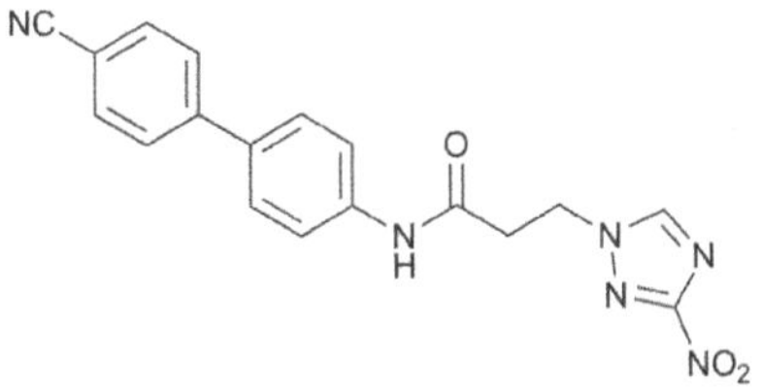

(71)
IC$_{50}$ *T. b. r.* BSF = 91 nM, SI = 2527

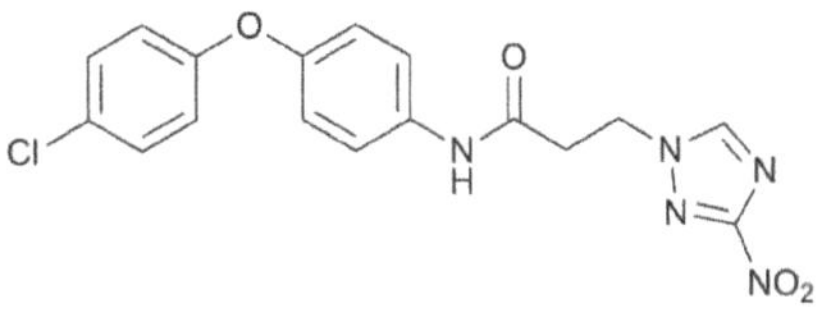

(70)
IC$_{50}$ *T. b. r.* BSF = 41 nM, SI = 418

Figure 17. Structures and anti-HAT activities of 3-nitrotriazole-based derivatives.

Other 3-nitro-1,2,4-triazole-based amides also known to display *in vivo* antichagasic activity were shown to possess excellent activity against BSF *T. b. rhodesiense* in the nanomolar range and with good to excellent selectivity indexes (Papadopoulou et al. 2016b). Compounds (**70**) and (**71**) (Figure 17) are good substrates for type I TbNTR but no correlation between anti-HAT activity and TbNTR-specific activity was observed.

Other nitroaromatics

Derivative (**72**) of anticancer aziridinyl nitrobenzamide CB1954 (**58**) was screened against BSF *T. b. brucei*, showing submicromolar activity (Figure 18). In the case of CB1954 (**58**), the two reduction metabolites identified and isolated by HPLC were screened for parasite-killing activity. Strangely, only 2-hydroxylamine showed significant levels of cytotoxicity against BSF *T. brucei* (IC$_{50}$ of 0.31 µM): no toxicity was observed with the 4-hydroxylamine derivative (Bot et al. 2010). 8-Nitroquinolones (**73a**, **73b**)(Figure 18), described by Verhaeghe et al., showed moderate activity toward BSF *T. b. brucei* (Pedron et al. 2018a). Related derivatives also showed antileishmanial activity. Interestingly, contrary to results previously obtained in this series, compound (**73b**) was inactive toward *L. infantum* and is not efficiently bioactivated by *T. brucei brucei* type I nitroreductase, which suggests the existence of an alternative mechanism of action (Pedron et al. 2018b). Other bicyclic derivatives belonging to the imidazo[1,2-*a*]pyridine series that also showed leishmanicidal activity were active toward *T. brucei*. Among them, compound (**74**) (Figure 18) showed the most promising activity with a selectivity index

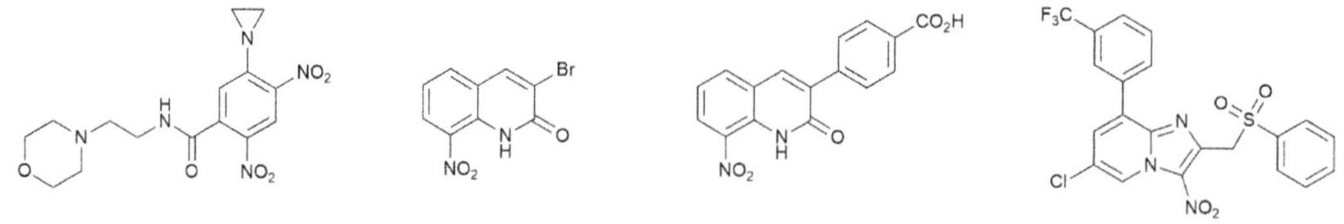

(72)
IC$_{50}$ *T. b. b.* BSF = 0.89 μM, SI = 701

(73a)
IC$_{50}$ *T. b. b.* BSF = 1.9 μM, SI = 92

(73b)
IC$_{50}$ *T. b. b.* BSF = 1.5 μM, SI = 80

(74)
IC$_{50}$ *T. b. b.* BSF = 40 nM, SI > 312

Figure 18. Structure and *in vitro* anti-*T. brucei* activity of aziridinyl dinitrobenzamide (**72**), 8-nitroquinolines (**73a, 73b**) and nitroimidazo[1,2-*a*]pyridine (**74**).

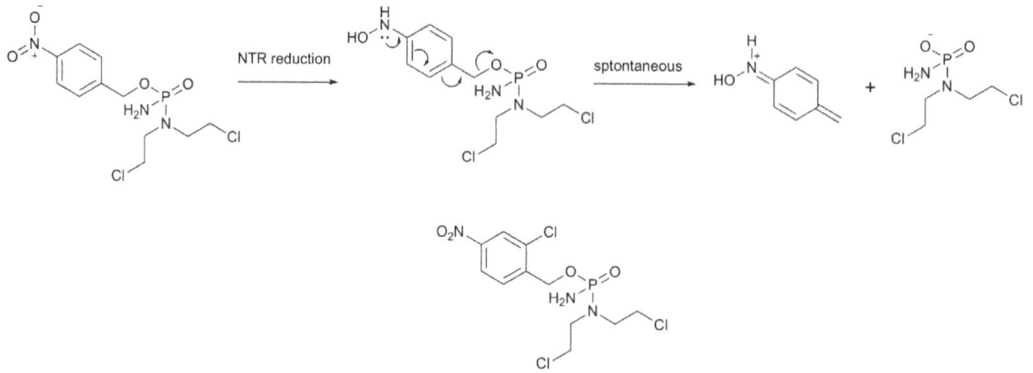

(75)
IC$_{50}$ *T.brucei* BSF = 8 nM, SI = 1250

Figure 19. Bioactivation, structures and *in vitro* anti-*T. brucei* activities of nitrobenzylphosphoramide mustards.

of 312 (HepG2 cells). The compound (**74**) was specifically bioactivated by type I TbNTR (Fersing et al. 2018).

Nitrobenzylphosphoramide mustards (NBPM) were designed to act as prodrug anticancer agents in gene-directed prodrug therapies (Jiang et al. 2006). After reduction by bacterial NTR, the NBPM hydroxylamine derivative rearranged to produce two potent alkylating centers: an aza-quinine methide and phosphoramide mustard. A series of NBPMs was screened to determine if bioactivation by trypanosomal type I NTR led to active and non-cytotoxic derivatives (against THP-1 cells). Interestingly, acyclic NBPMs (**75**) (Figure 19) were found to be active in the nanomolar range against BSF *T. brucei*, and 1,250-fold more toxic to the parasite than to THP-1 macrophages. *T. brucei* NTR plays a key role in parasite killing: heterozygous lines displayed resistance to the compounds, while parasites overexpressing the enzyme showed hypersensitivity (Hall et al. 2010).

Antileishmanial Nitroaromatic Compounds

Of the leishmaniases, only the lethal visceral form is discussed herein, mainly caused by *L. donovani* and *L. infantum*.

Nitroaryle derivatives

Previous work demonstrated the antileishmanial activity of several dinitroaniline sulfonamide compounds based on the herbicide oryzalin (**76**) (Figure 20) (Chan et al. 1991, Bhattacharya et al. 2004). Replacement of the sulfonamide of oryzalin (**76**) by a phenylsulfane group greatly enhanced its activity against *L. donovani* axenic amastigotes (Delfin et al. 2006, 2009). Compound (**77**) (Figure 20) at 25 mg/kg/day led to a 28% decrease in parasitemia *in vivo* in *L. donovani*-infected BALB/c mice for 5 days. The dinitrophenyle derivatives mechanism of action was believed to involve an increase in ROS generation in *Leishmania* parasites, dissipating the mitochondrial membrane potential (Delfín et al. 2009).

5-Nitroazoles derivatives

As with the Chagas disease, nifuroxazide derivatives were also tested against the kinetoplastid *L. donovani*. Although nifuroxazide (**29**) belongs to the family of 5-nitrofurans, far better results were obtained by replacing the furan ring by a thiophene ring. The antileishmanial activities obtained on the promastigote form of the parasite were below the micromolar value for two compounds (**78–79**) (Figure 21) (Rando et al. 2008). Similar activity was demonstrated by compound (**79**) based on the 5-nitrofuran ring against *L. infantum* promastigotes. With its two nitro groups, the mutagenicity of this compound may be questionable (Petri e Silva et al. 2016).

Nitrotriazoles

The 3-nitro-1,2,4-triazole-based derivatives are known for their promising activities against the kinetoplastids *T. brucei* and *T. cruzi*. These series also demonstrated activity against *L. donovani* axenic amastigotes, submicromolar activity being observed for compound **80** (Figure 22) (Papadopoulou et al. 2011).

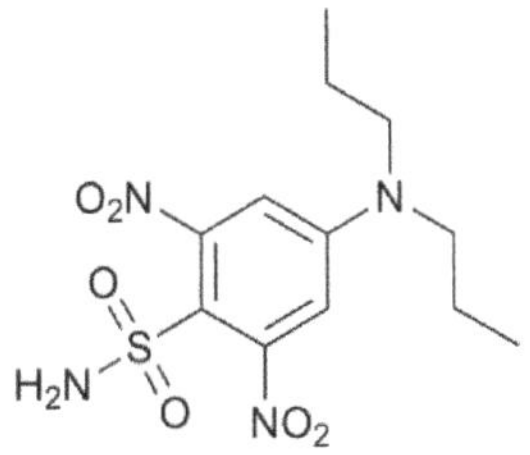

oryzalin (76)
IC$_{50}$ *L. dono.* axen. ama. = 65 µM

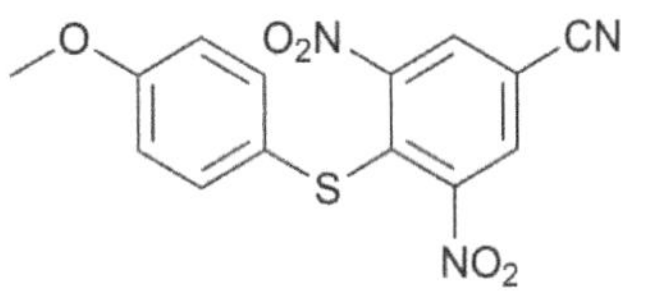

(77)
IC$_{50}$ *L. dono.* axen. ama. = 0.67 µM

Figure 20. Structures and *in vitro* anti-*L. donovani* activities of dinitrophenyle derivatives.

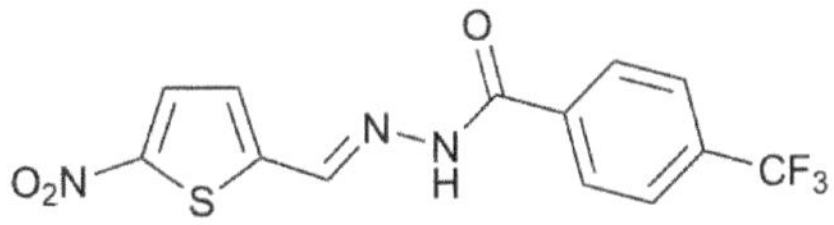

(78)
IC$_{50}$ *L. donovani* pro. = 0.41 µM

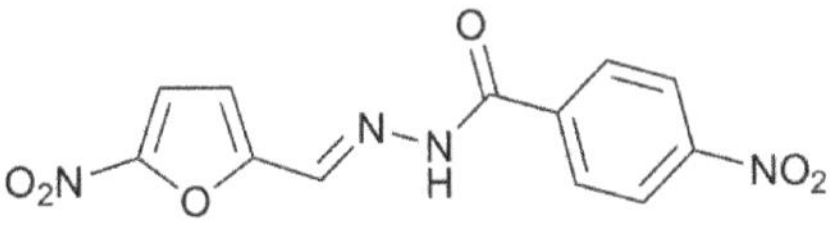

(79)
IC$_{50}$ *L. infantum* pro. = 0.58 µM

Figure 21. Structures and *in vitro* anti-*L. donovani* activities of nifuroxazide analogs (**78–79**).

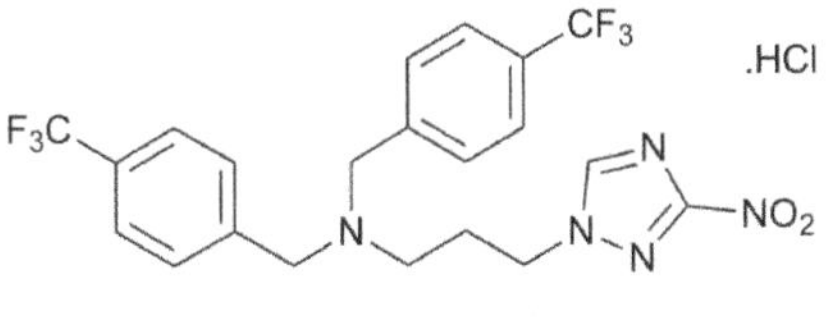

(79)
IC$_{50}$ *L. dono.* axen. ama. = 348 nM, SI = 264

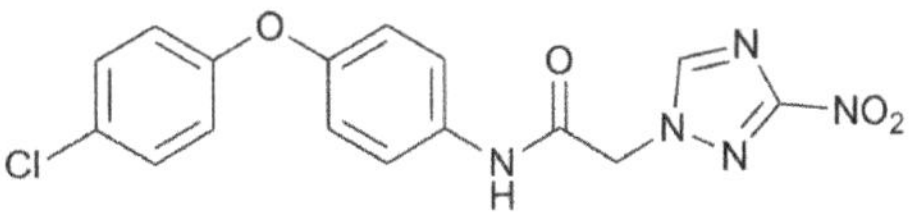

(50)
IC$_{50}$ *L. dono.* axen. ama. = 34 nM, SI = 853

Figure 22. Structure and *in vitro* anti-*L. donovani* activity of nitrotriazoles.

A series of 3-nitro-1*H*-1,2,4-triazole-based amides including an aryloxy-phenyl moiety showed a very promising *in vitro* antichagasic activity. Derivative (**50**) (Figure 22) also displayed nanomolar activity against *L. donovani* axenic amastigotes, ca. 4.8-fold more potent than miltefosine (**19**). Unfortunately, in infected macrophages, a more suitable model for drug screening since it takes into account host cell-mediated effects, compound (**50**) was only poorly active (IC$_{50}$ *L. dono.* ama. > 27 μM), suggesting either difficulties to cross the macrophage membrane or poor metabolic stability inside the macrophages (Papadopoulou et al. 2016a, b).

Nitrobicyclic aromatic

Apart from the antitubercular 5-nitroimidazooxazoles and 5-nitroimidazooxazines, a few nitrobicyclic aromatic derivatives were described as fighting kinetoplastid disease. However, the Vanelle team studied new nitrobicyclic aromatic compounds such as nitroquinoline derivatives. The SARs studied the position of the nitro group and the substitution at position C-2 of this nucleus. The best activity was observed with the 8-nitroquinolin-2-one (**81**) (Figure 23), which was active over a micromolar range against both *L. donovani* promastigote and amastigote forms of the parasite (miltefosine (**19**), IC$_{50}$ *L. dono* pro. = 3.1 μM, IC$_{50}$ *L. dono* ama. = 6.8 μM). Although similar activity was observed against *L. infantum* promastigotes, activity was lower against the *L. infantum* amastigote form, as with the reference drug miltefosine (**19**) (Paloque et al. 2012, Kieffer et al. 2015a).

A SAR study aimed to functionalize the position 4 by various substituents such as alkanes, alkynes, aryls, heteroaryls, *O*-aryls or *S*-aryls (Kieffer et al. 2015a, b). While the activity on promastigotes was slightly increased (**82–83**) (Figure 23), no improvement was made against the amastigote form of *L. donovani*. Although these derivatives were bicyclic, bioactivation was only due to type I LdNTR (Pedron et al. 2018).

Other nitrobicyclic systems were investigated in the 3-nitroimidazo[1,2-*a*]pyridine series. A SAR study highlighted an interesting hit molecule bearing bromine atoms at position 6 and 8. The presence of the nitro group is a prerequisite to the activity. Compound (**84**) (Figure 24) was active on both promastigote

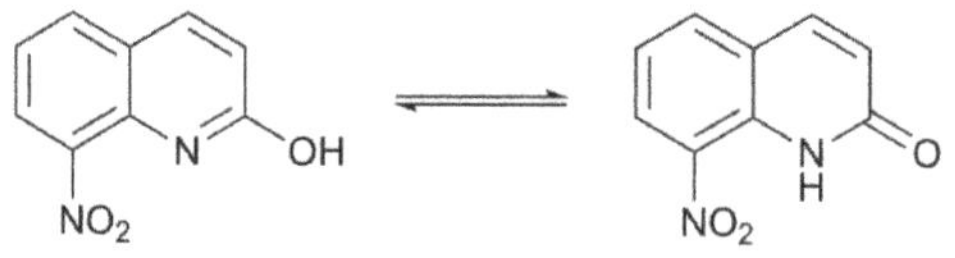

(81)
IC$_{50}$ *L. donovani* pro. = 6.6 μM, SI = 19
IC$_{50}$ *L. donovani* ama. = 6.5 μM
IC$_{50}$ *L. infantum* pro. = 7.6 μM
IC$_{50}$ *L. infantum* ama. = 14.0 μM

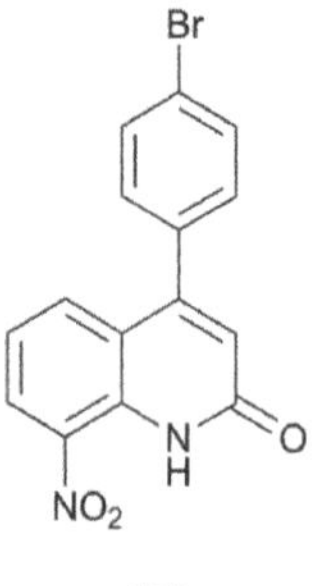

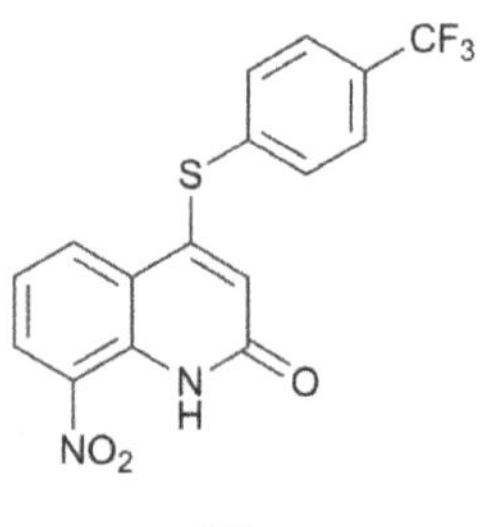

(82)
IC$_{50}$ *L. donovani* pro. = 3.3 μM

(83)
IC$_{50}$ *L. donovani* pro. = 3.8 μM

Figure 23. Structure and *in vitro* anti-leishmanial activities of nitroquinolinone (**81–83**).

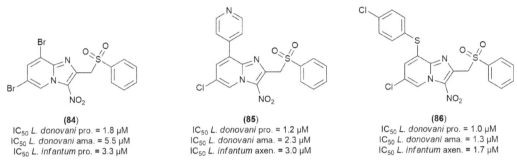

(84)
IC$_{50}$ *L. donovani* pro. = 1.8 μM
IC$_{50}$ *L. donovani* ama. = 5.5 μM
IC$_{50}$ *L. infantum* pro. = 3.3 μM

(85)
IC$_{50}$ *L. donovani* pro. = 1.2 μM
IC$_{50}$ *L. donovani* ama. = 2.3 μM
IC$_{50}$ *L. infantum* axen. = 3.0 μM

(86)
IC$_{50}$ *L. donovani* pro. = 1.0 μM
IC$_{50}$ *L. donovani* ama. = 1.3 μM
IC$_{50}$ *L. infantum* axen. = 1.7 μM

Figure 24. Structure and *in vitro* anti-leishmanial activity of nitroimidazopyridines (**84-86**).

and intramacrophagic amastigote forms of *L. donovani* (Castera-Ducros et al. 2013). Pharmacomodulation was pursued on this and recently afforded a more potent derivative (**85**) active on the amastigote stage of *L. donovani*, slightly more active than reference drug miltefosine (IC$_{50}$ *L. donovani* ama = 4.3 μM) and without cytotoxicity toward the macrophages. Like before, bicyclic imidazopyridine bioactivation was only due to type I LdNTR (Fersing et al. 2018). Recently, new pharmacomodulation led to the compound (**86**) more potent on the amastigote stage of *L. donovani*. Interestingly, (**86**) was active against the BSF of *T. brucei brucei* (IC$_{50}$ = 1.3 μM) and the epimastigote stage of *T. cruzi* (IC$_{50}$ = 2.2 μM) (Fersing et al. 2019). Moreover, (**86**) was the first compound in the series that was neither mutagenic nor genotoxic but presented a short microsomal half-life due to transformation into the sulfoxide metabolite that fortunately remains active and non-mutagenic. Finally, a preliminary *in vivo* toxicity study was conducted on swiss mice that were treated by intraperitoneal administration (50 μL) of molecule (**86**) at either 1 or 10 mg/kg for 5 days. There was neither sign of acute toxicity noted on living mice nor any sign of chronic toxicity in tissues (brain, liver, kidney, spleen, heart, lung, adipose tissues, and muscles) (Fersing et al. 2019).

Acknowledgments

The authors would like to thank Aix-Marseille University (AMU) and the "Centre National de la Recherche Scientifique" (CNRS) for their financial support. The authors also thank Romain Paoli-Lombardo for his kind reviewing.

References

Andrews, K.T., G. Fisher and T.S. Skinner-Adams. 2014. Drug repurposing and human parasitic protozoan diseases. Int. J. Parasitol. Drugs Drug Resist. 4: 95–111.

Angermaier, L. and H. Simon. 1983. On the reduction of aliphatic and aromatic nitro compounds by Clostridia, the role of ferredoxin and its stabilization. Hoppe-Seyler's Z Physiol. Chem. 364: 961–975.

Apted, F.I. 1960. Nitrofurazone in the treatment of sleeping sickness due to *Trypanosoma rhodesiense*. Trans. R Soc. Trop. Med. Hyg. 54: 225–228.

Aran, V.J., C. Fonseca-Berzal, A. Ibáñez-Escribano, N. Vela, J. Cumella, J.J. Nogal-Ruiz et al. 2018. Antichagasic, leishmanicidal and trichomonacidal activity of 2-Benzyl-5-nitroindazole-Derived amines. ChemMedChem. 13: 1246–1259.

Arancibia, R., A.H. Klahn, G.E. Buono-Core, E. Gutierrez-Puebla, A. Monge, M.E. Medina et al. 2011. Synthesis, characterization and anti-*Trypanosoma cruzi* evaluation of ferrocenyl and cyrhetrenyl imines derived from 5-nitrofurane. J. Organomet. Chem. 696: 3238–3244.

Arias, D.G., F.E. Herrera, A.S. Garay, D. Rodrigues, P.S. Forastieri, L.E. Luna et al. 2017. Rational design of nitrofuran derivatives: Synthesis and valuation as inhibitors of *Trypanosoma cruzi* trypanothione reductase. Eur. J. Med. Chem. 125: 1088–1097.

Ashtekar, D.R., R. Costa-Perira, K. Nagrajan, N. Vishvanathan, A.D. Bhatt and W. Rittel. 1993. *In vitro* and *in vivo* activities of the nitroimidazole CGI 17341 against *Mycobacterium tuberculosis*. Antimicrob. Agents Chemother. 37: 183–186.

Azam, A., M.N. Peerzada and K. Ahmad. 2015. Parasitic diarrheal disease: drug development and targets. Front. Microbiol. 6: 1183.

Bahia, M.T., I.M. de Andrade, T.A.F. Martins, Á.F. da, S. do Nascimento, L. de F. Diniz et al. 2012. Fexinidazole: a potential new drug candidate for Chagas disease. PLoS Negl. Trop. Dis. 6: e1870.

Bahia, M.T., A.F.S. Nascimento, A.L. Mazzeti, L.F. Marques, K.R. Gonçalves, L.W.R. Mota et al. 2014. Antitrypanosomal activity of fexinidazole metabolites, potential new drug candidates for Chagas disease. Antimicrob. Agents Chemother. 58: 4362–4370.

Baliani, A., G.J. Bueno, M.L. Stewart, V. Yardley, R. Brun, M.P. Barrett et al. 2005. Design and synthesis of a series of melamine-based nitroheterocycles with activity against Trypanosomatid parasites. J. Med. Chem. 48: 5570–5579.

Baliani, A., V. Peal, L. Gros, R. Brun, M. Kaiser, M.P. Barrett et al. 2009. Novel functionalized melamine-based nitroheterocycles: synthesis and activity against trypanosomatid parasites. Org. Biomol. Chem. 7: 1154–1166.

Bern, C., S.P. Montgomery, B.L. Herwaldt, A. Rassi, J.A. Marin-Neto, R.O. Dantas et al. 2007. Evaluation and treatment of Chagas disease in the United States: A systematic review. JAMA. 298: 2171–2181.

Bhattacharya, G., J. Herman, D. Delfín, M.M. Salem, T. Barszcz, M. Mollet et al. 2004. Synthesis and antitubulin activity of N1- and N4-substituted 3,5-dinitro sulfanilamides against African trypanosomes and *Leishmania*. J. Med. Chem. 47: 1823–1832.

Blumer, J.L., A. Friedman, L.W. Meyer, E. Fairchild, L.T. Webster and W.T. Speck. 1980. Relative importance of bacterial and mammalian nitroreductases for niridazole mutagenesis. Cancer Res. 40: 4599–4605.

Bot, C., B.S. Hall, N. Bashir, M.C. Taylor, N.A. Helsby and S.R. Wilkinson. 2010. Trypanocidal activity of aziridinyl nitrobenzamide prodrugs. Antimicrob. Agents Chemother. 54: 4246–4252.

Bot, C., B.S. Hall, G. Álvarez, R.D. Maio, M. González, H. Cerecetto et al. 2013. Evaluating 5-nitrofurans as trypanocidal agents. Antimicrob. Agents Chemother. 57: 1638–1647.

Brenk, R., A. Schipani, D. James, A. Krasowski, I.H. Gilbert, J. Frearson et al. 2008. Lessons learnt from assembling screening libraries for drug discovery for neglected diseases. ChemMedChem. 3: 435–444.

Broekhuysen, J., A. Stockis, R.L. Lins, J. De Graeve and J.F. Rossignol. 2000. Nitazoxanide: pharmacokinetics and metabolism in man. Int. J. Clin. Pharmacol. Ther. 38: 387–394.

Bryant, D.W., D.R. McCalla, M. Leeksma and P. Laneuville. 1981. Type I nitroreductases of *Escherichia coli*. Can. J. Microbiol. 27: 81–86.

Burden, E.J. and E. Racette. 1968. 2-Amino-5-(1-methyl-5-nitro-2-imidazolyl)-1,3,4-thiadiazole, a new antimicrobial agent. IX. Action against hemoflagellate infections in laboratory animals. Antimicrob. Agents Chemother. 8: 545–547.

Büscher, P., G. Cecchi, V. Jamonneau and G. Priotto. 2017. Human African trypanosomiasis. The Lancet. 390: 2397–2409.

Cabrera, E., M.G. Murguiondo, M.G. Arias, C. Arredondo, C. Pintos, G. Aguirre et al. 2009. 5-Nitro-2-furyl derivative actives against *Trypanosoma cruzi*: Preliminary *in vivo* studies. Eur. J. Med. Chem. 44: 3909–3914.

Carter, N.S. and A.H. Fairlamb. 1993. Arsenical-resistant trypanosomes lack an unusual adenosine transporter. Nature. 361: 173–176.

Castera-Ducros, C., L. Paloque, P. Verhaeghe, M. Casanova, C. Cantelli, S. Hutter et al. 2013. Targeting the human parasite Leishmania donovani: Discovery of a new promising anti-infectious pharmacophore in 3-nitroimidazo[1,2-*a*] pyridine series. Bioorg. Med. Chem. 21: 7155–7164.

Chan, M.M., R.E. Triemer and D. Fong. 1991. Effect of the anti-microtubule drug oryzalin on growth and differentiation of the parasitic protozoan *Leishmania mexicana*. Differentiation. 46: 15–21.

Chan-Bacab, M.J., E. Hernández-Núñez and G. Navarrete-Vázquez. 2009. Nitazoxanide, tizoxanide and a new analogue [4-nitro-*N*-(5-nitro-1,3-thiazol-2-yl)benzamide; NTB] inhibit the growth of kinetoplastid parasites (*Trypanosoma cruzi* and *Leishmania mexicana*) in vitro. J. Antimicrob. Chemother. 63: 1292–1293.

Charlton, R.L., B. Rossi-Bergmann, P.W. Denny and P.G. Steel. 2018. Repurposing as a strategy for the discovery of new anti-leishmanials: the-state-of-the-art. Parasitology. 145: 219–236.

Copeland, N.K. and N.E. Aronson. 2015. Leishmaniasis: treatment updates and clinical practice guidelines review. Curr. Opin. Infect. Dis. 28: 426–437.

Crozet, M.D., C. Botta, M. Gasquet, C. Curti, V. Rémusat, S. Hutter et al. 2009. Lowering of 5-nitroimidazole's mutagenicity: towards optimal antiparasitic pharmacophore. Eur. J. Med. Chem. 44: 653–659.

Darsaud, A., C. Chevrier, L. Bourdon, M. Dumas, A. Buguet and B. Bouteille. 2004. Megazol combined with suramin improves a new diagnosis index of the early meningo-encephalitic phase of experimental African trypanosomiasis. Trop. Med. Int. Health. 9: 83–91.

de Oliveira, I.M. 2010a. Nitroreductases: enzymes with environmental, biotechnological and clinical importance. pp. 1078–1086. *In*: A. Méndez-Vilas [ed.]. Formatex Research Center Vol. 2 (Current Research, Technology and Education. Topics in Applied Microbiology and Microbial Biotechnology).

de Oliveira, I.M., A. Zanotto-Filho, J.C.F. Moreira, D. Bonatto and J.A.P. Henriques. 2010b. The role of two putative nitroreductases, Frm2p and Hbn1p, in the oxidative stress response in *Saccharomyces cerevisiae*. Yeast. 27: 89–102.

Delfín, D.A., A.K. Bhattacharjee, A.J. Yakovich and K.A. Werbovetz. 2006. Activity of and initial mechanistic studies on a novel antileishmanial agent identified through *in silico* pharmacophore development and database searching. J. Med. Chem. 49: 4196–4207.

Delfín, D.A., R.E. Morgan, X. Zhu and K.A. Werbovetz. 2009. Redox-active dinitrodiphenylthioethers against *Leishmania*: Synthesis, structure–activity relationships and mechanism of action studies. Bioorg. Med. Chem. 17: 820–829.

Denny, W.A. and B.D. Palmer. 2010. The nitroimidazooxazines (PA-824 and analogs): structure-activity relationship and mechanistic studies. Future Med. Chem. 2: 1295–1304.

Diacon, A.H., R. Dawson, J. du Bois, K. Narunsky, A. Venter, P.R. Donald et al. 2012. Phase II dose-ranging trial of the early bactericidal activity of PA-824. Antimicrob. Agents Chemother. 56: 3027–3031.

DNDi. 2015. VL-2098. https://www.dndi.org/diseases-projects/portfolio/completed-projects/vl-2098/ (accessed 29/03/2018).

DNDi. 2016. Fexinidazole/Miltefosine Combination (VL). https://www.dndi.org/diseases-projects/portfolio/completedprojects/fexinidazole-vl/ (accessed 29/03/2018).

DNDi. 2018. Fexinidazole (Chagas). https://www.dndi.org/diseases-projects/portfolio/fexinidazole-chagas/ (accessed 29/03/2018).

DNDi. 2019a. Fexinidazole HAT. https://www.dndi.org/diseases-projects/portfolio/fexinidazole/ (accessed 12/03/2019.

DNDi. 2019b. DNDi-0690. https://www.dndi.org/diseases-projects/portfolio/dndi-0690/ (accessed 12/03/2019).

Dodd, M.C., W.B. Stillman, M. Roys and C. Crosby. 1944. The *in vitro* bacteriostatic action of some simple furan derivatives. J. Pharmacol. Exp. Ther. 82: 11–18.

Dodd, M.C., D.L. Cramer and W.C. Ward. 1950. The relationship of structure and antibacterial activity in the nitrofurans. J. Am. Pharm. Assoc. 39: 313–318.

Don, R. and J.-R. Ioset. 2014. Screening strategies to identify new chemical diversity for drug development to treat kinetoplastid infections. Parasitology. 141: 140–146.

Echeverría, C., V. Romero, R. Arancibia, H. Klahn, I. Montorfano, R. Armisen et al. 2016. The characterization of anti-*T. cruzi* activity relationships between ferrocenyl, cyrhetrenyl complexes and ROS release. Biometals. 29: 743–749.

Edwards, D.I. 1993. Nitroimidazole drugs-action and resistance mechanisms. I. Mechanisms of action. J. Antimicrob. Chemother. 31: 9–20.

Enanga, B., M. Keita, G. Chauvière, M. Dumas and B. Bouteille. 1998. Megazol combined with suramin: a chemotherapy regimen which reversed the CNS pathology in a model of human African trypanosomiasis in mice. Trop. Med. Int. Health. 3: 736–741.

Enanga, B., M.R. Ariyanayagam, M.L. Stewart and M.P. Barrett. 2003. Activity of megazol, a trypanocidal nitroimidazole, is associated with DNA damage. Antimicrob. Agents Chemother. 47: 3368–3370.

Evens, F., K. Niemegeers and A. Packchanian. 1957. Nitrofurazone therapy of *Trypanosoma gambiense* sleeping sickness in man. Am. J. Trop. Med. Hyg. 6: 665–678.

Fairlamb AH. 2003. Trends Parasitol. 19: 488.

Fairlamb, A.H. and S. Patterson. 2018. Current and future prospects of nitro-compounds as drugs for trypanosomiasis and leishmaniasis. Curr. Med. Chem. (in press) DOI: 10.2174/0929867325666180426164352.

Ferreira, H. and O. de. 1967. Treatment of Chagas' disease (acute phase) using Bayer 2502. Rev. Inst. Med. Trop. Sao Paulo. 9: 343–345.

Ferreira, H.D. 1976. Clinico-therapeutic trial with benzonidazole in Chagas' disease. Rev. Inst. Med. Trop. Sao Paulo. 18: 357–364.

Fersing, C., C. Boudot, J. Pedron, S. Hutter, N. Primas, C. Castera-Ducros et al. 2018. 8-Aryl-6-chloro-3-nitro-2-(phenylsulfonylmethyl)imidazo[1,2-*a*]pyridines as potent antitrypanosomatid molecules bioactivated by type 1 nitroreductases. Eur. J. Med. Chem. 157: 115–126.

Fersing, C., L. Basmaciyan, C. Boudot, J. Pedron, S. Hutter, A. Cohen et al. 2019. Nongenotoxic 3-Nitroimidazo[1,2-a] pyridines are NTR1 substrates that display potent *in vitro* antileishmanial activity. ACS Med Chem Lett. 10: 34–39.

Fonseca-Berzal, C., C.F.D. Silva, R.F.S. Menna-Barreto, M.M. Batista, J.A. Escario, V.J. Arán et al. 2016a. Biological approaches to characterize the mode of action of two 5-nitroindazolinone prototypes on *Trypanosoma cruzi* bloodstream trypomastigotes. Parasitology. 143: 1469–1478.

Fonseca-Berzal, C., A. Ibáñez-Escribano, F. Reviriego, J. Cumella, P. Morales, N. Jagerovic et al. 2016b. Antichagasic and trichomonacidal activity of 1-substituted 2-benzyl-5-nitroindazolin-3-ones and 3-alkoxy-2-benzyl-5-nitro-2H-indazoles. Eur. J. Med. Chem. 115: 295–310.

Francisco, A.F., S. Jayawardhana, M.D. Lewis, K.L. White, D.M. Shackleford, G. Chen et al. 2016. Nitroheterocyclic drugs cure experimental *Trypanosoma cruzi* infections more effectively in the chronic stage than in the acute stage. Sci. Rep. 6: 35351.

Franco, J.R., P.P. Simarro, A. Diarra and J.G. Jannin. 2014. Epidemiology of human African trypanosomiasis. Clin. Epidemiol. 6: 257–275.

Furtado, T.A. and A.C. Viegas. 1967. Therapeutic trials in American in mucocutaneous leishmaniasis. IV. Hydroxyethylmethyl-nitro-imidazole. An. Bras. Dermatol. 42: 47–55.

García-Hernández, R., J.I. Manzano, S. Castanys and F. Gamarro. 2012. *Leishmania donovani* develops resistance to drug combinations. PLoS Negl. Trop. Dis. 6: e1974.

Gler, M.T., V. Skripconoka, E. Sanchez-Garavito, H. Xiao, J.L. Cabrera-Rivero, D.E. Vargas-Vasquez et al. 2012. Delamanid for multidrug-resistant pulmonary tuberculosis. N. Engl. J. Med. 366: 2151–2160.

Goldman, P. 1982. The development of 5-nitroimidazoles for the treatment and prophylaxis of anaerobic bacterial infections. J. Antimicrob. Chemother. 10 Suppl. A: 23–33.

Grunberg, E. and E.H. Titsworth. 1973. Chemotherapeutic properties of heterocyclic compounds: monocyclic compounds with five-membered rings. Annu. Rev. Microbiol. 27: 317–346.

Gupta, S., V. Yardley, P. Vishwakarma, R. Shivahare, B. Sharma, D. Launay et al. 2015. Nitroimidazo-oxazole compound DNDI-VL-2098: an orally effective preclinical drug candidate for the treatment of visceral leishmaniasis. J. Antimicrob. Chemother. 70: 518–527.

Gupta, R., C.D. Wells, N. Hittel, J. Hafkin and L.J. Geiter. 2016. Delamanid in the treatment of multidrug-resistant tuberculosis. Int. J. Tuberc. Lung Dis. 20: 33–37.

Hall, B.S., X. Wu, L. Hu and S.R. Wilkinson. 2010. Exploiting the drug-activating properties of a novel trypanosomal nitroreductase. Antimicrob. Agents Chemother. 54: 1193–1199.

Hall, B.S., C. Bot and S.R. Wilkinson. 2011. Nifurtimox activation by trypanosomal type I nitroreductases generates cytotoxic nitrile metabolites. J. Biol. Chem. 286: 13088–13095.

Hall, B.S. and S.R. Wilkinson. 2012. Activation of benznidazole by trypanosomal type I nitroreductases results in glyoxal formation. Antimicrob. Agents Chemother. 56: 115–123.

Hanaki, E., M. Hayashi and M. Matsumoto. 2017. Delamanid is not metabolized by Salmonella or human nitroreductases: A possible mechanism for the lack of mutagenicity. Regulatory Toxicology and Pharmacology. 84: 1–8.

Jennings, F.W. and G.M. Urquhart. 1983. The use of the 2 substituted 5-nitroimidazole, Fexinidazole (Hoe 239) in the treatment of chronic *T. brucei* infections in mice. Z. Parasitenkd. 69: 577–581.

Jiang, Y., J. Han, C. Yu, S.O. Vass, P.F. Searle, P. Browne et al. 2006. Design, synthesis, and biological evaluation of cyclic and acyclic nitrobenzylphosphoramide mustards for *E. coli* nitroreductase activation. J. Med. Chem. 49: 4333–4343.

Jiricek, J., S. Patel, T.H. Keller, C.E. Barry and C.S. Dowd. 2008. Nitroimidazole Compounds. U.S. Patent # 12,097,976.

Junior, P.A.S., I. Molina, S.M.F. Murta, A. Sánchez-Montalvá, F. Salvador, R. Corrêa-Oliveira et al. 2017. Experimental and clinical treatment of Chagas disease: A review. Am. J. Trop. Med. Hyg. 97: 1289–1303.

Kaiser, M., M.A. Bray, M. Cal, B. Bourdin Trunz, E. Torreele and R. Brun. 2011. Antitrypanosomal activity of fexinidazole, a new oral nitroimidazole drug candidate for treatment of sleeping sickness. Antimicrob. Agents Chemother. 55: 5602–5608.

Khan, A.H. and W.C. Ross. 1969. Tumour-growth inhibitory nitrophenylaziridines and related compounds: structure-activity relationships. Chem. Biol. Interact. 1: 27–47.

Kieffer, C., A. Cohen, P. Verhaeghe, S. Hutter, C. Castera-Ducros, M. Laget et al. 2015a. Looking for new antileishmanial derivatives in 8-nitroquinolin-2(1*H*)-one series. Eur. J. Med. Chem. 92: 282–294.

Kieffer, C., A. Cohen, P. Verhaeghe, L. Paloque, S. Hutter, C. Castera-Ducros et al. 2015b. Antileishmanial pharmacomodulation in 8-nitroquinolin-2(1*H*)-one series. Bioorg. Med. Chem. 23: 2377–2386.

Knox, R.J., P.J. Burke, S. Chen and D.J. Kerr. 2003. CB 1954: From the walker tumor to NQO2 and VDEPT. Curr. Pharm. Des. 9: 2091–2104.

Koder, R.L., C.A. Haynes, M.E. Rodgers, D.W. Rodgers and A.-F. Miller. 2002. Flavin thermodynamics explain the oxygen insensitivity of enteric nitroreductases. Biochemistry. 41: 14197–14205.

Koniordou, M., S. Patterson, S. Wyllie and K.S eifert. 2017. Snapshot profiling of the antileishmanial potency of lead compounds and drug candidates against intracellular leishmania donovani amastigotes, with a focus on human-derived host cells. Antimicrob. Agents Chemother. 61: e01228–16.

Liévin-Le Moal, V. and P.M. Loiseau. 2016. Leishmania hijacking of the macrophage intracellular compartments. FEBS J. 283: 598–607.

Main, R.J. 1947. The nitrofurans—a new type of antibacterial agent. J. Am. Pharm. Assoc. 36: 317–320.

Matsumoto, M., H. Hashizume, T. Tomishige, M. Kawasaki, H. Tsubouchi, H. Sasaki et al. 2006. OPC-67683, a Nitro-Dihydro-Imidazooxazole derivative with promising action against tuberculosis *In Vitro* and in mice. PLOS Medicine. 3: e466.

McCann, J., N.E. Spingarn, J. Kobori and B.N. Ames. 1975. Detection of carcinogens as mutagens: bacterial tester strains with R factor plasmids. Proc. Natl. Acad. Sci. USA. 72: 979–983.

Mesu, V.K.B.K., W.M. Kalonji, C. Bardonneau, O.V. Mordt, S. Blesson, F. Simon et al. 2018. Oral fexinidazole for late-stage African *Trypanosoma brucei gambiense* trypanosomiasis: a pivotal multicentre, randomised, non-inferiority trial. Lancet. 391: 144–154.

Moraes, C.B., M.A. Giardini, H. Kim, C.H. Franco, A.M. Araujo-Junior, S. Schenkman et al. 2014. Nitroheterocyclic compounds are more efficacious than CYP51 inhibitors against *Trypanosoma cruzi*: implications for Chagas disease drug discovery and development. Sci. Rep. 4: 4703.

Molyneux, D.H., L. Savioli and D. Engels. 2017. Neglected tropical diseases: progress towards addressing the chronic pandemic. The Lancet. 389: 312–325.

Mukherjee, T. and H. Boshoff. 2011. Nitroimidazoles for the treatment of TB: past, present and future. Future Med. Chem. 3: 1427–1454.

Mukkavilli, R., J. Pinjari, B. Patel, S. Sengottuvelan, S. Mondal, A. Gadekar et al. 2014. *In vitro* metabolism, disposition, preclinical pharmacokinetics and prediction of human pharmacokinetics of DNDI-VL-2098, a potential oral treatment for Visceral Leishmaniasis. Eur. J. Pharm. Sci. 65: 147–155.

Nagarajan, K., R.G. Shankar, S. Rajappa, S.J. Shenoy and R. Costa-Pereira. 1989. Nitroimidazoles XXI 2,3-dihydro-6-nitroimidazo [2,1-*b*] oxazoles with antitubercular activity. Eur. J. Med. Chem. 24: 631–633.

Navarro, M., T. Lehmann, E.J. Cisneros-Fajardo, A. Fuentes, R.A. Sánchez-Delgado, P. Silva et al. 2000. Toward a novel metal-based chemotherapy against tropical diseases: Part 5. Synthesis and characterization of new Ru(II) and Ru(III) clotrimazole and ketoconazole complexes and evaluation of their activity against *Trypanosoma cruzi*. Polyhedron. 19: 2319–2325.

Neal, R.A., J. van Bueren and G. Hooper. 1988. The activity of nitrofurazone and furazolidone against Leishmania donovani, *L. major* and *L. enriettii in vitro* and *in vivo*. Ann. Trop. Med. Parasitol. 82: 453–456.

Nogueira Silva, J.J., W.R. Pavanelli, F.R. Salazar Gutierrez, F.C. Alves Lima, A.B. Ferreira da Silva, J. Santana Silva et al. 2008. Complexation of the anti-*Trypanosoma cruzi* drug benznidazole improves solubility and efficacy. J. Med. Chem. 51: 4104–4114.

O'Shea, I.P., M. Shahed, B. Aguilera-Venegas and S.R. Wilkinson. 2016. Evaluating 5-nitrothiazoles as trypanocidal agents. Antimicrob. Agents Chemother. 60: 1137–1140.

Olmo, F., F. Gómez-Contreras, P. Navarro, C. Marín, M.J.R. Yunta, C. Cano et al. 2015. Synthesis and evaluation of *in vitro* and *in vivo* trypanocidal properties of a new imidazole-containing nitrophthalazine derivative. Eur. J. Med. Chem. 106: 106–119.

Packchanian, A. 1955. Chemotherapy of African sleeping sickness. I. Chemotherapy of experimental *Trypanosoma gambiense* infection in mice (Mus musculus) with nitrofurazone. Am. J. Trop. Med. Hyg. 4: 705–711.

Packchanian, A. 1957. Chemotherapy of experimental Chagas' disease with nitrofuran compounds. Antibiot. Chemother. (Northfield). 7: 13–23.

Palace-Berl, F., S.D. Jorge, K.F.M. Pasqualoto, A.K. Ferreira, D.A. Maria, R.R. Zorzi et al. 2013. 5-Nitro-2-furfuriliden derivatives as potential anti-*Trypanosoma cruzi* agents: Design, synthesis, bioactivity evaluation, cytotoxicity and exploratory data analysis. Bioorg. Med. Chem. 21: 5395–5406.

Palace-Berl, F., K.F.M. Pasqualoto, S.D. Jorge, B. Zingales, R.R. Zorzi, M.N. Silva et al. 2015. Designing and exploring active N'-[(5-nitrofuran-2-yl) methylene] substituted hydrazides against three *Trypanosoma cruzi* strains more prevalent in Chagas disease patients. Eur. J. Med. Chem. 96: 330–339.

Palace-Berl, F., K.F.M. Pasqualoto, B. Zingales, C.B. Moraes, M. Bury, C.H. Franco et al. 2018. Investigating the structure-activity relationships of *N*'-[(5-nitrofuran-2-yl) methylene] substituted hydrazides against *Trypanosoma cruzi* to design novel active compounds. Eur. J. Med. Chem. 144: 29–40.

Paloque, L., P. Verhaeghe, M. Casanova, C. Castera-Ducros, A. Dumètre, L. Mbatchi et al. 2012. Discovery of a new antileishmanial hit in 8-nitroquinoline series. Eur. J. Med. Chem. 54: 75–86.

Papadopoulou, M.V. and W.D. Bloomer. 1993. Nitroheterocyclic-linked acridines as DNA-targeting bioreductive agents. Drugs of the Future. 18: 231–238.

Papadopoulou, M.V., B.B. Trunz, W.D. Bloomer, C. McKenzie, S.R. Wilkinson, C. Prasittichai et al. 2011. Novel 3-Nitro-1H-1,2,4-triazole-based aliphatic and aromatic amines as anti-Chagasic agents. J. Med. Chem. 54: 8214–8223.

Papadopoulou, M.V., W.D. Bloomer, H.S. Rosenzweig, E. Chatelain, M. Kaiser, S.R. Wilkinson et al. 2012. Novel 3-Nitro-1H-1,2,4-triazole-based amides and sulfonamides as potential antitrypanosomal agents. J. Med. Chem. 55: 5554–5565.

Papadopoulou, M.V., W.D. Bloomer, H.S. Rosenzweig, R. Ashworth, S.R. Wilkinson, M. Kaiser et al. 2013a. Novel 3-nitro-1H-1,2,4-triazole-based compounds as potential anti-Chagasic drugs: *in vivo* studies. Future Med. Chem. 5: 1763–1776.

Papadopoulou, M.V., W.D. Bloomer, H.S. Rosenzweig, M. Kaiser, E. Chatelain and J.-R. Ioset. 2013b. Novel 3-nitro-1H-1,2,4-triazole-based piperazines and 2-amino-1,3-benzothiazoles as antichagasic agents. Bioorg. Med. Chem. 21: 6600–6607.

Papadopoulou, M.V., W.D. Bloomer, H.S. Rosenzweig, S.R. Wilkinson and M. Kaiser. 2014. Novel nitro(triazole/imidazole)-based heteroarylamides/sulfonamides as potential antitrypanosomal agents. Eur. J. Med. Chem. 87: 79–88.

Papadopoulou, M.V., W.D. Bloomer, G.I. Lepesheva, H.S. Rosenzweig, M. Kaiser, B. Aguilera-Venegas et al. 2015a. Novel 3-Nitrotriazole-based amides and carbinols as bifunctional antichagasic agents. J. Med. Chem. 58: 1307–1319.

Papadopoulou, M.V., W.D. Bloomer, H.S. Rosenzweig, I.P. O'Shea, S.R. Wilkinson, M. Kaiser et al. 2015b. Discovery of potent nitrotriazole-based antitrypanosomal agents: *In vitro* and *in vivo* evaluation. Bioorg. Med. Chem. 23: 6467–6476.

Papadopoulou, M.V., W.D. Bloomer, H.S. Rosenzweig, I.P. O'Shea, S.R. Wilkinson and M. Kaiser. 2015c. 3-Nitrotriazole-based piperazides as potent antitrypanosomal agents. Eur. J. Med. Chem. 103: 325–334.

Papadopoulou, M.V., W.D. Bloomer, H.S. Rosenzweig, S.R. Wilkinson, J. Szular and M. Kaiser. 2016a. Antitrypanosomal activity of 5-nitro-2-aminothiazole-based compounds. Eur. J. Med. Chem. 117: 179–186.

Papadopoulou, M.V., W.D. Bloomer, H.S. Rosenzweig, S.R. Wilkinson, J. Szular and M. Kaiser. 2016b. Nitrotriazole-based acetamides and propanamides with broad spectrum antitrypanosomal activity. Eur. J. Med. Chem. 123: 895–904.

Papadopoulou, M.V., W.D. Bloomer, H.S. Rosenzweig and M. Kaiser. 2017. The antitrypanosomal and antitubercular activity of some nitro(triazole/imidazole)-based aromatic amines. Eur. J. Med. Chem. 138: 1106–1113.

Patterson, S., S. Wyllie, L. Stojanovski, M.R. Perry, F.R.C. Simeons, S. Norval et al. 2013. The R enantiomer of the antitubercular drug PA-824 as a potential oral treatment for visceral Leishmaniasis. Antimicrob. Agents Chemother. 57: 4699–4706.

Patterson, S. and S. Wyllie. 2014. Nitro drugs for the treatment of trypanosomatid diseases: past, present, and future prospects. Trends Parasitol. 30: 289–298.

Patterson, S., S. Wyllie, S. Norval, L. Stojanovski, F.R. Simeons, J.L. Auer et al. 2016. The anti-tubercular drug delamanid as a potential oral treatment for visceral leishmaniasis. Elife. 5: e09744.

Paula, F.R., S.D. Jorge, L.V. de Almeida, K.F.M. Pasqualoto and L.C. Tavares. 2009. Molecular modeling studies and *in vitro* bioactivity evaluation of a set of novel 5-nitro-heterocyclic derivatives as anti-*T. cruzi* agents. Bioorg. Med. Chem. 17: 2673–2679.

Pedron, J., C. Boudot, S. Hutter, S. Bourgeade-Delmas, J.-L. Stigliani, A. Sournia-Saquet et al. 2018a. Novel 8-nitroquinolin-2(1H)-ones as NTR-bioactivated antikinetoplastid molecules: Synthesis, electrochemical and SAR study. Eur. J. Med. Chem. 155: 135–152.

Pedron, J., C. Boudot, S. Bourgeade-Delmas, A. Sournia-Saquet, L. Paloque, M. Rastegari et al. 2018b. Antitrypanosomatid pharmacomodulation at position 3 of the 8-Nitroquinolin-2(1H)-one scaffold using palladium-catalysed cross-coupling reactions. ChemMedChem. 13: 2217–2228.

Pérez-Molina, J.A. and I. Molina. 2018. Chagas disease. The Lancet. 391: 82–94.

Peterson, F.J., R.P. Mason, J. Hovsepian and J.L. Holtzman. 1979. Oxygen-sensitive and -insensitive nitroreduction by *Escherichia coli* and rat hepatic microsomes. J. Biol. Chem. 254: 4009–4014.

Petri e Silva, S.C.S., F. Palace-Berl, L.C. Tavares, S.R.C. Soares and J.A.L. Lindoso. 2016. Effects of nitro-heterocyclic derivatives against *Leishmania infantum* promastigotes and intracellular amastigotes. Exp. Parasitol. 163: 68–75.

Pollastri, M.P. 2018. Fexinidazole: A new drug for african sleeping sickness on the horizon. Trends Parasitol. 34: 178–179.

Priotto, G., C. Fogg, M. Balasegaram, O. Erphas, A. Louga, F. Checchi et al. 2006. Three drug combinations for late-stage *Trypanosoma brucei gambiense* sleeping sickness: a randomized clinical trial in Uganda. PLoS Clin. Trials. 1: e39.

Priotto, G., S. Kasparian, W. Mutombo, D. Ngouama, S. Ghorashian, U. Arnold et al. 2009. Nifurtimox-eflornithine combination therapy for second-stage African *Trypanosoma brucei gambiense* trypanosomiasis: a multicentre, randomised, phase III, non-inferiority trial. The Lancet. 374: 56–64.

Race, P.R., A.L. Lovering, R.M. Green, A. Ossor, S.A. White, P.F. Searle et al. 2005. Structural and mechanistic studies of *Escherichia coli* nitroreductase with the antibiotic nitrofurazone. Reversed binding orientations in different redox states of the enzyme. J. Biol. Chem. 280: 13256–13264.

Raether, W. and H. Seidenath. 1983. The activity of fexinidazole (HOE 239) against experimental infections with *Trypanosoma cruzi*, trichomonads and *Entamoeba histolytica*. Ann. Trop. Med. Parasitol. 77: 13–26.

Rando, D.G., M.A. Avery, B.L. Tekwani, S.I. Khan and E.I. Ferreira. 2008. Antileishmanial activity screening of 5-nitro-2-heterocyclic benzylidene hydrazides. Bioorg. Med. Chem. 16: 6724–6731.

Rodríguez, J., V.J. Arán, L. Boiani, C. Olea-Azar, M.L. Lavaggi, M. González et al. 2009a. New potent 5-nitroindazole derivatives as inhibitors of *Trypanosoma cruzi* growth: synthesis, biological evaluation, and mechanism of action studies. Bioorg. Med. Chem. 17: 8186–8196.

Rodríguez, J., A.G erpe, G. Aguirre, U. Kemmerling, O.E. Piro, V.J. Arán et al. 2009b. Study of 5-nitroindazoles anti-*Trypanosoma cruzi* mode of action: electrochemical behaviour and ESR spectroscopic studies. Eur. J. Med. Chem. 44: 1545–1553.

Rodriques Coura, J. and S.L. de Castro. 2002. A critical review on Chagas disease chemotherapy. Mem. Inst. Oswaldo Cruz. 97: 3–24.

Roldán, M.D., E. Pérez-Reinado, F. Castillo and C. Moreno-Vivián. 2008. Reduction of polynitroaromatic compounds: the bacterial nitroreductases. FEMS Microbiol. Rev. 32: 474–500.

Romero, A.H., J. Rodríguez, Y. García-Marchan, J. Leañez, X. Serrano-Martín and S.E. López. 2017. Aryl- or heteroaryl-based hydrazinylphthalazine derivatives as new potential antitrypanosomal agents. Bioorg. Chem. 72: 51–56.

Rosenzweig, H.S., M.V. Papadopoulou and W.D. Bloomer. 2005. Interaction of strong DNA-intercalating bioreductive compounds with topoisomerases I and II. Oncol. Res. 15: 219–231.

Sánchez-Moreno, M., F. Gómez-Contreras, P. Navarro, C. Marín, F. Olmo, M.J.R. Yunta et al. 2012. Phthalazine derivatives containing imidazole rings behave as Fe-SOD inhibitors and show remarkable anti-*T. cruzi* activity in immunodeficient-mouse mode of infection. J. Med. Chem. 55: 9900–9913.

Sasaki, H., Y. Haraguchi, M. Itotani, H. Kuroda, H. Hashizume, T. Tomishige et al. 2006. Synthesis and antituberculosis activity of a novel series of optically active 6-nitro-2,3-dihydroimidazo[2,1-*b*]oxazoles. J. Med. Chem. 49: 7854–7860.

Seneca, H., P.M. Peer and J.W. Regan. 1964. Chemotherapy of experimental *Trypanosoma cruzi* infection in mice with L-furaltadone. Exp. Parasitol. 15: 479–484.

Shultz, M.D. 2013. Setting expectations in molecular optimizations: Strengths and limitations of commonly used composite parameters. Bioorg. Med. Chem. Lett. 23: 5980–5991.

Simarro, P.P., G. Cecchi, J.R. Franco, M. Paone, A. Diarra, J.A. Ruiz-Postigo et al. 2012. Estimating and mapping the population at risk of sleeping sickness. PLoS Negl. Trop. Dis. 6: e1859.

Sokolova, A.Y., S. Wyllie, S. Patterson, S.L. Oza, K.D. Read and A.H. Fairlamb. 2010. Cross-resistance to nitro drugs and implications for treatment of human African trypanosomiasis. Antimicrob. Agents Chemother. 54: 2893–2900.

Spain, J.C. 1995. Biodegradation of nitroaromatic compounds. Annu. Rev. Microbiol. 49: 523–555.

Stover, C.K., P. Warrener, D.R. VanDevanter, D.R. Sherman, T.M. Arain, M.H. Langhorne et al. 2000. A small-molecule nitroimidazopyran drug candidate for the treatment of tuberculosis. Nature. 405: 962–966.

Strauss, M.J. 1979. The nitroaromatic group in drug design. Pharmacology and toxicology (for Nonpharmacologists). Ind. Eng. Chem. Prod. Res. Dev. 18: 158–166.

Thompson, A.M., P.D. O'Connor, A. Blaser, V. Yardley, L. Maes, S. Gupta et al. 2016. Repositioning antitubercular 6-Nitro-2,3-dihydroimidazo[2,1-*b*][1,3]oxazoles for neglected tropical diseases: Structure-activity studies on a preclinical candidate for visceral leishmaniasis. J. Med. Chem. 59: 2530–2550.

Thompson, A.M., P.D. O'Connor, A.J. Marshall, V. Yardley, L. Maes, S. Gupta et al. 2017. 7-Substituted 2-Nitro-5,6-dihydroimidazo[2,1-*b*][1,3]oxazines: Novel antitubercular agents lead to a new preclinical candidate for visceral leishmaniasis. J. Med. Chem. 60: 4212–4233.

Thompson, A.M., P.D. O'Connor, A.J. Marshall, A. Blaser, V. Yardley, L. Maes et al. 2018. Development of (6*R*)-2-Nitro-6-[4-(trifluoromethoxy)phenyl]-6,7-dihydro-5*H*-imidazo[2,1-*b*][1,3]oxazine (DNDI-8219): A new lead for visceral leishmaniasis. J. Med. Chem. 61: 2329–2352.

Torreele, E., B. Bourdin Trunz, D. Tweats, M. Kaiser, R. Brun, G. Mazué et al. 2010. Fexinidazole—a new oral nitroimidazole drug candidate entering clinical development for the treatment of sleeping sickness. PLoS Negl. Trop. Dis. 4: e923.

Trochine, A., D.J. Creek, P. Faral-Tello, M.P. Barrett and C. Robello. 2014. Benznidazole biotransformation and multiple targets in *Trypanosoma cruzi* revealed by metabolomics. PLoS Negl. Trop. Dis. 8: e2844.

Tweats, D., B. Bourdin Trunz and E. Torreele. 2012. Genotoxicity profile of fexinidazole—a drug candidate in clinical development for human African trypanomiasis (sleeping sickness). Mutagenesis. 27: 523–532.

Van den Kerkhof, M., D. Mabille, E. Chatelain, C.E. Mowbray, S. Braillard, S. Hendrickx et al. 2018. *In vitro* and *in vivo* pharmacodynamics of three novel antileishmanial lead series. Int. J. Parasitol. Drugs Drug Resist. 8: 81–86.

Vega, M.C., M. Rolón, A. Montero-Torres, C. Fonseca-Berzal, J.A. Escario, A. Gómez-Barrio et al. 2012. Synthesis, biological evaluation and chemometric analysis of indazole derivatives. 1,2-Disubstituted 5-nitroindazolinones, new prototypes of antichagasic drug. Eur. J. Med. Chem. 58: 214–227.

Voak, A.A., V. Gobalakrishnapillai, K. Seifert, E. Balczo, L. Hu, B.S. Hall et al. 2013. An essential type I nitroreductase from *Leishmania major* can be used to activate leishmanicidal prodrugs. J. Biol. Chem. 288: 28466–28476.

Walsh, J.S., R. Wang, E. Bagan, C.C. Wang, P. Wislocki and G.T. Miwa. 1987. Structural alterations that differentially affect the mutagenic and antitrichomonal activities of 5-nitroimidazoles. J. Med. Chem. 30: 150–156.

Weiss, M.G. 2008. Stigma and the social burden of neglected tropical diseases. PLOS Neglected Tropical Diseases. 2: e237.

Whitmore, G.F. and A.J. Varghese. 1986. The biological properties of reduced nitroheterocyclics and possible underlying biochemical mechanisms. Biochem. Pharmacol. 35: 97–103.

WHO | Investing to overcome the global impact of neglected tropical diseases, 2015. WHO [Internet]. [cited 2018 Mar 15]. Available from: http://www.who.int/neglected_diseases/9789241564861/en/.

Wilkinson, S.R., M.C. Taylor, D. Horn, J.M. Kelly and I. Cheeseman. 2008. A mechanism for cross-resistance to nifurtimox and benznidazole in trypanosomes. Proc. Natl. Acad. Sci. USA. 105: 5022–5027.

Williamson, J. 1962a. Chemotherapy and chemoprophylaxis of African trypanosomiasis. Exp. Parasitol. 12: 274–322.

Williamson, J. 1962b. Chemotherapy and chemoprophylaxis of African trypanosomiasis. Exp. Parasitol. 12:323–367.

Willyard, C. 2013. Neglected diseases see few new drugs despite upped investment. Nature Medicine. 19: 2.

Winkelmann, E. and W. Raether. 1978. Chemotherapeutically active nitro compounds. 4. 5-Nitroimidazoles (Part III). Arzneimittelforschung. 28: 739–749.

Wyllie, S., S. Patterson, L. Stojanovski, F.R.C. Simeons, S. Norval, R. Kime et al. 2012. The anti-trypanosome drug fexinidazole shows potential for treating visceral leishmaniasis. Sci. Transl. Med. 4: 119re1.

Wyllie, S., S. Patterson and A.H. Fairlamb. 2013. Assessing the essentiality of *Leishmania donovani* nitroreductase and its role in nitro drug activation. Antimicrob. Agents Chemother. 57: 901–906.

Wyllie, S., B.J. Foth, A. Kelner, A.Y. Sokolova, M. Berriman and A.H. Fairlamb. 2016a. Nitroheterocyclic drug resistance mechanisms in *Trypanosoma brucei*. J. Antimicrob. Chemother. 71: 625–634.

Wyllie, S., A.J. Roberts, S. Norval, S. Patterson, B.J. Foth, M. Berriman et al. 2016b. Activation of bicyclic nitro-drugs by a Novel Nitroreductase (NTR2) in *Leishmania*. PLOS Pathogens. 12: e1005971.

Zhou, L., H. Ishizaki, M. Spitzer, K.L. Taylor, N.D. Temperley, S.L. Johnson et al. 2012. ALDH2 Mediates 5-Nitrofuran activity in multiple species. Chem. Biol. 19: 883–892.

Zhou, L., G. Stewart, E. Rideau, N.J. Westwood and T.K. Smith. 2013. A Class of 5-Nitro-2-furancarboxylamides with potent trypanocidal activity against *Trypanosoma brucei in vitro*. J. Med. Chem. 56: 796–806.

Zulfiqar, B., T.B. Shelper and V.M. Avery. 2017. Leishmaniasis drug discovery: recent progress and challenges in assay development. Drug Discovery Today. 22: 1516–1531.

Chapter **13**

New Biological Targets for the Treatment of Leishmaniasis

Fabrizio Carta,[1] *Andrea Angeli,*[1] *Christian D.-T. Nielsen,*[2] *Claudiu T. Supuran*[1] and *Agostino Cilibrizzi*[3,*]

Introduction

The protozoan parasites of genus *Leishmania* are the causative agents of leishmaniasis, a potentially fatal disease which is endemic in 98 countries and represents a serious health problem worldwide. It is estimated that about 0.9–1.3 million new cases of leishmaniasis occur annually, leading to 20000–30000 deaths, with approximately 350 million individuals at risk of infection (Njoroge et al. 2014, Pace 2014, WHO 2016).

Through geographical distribution, more than 20 different *Leishmania* species have been reported to date, including *L. major, L. donovani, L. braziliensis, L. infantum, L. amazonensis, L. mexicana* and *L. chagasi,* to name a few. However, four main forms of leishmaniasis syndromes are clinically recognized: cutaneous leishmaniasis, mucocutaneous leishmaniasis, visceral leishmaniasis (commonly known as kala-azar or fatal black fever) and post-kala-azar dermal leishmaniasis (Grimaldi et al. 1991, Nagle et al. 2014).

Leishmaniasis is transmitted by the bite of female phlebotomine sand-flies (i.e., vectors). The parasites multiply in the vector's digestive tract and they are transmitted to the mammalian host during insect blood feeding. Inside the vectors, the *Leishmania* parasites are in the promastigote forms, existing extracellularly and appearing long with flagella. By contrast, the amastigote forms that are found in the mammalian hosts are located intracellularly and appear spherical without flagella (Chang 1990, Green et al. 1990, Ritting and Bogdan 2000).

Currently, there is no vaccine against leishmaniasis and the therapeutic approach is narrow, mainly due to the small number of drugs available. Clinically used agents include amphotericin-B, miltefosine (i.e., hexadecylphosphocholine, HePC) and paromomycin (Figure 1), which show a number of limitations, including host toxicity, emerging drug resistance, suboptimal dose regimens as well as high costs (Croft et

[1] NEUROFARBA Department, Sezione di Scienze Farmaceutiche, University of Florence, Via Ugo Schiff 6, 50019 Sesto Fiorentino, Italy.

[2] Department of Chemistry, Imperial College London, South Kensington, London SW7 2AZ, UK.

[3] Institute of Pharmaceutical Science, King's College London, 150 Stamford Street, London SE1 9NH, UK.

* Corresponding author: agostino.cilibrizzi@kcl.ac.uk

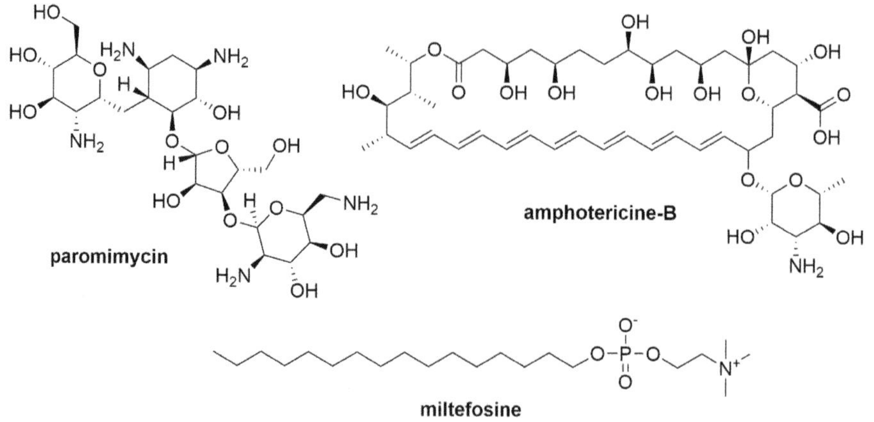

Figure 1. Chemical structures of three drugs currently used for the treatment of leishmaniasis.

al. 2006, Croft and Olliaro 2011). In particular, a selective mechanism of action towards the parasite remains the main clinical challenge for the majority of anti-*Leishmania* agents in use and/or under development (Andrews et al. 2012a, 2014).

In this context, there are two major pathways towards improved leishmaniasis treatment. Firstly, the development of novel drug candidates represents a valuable resource to improve current therapies (Lima and Barreiro 2005, Nagle et al. 2014). Furthermore, identifying, understanding, rationalizing, and predicting new biological targets (which are specific to *Leishmania* parasites) offer an opportunity for medical research (Chawla and Madhubala 2010), in order to develop tailored approaches against this disease. Secondly, a recently adopted drug discovery strategy in the field of parasitic infection is the so-called 'repurposing strategy', which focuses on the development and validation of novel uses for existing drugs (i.e., already validated in humans). Clinically approved drugs are attracting interest for repurposing in the treatment of neglected tropical diseases, since this is believed to shorten the time required to introduce the agent into the market, as well as to reduce the associated costs when compared to the *de novo* processes of drug discovery and marketing (Aubé 2012, Andrews et al. 2014, Njoroge et al. 2014).

Overall, this chapter provides an overview of novel enzyme targets which have been recently identified as biological junctions in leishmaniasis, namely histone deacetylases, carbonic anhydrases, topoisomerases and phosphodiesterases. Relevant medicinal chemistry studies in the search of new therapeutic hit compounds and treatments are also detailed. The last sections focus on novel drug discovery strategies and new uses of marketed drugs, i.e., the 'repurposing strategy', specifically within the context of neglected diseases. Rather than providing an exhaustive and comprehensive review of the extensive literature, the main aim of this chapter is to highlight key aspects that could drive future medicinal chemistry and clinical research in the field of anti-*Leishmania* agents.

Histone Deacetylases (HDACs)

Histones are ubiquitous proteins, reflecting their well-known versatility of function and critical role played in regulating chromatin assembly. They consist of a highly conserved central domain, whereas the hydrophilic *N*- and *C*-terminus exhibit a lower sequence conservation and are also extensively post-translationally modified. Due to this sequence variation at both the amino- and carboxy-terminal domains, histones represent potential diagnostic and/or therapeutic targets for medicinal chemistry investigation. In this regard, the search for molecules that specifically recognize and/or interfere with *Leishmania* histones is of great interest. Successful identification of such molecules would facilitate highly specific treatment.

Histone deacetylases (HDACs; EC 3.5.1.98) are a class of enzymes that remove the acetyl group from ε-*N*-acetyl lysine amino acids residues in histones. This reported post-translational modification (Cairns 2001) crucially contributes to the regulation of essential biological processes in eukaryotes, such as transcriptional events (Heintzman et al. 2009), cell cycle progression (Montenegro et al. 2015) and apoptosis (Bose et al. 2014, Zhang and Zhong 2014). In addition to histones, HDACs bind to and deacetylate a variety of other non-histone biological targets (by acting as 'lysine deacetylases', i.e., KDACs; EC 3.5.1.17), including transcription factors and cellular proteins involved in the control of cell growth, differentiation and death (Glozak and Seto 2007). The high variety of HDAC substrates is also reflected in phylogenetic analysis studies, proving that the evolution of these enzymes preceded the evolution of the histones themselves, thus suggesting that primary HDAC targets may not be the histones (Gregoretti et al. 2004).

On the basis of structural differences, HDACs are grouped into two main families, in turn composed by a number of subfamilies: (1) zinc-dependent histone deacetylases, generically referred as histone deacetylases or metal-dependent histone deacetylases, i.e., class I (HDACs 1, 2, 3 and 8), class IIa (HDACs 4, 5, 7, 9), class IIb (HDACs 6, 10) and class IV (HDAC11); (2) NAD-dependent histone deacetylases (also named sirtuins, SIRT), i.e., class III HDAC.

The *Leishmania* genome contains multiple genes putatively encoding both class I/II (zinc dependent) and class III (SIRT) HDAC homologues (Andrews et al. 2012a), which are essential (mainly the sirtuins) for the parasite growth, verified by both *in vitro* and *in vivo* experiments (Azzi et al. 2009, Coleman et al. 2014). Importantly, it has been demonstrated that protozoan HDACs have a low level of homology compared to human proteins (Andrews et al. 2012a, b) and highlight significant differences in the catalytic domains (Marek et al. 2013, Melesina et al. 2015). These discrepancies make *Leishmania* HDACs attractive targets for the development of selective antiparasitic drugs.

Class I/II HDAC Leishmanial inhibitors

The active site of typical metal-dependent HDACs (i.e., class I/II and IV) has a zinc ion buried at the bottom of a narrow hydrophobic pocket, coordinated to two aspartates (D178 and D277), a histidine (H180) and a water molecule (Figure 2). Other important residues include two histidines (H142 and H143), which are in turn coordinated to two aspartates (D176 and D183). These four outer residues (H142, H143, D176 and D183) are identical in the four class I human HDAC isoforms, while D183 is replaced by a glutamine or asparagine in class II and IV HDACs, respectively.

The catalytic cycle of zinc-dependent HDACs proceeds through a zinc-hydroxide/water promoted mechanism similar to other Zn^{2+}-metalloenzymes reported in the literature (Matthews 1988). As shown in Figure 2, the substrate is located within the catalytic site and properly oriented by means of coordination to both the Zn (II) and a tyrosine residue (i.e., Y306) (Gantt et al. 2010). Nucleophilic attack towards the substrate carbonyl moiety (I) is reported as the rate-determining step in the catalytic process (Dowling at al. 2008) and affords the *gem*-diol (II). This rearranges to the corresponding acetate (III) (i.e., HDAC-acetate complex) (Nielsen et al. 2005) that can subsequently exit through an internal enzyme channel (Haider et al. 2011).

Several hydroxamic acid-based class I/II HDAC inhibitors in clinical use (e.g., vorinostat, romidepsin, belinostat and panobinostat, Figure 3) have been tested as leads to identify *Leishmania*-selective agents (Chua et al. 2017).

The subtle interplay between active compounds and the corresponding different HDAC isoforms in the parasite highlight the aforementioned opportunity for medical research to disentangle structure-activity relationships (SARs). For example, none of the four hydroxamates in Figure 3 showed any activity on *L. amazonensis* promastigotes, while they all show (limited) efficacy on *L. donovani* axenic amastigotes. Furthermore, weak activity was observed for belinostat, panobinostat and vorinostat on *L. donovani* promastigotes (20–35% inhibition at 20 mM) and no inhibition of the growth was achieved using romidepsin. As such, more intensive research has been conducted to develop new and structurally different inhibitors with an improved activity profile. To this end, Oyelere and colleagues have reported a library of hydroxamic acid-based compounds as class I/II HDAC inhibitors (e.g., **1**, **2** and **3** in Figure 4) (Guerrant et al. 2010, Mwakwari et al. 2010, Patil et al. 2010). Biological evaluations demonstrated antimalarial and anti-leishmanial activity for these triazole-linked agents. In parallel, SAR studies showed that the length of the aliphatic linker (i.e., the distance between the triazole and the hydroxamic acid

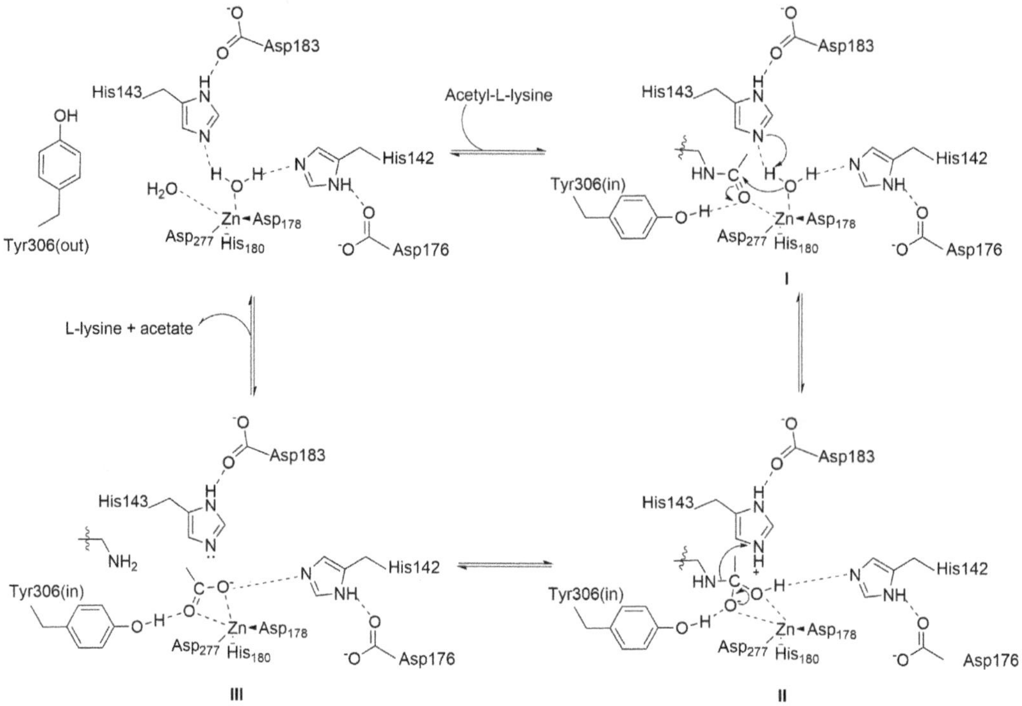

Figure 2. General mechanism of zinc-dependent histone deacetylases.

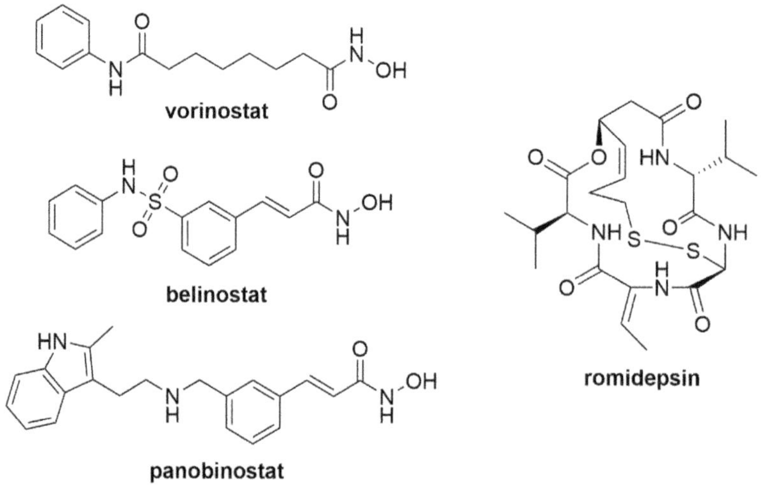

Figure 3. Chemical structures of clinically used hydroxamic acid-based HDAC inhibitors.

function) is a major structural determinant for inhibitory effects on the parasites, with chain of eight or nine methylene units producing the highest anti-leishmanial activity.

The same research group also developed a new class of non-hydroxamate HDAC ligands based on the 3-hydroxypyridine-2-thione scaffold (e.g., **4** and **5** in Figure 4), as selective inhibitors for human HDAC 6 and/or HDAC 8. Overall, these analogues demonstrated a potent inhibition of the viability for *L. donovani* amastigote and promastigote forms, while only limited activity was found on human HDAC 6 and HDAC 8 for some compounds within the series. Accurate analysis of biological activity highlights the possible role that human HDAC 6 and HDAC 8 inhibitors can have as anti-leishmanial agents. Comparison with

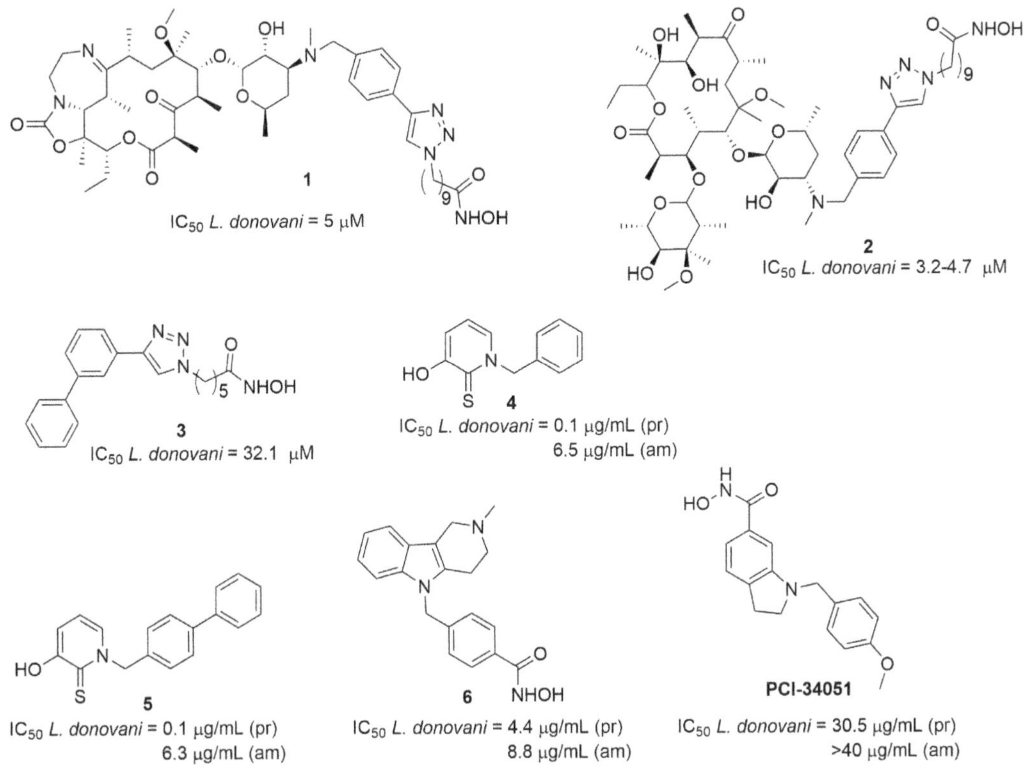

Figure 4. Representative class I/II HDAC inhibitors with anti-leishmanial activity. pr = promastigote, am = amastigote.

tubastatin A (**6**) and PCI-34051 (Figure 4) (i.e., two well-known HDAC 6 and HDAC 8 reference inhibitors) has been carried out to determine parasite selective effects. Tubastatin A showed high cytotoxicity on both the extracellular and intracellular stages of *L. donovani* while PCI-34051 proved nontoxic. This result suggests that HDAC 6 isoform can be a selective target for a more focused therapeutic strategy to treat leishmaniasis (Sodji et al. 2014).

Class III HDAC Leishmania inhibitors

To date, only a small number of sirtuin inhibitors (SIRTi) have been developed to specifically target *Leishmania* parasites. Representative hits are shown in Figure 5. In 2005, Vergnes et al. first explored the effect of sirtuin type 2 (SIRT2) inhibitors on *Leishmania* viability (Vergnes et al. 2005). Compound **8** (i.e.,'sirtinol') showed dose dependent inhibition of *L. infantum* axenic amastigote proliferation for a range of concentrations higher than 15 μM. In contrast, the agent was completely devoid of activity toward *L. infantum* promastigotes. Although unexpected, this observed difference for the sensitivity of promastigote and amastigote forms to sirtinol treatment might reflect a different conformational state and/or activity of the SIRT2 protein between the two stages of the parasite.

Nicotinamide derivative **9** (Figure 5) has also been shown effective in decreasing *L. infantum* axenic amastigote growth *in vitro* (Kadam et al. 2008); however, substantial lack of parasite selectivity was found due to a similar inhibition potency on human sirtuin type 1 (SIRT1) enzyme. In addition, Tavares and colleagues reported the *in vitro* anti-leishmanial activity of 12 bisnaphthalimidopropyl (BNIP) derivatives (e.g., **10** in Figure 5) having different length and nature of the central alkyl chains that link the two naphthalimidopropyl moieties (i.e., 4–12 methylene groups and 2–4 nitrogen atoms). All BNIP derivatives were able to inhibit *L. infantum* cytosolic SIR2-related protein 1 (LiSir2rp1) with IC_{50} values in the range of 5.7–54.7 μM and some of the compounds produced a selective inhibitory effect over the human SIRT1

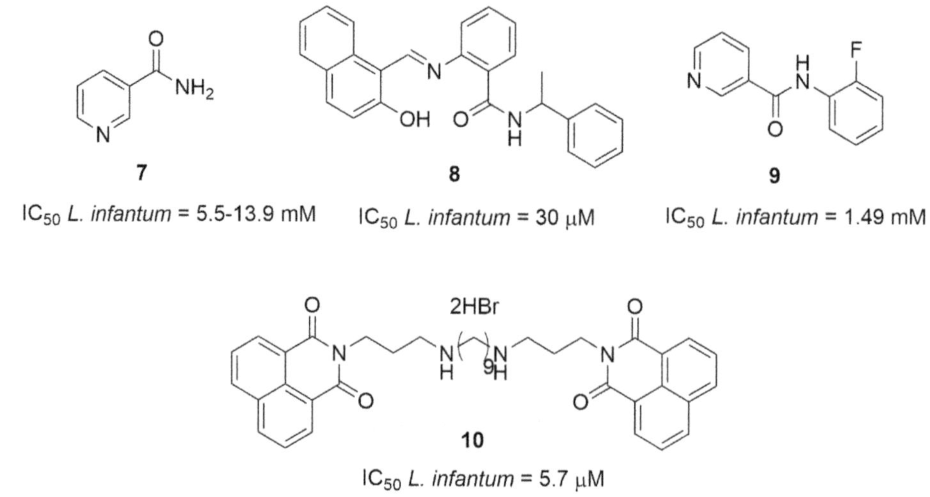

7

IC$_{50}$ *L. infantum* = 5.5-13.9 mM

8

IC$_{50}$ *L. infantum* = 30 µM

9

IC$_{50}$ *L. infantum* = 1.49 mM

10

IC$_{50}$ *L. infantum* = 5.7 µM

Figure 5. Representative class III HDAC inhibitors with anti-leishmanial activity.

(Tavares et al. 2010). The potency and selectivity of inhibition for these analogues varied on the base of net charges and length of the linker group. BNIP diamine derivatives with 4–7 methylene units in the spacer were both less active and less selective than BNIP containing 8–12 methylene units. In contrast, the introduction of additional positively charged amine functions in the linker did not improve either potency or selectivity. Compound **10** (Figure 5) with a linker of nine methylene units is the most active analogue with an IC$_{50}$ value of 5.7 µM on LiSir2rp1 and a 17-fold selectivity over human SIRT1. Furthermore, a number of BNIP derivatives in the series were also able to inhibit the intracellular development of *L. infantum* amastigotes *in vitro* (IC$_{50}$ values ~ 1–10 µM) (Tavares et al. 2010).

Carbonic Anhydrases

Carbonic anhydrases (CAs, EC 4.2.1.1) belong to a superfamily of metalloenzymes which are present through most living organisms. They are encoded by seven evolutionarily unrelated gene families and are classified using the Greek letters α-, β-, γ-, δ-, ζ- η- and θ- (Supuran 2017). All these enzymes reversibly catalyze the hydration of carbon dioxide ($CO_2 + H_2O \leftrightarrows HCO_3^- + H^+$) by means of a 'ping-pong mechanism' as highlighted in Figure 6, which reports as a model the catalytic pathway for the ubiquitous human (h) CA II isoform (Supuran 2008).

The catalytic cycle begins with the nucleophilic attack of the zinc-bound hydroxide species **b** towards the CO_2 substrate properly located within a hydrophobic pocket. The bicarbonate adduct **c** formed is subsequently displaced by a water molecule to afford the inactive enzyme (adduct **d**). The regeneration of the zinc hydroxide species **a** requires a proton transfer reaction to occur. This transformation is the rate-determining step of the entire CA catalytic cycle and is usually assisted by a His residue, which is located at the centre of the enzyme catalytic pocket (i.e., active site) and acts as 'proton shuttle' (Supuran 2008).

The biological function of CAs is not limited to the hydration of CO_2. For instance, these enzymes are also involved in many crucial biological processes connected with pH and CO_2 homoeostasis/sensing, biosynthetic reactions (such as gluconeogenesis, lipogenesis and ureagenesis), respiration and transport of CO_2/bicarbonate, electrolyte secretion in a variety of tissues/organs, as well as bone resorption, calcification, tumorigenicity and many other physiological or pathological conditions (thoroughly studied in vertebrates and some pathogens). Many CAs within vertebrates, nematodes, fungi, protozoa and bacteria are established drug targets (Supuran 2008, 2011, 2017, Neri and Supuran 2011), since interfering with their activity leads to valuable pharmacological effects.

The genome of *Leishmania* species encode for one α- and one β-CA. Currently, only the β-CA from *L. donovani* (LdcCA) has been successfully expressed, purified and characterized (Syrjänen et al. 2013).

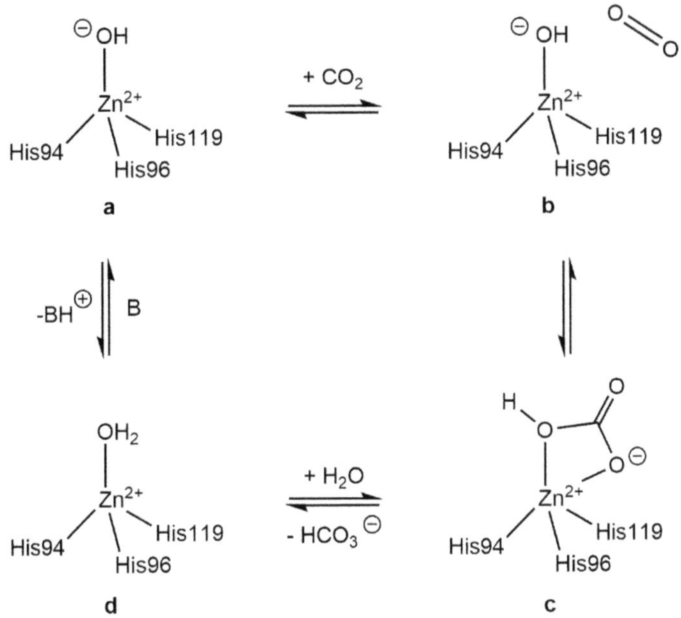

Figure 6. Catalytic mechanism of CO_2 hydration.

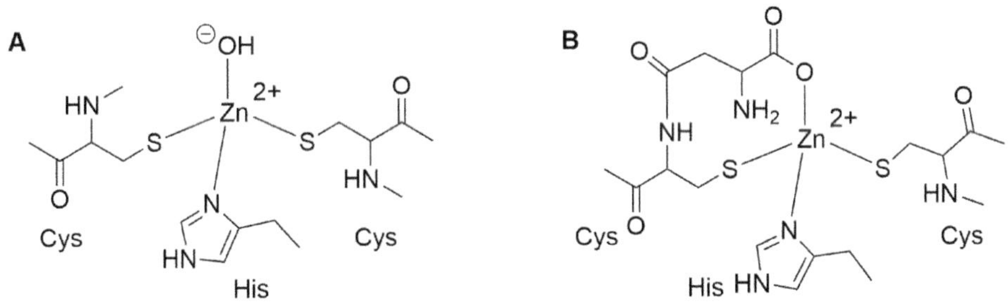

Figure 7. Metal ion coordination pattern in type I β-Cas (i.e., opened active site **A**) and type II β-CAs (i.e., closed active site, with an aspartate residue as the fourth zinc ligand **B**).

Since β-CAs are absent in vertebrates, the development of parasite specific β-CA inhibitors clearly paves the way to efficiently tackle leishmaniasis.

A pioneering crystallographic study on β-CA showed that two different metal ion coordination patterns (i.e., type I and II) are possible for this enzyme (Suarez Covarrubias et al. 2005). As depicted in Figure 7A, type I β-CA has the Zn(II) complexed by two Cys and one His residues with water/hydroxide as the fourth ligand. Differently, an Asp residue represents the fourth ligand in type II β-CA (Figure 7B). The latter coordination pattern makes the enzyme devoid of any catalytic activity due to the absence of the nucleophilic water molecule/hydroxide ion necessary for the cycle to happen. The exposure of β-CAs to pH values > 8.3 produces a switch from type II to type I coordination pattern by engaging a highly conserved Arg residue. In particular, such a residue can form ionic interactions with the coordinated Asp residue in type II β-CAs, thus allowing an incoming water molecule to take its place as the fourth zinc ligand and yield the enzymatically active type I β-CA (Suarez Covarrubias et al. 2005).

Clearly, coordination and subsequent loss of catalytic activity is a potential mode of inhibition for CAs. Indeed, primary sulfonamides and other inorganic metal complexing anions are commonly known to inhibit CAs by this coordination, therefore representing the most investigated classes of CA inhibitors (CAIs) (Supuran 2008, 2016a, b). In recent years, several other chemical moieties have been introduced in selected scaffolds and explored for their ability to interfere with the catalytic activity of various CA families (De Simone et al. 2013). These address the CA isoform selectivity issue (i.e., α-CAs vs β-CAs) which is the blue print for the development of efficient CA-based agents for pharmacological approaches in the treatment of leishmaniasis. A selection of the most striking contributions in the development of CA-inhibitors as anti-*Leishmania* agents is reported in the following sections.

Sulfonamides

According to literature reports, classical sulfonamide-based CAIs exhibit very different inhibition profiles on LdcCA *in vitro*, in comparison to mammalian and human expressed CAs. For instance, most of the clinically used CAIs of the sulfonamide type showed weak or ineffective inhibition activity against the protozoan isoenzyme. Only the five-membered heterocyclic sulfonamides (i.e., acetazolamide, **AZA**, and methazolamide, **MZA**, in Figure 8) were effective LdcCA inhibitors with K_I values of 87.1 and 91.7 nM, respectively. Moreover, better results were obtained with the bicyclic ethoxyzolamide (**EZA**) and hydrochlorothiazide (**HCT**) (Figure 8), having K_I values in the range of 50.2–51.5 nM (Syrjänen et al. 2013).

Recently, Carta and collaborators reported PAMAM dendrimers functionalized with aromatic sulfonamides, which showed excellent inhibitory activity against LdcCA isoform (Carta et al. 2015a, b, c). Among the various "generations", the so-reported "G2" (Figure 9) had an activity of 34.8 nM (K_I), being almost 3-fold more potent than acetazolamide as LdcCA inhibitor. However, the other "generations" also showed a potent profile of inhibition on this enzyme with K_I spanning from 75.4 to 90.7 nM (Carta et al. 2015a, b, c).

Other research groups have also investigated sulfonamide-based compounds as antiparasitic agents. For instance, Galiana-Roselló et al. synthetized *N*-naphthalenesulfonamide derivatives **11a–c** (Figure 10) which determined a potent inhibition on the promastigote form of four *Leishmania* species (i.e., *L. infantum*, *L. braziliensis*, *L. guyanensis*, and *L. amazonensis*). Subsequently, *in vivo* studies demonstrated that these compounds are also active on the amastigote form of *L. amazonensis* and *L. infantum*, with additional anti-nuclear and/or anti-tubulin effects on *L. infantum* promastigote stages (Galiana-Roselló et al. 2013).

Various reports have recently hypothesized relevance for the trace element selenium to be effective in leishmaniasis treatment. The increased concentration of this chalcogen in plasma has been indeed recognized as a new defensive strategy against *Leishmania* infection (Araujo et al. 2008, Culha et al. 2008). In this regard, the sulphonamide moieties and a di-selenide linker were jointly incorporated into derivatives **12a–d** (Figure 11) by Baquedano and collaborators (Baquedano et al. 2014). These agents exhibited potent antiparasitic activity *in vitro* against *L. infantum*, with a selectivity index (i.e., quantity of compound that is active against the pathogen but is not toxic towards the host cell) higher than that of miltefosine and edelfosine (i.e., reference drugs used as controls in the tests).

Thiols

The thiolate group (i.e., thiol in the ionized anionic form) is widely known to biologically act as a good zinc-binding group (similar to SO_2NH^-), such a feature being essential to generate effective CA inhibitors (Supuran 2016b). In this regard, Abdel-Hamid et al. reported a group of urea-based 1,3,4-thiadiazole-5-mercapto derivatives (**13a–l** in Figure 12) as human CA I and II inhibitors with moderate potency (Abdel-Hamid et al. 2007). Among them, the simple semicarbazido derivative **13a** firstly demonstrated a valuable LdcCA inhibition (K_I of 74.1 nM). Similarly, the Schiff base analogues **13b–f** and **13h** (Figure 12)

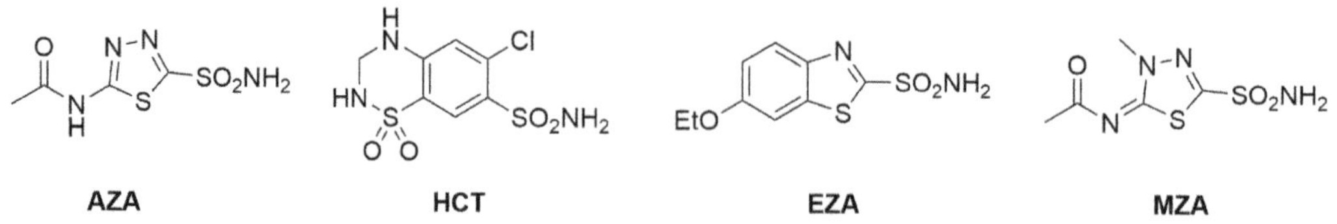

| AZA | HCT | EZA | MZA |

Figure 8. Clinically used CAIs of the sulfonamide type with antiparasitic activity.

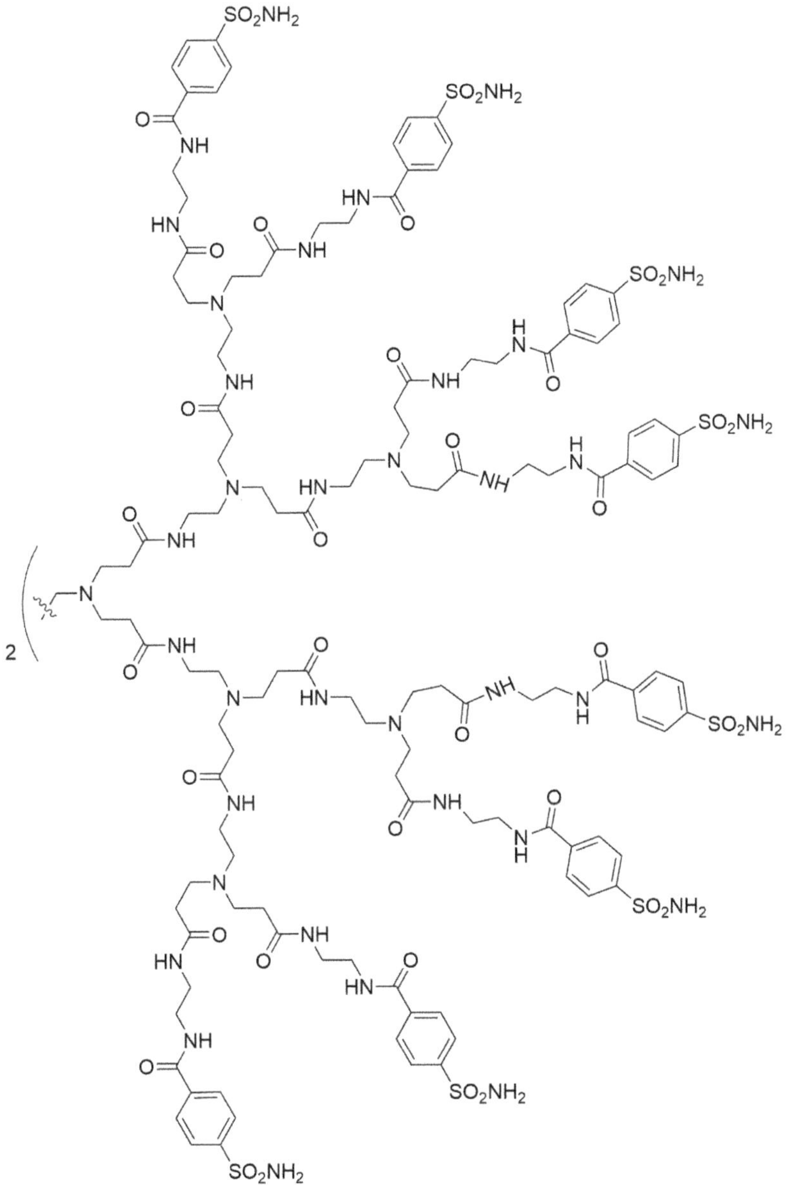

Figure 9. Structure of PAMAM-based G2 dendrimer (functionalized with aromatic sulfonamides) investigated as LdcCA inhibitor.

proved highly powerful as inhibitors of the protozoan enzyme, with inhibition constants in the range of 13.4–40.1 nM (Syrjänen et al. 2013). The different inhibition profile found for this group of anti-*Leishmania* agents toward LdcCA, in comparison to mammalian CAs (i.e., type I and II) and other protozoan CA isoforms, suggested possible specificity in the mechanism of action (Vermelho et al. 2017). This prompted the use of analogues **13a–l** in *in vivo* experiments with promastigote forms of *L. chagasi* and *L. amazonensis*. Compound **13e** (Figure 12) demonstrated the highest inhibition values with a decrease of promastigote growth of 100% in *L. chagasi* and 97% in *L. amazonensis*. The anti-leishmanial properties of CA inhibitor **13e** were observed with the appearance of electron-dense granules in the cytoplasm and in the flagellar pocket, as well as the presence of many vesicles and the formation of autophagic structures in the cytoplasm.

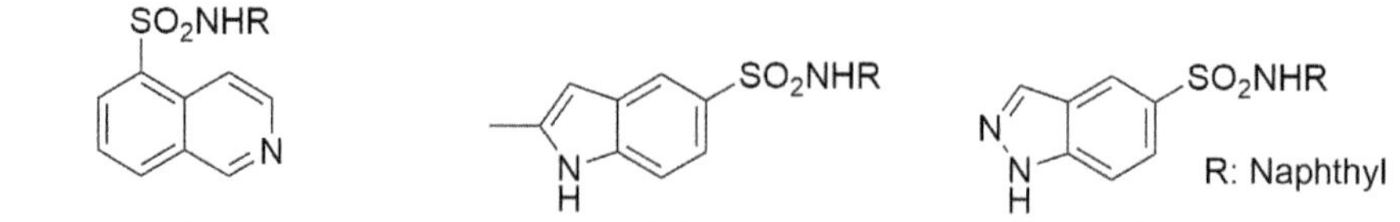

11a
IC$_{50}$ *L. infantum* = 20.3 μM

11b
IC$_{50}$ *L. infantum* = 11.9 μM

11c
IC$_{50}$ *L. infantum* = 37.3 μM

R: Naphthyl

Figure 10. Representative N-naphthalenesulfonamides as anti-leishmania agents.

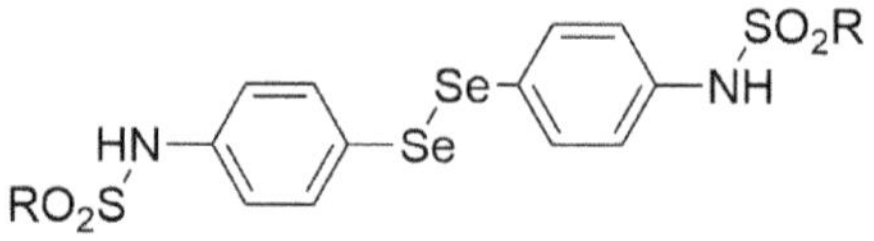

12a: R= 4-methylphenyl   IC$_{50}$ *L. infantum* = 1.40 μM
12b: R= 4-methoxyphenyl   IC$_{50}$ *L. infantum* = 1.30 μM
12c: R= 2-chlorophenyl   IC$_{50}$ *L. infantum* = 1.17 μM
12d: R= 8-quinolinyl   IC$_{50}$ *L. infantum* = 0.83 μM

Figure 11. Diselenide-based sulfonamides as anti-leishmania agents.

13a

13b: R= H
13c: R= 4-F
13d: R= 4-Cl
13e: R= 3-Br
13f: R= 3-MeO

13g

13h

13i: R= H
13l: R= Br

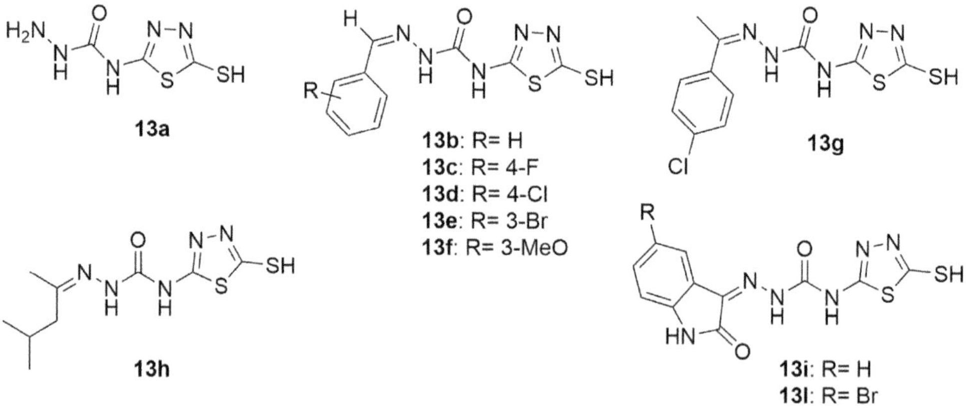

Figure 12. Urea-based 1,3,4-thiadiazole-2-thiols as carbonic anhydrases inhibitors.

A recent contribution by da Silva-Cardoso et al. reports a small series of acetazolamide and benzene sulphonamide containing compounds (**14a–f** in Figure 13) which showed *in vitro* inhibition against LdcCA in the low nanomolar range. However, no activity was observed for these analogues when tested *in vivo* on *L. infantum* and *L. amazorensis* promastigote strains. In contrast, formulation of such compounds as nanoemulsions (NEs) in clove oil resulted in effective anti-leishmanial activity (da Silva-Cardoso et al. 2018). This research suggests a winning strategy for the effective administration of drugs, since the low penetration of compounds through membranes often represents a major hurdle for the development of effective pharmacologic treatments, also in the case of leishmaniasis.

Metal dithiocarbamates

Three hitherto unexplored metal dithiocarbamates, namely maneb, zineb and propineb (Figure 14), demonstrated a strong anti-leishmanial activity on CA of *L. major* promastigotes, by inhibiting the parasite growth at sub-micromolar concentrations and in a dose-dependent fashion.

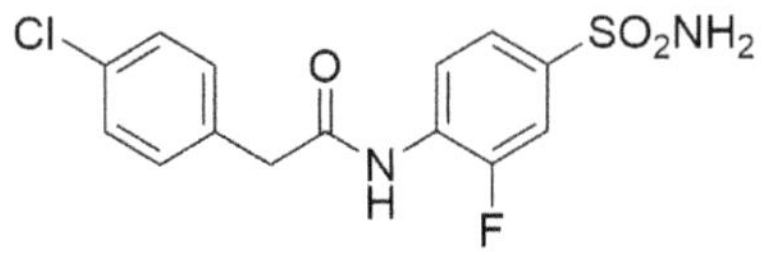

14a (8.3 nM)

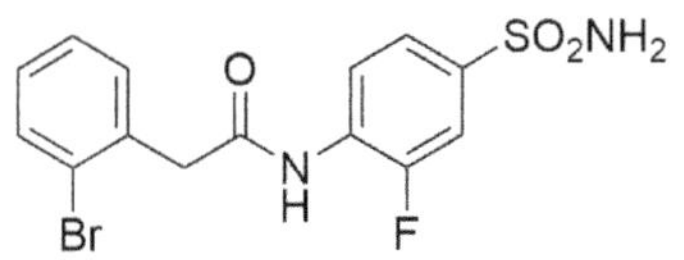

14b (5.4 nM)

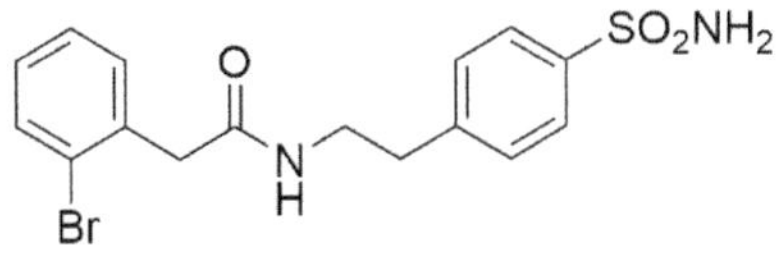

14c (3.9 nM)

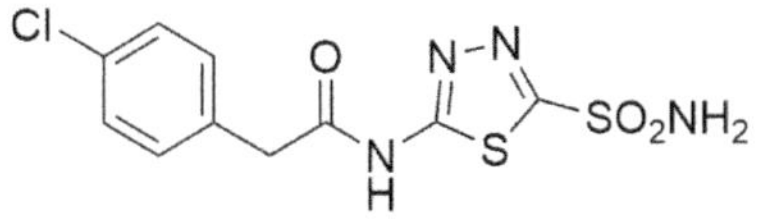

14d (3.3 nM)

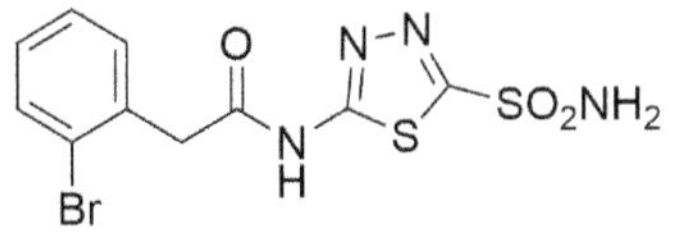

14e (4.1 nM)

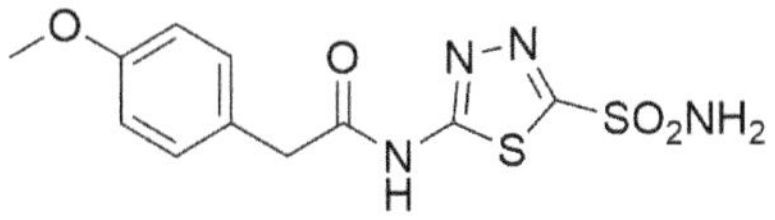

14f (3.7 nM)

Figure 13. Sulfonamides administered as nanoemulsions.

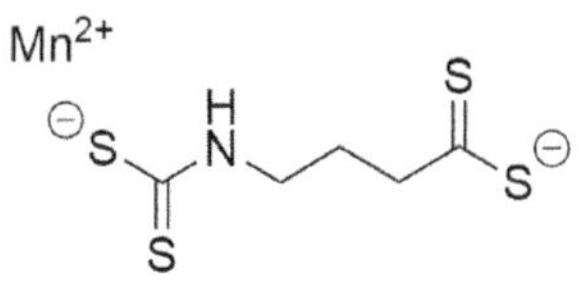

maneb

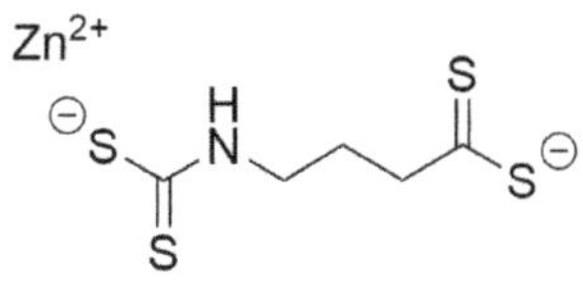

zineb

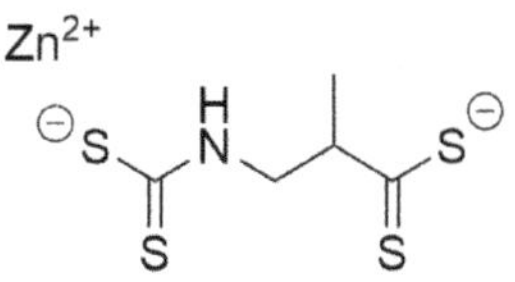

propineb

Figure 14. Chemical structures of metal dithiocarbamate complexes (i.e., presented as monomeric units).

Specifically, the treatment with maneb, zineb and propineb (also known as coordination polymeric complexes) produced morphological deformities and pronounced cell death in *Leishmania* parasites, with 50% lethal dose (LD_{50}) values of 0.56 μM, 0.61 μM and 0.27 μM, respectively (Pal et al. 2015).

Benzoxaboroles

As mentioned above, β-CA of *L. donavani* (LdcCA) has been reported to be efficiently inhibited by sulfonamides and heterocyclic thiols. Considering the druggability of protozoans CAs, Nocentini at al. designed a new generation of CAIs based on the benzoxaborole scaffold. This new family of inhibitors was shown to act *via* a new binding mode and to be effective against human α-CA as well as β-CA from pathogenic fungi (Alterio et al. 2016, Nocentini et al. 2017). Encouraged by these results, as well as the interesting profile of the trypanocidal orally active benzoxaborole compound SCYX-7158 (Figure 15) (Jacobs et al. 2011a, b) which entered Phase IIb/III trials in 2016 for the treatment of African trypanosomiasis, the authors evaluated inhibitory activities of a series of 6-substituted urea/thiourea benzoxaboroles (**15a–e** in Figure 15) against LdcCA in order to detect possible candidates for antiprotozoans studies.

Substitution of the urea function (**15a, b**) with a thiourea bioisosteric group (**15c–e**) did not significantly affect the inhibitory potency. Derivatives **15a–e** (Figure 15) exhibited micromolar inhibition, showing a pronounced selectivity for LdcCA *versus* other protozoan CAs. Moreover, compound **15e** also displayed excellent LdcCA selectivity over the human isoform hCA II. Thus, the benzoxaborole chemotype offers interesting opportunities for CA targeting in pathogenic protozoans eliciting leishmaniasis, thus warranting further development (Nocentini et al. 2018).

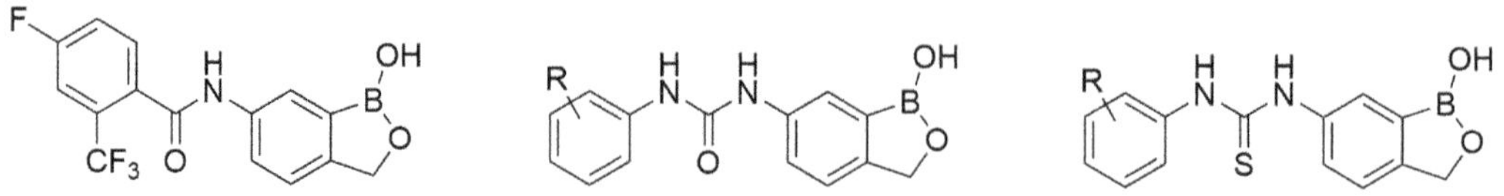

SCYX-7158

15a: R= 4-COCH$_3$
15b: R= 4-Cl

15c: R= 4-OCH$_3$
15d: R= 4-F
15e: R= 4-NO$_2$

Figure 15. The most relevant benzoxaborole compounds **15a-e** and SCYX-7158.

Borylation

As discussed above, boron-containing drugs have been reported to exhibit valuable properties and activities against protozoans causing neglected tropical diseases, including leishmaniasis (Jacobs et al. 2011b). The presence of a boron atom in the structure has been often found essential for antiprotozoal activity (Colotti et al 2018). Furthermore, various boronic acid-based agents have been shown effective agents against several Leishmania parasites (Brun et al. 2011, Adamczyk-Woźniak et al. 2015, Hai and Christianson 2016). Within this context, a general overview of recently reported catalytic strategies to perform efficient borylation reactions, worthy of consideration when synthesising boron-containing agents of biological interest (e.g., benzoxaboroles discussed in paragraph 3.4) is presented herein.

Since the advent of Suzuki cross coupling reaction, a sustained effort of synthetic chemists has been the insertion of boron in organic scaffolds. While initially the insertion of boron was simply viewed as the nucleophilic component for Pd catalysed cross coupling reactions, more recently boronic acids have been reported as valuable bioisosteres for carboxylic acids, attracting attention in biological and medicinal chemistry context (Mak et al. 2011, Nishiyabu et al. 2011). Seminal contributions have recently demonstrated powerful methodologies to access borylated compounds in a straightforward stereoselective fashion from abundant feedstocks (Ingleson et al. 2015, Zhang et al. 2016, Fawcett et al. 2017, Li et al. 2017, Palmer et al. 2016, 2017). Such methodologies are useful as they allow the synthesis of compound libraries as well as late stage chemical diversification, which can in turn be exploited for SAR studies, in order to identify new potent hit compounds. While a complete survey of borylative methods is well outside the realms of relevance to this chapter, a few methodologies are highlighted below showcasing the importance of chemical synthesis to access scaffolds which may be of interest, as well as 'scaffold diversity' for successful biological targeting and exploration of new areas of the 'chemical space' (Isidro-Llobet et al. 2011). In particular, a number of procedures that can facilitate the production of specific borylated compounds are reported along with a list of considerations and practical aspects for the optimization of synthetic methods, which are generally necessary to achieve the quality and amount of compound required for biological investigation.

In the last decade, there has been high interest in the synthetic chemistry community to shift away from precious metal catalysis (i.e., rhodium, platinum and iridium). In this regard, Palmer et al. (2016) have used cobalt as a nontoxic, earth abundant first row transition metal, and viable substitute for more precious metals. Indeed, Co is cheap and it allows unprecedentedly explored chemical transformations. A demonstration of this is the Co catalyzed benzylic borylation methodology recently reported by Palmer et al. (2016). While precious (and non-precious) metals have been known to undergo sp^2 C-H borylation, benzylic borylation is an underdeveloped methodology. Furthermore, polybenzylic borylation had never been reported nor directing group free homobenzylic diborylation (data not shown). Tuning equivalents of Co catalyst (Figure 16) and B$_2$pin$_2$ (i.e., bis(pinacolato)diboron) as the borylating reagent led to varying degrees of borylation of toluene (Figure 16A).

Nickel is another earth abundant metal that has received intense research as a potential replacement for precious metals. Altering the ligand scaffold (substitution of a cyclohexyl for a bulkier pinene derived motif) facilitated a one-pot three-step triborylation-conjugate addition-alkylation in increased yields compared to the original Co system (Figure 16B) (Palmer et al. 2017). This highlights the power of

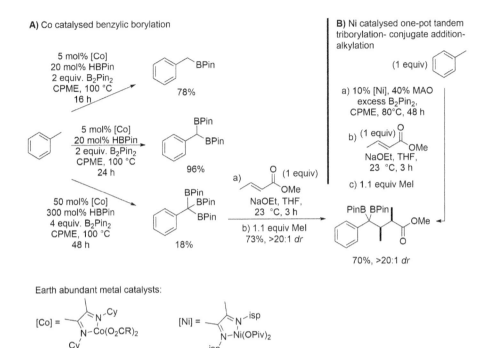

Figure 16. Chiriks polybenzylic borylation using (A) Co (Palmer et al. 2016) and (B) Ni (Palmer et al. 2017). THF = tetrahydrofuran; BPin = boronic acid pinacol; B_2Pin_2 CPME = bis(pinacolato)diboron cyclopentylmethyl ether; MAO = methylaluminoxane; Cy = cyclohexyl; Piv = pivaloyl; isp= (1*R*,2*R*,3*R*,5*S*)-(–)-isopinocampheylamine.

earth abundant catalysts in revealing novel reactivity and the rapid formation of complexity in a highly stereocontrolled manner.

A further extension of stereocontrol is enantioselectivity. Enantioselectivity and the resultant 3D orientation in space are key in biological structures (see section 7) and are often at the forefront of any synthetic approach. Morken and co-workers have recently utilized a well-known boron reactivity (1,2 migration of boronates) coupled with a metal induced 1,2-metallate rearrangement to yield a conjunctive coupling partner *via* the union of two nucleophilic reagents (Figure 17) (Zhang et al. 2016).

The application of a chiral ferrocene-based ligand (i.e., 'MandyPhos') facilitated chirality transfer yielding the products in high enantioselectivity. Notably, alkyl lithium reagents well as vinyl triflates could be used as in the 1,2 metallate rearrangement. To allow facile workup, the boron containing product was oxidized to the alcohol prior to isolation; however, the boron containing product could also be isolated in slightly diminished yields.

Finally, almost simultaneously the groups of Baran and Aggarwal reported a decarboxylative borylation methodology (Figures 18A and B) (Fawcett et al. 2017, Li et al. 2017). The power of this methodology lies in the ubiquity of the carboxylic acid group in nature as well as the chemoselectivity of the transformation.

Indeed, the medicinal properties of boronic acids were highlighted by the comparison of a native peptide with the borylated analogue as human neutrophil elastase (HNE) inhibitors (Figure 18B). In this case, the parent carboxylic acid demonstrated no activity while the boronic acid (obtained in 48% yield) displayed an IC_{50} of 0.27 nM (Li et al. 2017).

Both methodologies rely upon the activation of the carboxylic acid moiety to a redox active ester which could be isolated or reacted *in situ*. Even though the mechanism proceeds *via* a radical pathway (confirmed by Aggarwal's studies employing radical clock experiments), the methodology could functionalize a variety of complex natural products, demonstrating exquisite control not often associated with traditional radical chemistry (Figures 18A and B). Of note, a borono-vancomycin analogue was obtained as a single diastereomer from vancomycin (Li et al. 2017).

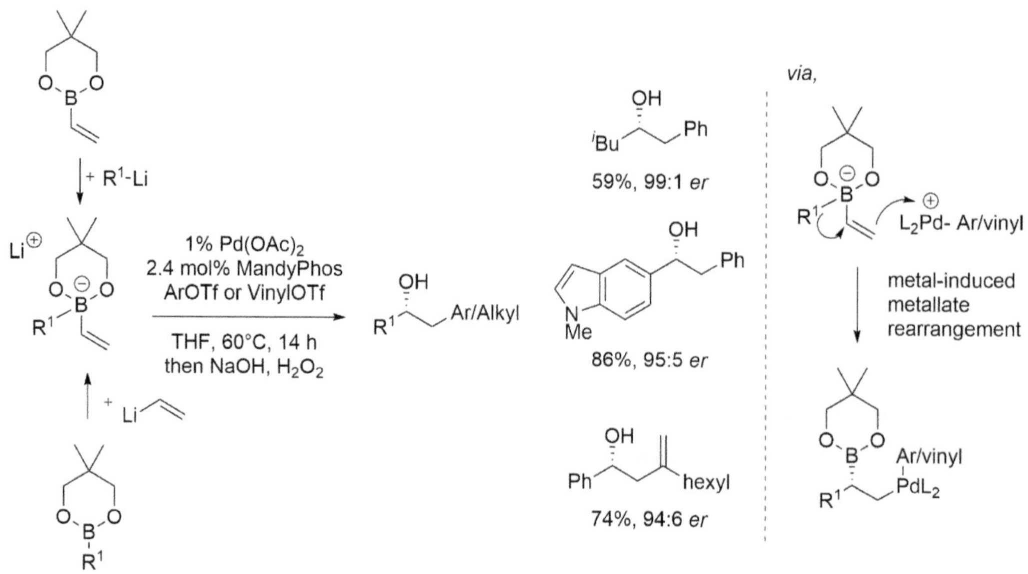

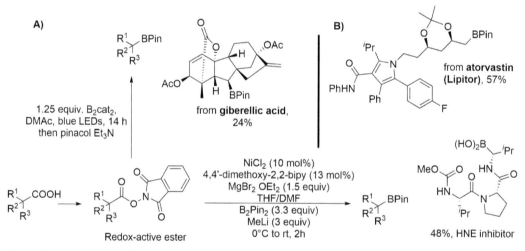

Figure 17. Morken's enantioselective conjunctive cross coupling. THF = tetrahydrofuran; Tf = triflate; L = ligand.

Figure 18. Aggarwal (A) and Baran's (B) decarboxylative borylations. THF = tetrahydrofuran; DMF = dimethylformamide; B_2Pin_2 = bis(pinacolato)diboron; DMAc = N,N-dimethylacetamide.

These examples above showcase the power of synthetic methodology to shortcut and rapidly diversify natural (and unnatural) products. They demonstrate strides taken by the synthetic chemistry community towards enabling boronic acid installation as an afterthought, as opposed to arduous boronic acid centred retrosynthesis (Li et al. 2017). The strategic value of such processes cannot be underestimated. The authors look forward to more synthetic shortcuts to boronic acids as well as alternate functionalities which are (or are bioisosteric) with those recurrent in drugs.

Topoisomerases

DNA topoisomerases (TOPs) are involved at many different levels in DNA metabolic processes and are validated targets for antibacterial and anticancer therapies (Pommier et al. 2010). TOPs play a pivotal role in the modulation of dynamic nature of DNA secondary or higher order structures, supporting essential functions inside the cells, with regard to nucleic acid metabolism processes, such as replication, transcription, recombination and repair (Bjornsti and Wang 1987, Stewart et al. 1997). Based on the number of DNA strands cleaved, these enzymes are classified as type IA-, IB- (EC 5.99.1.2) and II-DNA (EC 5.99.1.3) topoisomerases (Champoux 2001).

Recently, TOP IB has emerged as a valuable target in anti-leishmaniasis therapy (Reguera et al. 2006), due to two main factors. Primarily, there is an increased expression of TOP IB during the division cycle of rapidly growing leishmanial protozoa. Secondly, *Leishmania* TOP IB isoform contains structural features which are not found in the same enzyme subtype of the mammalian host (Balana-Fouce et al. 2014, D'Annessa et al. 2015). This latter scenario is analogous to the aforementioned absence of β-CA within vertebrates, in order to favour drug selectivity. Specifically, *Leishmania* TOP IB displays two non-conserved regions (i.e., at the C-terminus of the large protomer and at the N-terminus of the small protomer), which are crucial for enzyme assembly and can be exploited to confer selectivity to topoisomerase inhibitors (Reguera et al. 2006, Prada et al. 2012). Similarly, subtype distinctive features are also present in other trypanosomatids of medical interest, i.e., *Trypanosoma brucei* (Bodley et al. 2003) and *Rypanosoma cruzi* (Zuma et al. 2014), rendering TOP enzymes remarkably important for wide drug discovery approaches in the field of neglected diseases.

In this context, Ubeira's group synthesized different oxoisoaporphine derivatives with potent anti-leishmanial effects *in vitro* against *L. amazonensis* amastigotes (Sobarzo-Sánchez et al. 2013). Among them, compounds **16** and **17** (Figure 19) were additionally selected to evaluate *in vitro* activity on the promastigote stages of four leishmanial species (i.e., *L. infantum*, *L. amazonensis*, *L. braziliensis* and *L. guyanensis*), as representative examples of the four main clinical forms generating disease states.

Oxoisoaporphine analogues **16** and **17** demonstrated anti-leishmanial activity on all four species tested and exhibited high selectivity indexes in comparison to miltefosine, proposing their further evaluation in *in vivo* models of Leishmaniasis (i.e., BALB/c mice infected with *L. infantum*) (Sobarzo-Sánchez et al. 2013). Disappointingly, **17** was found to be ineffective *in vivo*, as the resultant reduction of *Leishmania* amastigotes in liver and spleen was minimal and did not show differences with the untreated control. In contrast, treatment with compound **16** caused a significant reduction of the parasite burden in the spleen and livers of BALB/c mice, with maximum efficacy by using a dose of 10 mg/kg (i.e., 99% reduction of parasites in livers).

Recently, Velásquez et al. (2017) designed the binuclear cycloplatinate complex **18** (Figure 19) as a new therapeutic agent for anti-protozoan treatment through TOP IB inhibition. Compound **18** was synthesized

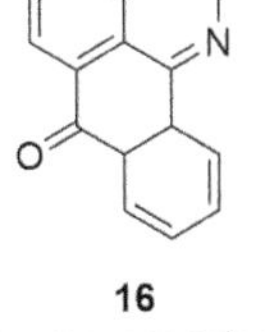

16
IC$_{50}$ *L. amazonensis* = <0.05 µg/mL

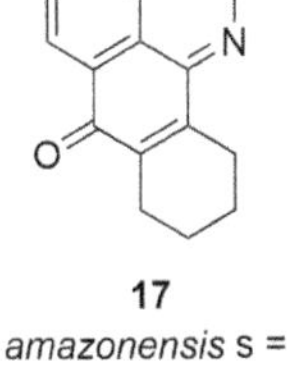

17
IC$_{50}$ *L. amazonensis* s = <0.025 µg/mL

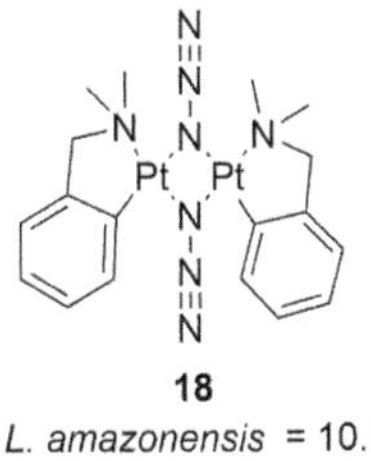

18
IC$_{50}$ *L. amazonensis* = 10.1-13.2 µM

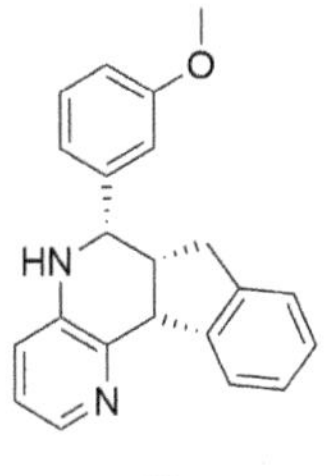

19
IC$_{50}$ *L. infantum* = 0.54-5.4 µM

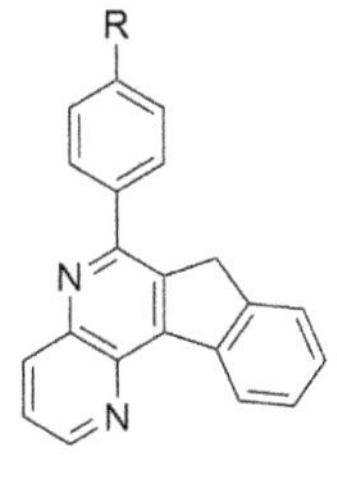

20: R= F   IC$_{50}$ *L. infantum* = 0.74-34.4 µM
21: R= OMe IC$_{50}$ *L. infantum* = 5.8 µM

Figure 19. Topoisomerase inhibitors with anti-leishmanial activity.

and investigated for inhibitory activity against *L. amazonensis* promastigote stages, showing an IC_{50} of 13.2 µM (Velásquez et al. 2017). The potency of this compound on intracellular amastigote forms (i.e., the clinically most relevant life-cycle stages of *Leishmania* parasites) was 10.1 µM with a selectivity index of 49.9, demonstrating higher efficacy in lowering the number of amastigotes in infected macrophages (i.e., 68.5% reduction). The performance of **18** has been further explored *in vivo* using a model of cutaneous leishmaniasis. Specifically, the treatment of *L. amazonensis*-infected mice with 0.35 mg/kg/d of the Pt-based complex produced a significant reduction of the parasite presence in foot lesions (80%, as determined from the LDU, i.e., Leishman Donovan units = number of intracellular amastigotes/1000 host cell nuclei × organ weight (mg)) (Velásquez et al. 2017).

Lastly, indeno-1,5-naphthyridine derivatives **19–21** (Figure 19) have also been reported as TOP IB inhibitors, exhibiting a significant activity (i.e., submicromolar range) on *L. infantum* isoform (Tejería et al. 2016). These analogues demonstrated selective and stage-specific anti-proliferative effects on amastigote over promastigote forms. In the tests, compounds **19–21** additionally behaved as selective inhibitors of *Leishmania* TOP IB over the human subtype, highlighting the potential role of this enzyme to mediate putative anti-leishmanial actions (Tejería et al. 2016).

Phosphodiesterases

Phosphodiesterases (PDEs) regulate the cellular concentration of cAMP and cGMP, which are key secondary messengers for many biological processes (Biagini et al. 2010, Giovannoni et al. 2011). The human genome contains more than twenty PDE genes that are grouped into 11 families (i.e., PDE 1-11). In comparison, a lower number of PDE genes have been identified in protozoal parasite. As an example, in the genome of *L. major* only five PDE genes have been found and characterized, encoding five related PDEs, i.e., LmjPDEA, LmjPDEB1, LmjPDEB2, LmjPDEC, and LmjPDED. Among these, LmjPDEB1 and LmjPDEB2 are adjacently situated on chromosome 15 and share extensive similarity in their overall structure (Savai et al. 2010, Shakur et al. 2011). Additionally, a highly specific cAMP phosphodiesterase from *L. mexicana* has been characterized and purified, showing low sensitivity for selective and non-selective human PDE inhibitors (Rascón et al. 2000). A similar inefficacy by human PDE inhibitors has been also described for two PDEs cloned from other members of the *Trypanosomatidae* family (i.e., TbPDE2A and TbPDE2B from *Trypanosoma brucei*, the causing agent of sleeping sickness) (Zoraghi et al 2001, Rascón et al. 2002).

Early reports demonstrated that non-specific PDE inhibitors (e.g., caffeine, theophylline, papaverine, dipyridamole and allopurinol) are very weak inhibitors of *Leishmania* PDEs. However, these agents were shown to inhibit the transformation of amastigotes to promastigotes as well as the proliferation of promastigotes in *L. donovani* and *L. tropica* (Walter et al. 1987, Kamau et al. 2001, Seebeck et al. 2001). Cibacron blue (Figure 20), a well-known PDE ligand, proved to be one of the most potent inhibitor of *L. mexicana* PDE (IC_{50}= 8 µM) (Hanggi and Carr 1985, Burton et al. 1988). Similarly, three human PDE inhibitors (i.e., dipyridamole, etazolate and trequinisin, Figure 20) inhibit the proliferation of *L. major* promastigotes and *L. infantum* amastigotes with EC_{50} values in the micromolar range (e.g., 45–58 µM inhibition for the three agents on *L. major* promastigotes, 10 µM inhibition for trequinisin on *L. infantum* amastigotes) (Johner et al. 2006).

In this context, Dal Piaz and colleagues developed a library of *Leishmania* PDE inhibitors based on the isoxazolo[3,4-*d*]pyridazin-3(2*H*)-one scaffold (Dal Piaz et al. 2002). These agents (e.g., compounds **22–25** in Figure 21) were designed as derivatives of previously identified mammalian PDE inhibitors (Dal Piaz et al. 1997, 1998), showing valuable activity profiles when tested at 100 µM concentration for their ability to inhibit phosphodiesterase activity of *L. mexicana* PDE subtype (Rascón et al. 2000). Although none of the tested compounds showed a similar level of activity in comparison with Cibacron blue (used as a control in the tests), the study led to the identification of relevant SARs for this class of *Leishmania* PDE inhibitors (Dal Piaz et al. 2002). From the study, compounds **22–24** (i.e., isoxazolopyridazinone-based agents) and **25** (i.e., pyridazinone analogue) (Figure 21) were the most active terms of the series, determining an inhibition of *L. mexicana* PDE of 58.7, 55.4, 51.8 and 51.9%, respectively.

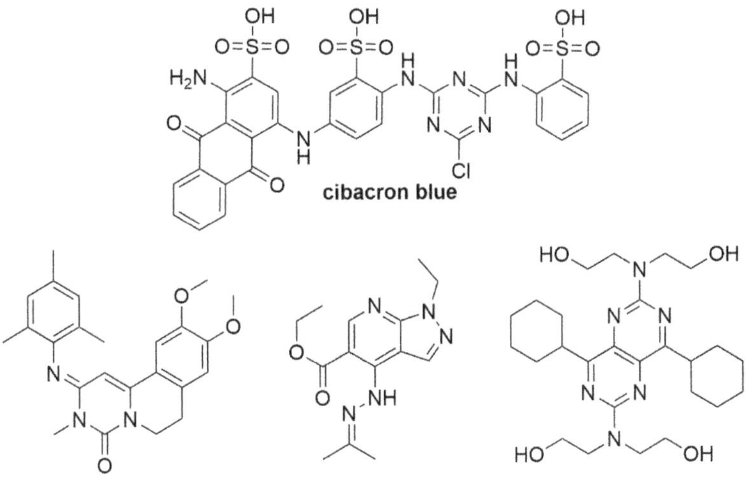

trequinisin etazolate dipyridamole

Figure 20. Cibacron blue and human PDE inhibitors active on *L. major* and *L. infantum*.

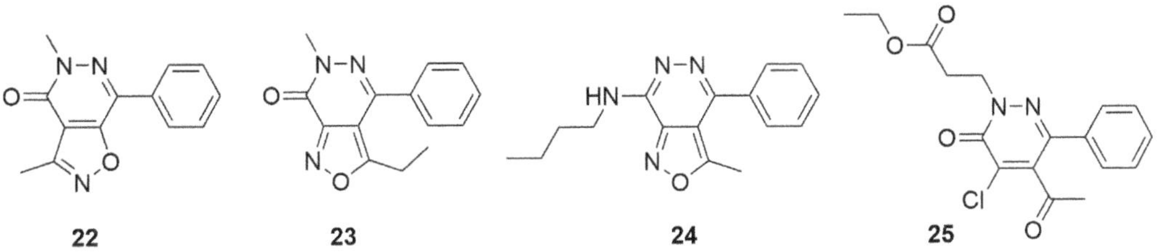

22 23 24 25

Figure 21. Isoxazolo[3,4-*d*]pyridazin-3(2*H*)-one as *L. mexicana* PDE inhibitors.

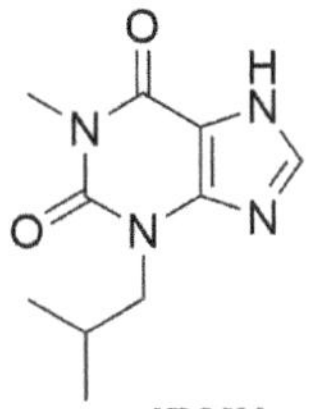

IBMX

Figure 22. 3-Isobutyl-1-methylxanthine (IBMX).

Recently, the nonspecific PDE ligand IBMX (i.e., 3-isobutyl-1-methylxanthine, Figure 22) showed an inhibition activity of 580 nM against LmjPDEB1. The co-crystallization of the catalytic domain of LmjPDEB1 bound to IBMX has been also reported, highlighting the presence of a characteristic pocket within the enzyme structure, which is not present in human PDEs and can be exploited for the design of parasite selective inhibitors as anti-*Leishmania* agents (Wang et al. 2007, Seebeck et al. 2011). This demonstrates the feasibility of discovering potent and selective PDE inhibitors that could be therapeutically useful to modulate cAMP levels and proliferation in *Leishmania* parasites and, possibly, other trypanosomatids.

Recent Drug Discovery Strategies to Identify New Anti-Leishmanial Agents

Leishmaniasis is recognized as one of the six major tropical diseases by the World Health Organization (WHO) (Frezard et al. 2009). To date, the efficacy of anti-*Leishmania* treatment has been shown to depend on both host and parasite factors, with certain therapies and regimens effective only against particular *Leishmania* species and/or strains (Nagle et al. 2014). Thus, WHO highlights that *"clinical research to evaluate new drugs and combinations of drugs to reduce the duration of treatment for all clinical forms of leishmaniasis remains a high priority"* [...], and *"efforts should be made to improve access to medicines and reduce their cost"* [...] (WHO 2010, Kaneko 2011).

In line with this, the number of intellectual property applications centred on leishmaniasis research has dramatically risen in the last ten years. The majority of patents reporting therapeutic approaches to treat leishmaniasis are filed in the US (47.2%), followed by Brazil (9.4%), Spain (6.6%), Denmark (6%), France (6%) and India (6%) (Machado-Silva et al. 2015). Interestingly, the percent of documents reporting new molecules with leishmanicidal activity is equally shared with those relating to the re-use of already existing drugs in leishmaniasis treatment (i.e., 'repurposing strategy').

In the following sections, we analyze experimental evidences for two new classes of molecules (i.e., quinone and phosphorus-containing derivatives) which have been patented as possible anti-*Leishmania* drug candidates.

Quinone derivatives

A large number of quinone-based agents, both natural (i.e., isolated from plants or animals) and synthetic, show a range of biological or pharmacological properties, including antiparasitic and anti-leishmanial activities (Liu 2011). In 2008, Fuchino et al. reported a library of 1,4-naphtoquinone-based anti-protozoal agents isolated by extraction from *Angelica radix* or *Lithospermi radix*, which were particularly effective as anti-leishmanial agents (e.g., compounds **26–28**, Figure 23) with limited side effects (Fuchino et al. 2008). The pharmacological activity of these agents was established on 26 patients and clinical observations concerning size and condition of lesions confirmed their effectiveness in the treatment of cutaneous leishmaniasis (Fuchino et al. 2008).

In a different study, Bakare et al. reported a novel series of synthetic 1,4-naphthoquinone derivatives with potent activity against *L. donovani*. Among them, compounds **29–32** (Figure 24) exhibited low cytotoxicity and high efficacy compared to traditionally used drugs during treatment at various stages of parasite infections (Bakare et al. 2013).

The data in Table 1 report the IC_{50} values of compounds **29–32** to demonstrate their efficacy in inhibiting *Leishmania* proliferation, in comparison to amphotericin-B (used as the control). Noteworthy, naphthoquinone **32**, with an IC_{50} value of 48 pM, has the higher anti-leishmanial efficacy and selectivity on promastigotes. In contrast, the other imido-naphthoquinone analogues **29–31** produced similar inhibition values as the control drug for the same stage (i.e., 4.4–7.0 μM for **29–31** and 5.6 μM for amphotericin-B) (Bakare et al. 2013). *L. donovani* amastigotes were also significantly inhibited by compounds **29–32**, with IC_{50} values ranging from 1.19 to 18.85 μM (Table 1). In general, the lower IC_{50} values of naphthoquinones **29–32** compared to IC_{50} value of amphotericin-B suggest that these compounds are more effective in inhibiting the growth of *L. donovani* amastigotes *in vitro* (Bakare et al. 2013). In particular, amphotericin-B has a lower selectivity index than all the screened compounds for both amastigotes and promastigotes forms (i.e., 0.05 and 0.22, respectively; Table 1) of the parasites. Furthermore, by evaluating cytotoxic effects on mouse fibroblasts, compounds **29–32** showed only minor toxicity effects compared to the control drug, as a direct consequence of the overall lower IC_{50} values (Table 1). Additional *in vivo* tests performed with naphthoquinones **29–32** at three different concentrations (i.e., 5 mg/kg, 20 mg/kg and 50 mg/kg) show a good reduction of the parasite growth, as demonstrated by the suppression of splenic and liver parasite burden after treatment (Bakare et al. 2013).

Several natural quinone-based anti-leishmanial agents have been recently isolated by Kimura et al. from *Sargassum yamadae* extracts, a brown alga belonging to *Sargas saceae* family (Freile-Pelegrin et al. 2008, Kimura et al. 2014). Compounds **33a–c** (Figure 25) are representative analogues of this family of natural compounds which demonstrated a good inhibition of *L. major* growth rate *in vitro*. Additionally, **33c** was used in a *Leishmania* mouse model to investigate the *in vivo* behaviour and possible therapeutic effects. From the whole study, it was confirmed that **33c** exhibits an anti-leishmanial activity equal to amphotericin-B both *in vitro* and *in vivo* (Kimura et al. 2014).

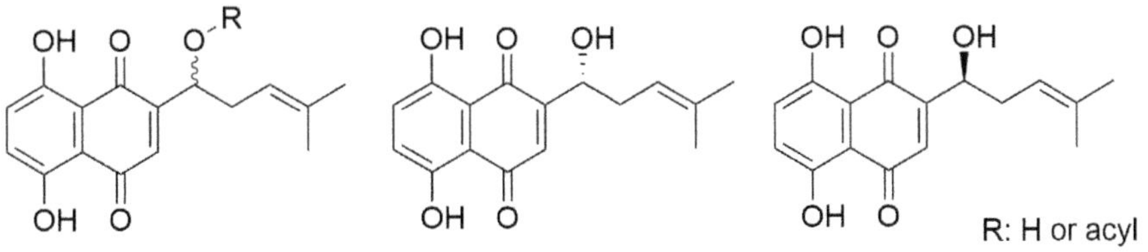

26 **27** **28**

Figure 23. Natural naphthoquinones with anti-leishmanial activity.

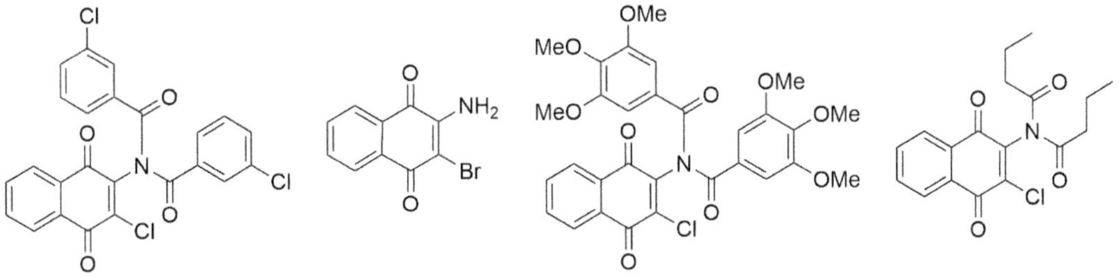

29 **30** **31** **32**

Figure 24. Synthetic 1,4-naphthoquinones with anti-leishmanial activity.

Table 1. IC_{50} values and selectivity index (SI) of naphthoquinones **29–32** on *L. donovani.*

	IC_{50} (mM)			SI Values	
	Promastigotes	Amastigotes	Fibroblasts	Promastigotes	Amastigotes
29	6.82 ± 2.3	1.19 ± 1.1	168.1 ± 7.91	24.65 ± 12.51	141.26 ± 56.8
30	4.4 ± 0.4	2.07 ± 1.0	14197.35 ± 0.84	3301.71 ± 321.1	6858.62 ± 3975.5
31	7.0 ± 1.0	1.69 ± 0.02	4.83 ± 1.5	0.69 ± 1.21	2.84 ± 0.04
32	0.000048 ± 0.004	18.85 ± 19.7	2.94 ± 0.001	612150.00 ± 438	0.16 ± 0.09
amphotericin-B	5.26 ± 0.9	22.26 ± 0.001	1.18 ± 0.2	0.22 ± 0.004	0.05 ± 0.001

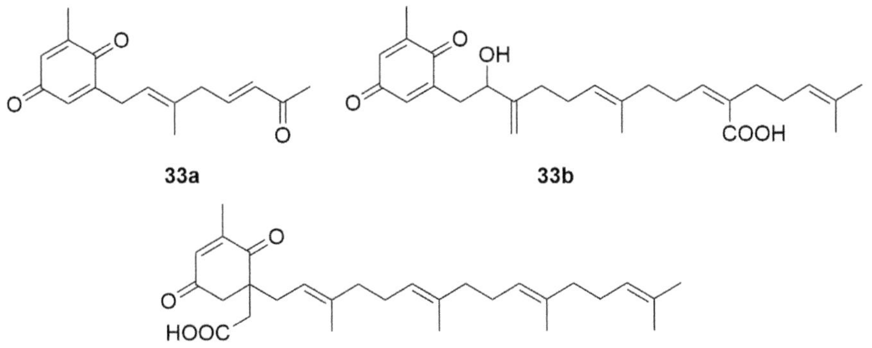

33a **33b** **33c**

Figure 25. Anti-leishmanial agents **33a–c** isolated from *Sargassum yamadae* extract.

Phosphorus-containing derivatives

Although initially developed as an antitumour agent, miltefosine (hexadecylphosphocholine, Figure 1) is an alkyllysophospholipid widely in use in current anti-leishmanial chemotherapy, showing good bioavailability as well as effectiveness toward both visceral and cutaneous leishmaniasis (Croft et al. 1987). However, the development of resistance has been reported owing to the long half-life in humans (i.e., 100–200 h) and low therapeutic ratio. Moreover, miltefosine has been found to be a teratogen in animals (Herwaldt 1999), being unsuitable for treatment during pregnancy. Furthermore, it has been shown to not give appreciable efficacy when administered to HIV-coinfected *Leishmania* patients. The limited efficacy of miltefosine against other non-Indian visceral leishmaniasis and the worldwide diffused range of cutaneous leishmaniasis syndromes are also major issues that limit the use of this drug.

In this context, Calogeropoulou et al. reported the synthesis and biological evaluation of substituted ether phospholipids, incorporating different alkyl and adamantylidene (or cyclohexylidene) groups in the lipid portion, with a quaternary ammonium moiety as polar head groups (compounds **34a–d** in Figure 26). In the study, compounds **34a–d** were profiled for their activity on *L. infantum* and *L. donovani* and showed inhibitory effects on the parasite growth. Although these agents had very different selectivity profiles, **34d** produced a potent inhibition (with high selectivity) on *L. donovani* over *L. infantum* (Calogeropoulou et al. 2006). Five years later, Hu and collaborators reported two series of phosphoramide-based nitrogen mustards (Figure 26) as potent anti-leishmanial agents—i.e., the acyclic compounds **35a–c** and the cyclic analogues **36a, b** (cyclophosphamide-like structures). These agents are prodrugs that remain inactive until activated by a group of oxidoreductases (i.e., nitroreductases, NTRs) selectively expressed in trypanosomes over different eukaryotes (Hu et al. 2011).

The nitroaromatic group has specifically been incorporated in the molecules as the trigger for this reductive activation. The reduction of the nitro group to the corresponding hydroxylamine derivative, by the NTR catalyzed reaction, leads to the fragmentation of the structure and consequent release of the requisite toxic moieties (e.g., mustards, nitro radical anions and hydroxylamine-based species) (Chen and Hu 2009). Overall, compounds **35a–c** and **36a, b** (Figure 26) resulted potent trypanocidal agents, although phosphoramide derivatives with a linear chain had a better inhibition profile against *L. major*

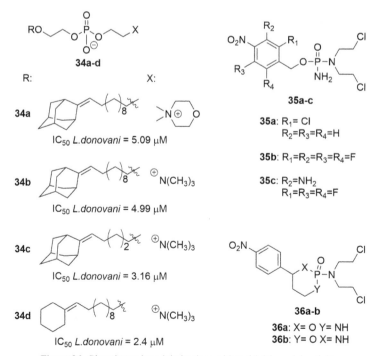

Figure 26. Phosphorus-based derivatives with anti-leishmanial activity.

(Hu et al. 2011). Therefore, Hu and collaborators propose to leverage the activity of NTR leishmanial isoform for drug development in two ways: (1) as an activator of new nitroaromatic/quinone-based prodrugs, (2) through the use of modulators for this enzyme target. These two approaches could also be complementary in a combined targeting strategy. For instance, *L. major* strains showing resistance to drug inhibitors of LmNTR (i.e., *L. major* nitroreductase, a flavin mononucleotide-containing nitroreductase) could theoretically be sensitive or even hypersensitive to prodrugs, which would therefore be activated by this leishmanial enzyme (Chen and Hu 2009).

Drug Repurposing Strategies in the Treatment of Leishmaniasis

We present here examples of researches carried out in the field of 'new uses for old drugs' as potential option for the treatment of leishmaniasis. While *de novo* identification of compounds in drug discovery campaigns is the traditional success story, the high cost and low successful output has led to the increasing requirement of alternative methods to present drugs in the market. One such example is the 'repurposing strategy' (Njoroge et al. 2014). Strictly, three possible situations are in existence:

- 'Drug repurposing'—when an approved drug is found to have activity against another disease. Dosing programmes may be altered but, crucially, a key aspect of repurposing is the lack of further structural modifications to the drug. This has an important implication in that the approved chemical agent has already been studied in terms of toxicity as well as pharmokinetics. As such, a free pass is often obtained up to, and often including, phase I clinical trials.

- 'Drug repositioning'—when a current drug serves as lead compound for further modifications to yield active derivatives in another disease. Clearly, such new 'chemical entity' will be subject to new testing. However, the ability to start 'downstream' and conduct SAR studies on an identified 'privileged structure' is still a powerful shortcut to new medicines (see borylation strategies in section 3.4.1, as an e.g., of synthetic shortcuts for late stage diversification).

- 'Drug rescue'—when a drug is 'resurrected' from unsuccessful campaigns to be used in an alternate disease.

More generally, the 'repurposing strategy' may be viewed as any approach which adapts current pharmacopheia for alternative uses (Aubé 2012). For simplicity, in this section we refer to 'repurposing' to encompass all the three situations reported above.

While 'repurposing' is on the rise, arguably it has been coming for a long time. As remarked by 1988 Nobel laureate James Black, "the most fruitful basis for the discovery of a new drug is to start with an old drug" (Chong and Sullivan 1989). In a simple cost-benefit analysis, drug repurposing sits favourably in the eyes of the pharmaceutical industry being low cost and high benefit. The advantage for such a 'repurposing' approach includes a reduction in time to the market and related cost (in terms of development of new compounds but also toxicology studies).

While there are numerous examples of successful repurposing, from acriscorin (i.e., antifungal to antimalarial) (Shahinas et al. 2010) to zafirlukast (i.e., asthma to NF-$_\kappa$B inhibitor) (Miller et al. 2010), perhaps the most telling is the case of thalidomide, universally taught in schools as it impresses upon students the importance of stereochemistry and the 3D nature of drug-biological target interactions. While one enantiomer indeed corrected the morning sickness of the patient mother, the other enantiomer led to severe birth defects in the child. Furthermore, the pitfalls of racemisation *in vivo* are revealed. What is perhaps less well documented is the revival of thalidomide. In a desperate attempt to sedate a critically ill patient suffering from erthyema nodosum leprosum (ENL, a painful complication of leprosy), Jacob Sheskin (a dermatologist working with leprosy patients) administered two pills of thalidomide (Sheskin 1975, Greenstone 2011). What followed after the patient's night of sleep and remarkable recovery was a WHO sponsored follow up study in which 99% of patients enjoyed complete remission within two weeks. This in turn led to the general adoption of thalidomide as an effective medicine for ENL (Brynner and Stephens 2001, Silverman 2002, Ashburn and Thor 2004). Furthermore, thalidomide (rebranded as Thalidomid®) has additionally been shown to be an inhibitor of angiogenesis (D'Amato et al. 1994) and is currently used to treat myeloma. Its successors, namely Revlimid® (i.e., lenalidomide) and Pomalyst®

(i.e., pomalidomide), made $6.97 billion for Celgene in 2015 (Kumar et al. 2014, Larocca et al. 2017, Büyükkaramikli et al. 2018).

In general, identification for 'repurposing' is centred on five main principles. Firstly, similarities in cell biology may be translatable. For example, exploiting similarities in haemoglobin degradation between schistoma and plasmodia has led to treatment through repurposing (Keiser and Utzinger 2012). Secondly, similarities in drug targets may be leveraged to yield downstream active scaffolds which in turn may be modified for increased potency (i.e., central to drug repositioning). Thirdly, genome information may be exploited. Utilising knowledge of genome homology between potential and validated targets offers an abbreviated path to successful drug candidates. Fourthly, docking studies are proving to be efficient preliminary filters in highlighting candidates through *in silico* evaluation. However, a cumbersome pre-requisite to such *in silico* screening is accurate 3D data of both the drug and the target (Kharkar et al. 2014). Finally, 'non-hypothesis screening' is a powerful approach to drug repurposing, repositioning and rescue. The initial excitement of high-throughput screening (HTS) led to an investment of over $100 million, which unfortunately overall had little difference on the community (Horrobin 2001, Glassman and Sun 2004). However, the thought process and technology itself can be 'repurposed' for the HTS of old drugs in known diseases.

An example of the application of HTS for repurposing in the context of anti-parasitic research is the study by Witschel and collaborators (Witschel et al. 2012). In this 2012 study, 600 agrochemicals were screened for anti-plasmodial, anti-trypanosomal and anti-leishmanial activities. Among them, zoxamide and tolyfluanid (Figure 27) showed submicromolar activity against *L. donovani*. It is notable that tolyfluanid contains the sulfonamide group, a structural function required for the activity of several carbonic anhydrase inhibitors (*vide supra*, section 3.1).

In contrast, a successful example of 'classic' repurposing for *Leishmania* was reported in 2007 by Uliana and co-workers (2007), who disclosed the use of tamoxifen (i.e., a triphenylethylene-based compound, Figure 28) to treat *Leishmania* (Miguel et al. 2007). In this case, tamoxifen (known to be an oestrogen receptor modulator used in the treatment and prevention of breast cancer) was found to be a potent inhibitor of the growth of several *Leishmania* species (IC$_{50}$ values ranging from 9.0 to 20.2 μM).

The repurposing of tamoxifen in leishmaniasis testifies the importance of understanding the mechanism of drug activity as well as the unintended consequences which in turn may be utilised when the drug is repurposed. Central to the initial hypothesis of tamoxifen efficacy in leishmaniasis treatment was the compilation of two pieces of information. Firstly, the parasitophorus vacuoles enclose a highly acidic environment. Secondly, previous work by Altan and co-workers (Altan et al. 1999) showed that tamoxifen

zoxamide   **tolylfluanid**

Figure 27. Anti-leishmanial agents identified by high-throughput screening of 600 known agrochemicals.

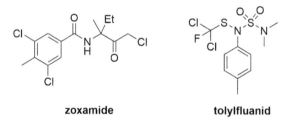

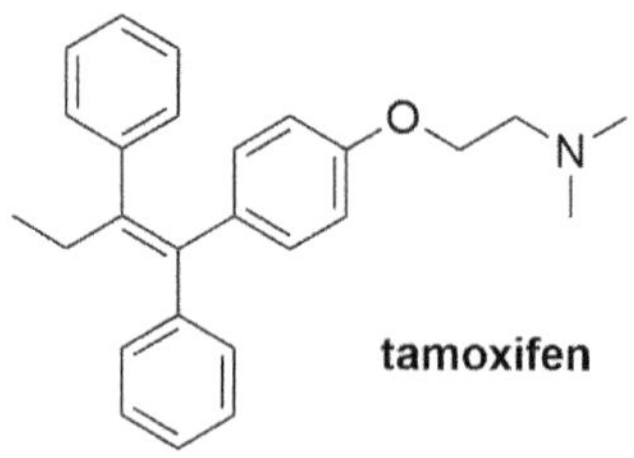

tamoxifen

Figure 28. Triphenylethylene-based structure of tamoxifen.

was able to reverse adriamycin resistance inhibiting the acidification of organelles in several breast cancer cell lines (by a mechanism which did not involve the oestrogen receptor). By following these evidences, Uliana et al. (2007) confirmed the activity of tamoxifen for the treatment of cutaneous and visceral leishmaniasis in rodents, caused by *L. braziliensis* and *L. chagasi*, respectively (Miguel et al. 2007). In the case of *L. braziliensis* infected mice, tamoxifen demonstrated significant reductions in lesion sizes as well as 99% decrease in parasite burden. *L. chagasi* infected hamsters had 95–98% reduction in spleen parasite burden. However, the most relevant outcome was that all animals treated with tamoxifen survived, whereas control animals (i.e., mice where the treatment was interrupted) died after 11 weeks.

Most recently, a study regarding the combined use of tamoxifen and miltefosine was also undertaken by Uliana and colleagues (Miguel et al. 2009). While the combination of tamoxifen and miltefosine at dosages corresponding to half the ED_{50} were more effective than either monotherapies, at higher dosages the combined therapy had the same effect as miltefosine monotherapy (Miguel et al. 2009). However, tamoxifen was able to retard and suppress the growth of parasites treated with miltefosine, indicating the ability to oppose the common resistance encountered with the use of this drug (see '*Phosphorus-based scaffolds*' in section 6.2).

In summary, the reinvention of old drugs for new purposes has already shown promise in the treatment of a panoply of diseases, including leishmaniasis. Clearly, the 'repurposing strategy' can serve as a useful 'stop-gap'. Ultimately, it is the recycling of invention, predicated upon knowledge of drug, biological target or disease activity (or through pure chance in the case of non-hypothesis guided HTS).

Conclusions

There has been significant progress in the treatment of leishmaniasis during the past ten years and the use of drugs, such as amphotericin-B, paromomycin and miltefosine, has improved clinical approaches on patients in endemic areas (mainly in the case of visceral leishmaniasis). Despite the recent progress, effective treatments are still urgently needed, in order to overcome issues such as poor selectivity, short acting and oral bioavailability of drug candidates, as well as resistance and expensive hospitalization of patients.

In this context, the validation of new biological targets (to interfere with and/or modulate) is of critical importance for leishmaniasis research, representing a valuable approach to help in the development of new therapies. Target-oriented strategies may also increasingly contribute to the discovery of new agents which overcome the aforementioned limitations of drugs currently used in the clinics. In parallel, the successes of the 'repurposing strategy' demonstrate the need for highly diversified screening of known drugs. Despite the immense potential for drug repurposing, continued de novo identification is still of paramount importance, for both. To borrow a sporting analogy from Aube, successful repurposing represents capitalising on an opponent's mistake—i.e., a free hit. While potentially key within that fixture, a successful team cannot only rely upon these opportunities and must instead have a diversified strategy to ensure long term success (Aubé 2012). Therefore, we look forward to the successful capitalisation of such free hits as well as strategies which incorporate numerous research avenues (e.g., antisense, pharmacogenomics, HTS and combinatorial chemistry, to name a few) towards overall better healthcare for all.

For instance, phenotypic HTS (De Ryckera et al. 2013, Reguera et al. 2014, Nühs et al. 2015, Peña et al. 2015, Ortiz et al. 2017), genomic (Cantacessi et al. 2015, Khanra et al. 2017, Valdivia et al. 2017) and proteomic (de Jesus et al. 2014, Pawar et al. 2014, da Silva Santos et al. 2015, Veras and Bezerra de Menezes 2016) techniques have already implemented the discovery and validation of drug targets in neglected diseases, by also highlighting similarities between known and new targets. In line with this, drug discovery and development in leishmaniasis research will highly benefit from more multidisciplinary collaborative approaches to maximize available resources and knowledge. Analogous to the attempt to meet increasing global energy demand, the solution lies within pulling together a variety of sources. The evolution of disease and the individuals suffering from these diseases is constant; therefore, the armoury for treatment must constantly evolve.

References

Abdel-Hamid, M.K., A.A. Abdel-Hafez, N.A. El-Koussi, N.M. Mahfoouz, A. Innocenti and C.T. Supuran. 2007. Design, synthesis and docking studies of new 1,3,4-thiadiazole-2-thione derivatives with carbonic anhydrase inhibitory activity. Bioorg. Med. Chem. 15: 6975–6984.

Adamczyk-Woźniak, A., K.M. Borys and A. Sporzyński. 2015. Recent developments in the chemistry and biological applications of benzoxaboroles. Chem. Rev. 115: 5224–5247.

Altan, N., Y. Chen, M. Schindler and S.M. Simon. 1999. Tamoxifen inhibits acidification in cells independent of the estrogen receptor. Proc. Natl. Acad. Sci. U.S.A. 96: 4432–4437.

Alterio, V., R. Cadoni, D. Esposito, D. Vullo, A.D. Fiore, S.M. Monti et al. 2016 Benzoxaborole as a new chemotype for carbonic anhydrase inhibition. Chem. Commun. 52: 11983–11986.

Andrews, K.T., A. Haque and M.K. Jones. 2012a. HDAC inhibitors in parasitic diseases. Immunol. Cell Biol. 90: 66–77.

Andrews, K.T., T.N. Tran and D.P. Fairlie. 2012b. Towards histone deacetylase inhibitors as new antimalarial drugs. Curr. Pharm. Des. 18: 3467–3479.

Andrews, K.T., G. Fisher and T.S. Skinner-Adams. 2014. Drug repurposing and human parasitic protozoan diseases. Int. J. Parasitol. Drugs Drug Resist. 4: 95–111.

Araujo, A.P., O.G.F. Rocha, W. Mayrink and G.L.L. Machado-Coelho. 2008. The influence of copper, selenium and zinc on the response to the Montenegro skin test in subjects vaccinated against American cutaneous leishmaniasis. Trans. R. Soc. Trop. Med. Hyg. 102: 64–69.

Ashburn, T.T. and K.B. Thor. 2004. Drug repositioning: identifying and developing new uses for existing drugs. Nat. Rev. Drug Discov. 3: 673–683.

Aubé, J. 2012. Drug repurposing and the medicinal chemist. ACS Med. Chem. Lett. 3: 442–444.

Azzi, A., C. Cosseau and C. Grunau. 2009. Schistosoma mansoni: developmental arrest of miracidia treated with histone deacetylase inhibitors. Exp. Parasitol. 121: 288–291.

Bakare, O., Y. Brandy and C. Manka. 2013. Methods for treating leishmaniasis. W.O. # 2013074930.

Balana-Fouce, R., R. Alvarez-Velilla, C. Fernandez-Prada, C. García-Estrada and R.M. Reguera. 2014. Trypanosomatids topoisomerase revisited. New structural findings and role in drug discovery. Int. J. Parasitol. Drugs Drug Resist. 4: 326–337.

Baquedano, Y., E. Moreno, S. Espuelas, P. Nguewa, M. Font, K.J. Gutierrez et al. 2014. Novel hybrid selenosulfonamides as potent antileishmanial agents. Eur. J. Med. Chem. 74: 116–123.

Biagini, P., C. Biancalani, A. Graziano, N. Cesari, M.P. Giovannoni, A. Cilibrizzi et al. 2010. Functionalized pyrazoles and pyrazolo[3,4-*d*]pyridazinones: synthesis and evaluation of their phosphodiesterase 4 inhibitory activity. Bioorg. Med. Chem. 18: 3506–3517.

Bjornsti, M.A. and J.C. Wang. 1987. Expression of yeast DNA topoisomerase I can complement a conditional-lethal DNA topoisomerase I mutation in Escherichia coli. Proc. Natl. Acad. Sci. U.S.A. 84: 8971–8975.

Bodley, A.L., A.K. Chakraborty, S. Xie, C. Burri and T.A. Shapirom. 2003. An unusual type IB topoisomerase from African trypanosomes. Proc. Natl. Acad. Sci. U.S.A. 100: 7539–7544.

Bose, P., Y. Dai and S. Grant. 2014. Histone deacetylase inhibitor (HDACI) mechanisms of action: emerging insights. Pharmacol. Ther. 143: 323–336.

Brynner, R. and T. Stephens. 2001. Dark Remedy: the impact of thalidomide and its revival as a vital medicine. Perseus Publishing, Cambridge.

Burton, S.J., S.S. McLoughlin, C.V. Stead and C.R. Lowe. 1988. Design and applications of biomimetic antraquinone dyes. I. Synthesis and characterization of terminal ring of C.I. reactive blue 2. J. Chromatogr. 435: 127–137.

Büyükkaramikli, N.C., S. de Groot, D. Fayter, R. Wolff, N. Armstrong, L. Stirk et al. 2018. Pomalidomide with dexamethasone for treating relapsed and refractory multiple myeloma previously treated with lenalidomide and bortezomib: an evidence review group perspective of an NICE single technology appraisal. Pharmacoeconomics. 36: 145–159.

Brun, R., R. Don, R.T. Jacobs, M.Z. Wang and M.P. Barrett. 2011. Development of novel drugs for human African trypanosomiasis. Future Microbiol. 6: 677–691.

Cairns, B.R. 2001. Emerging roles for chromatin remodeling in cancer biology. Trends Cell Biol. 11: S15–S21.

Calogeropoulou, T., M. Koufaki, N. Avlonitis and A. Makriyannis. 2006. Antiprotozoal ring-substituted phospholipids. U.S. Patent # 20060105998.

Cantacessi, C., F. Dantas-Torres, M.J. Nolan and D. Otranto. 2015. The past, present, and future of Leishmania genomics and transcriptomics. Trends Parasitol. 31: 100–108.

Carta, F., S.M. Osman, D. Vullo, A. Gullotto, J.Y. Winum, Z. AlOthman et al. 2015a. Poly(amidoamine) dendrimers with carbonic anhydrase inhibitory activity and antiglaucoma action. J. Med. Chem. 58: 4039–4045.

Carta, F., S.M. Osman, D. Vullo, Z. AlOthman, S. Del Prete, C. Capasso et al. 2015b. Poly(amidoamine) dendrimers show carbonic anhydrase inhibitory activity against α-, β-, γ- and η-class enzymes. Bioorg. Med. Chem. 23: 6794–6798.

Carta, F., S.M. Osman, D. Vullo, Z. AlOthmanc and C.T. Supuran. 2015c. Dendrimers incorporating benzenesulfonamide moieties strongly inhibit carbonic anhydrase isoforms I–XIV. Org. Biomol. Chem. 13: 6453–6457.

Champoux, J.J. 2001. DNA topoisomerases: structure, function, and mechanism. Annu. Rev. Biochem. 70: 369–413.

Chang, K.P. 1990. Cell biology of Leishmania. pp. 79–90. *In*: D.W. Wyler [ed.]. Modem Parasite Biology Cellular, Immunological and Molecular Aspects. Freeman, New York.

Chawla, B. and R. Madhubala. 2010. Drug targets in Leishmania. J. Parasit. Dis. 34: 1–13.

Chen, Y. and L. Hu. 2009. Design of anticancer prodrugs for reductive activation. Med. Res. Rev. 29: 29–64.

Chong, C.R. and D.J. Sullivan. 1989. New uses for old drugs. Infect. Dis. Clin. North Am. 3: 653–664.

Chua, M.J., M.S. Arnold, W. Xu, J. Lancelot, S. Lamotte, G.F. Späth et al. 2017. Effect of clinically approved HDAC inhibitors on Plasmodium, *Leishmania* and Schistosoma parasite growth. Int. J. Parasitol. Drugs Drug Resist. 7: 42–50.

Coleman, B.I., K.M. Skillman, R.H.Y. Jiang, L.M. Childs, L.M Altenhofen, M. Ganter et al. 2014. A plasmodium falciparum histone deacetylase regulates antigenic variation and gametocyte conversion. Cell Host Microbe. 16: 177–186.

Colotti, G., A. Fiorillo and A. Ilari. 2018. Metal- and metalloid-containing drugs for the treatment of trypanosomatid diseases. Front. Biosci. 23: 954–966.

Croft, S.L., R.A. Neal, W. Pendergast and J.H. Chan. 1987. The activity of alkylphosphocholines and related derivatives against *Leishmania donovani*. Biochem. Pharmacol. 36: 2633–2636.

Croft, S.L., S. Sundar and A.H. Fairlamb. 2006. Drug resistance in leishmaniasis. Clin. Microbiol. Rev. 19: 111⁻126.

Croft, S.L. and P. Olliaro. 2011. Leishmaniasis chemotherapy–challenges and opportunities. Clin. Microbiol. Infect. 17: 1478⁻1483.

Culha, G., E. Yalin and K. Sanguen. 2008. Alterations in serum levels of trace elements in Cutaneous leishmaniasis patients in endemic region of Hatay. Asian J. Chem. 20: 3104–3108.

da Silva-Cardoso, V., A.B. Vermelho, E. Ricci Jr., I. Almeida-Rodrigues, A.M. Mazotto and C.T. Supuran. 2018. Antileishmanial activity of sulphonamide nanoemulsions targeting the β-carbonic anhydrase from Leishmania species. J. Enzyme Inhib. Med. Chem. 33: 850–857.

Dal Piaz, V., M.P. Giovannoni, M.C. Castellana, J.M. Palacios, J. Beleta, T. Domenech et al. 1998. Heterocyclic-fused pyridazinones as potent and selective PDE IV inhibitors: further structure–activity relationships and molecular modeling studies. Eur. J. Med. Chem. 33: 789–797.

Dal Piaz, V., M.P. Giovannoni, M.C. Castellana, J.M. Palacios, J. Beleta and T. Domenech. 1997. Novel heterocyclic-fused pyridazinones as potent and selective phosphodiesterase IV inhibitors. J. Med. Chem. 40: 1417–1421.

Dal Piaz, V., A. Rascón, M.E. Dubra, M.P. Giovannoni, C. Vergelli and M.C. Castellana. 2002. Isoxazolo[3,4-*d*] pyridazinones and analogues as *Leishmania mexicana* PDE inhibitors. Il Farmaco. 57: 89–96.

D'Amato, R.J., M.S. Loughnan, E. Flynn and J. Folkman. 1994. Thalidomide is an inhibitor of angiogenesis. Proc. Nat. Acad. Sci. U.S.A. 91: 4082–4085.

D'Annessa, I., S. Castelli and A. Desideri. 2015. Topoisomerase 1B as a target against leishmaniasis. Mini Rev. Med. Chem. 15: 203–210.

da Silva Santos, C., S. Attarha, R.K. Saini, V. Boaventura, J. Costa, R. Khouri et al. 2015. Proteome profiling of human cutaneous leishmaniasis lesion. J. Invest. Dermatol. 135: 400–410.

de Jesus, J.B., C. Mesquita-Rodrigues and P. Cuervo. 2014. Proteomics advances in the study of Leishmania parasites and leishmaniasis. Subcell. Biochem. 74: 323–349.

De Ryckera, M., I. Hallyburtona, J. Thomas, L. Campbell, S. Wyllieb, D. Joshia et al. 2013. Comparison of a high-throughput high-content intracellular Leishmania donovani assay with an axenic amastigote assay. Antimicrob. Agents Chemother. 57: 2913–2922.

De Simone, G., V. Alterio and C.T. Supuran. 2013. Exploiting the hydrophobic and hydrophilic binding sites for designing carbonic anhydrase inhibitors. Expert. Opin. Drug Discov. 8: 793⁻810.

Dowling, D.P., S.L. Gantt, S.G. Gattis, C.A. Fierke and D.W. Christianson. 2008. Structural studies of human histone deacetylase 8 and its site-specific variants complexed with substrate and inhibitors. Biochemistry. 47: 13554–13563.

Fawcett, A., J. Pradeilles, Y. Wang, T. Mutsuga, E.L. Myers and V.K. Aggarwal. 2017. Photoinduced decarboxylative borylation of carboxylic acids. Science. 357: 283–286.

Freile-Pelegrin, Y., D. Robledo, M.J. Chan-Bacab and B.O. Ortega-Morales. 2008. Antileishmanial properties of tropical marine algae extracts. Fitoterapia. 79: 374–377.

Frezard, F., C. Demicheli and R.R. Ribeiro. 2009. Pentavalent antimonials: new perspectives for old drugs. Molecules. 14: 2317–2336.

Fuchino, H., S. Sekita, M. Takahashi and M. Satake. 2008. Antiprotozoal agent. US Patent # 20080254136.

Galiana-Roselló, C., P. Bilbao-Ramos, M.A. Dea-Ayuela, M. Rolón, C. Vega, F. Bolás-Fernández et al. 2013. *In vitro* and *in vivo* antileishmanial and trypanocidal studies of new N-benzene- and N-baphthalenesulfonamide derivatives. J. Med. Chem. 56: 8984–8998.

Gantt, S.L., C.G. Joseph and C.A. Fierke. 2010. Activation and inhibition of histone deacetylase 8 by monovalent cations. J. Biol. Chem. 285: 6036–6043.

Giovannoni, M.P., A. Graziano, R. Matucci, M. Nesi, N. Cesari, C. Vergelli et al. 2011. Synthesis and evaluation as PDE4 inhibitors of pyrimidine-2,4-diones derivatives. Drug Dev. Res. 72: 274–288.

Glassman, R.H. and A.Y. Sun. 2004. Biotechnology: Identifying advances from the hype. Nat. Rev. Drug Discov. 3: 177–83.

Glozak, M.A. and E. Seto. 2007. Histone deacetylases and cancer. Oncogene. 26: 5420–5432.

Green, S.J., M.S. Jr Meltzer, J.B. Hibbs and C.A. Nacy. 1990. Activated macrophages destroy intracellular *Leishmania major* amastigotes by an L-arginine-dependent killing mechanism. J. Immunol. 144: 278–283.

Greenstone, G. 2011. The revival of thalidomide: from tragedy to therapy. BC Med. J. 53: 230–233.

Gregoretti, I.V., Y.M. Lee and H.V. Goodson. 2004. Molecular evolution of the histone deacetylase family: functional implications of phylogenetic analysis. J. Mol. Biol. 338: 17–31.

Grimaldi, G., D. Mc-Mahon-Pratt and T. Sun. 1991. Leishmaniasis and its etiologic agents in the New World: an overview. Prog. Clin. Parasitol. 2: 73–118.

Guerrant, W., S.C. Mwakwari, P.C. Chen, S.I. Khan, B.L. Tekwani and A.K. Oyelere. 2010. A structure-activity relationship study of the antimalarial and antileishmanial activities of nonpeptide macrocyclic histone deacetylase inhibitors. ChemMedChem, 5: 1232–1235.

Hai, Y. and D.W. Christianson. 2016. Crystal structures of Leishmania mexicana arginase complexed with α,α-disubstituted boronic amino-acid inhibitors. Acta Crystallogr. F Struct. Biol. Commun. 72(Pt 4): 300–306.

Haider, S., C.G. Joseph, S. Neidle, C.A. Fierke and M.J. Fuchter. 2011. On the function of the internal cavity of histone deacetylase protein 8: R37 is a crucial residue for catalysis. Bioorg. Med. Chem. Lett. 21: 2129–2132.

Hanggi, D. and P. Carr. 1985. Analytical evaluation of the purity of commercial preparations of Cibacron Blue F3GA and related dyes. Anal. Biochem. 149: 91–104.

Heintzman, N.D., G.C. Hon, R.D. Hawkins, P. Kheradpour, A. Stark, L.F. Harp et al. 2009. Histone modifications at human enhancers reflect global cell-type-specific gene expression. Nature. 459: 108–112.

Herwaldt, B. 1999. Miltefosine. The long-awaited therapy for visceral leishmaniasis. N. Engl. J. Med. 341: 1840–1842.

Horrobin, D.F. 2001. Realism in drug discovery—could cassandra be right? Nat. Biotechn. 19: 1099–1100.

Hu, L., S.R. Wilkinson, X. Wu and B.S. Hall. 2011. Compounds, compositions and methods for treatment of protozoan infections. W.O. # 2011066416.

Ingleson, M.J., M.L. Turner and D.L. Crossley. 2015. Borylated compounds. European Patent # 20150729916.

Isidro-Llobet, A., T. Murillo, P. Bello, A. Cilibrizzi, J.T. Hodgkinson, W.R.J.D. Galloway et al. 2011. Diversity-oriented synthesis of macrocyclic peptidomimetics. PNAS. 108: 6793–6798.

Jacobs, R.T., J.J. Plattner, B. Nare, S.A. Wring, D. Chen, Y. Freund et al. 2011a. Benzoxaboroles: a new class of potential drugs for human African trypanosomiasis. Future Med. Chem. 3: 1259–1278.

Jacobs, R.T., J.J. Plattner and M. Keenan. 2011b. Boron-based drugs as antiprotozoals. Curr. Opin. Infect. Dis. 6: 586–592.

Johner, A., S. Kunz, M. Linder, Y. Shakur and T. Seebeck. 2006. Cyclic nucleotide specific phosphodiesterases of *Leishmania major*. BMC Microbiol. 6: 25.

Kadam, R.U., J. Tavares, V.M. Kiran, A. Cordeiro, A. Ouaissi and N. Roy. 2008. Structure function analysis of *Leishmania* sirtuin: an ensemble of *in silico* and biochemical studies. Chem. Biol. Drug Des. 71: 501–506.

Kamau, S.W., R. Nunez and F. Grimm. 2001. Flow cytometry analysis of effect of allopurinol and the dinitroaniline compound (Chloralin) on the viability and proliferation of Leishmania infantum promastigotes. BMC Pharmacol. 1: 1.

Kaneko, T. 2011. Drugs for neglected diseases: part I. Future Med. Chem. 3: 1235–1237.

Keiser, J. and J. Utzinger. 2012. Antimalarials in the treatment of schistosomiasis. Curr. Pharm. Des. 18: 3531–3538.

Khanra, S., N.R. Sarraf, S. Lahiry, S. Roy and M. Manna. 2017. Leishmania genomics: a brief account. Nucleus. 60: 227–235.

Kharkar, P.S., S. Warrier and R.S. Gaud. 2014. Reverse docking: a powerful tool for drug repositioning and drug rescue. Future Med. Chem. 6: 333–342.

Kimura, J., S. Horie, H. Marushima, Y. Matsumoto, C. Sanjoba and Y. Osada. 2014. Anti-leishmanial compound and anti-leishmanial drug. U.S. Patent # 8809555.

Kumar, A., M. Porwal, A. Verma and A.K. Mishra. 2014. Impact of pomalidomide therapy in multiple myeloma: a recent survey. J. Chemother. 26: 321–327.

Larocca, A., R. Mina, F. Gay, S. Bringhen and M. Boccadoro. 2017. Emerging drugs and combinations to treat multiple myeloma. Oncotarget. 8: 60656–60672.

Li, C., J. Wang, L.M. Barton, S. Yu, M. Tian, D.S. Peters et al. 2017. Decarboxylative Borylation. Science. 356: 7355.

Lima, L.M. and E.J. Barreiro. 2005. Bioisosterism: a useful strategy for molecular modification and drug design. Curr. Med. Chem. 12: 23–49.

Liu, H. 2011. Extraction and Isolation of Compounds from Herbal Medicines in Traditional Herbal Medicine Research Methods. John Wiley and Sons, Inc.

Machado-Silva, A., P.P. Guimarães, C.A. Tavares and R.D. Sinisterra. 2015. New perspectives for leishmaniasis chemotherapy over current anti-leishmanial drugs: a patent landscape. Expert. Opin. Ther. Pat. 25: 247–260.

Mak, L.H., S.N. Georgiades, E. Rosivatz, G.F. Whyte, M. Mirabelli, R. Vilar et al. 2011. A small molecule mimicking a phosphatidylinositol (4,5)-bisphosphate binding pleckstrin homology domain. ACS Chem. Biol. 6: 1382–1390.

Marek, M., S. Kannan, A.T. Hauser, M. Moraes Mourao, S. Caby, V. Cura et al. 2013. Structural basis for the inhibition of histone deacetylase 8 (HDAC8), a key epigenetic player in the blood fluke Schistosoma mansoni. PLoS Pathog. 9: e1003645.

Matthews, B.W. 1988. Structural basis of the action of thermolysin and related zinc peptidases. Acc. Chem. Res. 21: 333–340.

Melesina, J., D. Robaa, R.J. Pierce, C. Romier and W. Sippl. 2015. Homology modeling of parasite histone deacetylases to guide the structure-based design of selective inhibitors. J. Mol. Graph. Model. 62: 342–361.

Miguel, D.C., J.K. Yokoyama-Yasunaka, W.K. Andreoli, R.A. Mortara and S.R. Uliana. 2007. Tamoxifen is effective against *Leishmania* and induces a rapid alkalinization of parasitophorous vacuoles harbouring Leishmania (Leishmania) Amazonensis Amastigotes. J. Antimicr. Chemother. 60: 526–534.

Miguel, D.C., R.C. Zauli-Nascimento, J.K. Yokoyama-Yasunaka, S. Katz, C.L. Barbiéri and S.R. Uliana. 2009. Tamoxifen as a potential antileishmanial agent: efficacy in the treatment of *Leishmania braziliensis* and *Leishmania chagasi Infections*. J. Antimicr. Chemother. 63: 365–368.

Miller, S.C., R. Huang, S. Sakamuru, S.J. Shukla, M.S. Attene-Ramos, P. Shinn et al. 2010. Identification of known drugs that act as inhibitors of NF-κB signaling and their mechanism of action. Biochem. Pharmacol. 79: 1272–1280.

Montenegro, M.F., L. Sanchez-del-Campo, M.P. Fernandez-Perez, M. Saez-Ayala, J. Cabezas-Herrera and J.N. Rodriguez-Lopez. 2015. Targeting the epigenetic machinery of cancer cells. Oncogene. 34: 135–143.

Mwakwari, S.C., W. Guerrant, V. Patil, S.I. Khan, B.L. Tekwani, Z.A. Gurard-Levin et al. 2010. Nonpeptide macrocyclic histone deacetylase inhibitors derived from tricyclic ketolide skeleton. J. Med. Chem. 53: 6100–6111.

Nagle, A.S., S. Khare, A.B. Kumar, F. Supek, A. Buchynskyy, C.J.N. Mathison et al. 2014. Recent developments in drug discovery for leishmaniasis and human african trypanosomiasis. Chem. Rev. 114: 11305–11347.

Neri, D. and C.T. Supuran. 2011. Interfering with pH regulation in tumours as a therapeutic strategy. Nat. Rev. Drug Discov. 10: 767–777.

Nielsen, T.K., C. Hildmann, A. Dickmanns, A. Schwienhorst and R. Ficner. 2005. Crystal structure of a bacterial class 2 histone deacetylase homologue. J. Mol. Biol. 354: 107–120.

Nishiyabu, R., Y. Kubo, T.D. James and J.S. Fossey. 2011. Boronic acid building blocks: tools for self assembly. Chem. Commun. 47: 1124–1150.

Njoroge, M., N.M. Njuguna, P. Mutai, D.S.B. Ongarora, P.W. Smith and K. Chibale. 2014. Recent approaches to chemical discovery and development against malaria and the neglected tropical diseases human African trypanosomiasis and schistosomiasis. Chem. Rev. 114: 11138–11163.

Nocentini, A., R. Cadoni, S. del Prete, C. Capasso, P. Dumy, P. Gratteri et al. 2017. Benzoxaboroles as efficient inhibitors of the b-carbonic anhydrases from pathogenic fungi: activity and modelling study. ACS Med. Chem. Lett. 8: 1194–1198.

Nocentini, A., R. Cadoni, P. Dumy, C.T. Supuran and J.Y. Winum. 2018. Carbonic anhydrases from *Trypanosoma cruzi* and *Leishmania donovani* chagasi are inhibited by benzoxaboroles. J. Enz. Inhib. Med. Chem. 33: 286–289.

Nühs, A., M. De Rycker, S. Manthri, E. Comer, C.A. Scherer, S.L. Schreiber et al. 2015. Development and validation of a novel leishmania donovani screening cascade for high-throughput screening using a novel axenic assay with high predictivity of leishmanicidal intracellular activity. Plos Negl. Trop. Dis. 9: e0004094.

Ortiz, D., W.A. Guiguemde, J.T. Hammill, A.K. Carrillo, Y. Chen, M. Connelly et al. 2017. Discovery of novel, orally bioavailable, antileishmanial compounds using phenotypic screening. Plos Negl. Trop. Dis. 11: e0006157.

Pace, D. 2014. Leishmaniasis. J. Infect. 69: S10–18.

Pal, D.S., D.K. Mondal and R. Datta. 2015. Identification of metal dithiocarbamates as a novel class of antileishmanial agents. Antimicrob. Agents Chemother. 59: 2144–2152.

Palmer, W.N., J.V. Obligacion, I. Pappas and P.J. Chirik. 2016. Cobalt-catalyzed benzylic borylation: enabling polyborylation and functionalization of remote, unactivated C(sp3)-H bonds. J. Am. Chem. Soc. 138: 766–769.

Palmer, W.N., C. Zarate and P.J. Chirik. 2017. Benzyltriboronates: building blocks for diastereoselective carbon-carbon bond formation. J. Am Chem. Soc. 139: 2589–2592.

Patil, V., W. Guerrant, P.C. Chen, B. Gryder, D.B. Benicewicz, S.I. Khan et al. 2010. Antimalarial and antileishmanial activities of histone deacetylase inhibitors with triazolelinked cap group. Bioorg. Med. Chem. 18: 415–425.

Pawar, H., A. Kulkarni, T. Dixit, D. Chaphekar and M.S. Patole. 2014. A bioinformatics approach to reanalyze the genome annotation of kinetoplastid protozoan parasite Leishmania donovani. Genomics. 104: 554–561.

Peña, I., M.P. Manzano, J. Cantizani, A. Kessler, J. Alonso-Padilla, A.I. Bardera et al. 2015. New compound sets identified from high throughput phenotypic screening against three kinetoplastid parasites: An Open Resource. Sci. Rep. 5: 8771.

Pommier, Y., E. Leo, H. Zhang and C. Marchand. 2010. DNA topoisomerases and their poisoning by anticancer and antibacterial drugs. Chem. Biol. 17: 421–433.

Prada, C.F., R. Alvarez-Velilla, R. Diaz-Gonzalez, C. Prieto, Y. Perez-Pertejo, R. Balana-Fouce et al. 2012. A pentapeptide signature motif plays a pivotal role in *Leishmania* DNA topoisomerase IB activity and camptothecin sensitivity. Biochim. Biophys. Acta. 1820: 2062–2071.

Rascón, A., M.E. Viloria, L. De-Chiara and M.E. Dubra. 2000. Characterization of cyclic AMP phosphodiesterases in *Leishmania Mexicana* and purification of a soluble form. Mol. Biochem. Parasitol. 106: 283–292.

Rascón, A., S. Soderling, J. Schaefer and J. Beavo. 2002. Cloning and characterization of cAMP specific phosphodiesterase (TbPDE2B) from *Trypanosoma brucei*. Proc. Natl. Acad. Sci. U.S.A. 99: 4714–4719.

Reguera, R.M., C.M. Redondo, R.G. de Prado, Y. Pérez-Pertejo and R. Balaña-Fouce. 2006. DNA topoisomerase I from parasitic protozoa: a potential target for chemotherapy. Biochim. Biophys. Acta, Gene Struct. Expression. 1759: 117131.

Reguera, R.M., E. Calvo-Álvarez, R. Álvarez-Velilla and R. Balaña-Fouce. 2014. Target-based *vs.* phenotypic screenings in Leishmania drug discovery: A marriage of convenience or a dialogue of the deaf? Int. J. Parasitol. Drugs Drug Resist. 4: 355–357.

Ritting, M.G. and C. Bogdan. 2000. *Leishmania* host–cell interaction: complexities and alternative views. Parasitol. Today. 16: 292–297.

Savai, R., S.S. Pullamsetti, G.A. Banat, N. Weissmann, H.A. Ghofrani, F. Grimminger et al. 2010. Targeting cancer with phosphodiesterase inhibitors Expert. Opin. Invest. Drugs. 19: 117–131.

Seebeck, T., K. Gong, S. Kunz, R. Schaub, T. Shalaby and R. Zoraghi. 2001. cAMP signalling in *Trypanosoma brucei*. Int. J. Parasitol. 31: 491–498.

Seebeck, T., G.J. Sterk and H. Ke. 2011. Phosphodiesterase inhibitors as a new generation of antiprotozoan drugs: exploiting the benefit of enzymes that are highly conserved between host and parasite. Future Med. Chem. 3: 1289–1236.

Shahinas, D., M. Liang, A. Datti and D.R. Pillai. 2010. A repurposing strategy identifies novel synergistic inhibitors of plasmodium falciparum heat shock protein 90. J. Med. Chem. 53: 3552–3557.

Shakur, Y., H.P. de Koning, H. Ke., J. Kambayashi and T. Seebeck. 2011. Therapeutic potential of phosphodiesterase inhibitors in parasitic diseases. Handb. Exp. Pharmacol. 204: 487–510.

Sheskin, J. 1975. Thalidomide in lepra reaction. Int. J. Dermatol. 14: 575–576.

Silverman, W.A. 2002. The schizophrenic career of a "monster drug". Pediatrics. 110: 404–406.

Sobarzo-Sánchez, E., P. Bilbao-Ramos, M. Dea-Ayuela, H. González-Díaz, M. Yañez, E. Uriarte et al. 2013. Synthetic oxoisoaporphine alkaloids: *in vitro*, *in vivo* and *in silico* assessment of antileishmanial activities. PLoS One. 8: e77560.

Sodji, Q., V. Patil, S. Jain, J.R. Kornacki, M. Mrksich, B.L. Tekwani et al. 2014. The antileishmanial activity of isoforms 6- and 8-selective histone deacetylase inhibitors. Bioorg. Med. Chem. Lett. 24: 4826–4830.

Stewart, L., G.C. Ireton and J.J. Champoux. 1997. Reconstitution of human topoisomerase I by fragment complementation. J. Molec. Biol. 269: 355–72.

Suarez Covarrubias, A., T.A. Larsson, M. Hogbom, J. Lindberg, T. Bergfors, C. Bjorkelid et al. 2005. Structure and function of carbonic anhydrases from Mycobacterium tuberculosis. J. Biol. Chem. 280: 18782–18789.

Supuran, C.T., A. Scozzafava and A. Casini. 2003. Carbonic anhydrase inhibitors. Med. Res. Rev. 23: 146–189.

Supuran, C.T. 2008. Carbonic anhydrases: novel therapeutic applications for inhibitors and activators. Nat. Rev. Drug Discov. 7: 168–181.

Supuran, C.T. 2011. Bacterial carbonic anhydrases as drug targets: towards novel antibiotics? Front. Pharmacol. 2: 34.

Supuran, C.T. 2016a. Structure and function of carbonic anhydrases. Biochem. J. 473: 2023–2032.

Supuran, C.T. 2016b. How many carbonic anhydrase inhibition mechanisms exist? J. Enzyme. Inhib. Med. Chem. 31: 345–360.

Supuran, C.T. 2017. Advances in structure-based drug discovery of carbonic anhydrase inhibitors. Exp. Opin. Drug Discov. 12: 61–88.

Syrjänen, L., A.B. Vermelho, A. Rodrigues Ide, S. Corte-Real, T. Salonen, P. Pan et al. 2013. Cloning, characterization, and inhibition studies of a β-carbonic anhydrase from *Leishmania donovani* chagasi, the protozoan parasite responsible for leishmaniasis. J. Med. Chem. 56: 7372–7381.

Tavares, J., A. Ouaissi, P.K.T. Lin, I. Loureiro, S. Kaur, N. Roy et al. 2010. Bisnaphthalimidopropyl derivatives as inhibitors of *Leishmania* SIR2 related protein 1. ChemMedChem. 5: 140–147.

Tejería, A., Y. Pérez-Pertejo, R.M. Reguera, R. Balaña-Fouce, C. Alonso, M. Fuertes et al. 2016. Antileishmanial effect of new indeno-1,5-naphthyridines, selective inhibitors of *Leishmania infantum* type IB DNA topoisomerase. Eur. J. Med. Chem. 124: 740–749.

Valdivia, H.O., L.V. Almeida, B.M. Roatt, J.L. Reis-Cunha, A.A. Sampaio Pereira, C. Gontijo et al. 2017. Comparative genomics of canine-isolated Leishmania (Leishmania) amazonensis from an endemic focus of visceral leishmaniasis in Governador Valadares, southeastern Brazil. Sci. Rep. 7: 40804.

Velásquez, A.M.A., W.C. Ribeiro, V. Venn, S. Castelli, M.S. Camargo, R.P. de Assis et al. 2017. Efficacy of a binuclear cyclopalladated compound therapy for cutaneous leishmaniasis in the murine model of infection with *Leishmania amazonensis* and its inhibitory effect on topoisomerase 1B. Antimicrob. Agents Chemother. 61: e00688–17.

Veras, P.S. and J.P. Bezerra de Menezes. 2016. Using proteomics to understand how leishmania parasites survive inside the host and establish infection. Int. J. Mol. Sci. 17: E1270.

Vergnes, B., L. Vanhille, A. Ouaissi and D. Sereno. 2005. Stage-specific antileishmanial activity of an inhibitor of SIR2 histone deacetylase. Acta Trop. 94: 107–115.

Vermelho, A.B., G.R. Capaci, I.A. Rodrigues, V.S. Cardoso, A.M. Mazotto and C.T. Supuran. 2017. Carbonic anhydrases from Trypanosoma and *Leishmania* as anti-protozoan drug targets. Bioorg. Med. Chem. 25: 1543–1555.

Walter, R.D., E. Buse and F. Ebert. 1987. Effect of cAMP on transformation and proliferation of *Leishmania* cells. Tropenmed. Parasit. 29: 439–447.

Wang, H., Z. Yan, J. Geng, S. Kunz, T. Seebeck and H. Ke. 2007. Crystal structure of the *Leishmania major* phosphodiesterase LmjPDEB1 and insight into the design of the parasite-selective inhibitors. Mol. Microbiol. 66: 1029–1038.

WHO Technical Report Series. 2010. Control of the leishmaniasis: report of a meeting of the WHO expert committee on the control of Leishmaniasis. World Health Organization; Geneva.

WHO Leishmaniasis Fact sheet 375, 2016. World Health Organization. Geneva, Switzerland.

Witschel, M., M. Rottmann, M. Kaiser and R. Brun. 2012. Agrochemicals against malaria, sleeping sickness, leishmaniasis and Chagas disease. PLoS Negl. Trop. Dis. 6: e1805.

Zhang, J. and Q. Zhong. 2014. Histone deacetylase inhibitors and cell death. Cell Mol. Life Sci. 71: 3885–3901.

Zhang, L., G.J. Lovinger, E.K. Edelstein, A.A. Szymaniak, M.P. Chierchia and J.P. Morken. 2016. Catalytic conjunctive cross-coupling enabled by metal-induced metallate rearrangement. Science. 351: 70–74.

Zoraghi, R., S. Kunz, K. Gong and T. Seebeck. 2001. Characterization of TbPDE2A, a novel cyclic nucleotide-specific phosphodiesterase from the protozoan parasite *Trypanosoma brucei*. J. Biol. Chem. 276: 11559–11566.

Zuma, A.A., I.C. Mendes, L.C. Reignault, M.C. Elias, W. de Souza, C.R. Machado et al. 2014. How *Trypanosoma cruzi* handles cell cycle arrest promoted by camptothecin, a topoisomerase I inhibitor. Mol. Biochem. Parasitol. 193: 93–100.

Chapter 14

Curcumin and Neglected Infectious Diseases

Francesca Mazzacuva[1] and *Agostino Cilibrizzi*[2,*]

Introduction

Curcuma species

The genus *Curcuma* belongs to the family of *Zingiberaceae* and consists of more than 100 definite species identified worldwide, although mainly distributed in tropical and subtropical regions all over Asia and Africa (Velayudhan et al. 1999). The plants are widely cultivated in southeast Asian countries and spontaneously grow in sandy and clay soils, from sea level to 1500 m, with high rainfall (1500–2000 mm) and temperatures of 18–30°C. *Curcuma* species are traditionally used for the treatment of several ailments. They mainly contain essential oils, a mixture of compounds known as curcuminoids and turmerin, a water-soluble antioxidant peptide (Aggarwal et al. 2003, Jagetia and Aggarwal 2007). Among the different species, *Curcuma longa* L. (Figure 1) has attracted considerable interest, being the main source of turmeric (i.e., rhizome), a culinary and medicinal spice which is particularly rich in curcuminoids (3–5% of raw plant) and essential oils (2–7% of raw plant).

Curcuma longa L. is a small herbaceous perennial plant and it bears on the root system many cylindrical rhizomes of 1 cm in diameter and 2.5–7.5 cm in length (Figure 1). The trunk grows from 60 cm to over 1 m and the leaves are usually 5 to 10, reaching over 90 cm in length. The bracts are characterized by a green bottom and a white or purple top, forming a series of pockets that contain large yellow-orange spike flowers.

Other species also well-known for their high content of curcuminoids are *Curcuma xanthorrhiza* L. (popularly utilized as a remedy against indigestion or rheumatism) (Ruslay et al. 2007), *Curcuma aromatic* L. (in use for the preparation of cosmetics in South Asia), *Curcuma zedoaria* L. (used in Chinese Traditional Medicine for the treatment of inflammation, pain and skin wounds or ulcers) and *Curcuma mangga* L. (traditionally employed against gastro-intestinal disorders) (Basnet and Skalko-Basnet 2011).

---

[1] Mass Spectrometry Facility, King's College London, Franklin-Wilkins Building, 150 Stamford Street, London SE1 9NH.
[2] Institute of Pharmaceutical Science, King's College London, Franklin-Wilkins Building, 150 Stamford Street, London SE1 9NH.
* Corresponding author: agostino.cilibrizzi@kcl.ac.uk

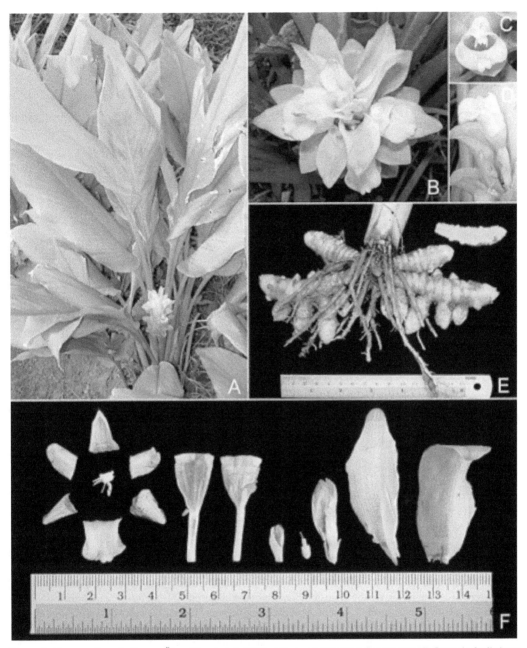

Figure 1. *Curcuma longa* L. (Leong-Škorničková et al. 2008): (A) plant habit; (B) inflorescence; (C) flower in fertile bract (front view); (D) flower in fertile bract (side view); (E) rhizome; (F) flower dissection.

Color version at the end of the book

Curcuminoids are a class of polyphenolic compounds poorly soluble in water (Figure 2), including curcumin (1) (i.e., 2–8% of turmeric by weight), demethoxycurcumin (2), bisdemethoxycurcumin (3) and cyclocurcumin (4), which are responsible for the yellow color of *Curcuma* rhizome. The term "curcuminoids" is currently included in the USP Pharmacists' Pharmacopoeia (i.e., the comprehensive handbook for pharmacist's practice in USA) to indicate any dietary supplement containing more than

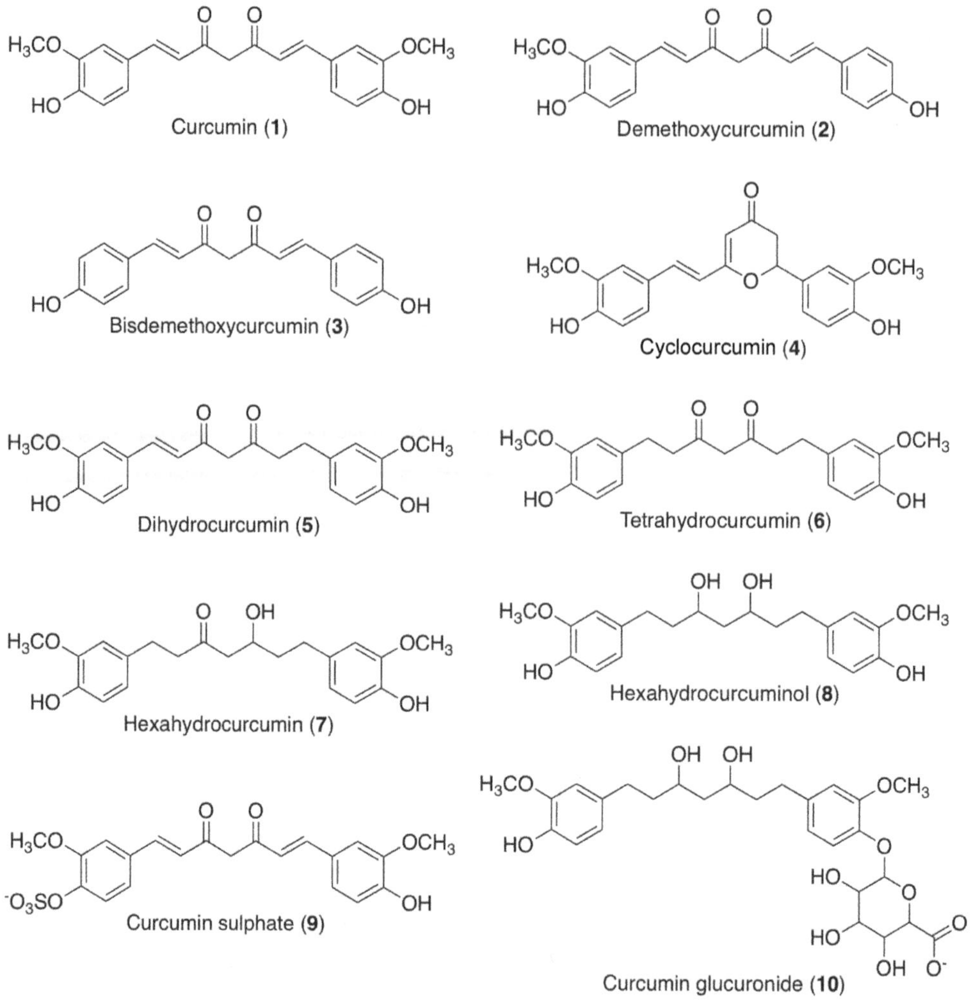

Figure 2. Relevant natural curcuminoids and curcumin metabolites.

95% of this class of polyphenols extracted from the rhizome of *Curcuma longa* L. (i.e., turmeric) (DSM 2009).

Differently, bisabolane sesquiterpenes (Ohshiro and Kuroyanagi 1990), such as turmerones (11–13) and curlone (14) (Figure 2), are the main components of the essential oil from turmeric. Additionally, other sesqiterpenic compounds are also present, including zingiberene (16), curcumenol (19) and curcumenone (20) (Figure 3) (Sharma et al. 2005). Two turmerones (i.e., aromatic turmerone and α-turmerone) and curlone have been reported as the principal determinant for antibacterial and antioxidant properties of this essential oil (Negi et al. 1999, Jayaprakasha et al. 2002). Furthermore, aromatic turmerone (11) has been recently found to possess anti-inflammatory and antioxidant activity *in vitro*, by interfering with NF-κB (nuclear factor kappa light chain enhancer of activated B cells) and other second messengers or signaling pathways involved in the inflammation process (Hucklenbroich et al. 2014).

Turmeric use in the history

The name turmeric comes from the Latin expression "*terra merita*" (i.e., "meritorious earth") and refers to the pigmented color of *Curcuma* grinded rhizome, which has widely been in use from ancient times as spice, food preservative and coloring agent (e.g., for the preparation of cosmetics in Hindu rituals

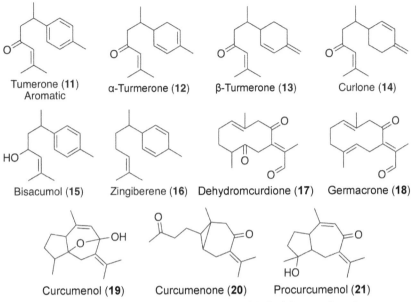

Figure 3. Relevant sesquiterpenes in the essential oil of *Curcuma longa* L.

and religious ceremonies). The first documented use of turmeric extracts is filed in the "Compendium of Materia Medica" of the Ming dynasty (A.D. 1590), a comprehensive medical herbology book in Traditional Chinese Medicine, listing plants, animals and minerals that were believed to have therapeutic properties. Moreover, the Traditional Ayurvedic Medicine and the Traditional Chinese Medicine report the administration of turmeric extracts for the treatment of various respiratory diseases, liver disorders and diabetic wounds (Araújo et al. 2001). Similarly, the Ayurvedic Pharmacopoeia of India recommends the use of *Curcuma longa* L. essential oil for the carminative, gastric and tonic effects (API 2001), while the Chinese Pharmacopoeia indicates that the extracts can help in pain relief (CPC 2010).

Despite the ancient use in India and other Asian countries, turmeric was introduced in Europe only in the 13th century by Marco Polo. Currently, it is worldwide used as spice and an annual growth rate of 10% in the demand has been estimated by the International Trade Centre of Geneva. India remains the world's largest producer and exporter, followed by China, Indonesia, Bangladesh and Thailand (Selvan et al. 2002).

Chemico-physical properties of curcumin

Curcumin (1) (also referred as 'diferuloylmethane', i.e., 1,7-bis-(4-hydroxy-3-methoxyphenyl)-1,6-heptadiene-3,5-dione) is commonly considered the most biologically active compound extracted from *Curcuma* species. It was isolated for the first time in 1815 by Vogel (Vogel and Pelletier 1815), although the crystalline form was obtained only 50 years later by Daybe (Daybe 1870). The exact structure, initially established by Lampe in 1913 (Lampe and Milobedzaka 1913) and conclusively confirmed by Roughley in 1973 (Roughley and Whiting 1973), is characterized by the presence of two *o*-methoxyphenols which are symmetrically linked through an α,β-unsaturated β-diketone spacer.

Curcumin (1) is a bright yellow powder with a melting point of 179–183°C (Tønnesen et al. 1986). It is poorly soluble in water, being approximately 11 ng/mL the maximum solubility reported in plain aqueous buffer at pH 5.5 (Tønnesen et al. 2002). In contrast, curcumin (1) is readily dissolved in organic solvents, such as methanol, ethanol or chloroform, and moderately soluble in hexane, cyclohexane and tetrahydrofuran. It exhibits a strong absorption in the UV-Vis region with a maximum in the range 408–434 nm, depending on the solvent used for the analysis (Mandeville et al. 2009). For instance, 420 nm has been reported as the absorption maximum (λ_{max}) in the majority of polar solvents, whereas

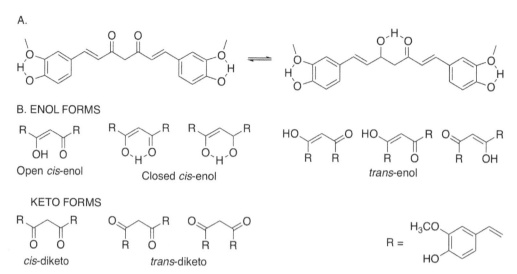

Figure 4. (A) Keto-enol tautomerism of curcumin (1); (B) representative *cis-trans* conformations for the keto-enol tautomeric forms.

430–434 nm in hydrogen bond acceptor and donor solvents (i.e., protic solvents), with the exception of methanol where the λ_{max} is 423–428 nm (Priyadarsini 2009).

The β-diketone function in the structure is responsible for the intramolecular hydrogen atom transfer leading to the typical keto/enol tautomers (Figure 4A). The two tautomeric forms have been reported to generate various *cis* and *trans* conformations in solution (Figure 4B) (Wright 2002, Kolev et al. 2005, Cornago et al. 2008). The relative abundance of specific keto and enol isomers can change on the basis of different temperatures, pH and polarity of the medium (or solvent).

Several studies focused on the determination of curcumin (1) structure in solution. The keto form has shown to be predominant in acidic and neutral aqueous media and in cell membranes (Wang et al. 1997). In these conditions, curcumin (1) is reported to act as a potent H donor (Jovanovich et al. 1999), due to the highly activated methylene in the linker. In contrast, at pH higher than 8 curcumin (1) mainly behaves as an electron donor, the enol being the prevalent form. These results have been also supported by NMR studies, indicating that curcumin (1) predominantly exists in the enol conformation in the majority of organic solvents, although the keto form may exist in equilibrium with the latter at low pH values (Payton et al. 2007). In parallel, X-ray crystal structure analyses indicate that the *cis*-enol form gives extra stabilization to the molecule in the solid state and allows improved conjugation between the π-electron systems of the two feruloyl residues (Parimita et al. 2007). This study confirms that the enol form is further stabilized by resonance-assisted hydrogen bonding, enol hydrogen being positioned between the two central oxygen atoms (Figure 4A). Furthermore, density functional theory (DFT) calculations also assist the hypothesis of an increased stability for the enol form (Galasso et al. 2008). Specifically, being planar (i.e., with the dihedral angle of 180°), the enol results are more stable than the nonplanar and twisted diketone form. This planar geometry produces a perfect resonance between the two phenolic rings, as the electron density can be distributed to the entire molecule.

The enolic structure of curcumin (1) is characterized by the presence of three ionisable protons: one from the enolic proton and two from the phenolic OH groups. Although different values have been attributed to the three acidity constants (Figure 5), it is now accepted that pKa ranges are between 9.5–10.7, 8.5–10.4 and 7.5–8.5, respectively (Priyadarsini 2009).

Biological and pharmacological properties of curcumin

Extensive research has been conducted within the past three decades focusing on the assessment of curcumin biological and pharmacological profile. The interaction with different molecular targets, including

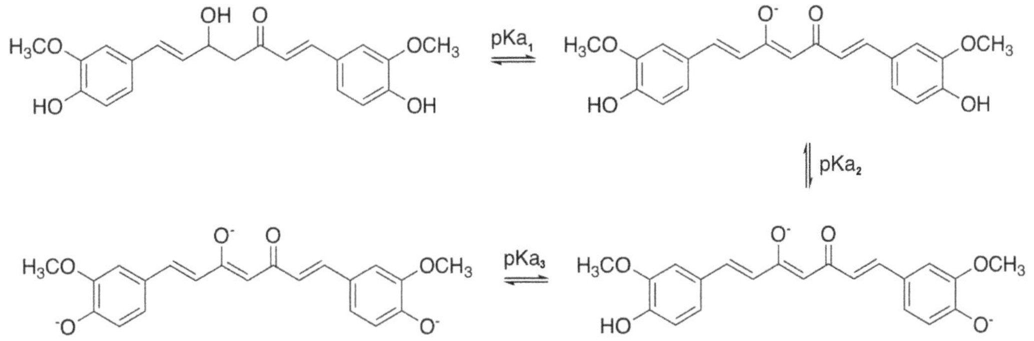

Figure 5. Prototropic equilibria of curcumin.

transcription and growth factors, enzymes, receptors and various second messengers has been proposed (Maheshwari et al. 2006, Anand et al. 2008). Several clinical studies have suggested a possible role in the treatment of various human diseases (Aggarwal et al. 2007a), such as inflammation (Masferrer et al. 1994, Sugiyama et al. 1996, Rao 2007), tumors (Basnet and Skalko-Basnet 2011, Song et al. 2011a), myocardial infarction (Nirmala and Puvanakrishnan 1996) and psoriasis (Heng et al. 2000, Pol et al. 2003, Aggarwal et al. 2007a, Kurd et al. 2008). Moreover, antioxidant, hypocholesterolemic, hepato- and nephro-protective properties have been also reported (Venkatesan and Rao 2000, Peschel et al. 2007, Basnet and Skalko-Basnet 2011).

Curcumin in Neglected Infectious Diseases

Several research groups have recently investigated the effects of curcumin (1) in relation to neglected parasitic diseases and a possible role in this context is supported by both *in vitro* and *in vivo* studies (Wink 2012, Padmanaban and Rangarajan 2016). For instance, the polyphenol demonstrated a more potent antifungal agent than fluconazole against *Paracoccidioides brasiliensis*, the causal agent of the neglected disease paracoccidioidomycosis (Martins et al. 2009). Although experimental data need further confirmation, the administration of curcumin (1) with currently used chemotherapeutic agents suggests the improvement of their therapeutic efficacy (Ndjonka et al. 2013).

Protozoan infections

Curcumin (1) has been reported as the most active antiprotozoal agent of turmeric (Ioset 2008). Overall, the idea of testing the antiprotozoal activity of curcumin (1) is a follow-up observation of inhibitory effects on *Plasmodium* parasites (Cui et al. 2007, Mimche et al. 2011). Natural compounds have been widely tested against malaria, in combination with traditionally used drugs or as monotherapy, for instance to find alternative clinical approaches and overcome the common issue of drug resistance. Curcumin (1) resulted particularly promising in the treatment of both chloroquine-sensitive and chloroquine-resistant *Plasmodium falciparum* strains (Cui et al. 2007). Although this polyphenol has been widely demonstrated as a powerful antioxidant agent (Toda et al. 1985, Fang et al. 2005), protecting healthy tissues and cells against oxidative stress, it has selectively shown pro-oxidant activity in *Plasmodium falciparum*, by promoting the production of reactive oxygen species (ROS). In parallel, the increase of ROS contributes to mitochondrial and nuclear DNA damage, as well as detrimental alterations of various enzymes and cellular organelles, with following parasite death.

For instance, Pérez-Arriaga et al. reported cytotoxic activity for curcumin (1) on *Giardia lamblia* trophozoite, by inhibiting the parasite growth, as well as inducing morphological alterations and apoptotic events (Pérez-Arriaga et al. 2006). Additionally, curcumin (1) has been found active against *Trichomonas vaginalis*, the protozoan causing trichomoniasis, a common sexually transmitted disease (Wachter et al. 2014). By testing different parasite strains, 100% eradication of all trichomonas cells was obtained after 24 hr incubation with curcumin (1) at 400 μg/mL concentration, with EC_{50} ranging from 73.0 to 105.8 μg/mL. A concentration 50-fold higher was also well tolerated by the human mucosa, proving the safety profile of the compound.

Chagas disease and African trypanosomiasis

The use of nitrocompounds (e.g., benznidazole (22) and nifurtimox (23), Figure 6) represents the common treatment in the event of infection from *Trypanosoma cruzi* (Muñoz et al. 2011, Diniz et al. 2013, Oliveira 2015), which is the etiological agent of Chagas disease. However, there is a lack of specific and effective therapies, since several disadvantages are associated to the use of nitrocompounds, including elevated toxicity (mainly due to the production of reactive oxygen and nitrogen species in the host through cytochrome P450 metabolism) and limited efficacy in the latest stages of the infection (i.e., once the parasites are diffused in multiple organs and tissues) (Rassi et al. 2010, Novaes et al. 2015).

With the aim to overcome the problems associated with current chemotherapeutical approaches, *Curcuma longa* L. extracts and curcumin (1) have been recently investigated against Chagas disease, as well as other parasitic infections (Cui et al. 2007, Das et al. 2008, Allam 2009, Mimche et al. 2011, Vathsala et al. 2012).

Nagajyothi and colleagues studied the effects of curcumin (1) in the early stage of *Trypanosoma cruzi* infection (Nagajyothi et al. 2011, 2012), demonstrating the prevention of parasite diffusion through a decreased expression of low density lipoprotein receptor (which is involved in host cell invasion). In particular, *in vivo* experiments with CD1 infected mice showed an improved animal survival after curcmin (1) administration. This effect has been associated with the reduction of infected heart tissue, as well as the decrease of macrophage infiltration and related inflammatory events in heart and liver (Nagajyothi et al. 2011, Padmanaban and Rangarajan 2016).

In a different study, the antiparasitic effects of curcumin (1) were evaluated in combination with benznidazole (22) (Figure 6), a typical drug also used in Chagas disease chemotherapy (Novaes et al. 2016). In mice acutely infected with *Trypanosoma cruzi*, the co-administration of benznidazole (22) and curcumin (1) revealed a significant decrease of parasite load, circulating levels of cytokines (e.g., INF-γ and interleukin 4) and myocardial inflammation, with a parallel reduction of the overall parasitemia. The combined therapy showed exceeding effects of benznidazole (22) monotherapy. In this study, curcumin (1) demonstrated not only improvement of the efficacy of benznidazole (22) but, most relevant, the allowing of the reduction of its therapeutic dose with a significant decrease of the overall toxicity.

Curcumin (1) also demonstrated cytotoxic effects *in vitro* against African trypanosomiasis (i.e., African sleeping sickness), with LD_{50} values of 4.77 μM and 46.52 μM for *Trypanosoma brucei brucei* (GUTat 3.1 clone) bloodstream and procyclic forms, respectively (Saleheen et al. 2002, Nose et al. 2006). Similarly,

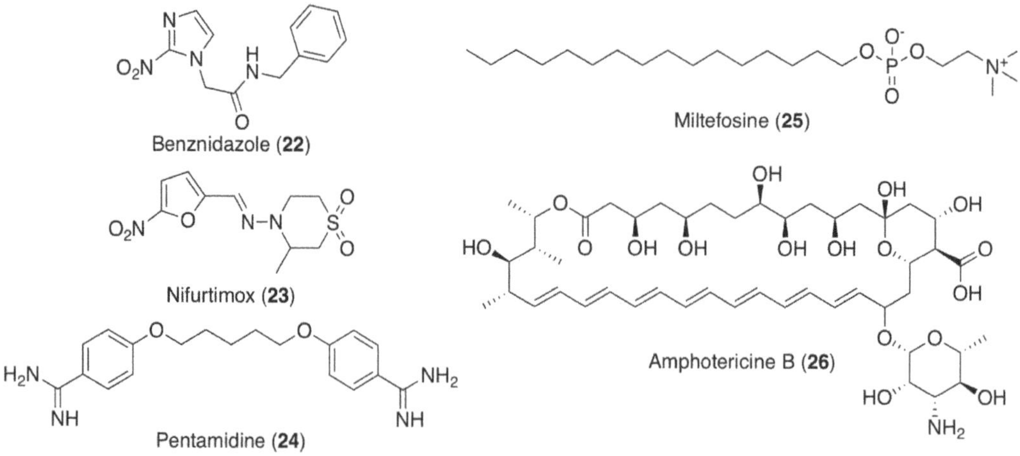

Figure 6. Antiparasitic and antiprotozoal agents in clinical use to treat various neglected diseases, including African trypanosomiasis and leishmaniasis.

demethoxycurcumin (2) and bisdemetoxycurcumin (3) (see section 1.1 and Figure 1) exhibited the same level of antitrypanosomal activity on this parasite species, with EC_{50} values in the low micromolar range (Changtam et al. 2010). All the curcuminoids tested in the study displayed a higher toxicity for *Tryoanosoma brucei brucei* than HEK cells (i.e., selectivity indexes ranging from 3- to 1500-fold) (Lim 2016).

Leishmaniasis

In India, where leishmaniasis is endemic, turmeric is traditionally used as spice in food and as relief formulations in the case of insect bites. In Traditional Indian Medicine (i.e., Ayurveda), curcumin (1) is largely known to have a wide spectrum of biological actions including immunomodulation and regulation of host defence mechanisms. Possible leishmanicidal effects have also been reported against a number of *Leishmania* species *in vitro*. However, the same antileishmanial activity is often not found in *in vivo* experiments, mainly due to the poor oral bioavailability, as a result of low solubility in water and low absorption (see section 6). In this regard, various curcumin-based formulations and nanoassemblies have been evaluated with the aim to increase the efficacy of the compound, showing good improvements of the effects against *Leishmania* parasites *in vivo* (see sections 7.2.1 and 7.2.5).

In 2002, Gomes et al. firstly reported that curcumin (1) was more effective than pentamidine (24) (i.e., a typically used drug, Figure 6) against *Leishmania amazonensis* (Gomes et al. 2002). Saleheen and co-worker also assessed the anti-proliferative effect of curcumin (1) against three additional strains, i.e., *Leishmania major*, *Leishmania tropica* and *Leishmania infantum*, proving effective leishmanicidal properties (Saleheen et al. 2002). In general, curcumin (1) showed low micromolar values of IC_{50} against promastigotes forms of these *Leishmania* strains. Additionally, the activity of curcumin (1) has been tested against axenic amastigote-like cells of *Leishmania major* (IC_{50} = 10 μM) and a cellular death of 100% was observed at 27 μM concentration (Saleheen et al. 2002). In a different study, curcumin (1) exhibited cytotoxicity effects against *Leishmania major* promastigotes *in vitro* with LD_{50} = 37.6 μM (Koide et al. 2002).

Demethoxycurcumin (2) (Figure 2) and various curcuminoids also demonstrated anti-leishmanial activity in the low micromolar range when tested against *Leishmania major* promastigotes and *Leishmania Mexicana* amastigotes. Das et al. studied the effect of curcumin (1) in relation to ROS and calcium homeostasis in *in vitro* models of leishmaniasis (Das et al. 2008), through flow cytometry experiments. Curcumin (1) demonstrated to arrest the cell cycle at G2/M phase in *Leishmania donovani*, the protozoan responsible for leishmaniasis visceral manifestations. Subsequently, the increase of ROS and the enhancement of calcium cytosolic levels in the parasite determine a change in permeability of membranes, which leads to the release of proapoptotic proteins (e.g., the cytochrome C) into the cytosol, with following nuclear alterations. Therefore, the authors have hypothesised that curcumin (1) action against *Leishmania donovani* is mediated by programmed cellular death.

In contrast, Chan et al. reported detrimental actions for the use of curcumin (1) during *Leishmania* infection. Specifically, an inhibitory effect on the action of endogenously produced nitric oxide (NO) is believed to exacerbate the pathogenesis of *Leishmania* parasites (Chan et al. 2005). In this regard, it is well-known that macrophages are activated to simultaneously produce oxygen radicals and NO, which are the two major weapons of infected host cells against the parasite. As an effective inhibitor of NO production and function (Hong et al. 2004, Chen et al. 2006), curcumin (1) is found to have a role in protecting promastigote and amastigote forms of *Leishmania donovani*, as well as promastigotes of *Leishmania major* (i.e., the cutaneous species) (Chan et al. 2005). In this scenario, the antioxidant and scavenging properties of curcumin (1) (Toda et al. 1985, Onoda and Inano 2000, Wright 2002) are found to suppress the action of NO, superoxide and peroxynitrite (which is formed from the reaction of NO with superoxide) against *Leishmania* parasites, by compromising the overall microbial defence of the host. Additionally, Adapala and Chan also reported that long-term and low-dose oral administration of curcumin (1) inhibits iNOS and limits the overall immune responses *in vivo*, including endogenous leishmanicidal mechanisms (Adapala and Chan 2008).

Lastly, an alternative approach has been recently adopted to investigate the photodynamic properties of curcumin (1) in eradicating *Leishmania* parasite (Pinto et al. 2016). Photodynamic therapy (PDT) has recently emerged as a promising alternative in various clinical settings, allowing local administration and limiting the appearance of side effects. In this context, *Leishmania major* and *Leishmania braziliensis* promastigotes have been incubated with curcumin (1) in serial dilutions (i.e., from 500 µg/mL up to 7.8 µg/mL) prior to light exposure. Confocal microscopy experiments confirmed the uptake by both *Leishmania* species and the treatment demonstrated significant effects on parasite viability. Noteworthy, the morphology of promastigotes was highly affected by the PDT, suggesting that curcumin (1) represents a promising photosensitizer agent to implement anti-*Leishmania* therapies.

Helminth infections

As single agents for monotherapy in helminth infections, curcumin (1) and other curcuminoids seem to possess only poor activity. In contrast, various combinations of them suggest possible synergistic effects with a high increase in nematocidal activity, as firstly demonstrated in studies with *Toxocara canis* (Kiuchi et al. 1993). For instance, the combination of *Curcuma longa* L. and *Zingiber officinalis* L. (both in the form of rhizome extracts) exhibited high antihelmintic properties, showing valuable vermicidal agents *in vitro* against *Pheretima posthuma* (Singh et al. 2011, Raul et al. 2012) and *Ascaridia galli* (Bazh and El-Bahy 2013).

In a recent study, Nayak and colleagues also used colorimetric *in vitro* tests to demonstrate the effect of curcumin (1) on *Setaria cervi* (Nayak et al. 2012), the causative agent of bovine filariasis. This parasite is recommended by the World Health Organization (WHO) as effective model to study the human parasite (i.e., *Wuchereria bancrofti*), due to the high similarities in nocturnal periodicity, antigenic patterns and metabolism (Saxena et al. 2016, Mukherjee et al. 2017). Specifically, a dose-dependent activation of pro-apoptotic genes and chromosomal DNA fragmentation have been observed for curcumin (1) in adult *Setaria* helminths. Moreover, the depletion of parasitic glutathione (GSH) level possibly contributes to curcumin-induced apoptosis, by increasing cellular oxidative stress (Nayak et al. 2012).

In the following sub-sections, we report a selection of studies on the effects of curcumin (1) against two common helminth infections, i.e., echinococcosis and schistosomiasis, where the activation of apoptotic pathways is believed to play an important role (Wink 2012, Nayak et al. 2012, de Paula Aguiar et al. 2016).

Echinococcosis

Ethanolic extracts of *Curcuma longa* L. and *Zingiber officinalis* L. (belonging to the same botanic family, |i.e., *Zingiberaceae*) have been tested as scolicidal combination in animal models of *Echinococcus granulosus* (Rajabloo et al. 2012, Almalki et al. 2017), a common agent causing zoonotic echinococcosis. Currently, the elective treatment for this helminth infection is the surgical excision. However, the pre-surgical injection of a scolicidal agent into the cysts is beneficial, in order to avoid dissemination of protoscolices and recurrence of the disease (Pensel et al. 2014). Promising results have been obtained after the co-administration of the two natural extracts, although it has not been established which are the active molecules or phytocomplexes responsible for this effect (Almaki et al. 2017, Siles-Lucas et al. 2018). In a different study, time- and concentration-dependent activity against *Echinococcus multilocularis* has been reported for curcumin (1) *in vitro* (Chu et al. 2016). Also in this case, the cellular mechanism has not been elucidated for this action, although the authors hypothesized that curcumin (1) can induce apoptotic events in infected cells.

Schistosomiasis

Several researches have focused on the identification of possible molecular and genetic mechanisms related to the observed anti-schistosomiasis activity of curcumin (1) (Ndjonka et al. 2013). For instance, *in vivo* experiments on murine models showed inhibition of *Schistosomiasis mansoni* growth and the reduction of parasite eggs. The decrease of inflammatory signs and hepatic manifestations (i.e., unbalanced enzymes activities and hepato-spleenomegaly) has been as well observed (El-Sherbiny et al. 2006, Allam 2009, Mahmoud and Elbessoumy 2013). Curcumin (1) administration is reported to restore the increased levels of transaminases, alkaline phosphatases, triglycerides and low-density lipoproteins (Mahmoud and

Elbessoumy 2014). An additional research has also demonstrated that curcumin (1) induces oxidative stress and inhibits glutathione S-transferase (GST) and superoxide dismutase in the parasite (de Paula Aguiar et al. 2016). Differently, a genetic study assessed the effect of curcumin (1) on the differential expression of several genes that are alternatively up- or down-regulated, supporting the hypothesis of a potential role for the compound in the treatments of schistosomiasis infections (Morais et al. 2013).

Viral infections: chikungunya and dengue virus

Curcumin (1) has also shown to reduce the infectivity of enveloped viruses, whereas no effects were observed in non-enveloped viruses (Mounce et al. 2017, Subudhi et al. 2018). In 2015, von Rhein et al. reported a number of *in cellulo* experiments showing that curcumin (1) has promising effects in inhibiting the infection by mosquito-borne Chikungunya virus (the causing agent of chikungunya fever), by blocking the entry of the lentiviral vector pseudotyped with the virus envelope proteins E2 and E1 (von Rhein et al. 2016). Therefore, the local application of curcumin (1) is prosed in this study as potential prophylactic treatment, in order to inhibit the systemic diffusion of the virus in the body. Moreover, direct treatment of virus-infected cells with curcumin (at 5 µM concentration) reduced the infectivity of Chikungunya and Zika viruses in a dose- and time-dependent fashion, including typical manifestations such as vesicular stomatitis, with no impact on cellular viability (Mounce et al. 2017). A number of curcuminoids were also tested and exhibited similar antiviral activity against enveloped viruses. The proposed mechanism of action relies on the possibility that curcumin (1) interferes with the binding of enveloped viruses to the cells (Mounce et al. 2017).

Similar results have been observed in the treatment of Dengue virus, as recently evaluated through an *in vitro* infection model (Padilla et al. 2014, Ichsyani et al. 2017). In particular, cells infected with Dengue virus type 2 were incubated with various concentrations of curcumin (1) for 24 hr. Treatment with 10, 15, and 20 µM were found to decrease the number of viral plaques and to produce an intracellular accumulation of viral proteins. Additionally, changes in cell and nuclear morphology, as well as alterations in the actin cytoskeleton, were also observed when curcumin (1) was used at a concentration of 20 µM, although these actions do not seem to determine direct effects on the production of viral particles. These data highlight the possible role of curcumin (1) in interfering with several cellular mechanisms, including the apoptosis process, in the event of Dengue virus and other viral infections (Padmanaban and Rangarajan 2016).

Bacterial infections: leprosy and trachoma

The use of curcumin (1) in the treatment of bacterial infections is well documented in Indian and Chinese Traditional Medicine (API 2001, CPC 2010, Raghav 2015) due to the recognized antibiotic properties. For instance, fresh juice from the rhizome, or paste and decoction prepared from turmeric, has been commonly used in the treatment of leprosy. Similarly, local and systemic administration of curcumin (1) also indicates possible beneficial effects against this disease (Snow 1995), which is transmitted from *Mycobacterium lepromatosis* or *Mycobacterium leprae* and affects the peripheral nerves and skin, determining a progressive debilitation.

Polyphenolic compounds have been also reported to inhibit *Chlamydia* growth through membrane disruption and restoration of host cell apoptosis or host immune system defence (Brown et al. 2016). Among the different species in *Chlamydiaceae* family, *Chlamydia trachomatis* and *Chlamydia pneumoniae* cause common human neglected diseases, while *Chlamydia abortus*, *Chlamydia psittaci* and *Chlamydia suis* represent zoonotic threats and can be endemic in human food sources. In this context, the neglected tropical disease trachoma is a leading cause of eye disease in the world (Hotez et al. 2007). The pathogenic vehicle for this condition is *Chlamydia trachomatis*, a sexually transmitted bacterium (Potroz and Cho 2015). In 2008, Bhengraj et al. developed the topical formulation 'BASANT', containing curcumin (1) in combination with other active natural compounds (i.e., aloe vera, amla, and reetha saponins), which showed promising antimicrobial activity against *Chlamydia trachomatis*, as well as various microorganisms, including other *Chlamydia* species, *Candida* species and *Neisseria gonorrhoeae* (Bhengraj et al. 2008).

Safety Profile of Curcumin

Although it cannot be assumed that dietary supplements are innocuous when administered as pharmaceutical formulations, curcumin (1) is commonly considered a highly safe agent. Indeed, turmeric- and curcumin-based preparations have been approved by the Food and Drug Administration (FDA), the Natural Health Products Directorate of Canada, the Joint Expert Committee of the Food and Agriculture Organization (FAO) and the WHO (NCI 1996). Curcumin (1) is also listed in the GRAS index (i.e., "Generally Regarded As Safe") of the FDA agency and in the international numbering system of coloring agents (code E100) for food additives. In this regard, a curcumin-based hydrogel patch has been developed for cosmetic purposes, resulting highly tolerated (irritation or toxicity not detected during the tests) (Kunnumakkara et al. 2008).

The first *in vivo* investigation with regards to the safety profile has been carried out in the late '70s, highlighting the lack of significant toxicity after oral administrations of 5 g/Kg of curcumin (1) to Sprague-Dawley rats (Wahlstrom and Blennow 1978). The vast majority of initial preclinical studies (mainly funded by the Prevention Division of the US National Cancer Institute) did not show any adverse effects in rats, dogs or monkeys treated for a period of 3 mon with to 3.5 g/Kg of curcumin (1) (NCI 1996). However, one report on the use of curcumin (1) as dietary supplement reported ulcerogenic activity in albino rats (Gupta et al. 1980), although this finding was not confirmed in later investigations. Additional preclinical tests also refer the lack of toxicity in mice and rats upon oral administration of curcumin (1) for 14 d, using a dose of 0.3 g/Kg or 1.2 g/Kg, respectively (Sharma et al. 2001, Perkins et al. 2002).

A clinical trial conducted on patients with pre-invasive malignant or high-risk pre-tumor conditions confirmed the absence of toxicity related to the administration of 8 g/day of curcumin for 3 mon (Cheng et al. 2001). Furthermore, the tolerability and efficacy of the daily administration of curcumin (1) at a regimen of 3.6 g/day for 4 mon was also demonstrated in patients with advanced colorectal cancer (Sharma et al. 2004).

Main Drawbacks Limiting Curcumin Therapeutic Use

Although various *in vitro* and *in vivo* studies suggest that curcumin (1) could be a suitable drug candidate for several human diseases (Aggarwal et al. 2003, 2007b), many drawbacks are limiting its use as a therapeutic agent.

Curcumin (1) demonstrates a highly unstable compound, being rapidly hydrolyzed and degraded at basic or physiological pH, whereas in acidic conditions the degradation is slightly slower (i.e., ~ 20% of total drug decomposes after 1 hour) (Wang et al. 1997). The photodegradation of curcumin (1) has been also reported after light exposure for both solution and solid samples (Chignell et al. 1994, Ansari et al. 2005), although the mechanisms of photodegradative reactions are not clear. The presence of the phenolic groups does not seem to have a role in this process. The degradation mainly proceeds through the breaking of the diketone linker, forming smaller phenolic compounds, such as vanillin (28) or ferulic acid (30) (Figure 7), which could potentially polymerize to form phenolic polymers (Canamares et al. 2006). Additional non-phenolic photodegradative products have been also identified and isolated, including benzaldehyde-, cinnamaldehyde-, benzochalcone- and flavanone-like analogues (Sundaryono et al. 2003).

Furthermore, poor aqueous solubility, relatively low bioavailability, rapid metabolism and slow cellular uptake are recognized as the principal limitations for oral or parenteral administration of curcumin (1) (Wahlstrom and Blennow 1978, Pan et al. 1999, Anand et al. 2007, Sharma et al. 2007). Topical applications are often hampered due to the insufficient aqueous solubility and the related low permeation through the stratum corneum, determining poor absorption. In addition, low bioavailability was widely demonstrated after intraperitoneal or intravenous injections (Pan et al. 1999, Perkins et al. 2002). Several studies also documented the presence of negligible plasma concentration of curcumin (1) after oral administration, due to the lack of absorption from the gut (Ravindranath and Chandrasekhara 1980, 1981a, b, 1982, Shoba et al. 1998).

In 1978, Wahlstrom and Blennow firstly reported that approximately 75% of curcumin (1) was excreted intact in the feces after the oral administration of 1 g/Kg of body weight, suggesting that the

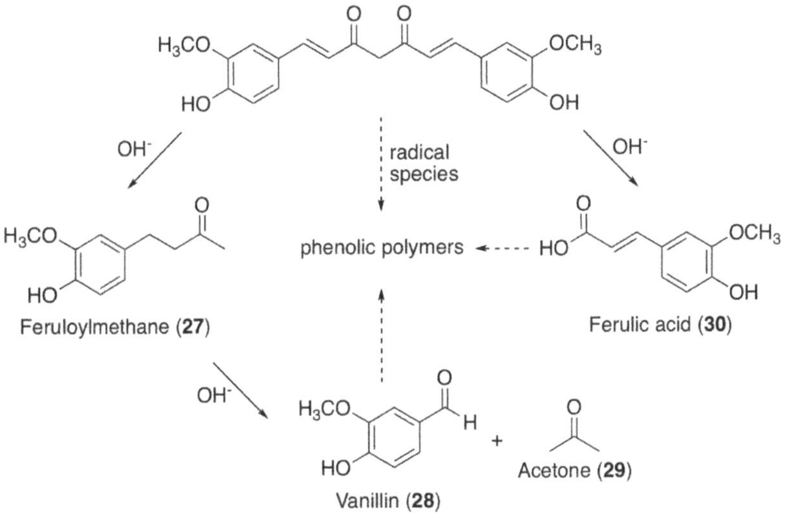

Figure 7. Degradation products of curcumin (1).

compound is poorly absorbed by the intestine (Wahlstrom and Blennow 1978). These findings have been also confirmed in animal studies by detecting curcumin metabolites, such as sulfate (9) and glucuronide (10) derivatives (Figure 2) and, in rat bile and urine (Ravindranath and Chandrasekhara 1980, Holder et al. 1978). Additionally, an investigation with liquid chromatography coupled to tandem mass spectrometry has estimated that the oral bioavailability of curcumin (1) in rats is about 1% (Yang et al. 2007). In a phase I clinical trial, curcumin (1) was used as a chemopreventive agent in patients with high-risk or pre-malignant lesions. Although the polyphenol showed good tolerability and the complete lack of treatment-related toxicity, only trace amounts could be detected in plasma (Cheng et al. 2001). Similarly, in a different clinical study conducted in patients with colorectal cancer, traces of intact curcumin (1) were detected in plasma samples after the oral administration of *Curcuma* extracts, while the presence of curcumin metabolites in faeces was easily observed (Sharma et al. 2001).

Strategies to improve curcumin bioavailability

Co-administration approaches

In the past three decades, several strategies have been adopted in order to increase curcumin (1) bioavailability, mainly by improving the solubility and stability of the compound, as well as decreasing the metabolic degradation. Initially, the co-administration with piperine (31) (Figure 8) demonstrated to limit the hepatic and intestinal metabolism of curcumin and, thus, increase its bioavailability (Shoba et al. 1998).

The rationale of using piperine (31) is related to its known inhibitory effects on hepatic and intestinal enzymes which perform glucuronic acid conjugations. In comparison to the administration of curcumin (1) alone, the co-administration with piperine (31) produced an improved serum concentration of the polyphenol, associated with longer half-life and decreased clearance, giving a final bioavailability 154% higher in rats and 2000% in human volunteers (Shoba et al. 1998). Despite these promising results, there are wide limitations for the use of piperine (31) in clinical context, mainly due to its gastro-intestinal side effects.

An analogous strategy has been proposed by Yue and colleagues (Yue et al. 2010, 2012). Specifically, the co-administration of curcumin (1) and turmerones (i.e., the main sesquiterpenes extracted from the essential oil of turmeric; see section 1.1 and analogues (11–13) in Figure 3) has been tested on CaCo-2 cells, chosen for their similarity to the absorptive intestinal human cells (Artursson and Karlsson 1991). This *in vitro* study demonstrated an improved uptake of curcumin (1) and the presence of turmerones

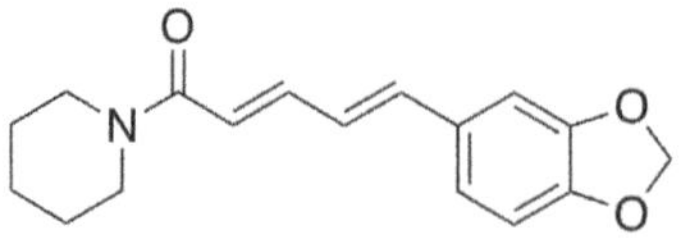

Piperine (**31**)

Figure 8. Chemical structure of piperine (31).

is reported to inhibit the activity of extruding membrane transporters in CaCo-2 cells. Specifically, the increased curcumin (1) uptake was more evident in the case of α-turmerone (12) (Figure 3), this compound being an inhibitor of glycoprotein P (i.e., the main transporter involved in multidrug resistance). In contrast, aromatic-turmerone (11) (Figure 3) showed to enhance the activity of the pump (Yue et al. 2012). Antiproliferative and immune-stimulating activities of turmerones were also confirmed in this study. The findings support previously published data on possible therapeutic effects of commercially available formulations (e.g., BCM-95®CG or Biocurcumax™) (Antony 2006, Antony et al. 2008, Shishu 2010), which contains curcumin and non-curcuminoid components of turmeric essential oil.

Drug delivery systems

In addition to co-administration strategies, several drug delivery systems have been tested to improve the stability and water solubility of curcumin (1), as well as enhance the overall bioavailability (Mazzacuva et al. 2011a, b). Moreover, to overcome the decomposition at the acidic pH of the stomach and the elevated liver metabolism are the main goals for curcumin (1) oral drug delivery systems. Differently, with regards to topic formulations, the highly lipophilic nature of curcumin (1) is not suited to an ease membrane permeation thorough the stratum corneum, in order to reach the lower skin layers.

A number of nanoparticles and nanosystems have been investigated, usually in accordance to the specific administration route of interest (Sweet and Singleton 2011, Dende et al. 2017). However, the formulations developed so far, with some exceptions, are too complicated or too expensive to be prepared on a large scale. Despite promising results, more efficient delivery vehicles are still a need in the field.

Liposomes: Liposomes are small spherical vesicles obtained by combining cholesterol and phospholipids (Akbarzadeh et al. 2013). They present one or more double layers of phospholipids which surround the aqueous *core*. On the base of the number of concentric bilayers, liposomes can be classified in mono-, uni- or multi-lamellar vesicles. They are widely used in the field of drug delivery due to their versatility of function (Mazzacuva et al. 2010, 2011a). Particularly, they can trap liposoluble molecules (as curcumin (1)) into the double layers and incorporate hydrophilic compounds into the aqueous *core*. Amphipathic compounds can also be efficiently carried with the hydrophobic side within the phospholipid tales and the hydrophilic part into the aqueous cavities (Koning and Storm 2003, Metselaar and Storm 2005, Ding et al. 2006, Johnston et al. 2007, Hua and Wu 2013).

The physical and chemical properties of liposomes, as well as their capability to target different cellular structures, can change on the basis of the method used for their preparation, the nature of their composition (i.e., specific phospholipids used), the percentage of cholesterol and the charges on the surface. For instance, saturated long chain phospholipids and high content of cholesterol have been reported to confer more rigidity and less permeability to the bilayer structure (Allen 1997, Gabizon et al. 1998, Sahoo and Labhasetwar 2003). Furthermore, the presence of specific molecules on the surface can modulate the diffusion properties and/or release of the content to a specific biological target or district (Omri et al. 2002, Schiffelers et al. 2001, Stano et al. 2004). Liposomes are also reported to improve the stability of entrapped compounds by preventing the enzymatic or pH-dependent hydrolysis (e.g., PEGylated liposomes are resistant to opsonization) (Mazzacuva et al. 2011a). *In vitro* studies recently demonstrated an increased bioavailability and reduced degradation for curcumin (1) upon inclusion into liposomal vesicles (Mahmud et al. 2016).

A sub-family of liposomal vesicles is Marinosomes®. They are prepared with natural marine lipid extracts containing a high polyunsaturated fatty acid (PUFA) ratio (Moussaoui et al. 2002). Recently, krill lipids-based liposomes loaded with curcumin (1) have been successfully tested as antiproliferative agents against lung cancer. A good stability of the system as well as a high antioxidant activity of the polyphenol have been demonstrated in HUVEC cells (Ibrahim et al. 2018) confirming the potential of this drug delivery system for clinical applications.

Phytosomes® (patented and commercialized by Indena) are an additional class of liposome-based oral drug delivery systems. Meriva® is the formulation of this type containing curcumin (1). Phytosomes are prepared by using a complex of curcumin (1) and soy lecithin (1:2 w/w) combined with two parts of microcrystalline cellulose. They have shown to improve curcumin (1) oral bioavailability and absorption of about 30-fold in comparison to unformulated curcumin (1) (Anand et al. 2007). Meriva® is currently employed as an oral anti-inflammatory formulation at a lower dosage than unformulated curcumin (1) (Farinacci et al. 2009, Belcaro et al. 2010a, b, Allegri et al. 2010, Steigerwalt et al. 2012, Appendino et al. 2011).

In the context of neglected diseases, liposomal encapsulated drugs showed a valuable strategy in the treatment of leishmaniasis, enhancing the efficacy of specific anti-*Leishmania* agents and related tissue absorptions, as well as reducing their side effects and clearance from the site of action (Ortega et al. 2017). In particular, turmerone-rich hexane fractions from *Curcuma longa* L. demonstrated an enhanced anti-leishmanial activity when included in liposomal formulations (Amaral et al. 2014). A dose dependent inhibition has been found toward *Leishmania amazonensis* promastigote forms upon treatment with LipoRHIC (i.e., one of the most active liposomal formulation reported). Specifically, a sub-inhibitory concentration of LipoRHIC (i.e., 2.75 µg/mL) produces evident morphological changes and the formation of holes in the plasmatic membrane of the parasite (Amaral et al. 2014).

Nanosuspensions: Nanosuspensions are sub-micron colloidal dispersions firstly developed by Müller and colleagues (Müller et al. 2001). They are usually prepared by bottom-up or top-down techniques (Liversidge et al. 1992, Liversidge and Cundy 1995, Nekkanti et al. 2012). In these systems, nano-sized drug particles are stabilized by small amounts of surfactant or polymeric materials (Patravale et al. 2004). One of the main advantages associated with nanosuspensions is the small particle size that can lead to a higher dissolution rate by increasing the surface area, thus improving the bioavailability of the drug (Rabinow 2004, Patel and Agrawal 2011). Nanosuspensions are considered versatile drug systems which allow several delivery routes, such as oral (Liversidge and Cundy 1995), parenteral (Peters et al. 2000), pulmonary (Jacobs and Müller 2002), ocular and topical (Pignatello et al. 2002) administration. They have been widely used to improve the bioavailability of curcumin (1). *In vitro* results suggest their potential as a nanocarrier for the polyphenol in clinical application (Gao et al. 2011, Li et al. 2016, Rahimi et al. 2017).

Microemulsions: Microemulsions are stable dispersions of oil in water (O/W) or water in oil (W/O) which are prepared and stabilized by means of surfactants. Curcumin-based microemulsions showed an increase of the bioavailability for the compound through local and transdermal administration in several pathological conditions, including scleroderma, psoriasis and skin cancer (Lin et al. 2009, Liu et al. 2011, Liu and Chang 2011, Wu et al. 2011). In a recent study, three curcumin (1) O/W microemulsions were developed by screening three different oils (i.e., olive oil, wheat germ oil, vitamin E) in combination with non-ionic surfactants as stabilizer (i.e., Cremophor EL, Tween 20, Tween 80 or Lecitin) (Bergonzi et al. 2014). The oral absorption of curcumin (1) was investigated *in vitro* through parallel artificial membrane permeability assay (PAMPA). The optimal formulation resulted as follows: 3.3 g/100 g of vitamin E, 53.8 g/100 g of Tween 20, 6.6 g/100 g of ethanol and 36.3 g/100 g of water, with 14.57 mg/mL maximum solubility of curcumin (1) and 70% of permeation through the artificial membrane. Chemical and physical stabilities of these systems were also evaluated, suggesting that both solubility and stability of curcumin (1) were improved, as well as its oral uptake.

Nanocrystals, micelles and mesoporous silica: Several techniques can be used for the preparation of nanocrystals (e.g., reactive crystallization, anti-solvent crystallization, supercritical fluid crystallization, high-pressure homogenization, high-gravity controlled precipitation) (Donsì et al. 2010, Rachmawati et al. 2013) and the use of surfactant agents is generally required as stabilizers (Wang et al. 2010). Curcumin (1) nanocrystals have been reported to increase the water dissolution of the compound (due to the higher specific surface area compared to curcumin (1) crystals) and they have been tested for pulmonary delivery of curcumin (1) *in vitro* and *in vivo* (Hu et al. 2015).

Micelles are formed by the spontaneous spherical re-arrangement of lipid molecules (i.e., 10–100 nm particle size) when introduced in aqueous solutions (Yallapu et al. 2010a, b). They have shown promising properties in order to improve the solubility of curcumin (1) (Liu et al. 2013, Raveendran et al. 2013). Similarly, curcumin-loaded mesoporous silica has also shown to potentiate the biological effects of curcumin (1), mainly by enhancing curcumin (1) cellular uptake (Kotcherlakota et al. 2016).

Nanoparticles: Various nanoparticle-based formulations have been investigated to overcome curcumin (1) limitations (Dhivya and Rajalakshmi 2017). Polymeric nanoparticles of curcumin are known to circulate in the bloodstream for a longer time, in comparison to unformulated curcumin (1). The polymers most commonly used for the preparation of this class of nanoassemblies are chitosan (Anitha et al. 2011, Das et al. 2010, Khalil et al. 2013b), poly(D,L-lactic-co-glycolic) acid (PLGA) (Yallapu et al. 2010b, Anand et al. 2010, Dende et al. 2017) and various polyethyleneglycoles (PEGs) (Song et al. 2011b).

Solid-lipid nanoparticles are colloidal drug delivery systems used as an alternative to polymeric nanoparticles, allowing an easier preparation and scale-up of the production (Khalil et al. 2013b). They are prepared by using lipids and surfactants as stabilizer. Several studies demonstrate that solid-lipid nanoparticles can improve curcumin (1) stability and solubility (Nair et al. 2011, Wang et al. 2013, Arora et al. 2015, Krausz et al. 2015, Jourghanian et al. 2016).

A third class of nanoparticles is represented by magnetic nanoparticles. They are usually employed to target a specific biological compartment, allowing the release of the drug *in situ* by applying an external magnetic field (Yang et al. 2009, Yallapu et al. 2011). Curcumin (1) magnetic nanoparticles have been recently tested in SKOV-3 cells (an ovarian cancer cell line) demonstrating pronounced therapeutic relevance (Mancarella et al. 2015).

Gold nanoparticles have also attracted high interest due to their safety and biocompatibility (Peng et al. 2009, Bessar et al. 2016). Curcumin (1) bioavailability showed improvements upon binding on the surface of gold nanoparticles (Singh et al. 2013). Moreover, flow cytometry and confocal microscopy experiments confirmed an increase in cellular internalization of the particles in various cell lines (e.g., HeLa, glioma and CaCo-2 cells) (Manju and Sreenivasan 2012).

In the context of leishmaniasis research, an oral nanoparticle-based formulation of curcumin (1) and PLGA has been developed and tested in a *Leishmania donovani*-hamster model (Tiwari et al. 2017). This nanoformulation exhibited significant leishmanicidal activity both *in vitro* and *in vivo*, suggesting its beneficial role in anti-leishmanial chemotherapy. Interestingly, co-administration of the 'nanotized curcumin' and miltefosine (25) (i.e., an oral drug for visceral leishmaniasis; Figure 6) exhibited synergistic effects on both promastigotes and amastigotes *in vitro*. An increased leishmanicidal activity *in vivo* has been also observed upon increased lymphocyte proliferation and production of toxic reactive oxygen/nitrogen species, as well as enhanced phagocytic activity (Tiwari et al. 2017).

Synthetic and Semi-synthetic Curcumin Analogues

Over the past few decades, medicinal chemists adopted a number of approaches to identify efficient curcumin-based derivatives with expanded structural diversity for various biological (Orlando et al. 2012, Thakur et al. 2014, Oliveira et al. 2015, Badavath et al. 2016), therapeutic (Sun et al. 2006, Kasinski et al. 2008, Di Martino et al. 2017a, b) and diagnostic (Zhang et al. 2015, Margar and Sekar 2016) applications. More potent and more stable analogues of curcumin (1) have been explored to establish SARs, to gain more information about the mechanisms of action and to overcome pharmacokinetic problems, with potential as drug candidates (Oliveira et al. 2015). These synthetic and semi-synthetic derivatives present a high potential in limiting *in vivo* drawbacks, demonstrating better stability and, in some cases, higher activity than the natural polyphenol (Shang et al. 2010), thus enhancing the overall pharmacological profile.

With regards to the research in the field of neglected disease, the simple derivative dimethylcurcumin (32) (Figure 9) resulted more potent than curcumin (1), by reducing of 66% the lesion size in *Leishmania amazonensis* infected mice at a *subcutaneous* dose of 20 mg/Kg/day (Araújo et al. 1999). The LD_{50} of

2.0 µg/mL is reported for this compound on promastigote forms of *Leishmania amazonensis* (Gomes et al. 2002). Additionally, the derivative (33) (i.e., 1*E*,4*Z*,6*E*)-5-hydroxy-1-(4-hydroxy-3-methoxyphenyl)-7-(4-methoxyphenyl)hepta-1,4,6-trien-3-one; Figure 9) was also tested in a model of *Leishmania amazonensis*, demonstrating high activity *in vivo* as anti-*Leishmania* agent (Alves et al. 2003, 2004).

A different library of curcumin-like synthetic analogues has also been investigated *in vitro* against *Leishmania amazonensis* promastigotes (Gomes et al. 2002), using pentamidine (24) (Figure 6) as control drug. (1*E*,4*Z*,6*E*)-5-Hydroxy-1,7-bis[3-methoxy-4-(prop-2-yn-1-yloxy)phenyl]hepta-1,4,6-trien-3-one (34) (Figure 9) was the most active compound of the series, being about ten times more efficient than curcumin (1). Cheikh-Ali and co-workers generated new curcumin-based derivatives by mono- or di-esterification of the phenolic groups in the structure with 1,1′,2-tris-norsqualenic acid (Cheikh-Ali et al. 2014). These "squalenoylcurcuminoids" (36, 37) (Figure 10) were formulated as stable and water-dispersible nanoassemblies, presenting a homogeneous size of the particles. Although these nanoformulated analogues were inactive against *Trypanosoma brucei brucei* trypomastigotes, they demonstrated a significant inhibition of *Leishmania donovani* promastigotes when compared to curcumin (1). Moreover, in *Leishmania donovani* axenic and intramacrophagic amastigotes, the squalenoyl-based analogues (36, 37) (Figure 10) showed activity in the range of miltefosine (25) (Figure 6) and good selectivity indexes, proposing as valuable candidates in preclinical study for the treatment of visceral leishmaniasis (Cheikh-Ali et al. 2014).

Changtam et al. studied a library of naturally occurring curcuminoids for the treatment of *Trypanosoma brucei* infections (Changtam et al. 2010). They initially exhibited low potency against the parasite. To

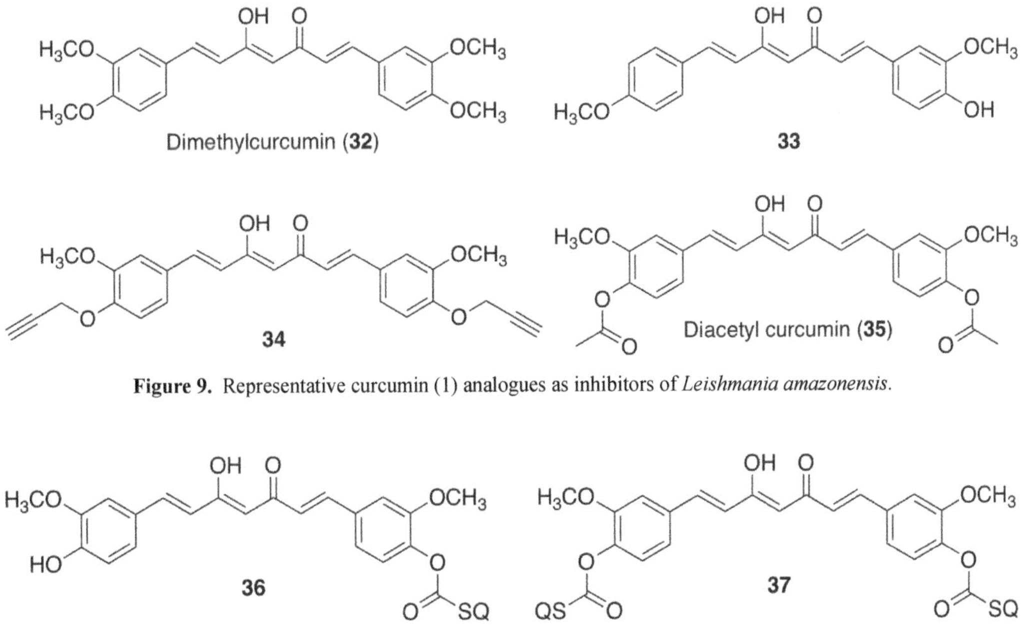

Figure 9. Representative curcumin (1) analogues as inhibitors of *Leishmania amazonensis*.

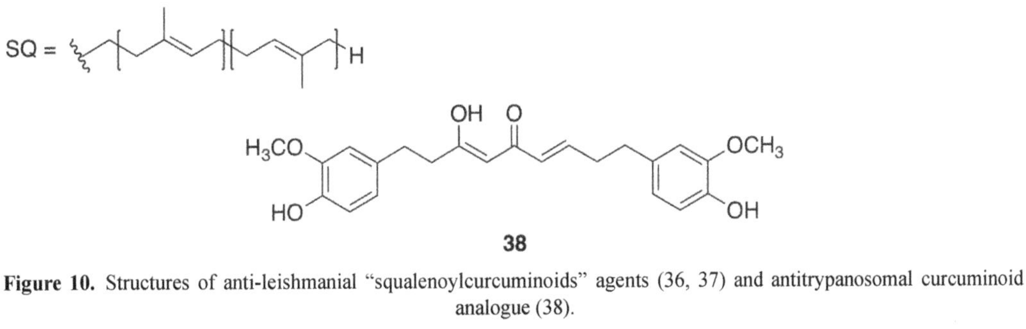

Figure 10. Structures of anti-leishmanial "squalenoylcurcuminoids" agents (36, 37) and antitrypanosomal curcuminoid analogue (38).

enhance the activity, several structural modifications were performed to generate 43 synthetic analogues that were tested as pure compounds or mixture of them. Thirteen curcumin derivatives in the series displayed sub-micromolar potency against *Trypanosoma brucei brucei*. (*E*)-1,7-Bis(4-hydroxy-3-methoxyphenyl) hept-4-en-3-one (38) (Figure 10) was the most active analogue with EC_{50} = 0.053 µM and a selectivity index of 453 for *Tryoanosoma brucei brucei* bloodstream forms *vs* human embryonic kidney (HEK) cells. An equal potency was also found against *Trypanosoma brucei brucei* strains resistant to diamidines and melaminophenyl arsenical drugs (Changtam et al. 2010).

On the other hand, curcumin (1) has shown to form relatively stable complexes with various metal ions (Figure 11), since the enol tautomer of the β-dike to function possesses wide chelating capabilities as monobasic bidentate ligand (Bernabé-Pineda et al. 2004, Priyadarsini 2014).

Generally, structures with ligand:metal stoichiometry of 2:1 (e.g., structure A in Figure 11) are found with various metals. In the case of iron(III), the 2:1 complex (39) (Figure 12) has been lately reported (Bicer et al. 2018), as well as a 3:1 complex (40) (Figure 12) with octahedral geometry (Khalil et al. 2013a). Moreover, Borsari et al. calculated that the stability constant for the formation of a curcumin-Fe(III) complex 1:1 (i.e., [curcumin-Fe-(OH)$_2$]) is comparable to that of desferrioxamine (i.e., log$K$ 29.1 *vs* 30.99), a clinically used iron chelator. However, the stability of the iron(III) complex with the curcuminoid diacetylcurcumin (35) (Figure 9) was higher than that of curcumin-Fe(III) complex (log$K$

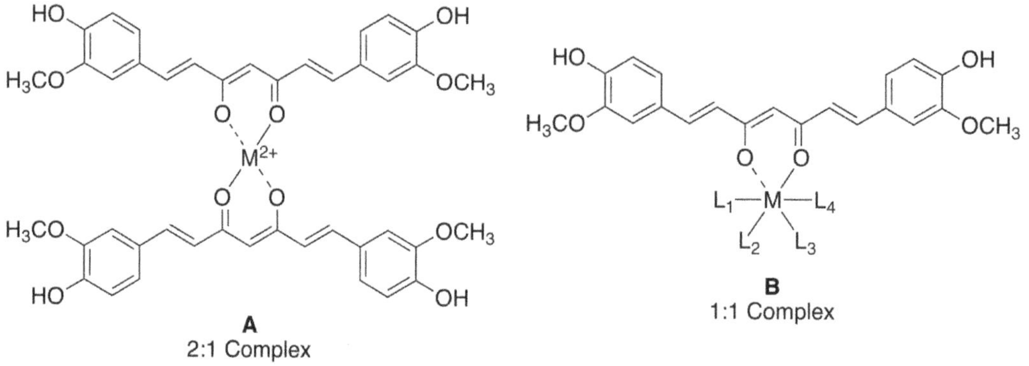

Figure 11. General structures of possible curcumin complexes with ligand:metal stoichiometry 2:1 (A) and 1:1 (B) (as 'mixed ligand complexes').

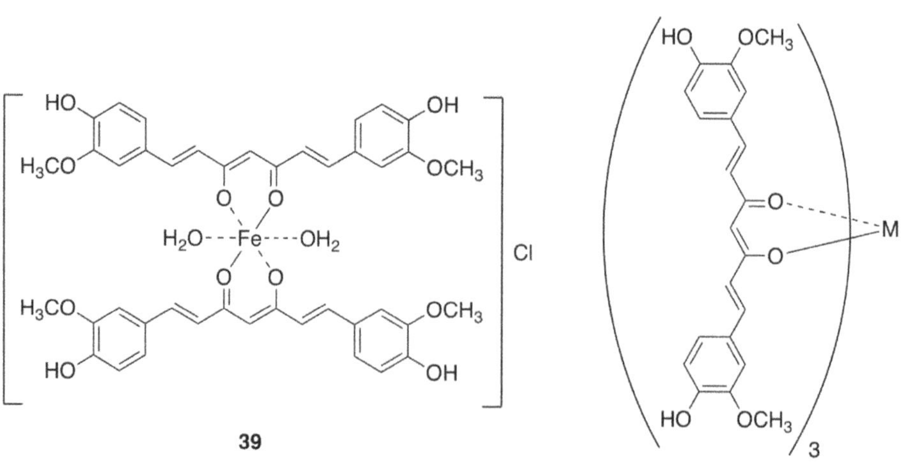

Figure 12. Curcumin-Fe(III) 2:1 complex (**39**) and 3:1 complexes with Fe(III) (**40**), In(III) (**41**) and Ga(III) (**42**).

30.1 *vs* 29.1) (Borsari et al. 2002). This property could be exploited to improve current therapies for iron-overload related diseases (Baum and Ng 2004), which are known to generate cellular free radicals *via* Fenton reaction (Cilibrizzi et al. 2018).

In a recent study, indium(III) (41) and gallium(III) (42) curcumin-based complexes (with ligand:metal stoichiometry of 3:1; Figure 12) showed higher anti-leishmanial activity in comparison to curcumin (1) and diacetylcurcumin (35) (Figure 9). IC_{50} values for the inhibition of the growth of *Leishmania major* promastigotes were found as follows: 38 µg/mL for curcumin (1), 26 µg/mL for indium-curcumin (41), 32 µg/mL for gallium-curcumin (42), 52 µg/mL for diacetylcurcumin (35) (Figure 9) and 20 µg/mL for amphotericin B (26) (i.e., control drug; Figure 6) (Fouladvand et al. 2013).

Conclusions

In this chapter, we present general aspects on curcumin (1) research, as well as a selection of studies where this polyphenol and its natural or synthetic analogues have been investigated in relation to neglected infectious diseases.

Over the past three decades, biological and pharmacological studies examined possible beneficial effects of curcumin (1), the most active compound extracted from the rhizome of *Curcuma longa* L. Anti-inflammatory, antioxidant, antibacterial, antimalarial, anti-HIV and anticancer activities have been proposed (Di Martino et al. 2017a, b). In parallel, toxicological studies demonstrated that this polyphenol is highly safe in both animal models and humans. Several mechanisms of action have been hypothesized due to its clear ability to modulate and interfere with a number of signalling pathways involved in physiological and pathological processes (Aggarwal et al. 2007c). Moreover, curcumin-based nanoformulations and nanosystems proved some efficacy in order to overcome well-known stability, solubility and pharmacokinetic issues.

Clearly, there has been a massive campaign of scientific reports on this natural compound, attempting to demonstrate a broad spectrum of health-promoting properties. The science behind curcumin (1) is massively abundant and the numbers are impressive. It is estimated that over 10,000 articles, 500 patents and 120 clinical trials (Padmanaban and Nagaraj 2017) have assessed possible pharmacological and/or biological actions. This gives an indication of the resources used by both academia and pharma industry in this field, in order to establish the 'secrets' behind the multiple biological actions hypothesized and reported for curcumin (1).

Although the mechanisms of action remain mostly undefined and the real efficacy in diseases is highly controversial (Nelson et al. 2017, Padmanaban and Nagaraj 2017), we cannot rule out the possibility that curcumin (1) might have beneficial effects on human health, associated to the low-toxic profile. Contextually, we cannot ignore that the possibility to act as a drug does not always apply to the variety of natural agents used in traditional medicine, for obvious reasons. To the best of our knowledge, there is no controversy about the interference of curcumin (1) with multiple signalling pathways and biochemical mechanisms (as demonstrated at least in *in vitro* experiments). Even if it is not established how it works, this natural product can still represent a promising lead compound for the development of new agents, occupying a privileged position in drug discovery context. There is certainly room for suitable 'structure-activity optimization efforts' to identify structurally related analogues with enhanced features for suitable clinical applications in neglected infectious diseases, as well as in other pathological conditions.

References

Adapala, N. and M.M. Chan. 2008. Long-term use of an antiinflammatory, curcumin, suppressed type 1 immunity and exacerbated visceral leishmaniasis in a chronic experimental model. Lab. Invest. 88: 1329–1339.

Aggarwal, B.B., A. Kumar and A.C. Bharti. 2003. Anticancer potential of curcumin: preclinical and clinical studies. Anticancer Res. 23: 363–398.

Aggarwal, B.B., I.D. Bhatt, H. Ichikawa, K.S. Ahn, G. Sethi, S.K. Sandur et al. 2007a. Curcumin: biological and medicinal properties. pp. 297–368. *In*: P.N. Ravindran, K. Nirmal Babu and K. Sivaraman [eds.]. Turmeric: The genus *Curcuma*. C.R.C. Press, New York, USA.

Aggarwal, B.B., C. Sundaram, N. Malani and H. Ichikawa. 2007b. Curcumin: the Indian solid gold. Adv. Exp. Med. Biol. 595: 1–75.

Aggarwal, B.B., Y.-J. Surh and S. Shishodia [eds.]. 2007c. The Molecular Targets and Therapeutic uses of Curcumin in Health and Disease. Springer US, New York, USA.

Akbarzadeh, A., R. Rezaei-Sadabady, S. Davaran, S.W. Joo, N. Zarghami, Y. Hanifehpour et al. 2013. Liposome: classification, preparation, and applications. Nanoscale Res. Lett. 8: 102.

Allam, G. 2009. Immunomodulatory effects of curcumin treatment on murine schistosomiasis mansoni. Immunobiology. 214: 712–727.

Allegri, P., A. Mastromarino and P. Neri. 2010. Management of chronic anterior uveitis relapses: efficacy of oral phospholipidic curcumin treatment. Long-term follow-up. Clin. Ophthalmol. 4: 1201–1206.

Allen, T.M. 1997. Liposomes. Opportunities in drug delivery. Drugs. 54: 8–14.

Almalki, E., E.M. Al-Shaebi, S. Al-Quarishy, M. El-Matboulic and A.-A.S. Abdel-Baki. 2017. *In vitro* effectiveness of *Curcuma longa* and *Zingiber officinale* extracts on *Echinococcus protoscoleces*. Saudi J. Biol. Sci. 24: 90–94.

Alves, L.V., R.M. Temporal, L. Cysne-Finkelstein and L.L. Leon. 2003. Efficacy of a diarylheptanoid derivative against *Leishmania amazonensis* in experimental murine cutaneous leishmaniasis. Mem. Inst. Oswaldo Cruz. 98: 553–555.

Alves, L.V., L. Cysne Finkelstein, R.M. Temporal, M.S. Genestra and L.L. Leon. 2004. An effective diaryl derivative against *Leishmania amazonensis* and its influence on the parasite X macrophage interaction. J. Enz. Inhib. Med. Chem. 19: 437–439.

Amaral, A.C.F., L.A. Gomes, J.R. de, A. Silva, J.L.P. Ferreira, A. de et al. 2014. Liposomal formulation of turmerone-rich hexane fractions from *Curcuma longa* enhances their antileishmanial activity. BioMed. Res. Int. 2014: 694934.

Anand, P., A.B. Kunnumakkara, R.A. Newman and B.B. Aggarwal. 2007. Bioavailability of curcumin: problems and promises. Mol. Pharm. 4: 807–818.

Anand, P., C. Sundaram, S. Jhurani, A.B. Kunnumakkara and B.B. Aggarwal. 2008. Curcumin and cancer: an "old-age" disease with an "age-old" solution. Cancer Lett. 267: 133–164.

Anand, P., H.B. Nair and B. Sung. 2010. Design of curcumin loaded PLGA nanoparticles formulation with enhanced cellular uptake, and increased bioactivity *in vitro* and superior bioavailability *in vivo*. Biochem. Pharmacol. 79: 330–338.

Anitha, A., S. Maya, N. Deepa, K.P. Chennazhi, S.V. Nair, H. Tamura et al. 2011. Efficient water soluble O-carboxy methyl chitosan nanocarrier for the delivery of curcumin to cancer cells. Carbohydr. Polym. 83: 452–461.

Ansari, M.J., S. Ahmad, K. Kohli, J. Ali and R.K. Khar. 2005. Stability-indicating HPTLC determination of curcumin in bulk drug and pharmaceutical formulations. J. Pharm. Biomed. Anal. 39: 132–138.

Antony, B. 2006. A composition to enhance the bioavailability of curcumin. EP # 1890546A1, US # 7883728B2, WO2006129323.

Antony, B., B. Merina, V.S. Iyer, N. Judy, K. Lennertz and S. Joyal. 2008. A pilot cross-over study to evaluate human oral bioavailability of BCM-95CG (Biocurcumax), a novel bioenhanced preparation of curcumin. Indian J. Pharm. Sci. 70: 445–449.

API. 2001. The ayurvedic pharmacopoeia of India, Part I. 2001. pp. 45–46. Ministry of Health and Family Welfare, Government of India. The Controller of Publications Civil Lines, New Delhi, India.

Appendino, G., G. Belcaro, U. Cornelli, R. Luzzi, S. Togni, M. Dugall et al. 2011. Potential role of curcumin phytosome (Meriva) in controlling the evolution of diabetic microangiopathy. A pilot study. Panminerva Med. 53: 43–49.

Araújo, C.A., L.V. Alegrio, D.C. Gomes, M.E. Lima, L. Gomes-Cardoso and L.L. Leon. 1999. Studies on the effectiveness of diarylheptanoids derivatives against *Leishmania amazonensis*. Mem. Inst. Oswaldo Cruz. 94: 791–794.

Araújo, M.C.P., L.M.G. Antunes and C.S. Takahashi. 2001. Protective effect of thiourea, a hydroxyl-radical scavenger, on curcumin-induced chromosomal aberrations in an *in vitro* mammalian cell system. Terat. Carcinogen. Mutagen. 21: 175–180.

Arora, R., A. Kuhad, I.P. Kaur and K. Chopra. 2015. Curcumin loaded solid lipid nanoparticles ameliorate adjuvant-induced arthritis in rats. Eur. J. Pain. 19: 940–952.

Artursson, P. and J. Karlsson. 1991. Correlation between oral drug absorption in humans and apparent drug permeability coefficients in human intestinal epithelial (Caco-2) cells. Biochem. Biophys. Res. Commun. 175: 880–885.

Badavath, V.N., İ. Baysal, G. Ucar, B.N. Sinha and V. Jayaprakash. 2016. Monoamine oxidase inhibitory activity of novel pyrazoline analogues: curcumin based design and synthesis. ACS Med. Chem. Lett. 7: 56–61.

Baum, L. and A. Ng. 2004. Curcumin interaction with copper and iron suggests one possible mechanism of action in Alzheimer's disease animal models. J. Alzheimer's Dis. 6: 367–377.

Bazh, E.K. and N.M. El-Bahy. 2013. *In vitro* and *in vivo* screening of anthelmintic activity of ginger and curcumin on *Ascaridia galli*. Parasitol. Res. 112: 3679–3686.

Belcaro, G., M.R. Cesarone, M. Dugall, L. Pellegrini, A. Ledda, M.G. Grossi et al. 2010a. Product-evaluation registry of Meriva®, a curcumin-phosphatidylcholine complex, for the complementary management of osteoarthritis. Panminerva Med. 52: 55–62.

Belcaro, G., M.R. Cesarone, M. Dugall, L. Pellegrini, A. Ledda, M.G. Grossi et al. 2010b. Efficacy and safety of Meriva®, a curcumin-phosphatidylcholine complex, during extended administration in osteoarthritis patients. Altern. Med. Rev. 15: 337–344.

Bessar, H., I. Venditti, L. Benassi, C. Vaschieri, P. Azzoni, G. Pellacani et al. 2016. Functionalized gold nanoparticles for topical delivery of methotrexate for the possible treatment of psoriasis. Colloids Surf. B Biointerfaces. 141: 141–147.

Basnet, P. and N. Skalko-Basnet. 2011. Curcumin: an anti-inflammatory molecule from a curry spice on the path to cancer treatment. Molecules. 16: 4567–4598.

Bergonzi, M.C., R. Hamdouch, F. Mazzacuva, B. Isacchi and A.R. Bilia. 2014. Optimization, characterization and *in vitro* evaluation of curcumin microemulsions. LWT-Food Sci. Technol. 59: 148–155.

Bernabé-Pineda, M., M.T. Ramírez-Silva, M. Romero-Romo, E. González-Vergara and A. Rojas-Hernández. 2004. Determination of acidity constants of curcumin in aqueous solution and apparent rate constant of its decomposition. Spectrochim. Acta A Mol. Biomol. Spectrosc. 60: 1091–1097.

Bhengraj, A.R., S.A. Dar, G.P. Talwar and A. Mittal. 2008. Potential of a novel polyherbal formulation BASANT for prevention of *Chlamydia trachomatis* infection. Int. J. Antimicrob. Agents. 32: 84–88.

Bicer, N., E. Yildiz, A.A. Yegani and F. Aksu. 2018. Synthesis of curcumin complexes with iron(III) and manganese(II), and effects of curcumin–iron(III) on Alzheimer's disease. New J. Chem. 42: 8098–8104.

Borsari, M., E. Ferrari, R. Grandi and M. Saladini. 2002. Curcuminoids as potential new iron-chelating agents: spectroscopic, polarographic and potentiometric study on their Fe(III) complexing ability. Inorg. Chim. Acta. 328: 61–68.

Brown, M.A., M.G. Potroz, S.-W. Teh and N.-J. Cho. 2016. Natural products for the treatment of *Chlamydiaceae* infections. Microorganisms. 4: E39.

Cañamares, M.V., J.V. Garcia-Ramos and S. Sanchez-Cortes. 2006. Degradation of curcumin dye in aqueous solution and on ag nanoparticles studied by ultraviolet-visible absorption and surface-enhanced Raman spectroscopy. Appl. Spectrosc. 60: 1386–1391.

Chan, M.M., N.S. Adapala and D. Fong. 2005. Curcumin overcomes the inhibitory effect of nitric oxide on Leishmania. Parasitol. Res. 96: 49–56.

Changtam, C., H.P. de Koning, H. Ibrahim, M.S. Sajid, M.K. Gould and A. Suksamrarn. 2010. Curcuminoid analogs with potent activity against *Trypanosoma* and *Leishmania* species. Eur. J. Med. Chem. 45: 941–956.

Cheikh-Ali, Z., J. Caron, S. Cojean, C. Bories, P. Couvreur, P.M. Loiseau et al. 2014. Squalenoylcurcumin nanoassemblies as water-dispersible drug candidates with antileishmanial activity. ChemMedChem. 10: 411–418.

Chen, J., X.Q. Tang, J.L. Zhi, Y. Cui, H.M. Yu, E.H. Tang et al. 2006. Curcumin protects PC12 cells against 1-methyl-4-phenylpyridinium ion-induced apoptosis by bcl-2-mitochondria-ROS-iNOS pathway. Apoptosis. 11: 943–953.

Cheng, A.L., C.H. Hsu, J.K. Lin, M.M. Hsu, Y.F. Ho, T.S Shen et al. 2001. Phase I clinical trial of curcumin, a chemopreventive agent, in patients with high-risk or pre-malignant lesions. Anticancer Res. 21: 2895–2900.

Chignell, C.F., P. Bilski, K.J. Reszka, A.G. Motten, R.H. Sik and T.A. Dahl. 1994. Spectral and photochemical properties of curcumin. Photochem. Photobiol. 59: 295–302.

Chu, X., H.-G. Yang, J.-X. Tang, X.-Y. Peng, Q.-K. Wang, L. Yang et al. 2016. Effect of curcumin on the growth of *Echinococcus multilocularis* protoscoleces. Journal of Pathogen Biology. 2016: 05.

Cilibrizzi, A., V. Abbate, Y.-L. Chen, Y. Ma, T. Zhou and R.C. Hider. 2018. Hydroxypyridinone (HOPO) journey into metal chelation. Chem. Rev. 118: 7657–7701.

Cornago, P., R.M. Claramunt, L. Bouissane, I. Alkorta and J. Elguero. 2008. A study of the tautomerism of β-dicarbonyl compounds with special emphasis on curcuminoids. Tetrahedron. 64: 8089–8094.

CPC. 2010. Chinese pharmacopoeia commission. chinese pharmacopoeia, Edition 1. 2010. pp. 247–248. China Medical Science and Technology Press, Beijing, China.

Cui, L., J. Miao and L. Cui. 2007. Cytotoxic effect of curcumin on malaria parasite *Plasmodium falciparum*: inhibition of histone acetylation and generation of reactive oxygen species. Antimicrob. Agents Chemother. 51: 488–494.

Das, R., A. Roy, N. Dutta and H.K. Majumder. 2008. Reactive oxygen species and imbalance of calcium homeostasis contributes to curcumin induced programmed cell death in *Leishmania donovani*. Apoptosis. 13: 867–882.

Das, R.K., N. Kasoju and U. Bora. 2010. Encapsulation of curcumin in alginate-chitosan-pluronic composite nanoparticles for delivery to cancer cells. Nanomedicine. 6: 153–160.

Daybe, F.V. 1870. Uber Curcumin. Den Farbstoff der Curcumawurzzel Ber. 3: 609.

Dende, C., J. Meena, P. Nagarajan, V.A. Nagaraj, A.K. Panda and G. Padmanaban. 2017. Nanocurcumin is superior to native curcumin in preventing degenerative changes in experimental cerebral malaria. Sci. Rep. 7: 10062.

de Paula Aguiar, D., M. Brunetto Moreira Moscardini, E. Rezende Morais, R. Graciano de Paula, P.M. Ferreira, A. Afonso et al. 2016. Curcumin generates oxidative stress and induces apoptosis in adult *Schistosoma mansoni* worms. PLoS One. 11: e0167135.

Di Martino, R.M.C., B. Luppi, A. Bisi, S. Gobbi, A. Rampa, A. Abruzzo et al. 2017a. Recent progress on curcumin-based therapeutics: a patent review (2012–2016). Part I: Curcumin. Exp. Opin. Ther. Pat. 27: 579–590.

Di Martino, R.M.C., A. Bisi, A. Rampa, S. Gobbi and F. Belluti. 2017b. Recent progress on curcumin-based therapeutics: a patent review (2012–2016). Part II: curcumin derivatives in cancer and neurodegeneration. Exp. Opin. Ther. Pat. 27: 953–965.

Ding, B.S., T. Dziubla, V.V. Shuvaev, S. Muro and V.R. Muzykantov. 2006. Advanced drug delivery systems that target the vascular endothelium. Mol. Interv. 6: 98–112.

Diniz, L.D.F., J.A. Urbina, I.M. De Andrade, A.L. Mazzeti, T.A. Martins, I.S. Caldas et al. 2013. Benznidazole and posaconazole in experimental Chagas disease: positive interaction in concomitant and sequential treatments. PLoS Negl. Trop. Dis. 7: e2367.

Dhivya, S. and A.N. Rajalakshmi. 2017. Curcumin nano drug delivery systems: a review on its type and therapeutic application. Pharma. Tutor. 5: 30–39.

Donsì, F., Y. Wang, J. Li and Q. Huang. 2010. Preparation of curcumin sub-micrometer dispersions by high-pressure homogenization. J. Agric. Food Chem. 58: 2848–2853.

DSM. 2009. Dietary Supplement Monographs. USP Pharmacists' Pharmacopeia, 2nd ed. The United States Pharmacopeial Convention, Rockville, MD, USA.

El-Sherbiny, M., M.M. Abdel-Aziz, K.A. Elbakry, E.A. Toson and A.T. Abbas. 2006. Schistosomicidal effect of curcumin. Trends Appl. Sci. Res. 1: 627–633.

Fang, J., J. Lu and A. Holmgren. 2005. Thioredoxin reductase is irreversibly modified by curcumin: a novel molecular mechanism for its anticancer activity. J. Biol. Chem. 280: 25284–25290.

Farinacci, M., B. Gaspardo, M. Colitti and B. Stefanon. 2009. Dietary administration of curcumin modifies transcriptional profile of genes involved in inflammatory cascade in horse leukocytes. Ital. J. Anim. Sci. 8: 84–86.

Fouladvand, M., A. Barazesh and R. Tahmasebi. 2013. Evaluation of *in vitro* antileishmanial activity of curcumin and its derivatives gallium curcumin, indium curcumin, and diacethyl-curcumin. Eur. Rev. Med. Pharmacol. Sci. 24: 3306–3308.

Gabizon, A., D. Goren, R. Cohen and Y. Barenholz. 1998. Development of liposomal anthracyclines: from basics to clinical applications. J. Control Release. 53: 275–279.

Galasso, V., B. Kovač, A. Modelli, M.F. Ottaviani and F. Pichierri. 2008. Spectroscopic and theoretical study of the electronic structure of curcumin and related fragment molecules. J. Phys. Chem. A. 112: 2331–2338.

Gao, Y., Z. Li, M. Sun, C. Guo, A. Yu, Y. Xi et al. 2011. Preparation and characterization of intravenously injectable curcumin nanosuspension. Drug Deliv. 18: 131–142.

Gomes, D. deC., L.V. Alegrio, M.E. de Lima, L.L. Leon and C.A. Araújo. 2002. Synthetic derivatives of curcumin and their activity against *Leishmania amazonensis*. Arzneimittelforschung. 52: 120–124.

Gupta, B., V.K. Kulshrestha, R.K. Srivastava and D.N. Prasad. 1980. Mechanisms of curcumin induced gastric ulcer in rats. Indian J. Med. Res. 71: 806–814.

Heng, M.C., M.K. Song, J. Harker and M.K. Heng. 2000. Drug-induced suppression of phosphorylase kinase activity correlates with resolution of psoriasis as assessed by clinical, histological and immunohistochemical parameters. Br. J. Dermatol. 143: 937–949.

Holder, G.M., J.L. Plummer and A.J. Ryan. 1978. The metabolism and excretion of curcumin (1,7-bis-(4-hydroxy-3-methoxyphenyl)-1,6-heptadiene-3,5-dione) in the rat. Xenobiotica. 8: 761–768.

Hong, J., M. Bose, J. Ju, J.-H. Ryu, X. Chen, S. Sang et al. 2004. Modulation of arachidonic acid metabolism by curcumin and related β-diketone derivatives: effects on cytosolic phospholipase A2, cyclooxygenases and 5-lipoxygenase. Carcinogenesis. 25: 1671–1679.

Hotez, P.J., D.H. Molyneux, A. Fenwick, J. Kumaresan, S. Ehrlich Sachs, J.D. Sachs et al. 2007. Control of neglected tropical diseases. New Eng. J. Med. 357: 1018–1027.

Hu, L., D. Kong, Q. Hu, N. Gao and S. Pang. 2015. Evaluation of high-performance curcumin nanocrystals for pulmonary drug delivery both *in vitro* and *in vivo*. Nanoscale Res. Lett. 10: 381.

Hua, S. and S.Y. Wu. 2013. The use of lipid-based nanocarriers for targeted pain therapies. Front. Pharmacol. 4: 143.

Hucklenbroich, J., R. Klein, B. Neumaier, R. Graf, G.R. Fink, M. Schroeter et al. 2014. Aromatic-turmerone induces neural stem cell proliferation *in vitro* and *in vivo*. Stem Cell Res. Ther. 5: 100.

Ibrahim, S., T. Tagami, T. Kishi and T. Ozeki. 2018. Curcumin marinosomes as promising nano-drug delivery system for lung cancer. Int. J. Pharm. 540: 40–49.

Ichsyani, M., A. Ridhanya, M. Risanti, H. Desti, R. Ceria, D.H. Putri et al. 2017. Antiviral effects of *Curcuma longa* L. against dengue virus *in vitro* and *in vivo*. IOP Conf. Series: Earth and Environmental Science. 101: 012005.

Ioset, J.-R. 2008. Natural products for neglected diseases: a review. Curr. Org. Chem. 12: 643–666.

Jacobs, C. and R.H. Müller. 2002. Production and characterization of a budesonide nanosuspension for pulmonary administration. Pharm. Res. 19: 189–194.

Jagetia, G.C. and B.B. Aggarwal. 2007. "Spicing up" of the immune system by curcumin. J. Clin. Immunol. 27: 19–35.

Jayaprakasha, G.K., L. Jagan Mohan Rao and K.K. Sakariah. 2002. Improved HPLC method for the determination of curcumin, demethoxycurcumin, and bisdemethoxycurcumin. J. Agric. and Food Chem. 50: 3668–3672.

Johnston, M.J., S.C. Semple, S.K. Klimuk, S. Ansell, N. Maurer and P.R. Cullis. 2007. Characterization of the drug retention and pharmacokinetic properties of liposomal nanoparticles containing dihydrosphingomyelin. Biochim. Biophys. Acta. 1768: 1121–1127.

Jourghanian, P., S. Ghaffari, M. Ardjmand, S. Haghighat and M. Mohammadnejad. 2016. Sustained release curcumin loaded solid lipid nanoparticles. Adv. Pharm. Bull. 6: 17–21.

Jovanovic, S.V., S. Steenken, C.W. Boone and Michael G. Simic. 1999. H-atom transfer is a preferred antioxidant mechanism of curcumin. J. Am. Chem. Soc. 121: 9677–9681.

Kasinski, A.L., Y. Du, S.L. Thomas, J. Zhao, S.-Y. Sun, F.R. Khuri et al. 2008. Inhibition of IκB kinase-nuclear factor-κB signaling pathway by 3,5-bis(2-flurobenzylidene)piperidin-4-one (EF24), a novel nonoketone analog of curcumin. Mol. Pharmacol. 74: 654–661.

Khalil, M.I., A.M. Al-Zahem and M.H. Al-Qunaibit. 2013a. Synthesis, characterisation, Mössbauer parameters and anti-tumor activity of Fe(III) curcumin complex. Bioinorg. Chem. Appl. 2013: 982423.

Khalil, N.M., A.C. de Mattos, T.C. Carraro, D.B. Ludwig and R.M. Mainardes. 2013b. Nanotechnological strategies for the treatment of neglected diseases. Curr. Pharm. Des. 19: 7316–7329.

Kiuchi, F., Y. Goto, N. Sugimoto, N. Akao, K. Kondo and Y. Tsuda. 1993. Nematocidal activity of turmeric: synergistic action of curcuminoids. Chem. Pharm. Bull. 41: 1640–1643.

Koide, T., M. Nose, Y. Ogihara, Y. Yabu and N. Ohta. 2002. Leishmanicidal effect of curcumin *in vitro*. Biol. Pharm. Bull. 25: 131–133.

Koning, G.A. and G. Storm. 2003. Targeted drug delivery systems for the intracellular delivery of macromolecular drugs. Drug Discov. Today. 8: 482–483.

Kolev, T.M., E.A. Velcheva, B.A. Stamboliyska and M. Spiteller. 2005. DFT and experimental studies of the structure and vibrational spectra of curcumin. Int. J. Quantum Chem. 102: 1069–1079.

Kotcherlakota, R., A.K. Barui, S. Prashar, M. Fajardo, D. Briones, A. Rodríguez-Diéguez et al. 2016. Curcumin loaded mesoporous silica: an effective drug delivery system for cancer treatment. Biomater. Sci. 4: 448–459.

Krausz, A.E., B.L. Adler, V. Cabral, M. Navati, J. Doerner, R.A. Charafeddine et al. 2015. Curcumin-encapsulated nanoparticles as innovative antimicrobial and wound healing agent. Nanomedicine. 11: 195–206.

Kurd, S.K., N. Smith, A. Van Voorhees, A.B. Troxel, V. Badmaev, J.T. Seykora et al. 2008. Oral curcuminoid C3 complex® in the treatment of moderate to severe psoriasis vulgaris: a prospective clinical trial. J. Am. Acad. Dermatol. 58: 625–631.

Kunnumakkara, A.B., P. Anand and B.B. Aggarwal. 2008. Curcumin inhibits proliferation, invasion, angiogenesis and metastasis of different cancers through interaction with multiple cell signaling proteins. Cancer Lett. 269: 199–225.

Lampe, V. and J. Milobedzka. 1913. Studien über curcumin. Ber. Dtsch. Chem. Ges. 46: 2235–2240.

Leong-Škorničková, J., O. Šída, S. Wijesundara and K. Marhold. 2008. On the identity of turmeric: the typification of *Curcuma longa* L. (Zingiberaceae). Bot. J. Linnean Soc. 157: 37–46.

Li, X., H. Yuan, C. Zhang, W. Chen, W. Cheng, X. Chen et al. 2016. Preparation and *in-vitro/in-vivo* evaluation of curcumin nanosuspension with solubility enhancement. J. Pharm. Pharmacol. 68: 980–988.

Lim, T.K. [ed.]. 2012. Edible Medicinal and Non-Medicinal Plants—Vol. 12. Springer International Publishing, Switzerland.

Lin, C.C., H.-Y. Lin, H.-C. Chenc, M.-W. Yua and M.-H. Lee. 2009. Stability and characterization of phospholipid-based curcumin-encapsulated microemulsions. Food Chem. 116: 923–928.

Liu, C.H. and F.Y. Chang. 2011. Development and characterization of eucalyptol microemulsions for topic delivery of curcumin. Chem. Pharm. Bull. 59: 172–178.

Liu, C.H., F.Y. Chang and D.K. Hung. 2011. Terpene microemulsions for transdermal curcumin delivery: effects of terpenes and cosurfactants. Colloids Surf. B. 82: 63–70.

Liu, L., L. Sun and Q. Wu. 2013. Curcumin loaded polymeric micelles inhibit breast tumor growth and spontaneous pulmonary metastasis. Int. J. Pharm. 443: 175–182.

Liversidge, G.G., K.C. Cundy, J.F. Bishop and D.A. Czekai. 1992. Surface modified drug nanoparticles. U.S. Patent. # US5145684A.

Liversidge, G.G. and K.C. Cundy. 1995. Particle size reduction for improvement of oral bioavailability of hydrophobic drugs: I. Absolute oral bioavailability of nanocrystalline danazol in beagle dogs. Int. J. Pharm. 125: 91–97.

Maheshwari, R.K., A.K. Singh, J. Gaddipati and R.C. Srimal. 2006. Multiple biological activities of curcumin: a short review. Life Sci. 78: 2081–2087.

Mahmoud, E.A. and A.A. Elbessoumy. 2013. Effect of curcumin on hematological, biochemical and antioxidants parameters in *Schistosoma Mansoni* infected mice. International Journal of Sciences. 3: 1–14.

Mahmoud, E.A. and A.A. Elbessoumy. 2014. Hematological and biochemical effects of curcumin in *Schistosoma Mansoni* infested mice. Assiut. Vet. Med. J. 60: 184–195.

Mahmud, M., A. Piwoni, N. Filipczak, M. Janicka and J. Gubernator. 2016. Long-circulating curcumin-loaded liposome formulations with high incorporation efficiency, stability and anticancer activity towards pancreatic adenocarcinoma cell lines *in vitro*. PLoS One. 11: e0167787.

Mancarella, S., V. Greco, F. Baldassarre, D. Vergara, M. Maffia and S. Leporatti. 2015. Polymer-coated magnetic nanoparticles for curcumin delivery to cancer cells. Macromol. Biosci. 15: 1365–1374.

Mandeville, J.S., E. Froehlich and H.A. Tajmir-Riahi. 2009. Study of curcumin and genistein interactions with human serum albumin. J. Pharm. Biomed. Anal. 49: 468–474.

Manju, S. and K. Sreenivasan. 2012. Gold nanoparticles generated and stabilized by water soluble curcumin-polymer conjugate: Blood compatibility evaluation and targeted drug delivery onto cancer cells. J. Colloid. Interface Sci. 368: 144–151.

Margar, S.N. and N. Sekar. 2016. Red and near-infrared emitting bis-coumarin analogues based on curcumin framework-synthesis and photophysical studies. J. Photochem. Photobiol. A Chem. 327: 58–70.

Martins, C.V.B., D.L. da Silva, A.T.M. Neres, T.F. Magalhães, G.A. Watanabe, L.V. Modolo et al. 2009. Curcumin as a promising antifungal of clinical interest. Journal of Antimicrob. Chemother. 63: 337–339.

Masferrer, J.L., B.S. Zweifel, P.T. Manning, S.D. Hauser, K.M. Leahy, W.G. Smith et al. 1994. Selective inhibition of inducible cyclooxygenase 2 *in vivo* is antiinflammatory and nonulcerogenic. Proc. Natl. Acad. Sci. USA. 91: 3228–3232.

Mazzacuva, F., C. Sinico and A.R. Bilia. 2010. Enhanced skin permeation of verbascoside-cyclodextrin complex loaded into liposomes. Planta Med. 76: P228.

Mazzacuva, F., B. Isacchi, M. Bergonzi, S. Arrigucci, S. Fallani, A. Novelli et al. 2011a. Development and evaluation of conventional and PEGylated curcumin liposomes, absorption and tissue distribution studies in mice. Planta Med. 77: PK15.

Mazzacuva, F., G. Guidelli, M. Bergonzi and A.R. Bilia. 2011b. Enhanced water solubility and stability of curcumin by microinclusion in natural and semi-synthetic cyclodextrins. Planta Med. 77: PK9.

Metselaar, J.M. and G. Storm. 2005. Liposomes in the treatment of inflammatory disorders. Expert. Opin. Drug Deliv. 2: 465–476.

Mimche, P.N., D. Taramelli and L. Vivas. 2011. The plant-based immunomodulator curcumin as a potential candidate for the development of an adjunctive therapy for cerebral malaria. Malar. J. 10(Suppl 1): S10.

Morais, E.R., K.C. Oliveira, L.G. Magalhãesc, É.B.C. Moreira, S. Verjovski-Almeida and V. Rodrigues. 2013. Effects of curcumin on the parasite *Schistosoma mansoni*: A transcriptomic approach. Mol. Biochem. Parasitol. 187: 91–97.

Mounce, B.C., T. Cesaro, L. Carrau, T. Vallet and M. Vignuzzi. 2017. Curcumin inhibits Zika and chikungunya virus infection by inhibiting cell binding. Antiviral Res. 142: 148–157.

Moussaoui, N., M. Cansell and A. Denizot. 2002. Marinosomes, marine lipid-based liposomes: physical characterization and potential application in cosmetics. Int. J. Pharm. 242: 361–365.

Mukherjee, S., S. Mukherjee, S. Bhattacharya and S.P. Sinha Babu. 2017. Surface proteins of *Setaria cervi* induce inflammation in macrophage through Toll-like receptor 4 (TLR4)-mediated signalling pathway. Parasite Immunol. 39: e12389.

Muller, R.H., C. Jacobs and O. Kayser. 2001. Nanosuspensions as particulate drug formulations in therapy. Rationale for development and what we can expect for thefuture. Adv. Drug Deliv. Rev. 47: 3–19.

Muñoz, M.J., L. Murcia and M. Segovia. 2011. The urgent need to develop new drugs and tools for the treatment of Chagas disease. Expert Rev. Anti Infect. Ther. 9: 5–7.

Nagajyothi, F., L.M. Weiss, D.L. Silver, M.S. Desruisseaux, P.E. Scherer, J. Herz et al. 2011. *Trypanosoma cruzi* utilizes the host low density lipoprotein receptor in invasion. PLoS Negl. Trop. Dis. 5: e953.

Nagajyothi, F., D. Zhao, L.M. Weiss and H.B. Tanowitz. 2012 Curcumin treatment provides protection against *Trypanosoma cruzi* infection. Parasitol. Res. 110: 2491–2499.

Nair, R., K.S. Arun Kumar, K. Vishnu Priya and M. Sevukarajan. 2011. Recent advances in solid lipid nanoparticle based drug delivery systems. J. Biomed. Sci. Res. 3: 368–384.

Nayak, A., P. Gayen, P. Saini, N. Mukherjee and S.P. Babu. 2012. Molecular evidence of curcumin-induced apoptosis in the filarial worm *Setaria cervi*. Parasitol. Res. 111: 1173–86.

NCI. National Cancer Institute, 1996. Clinical development plan: curcumin. J. Cell. Biochem. Suppl. 26: 72–85.

Ndjonka, D., L.N. Rapado, A.M. Silber, E. Liebau and C. Wrenger. 2013. Natural products as a source for treating neglected parasitic diseases. Int. J. Mol. Sci. 14: 3395–3439.

Negi, P.S., G.K. Jayaprakasha, L. Jagan, M. Rao and K.K. Sakariah. 1999. Antibacterial activity of turmeric oil: a byproduct from curcumin. J. Agric. Food Chem. 47: 4297–4300.

Nekkanti, V., V. Vabalaboina and R. Pillai. 2012. Drug nanoparticles—An overview. pp. 111–132. *In*: A.A. Hashim [ed.]. The Delivery of Nanoparticles. InTech, Rijeka, Croatia.

Nelson, K.M., J.L. Dahlin, J. Bisson, J. Graham, G.F. Pauli and M.A. Walters. 2017. The essential medicinal chemistry of curcumin. J. Med. Chem. 60: 1620⁻1637.

Nirmala, C. and R. Puvanakrishnan. 1996. Protective role of curcumin against isoproterenol induced myocardial infarction in rats. Mol. Cell Biochem. 159: 85–93.

Nose, M., T. Koide, Y. Ogihara, Y. Yabu and N. Ohta. 1998. Trypanocidal effects of curcumin *in vitro*. Biol. Pharm. Bull. 21: 643–645.

Novaes, R.D., E.C. Santos, M.C. Cupertino, D.S.S. Bastos, J.M. Oliveira, T.V. Carvalho et al. 2015. *Trypanosoma cruzi* infection and benznidazole therapy independently stimulate oxidative status and structural pathological remodeling of the liver tissue in mice. Parasitol. Res. 114: 2873–2881.

Novaes, R.D., M.V. Sartini, J.P. Rodrigues, R.V. Gonçalves, E.C. Santos, R.L. Souza et al. 2016. Curcumin enhances the anti-*Trypanosoma cruzi* activity of benznidazole-based chemotherapy in acute experimental Chagas disease. Antimicrob. Agents Chemother. 60: 3355–3364.

Ohshiro, M., M. Kuroyanagi and A. Ueno. 1990. Structures of sesquiterpenes from *Curcuma longa*. Phytochem. 29: 2201–2206.

Oliveira, A.S., E. Sousa, M.H. Vasconcelos and M. Pinto. 2015. Curcumin: A natural lead for potential new drug candidates. Curr. Med. Chem. 22: 4196–4232.

Omri, A., Z.E. Suntres and P.N. Shek. 2002. Enhanced activity of liposomal polymyxin B against *Pseudomonas aeruginosa* in a rat model of lung infection. Biochem. Pharmacol. 64: 1407–1413.

Onoda, M. and H. Inano. 2000. Effect of curcumin on the production of nitric oxide by cultured rat mammary gland. Nitric Oxide. 4: 505–515.

Orlando, R.A., A.M. Gonzales, R.E. Royer, L.M. Deck and D.L. Vander Jagt. 2012. A chemical analog of curcumin as an improved inhibitor of amyloid abeta oligomerization. Plos ONE. 7: e31869.

Ortega, V., S. Giorgio and E. de Paula. 2017. Liposomal formulations in the pharmacological treatment of leishmaniasis: a review. J. Liposome Res. 27: 234–248.

Padilla-S. L., A. Rodríguez, M.M. Gonzales, J.C. Gallego-G. and J.C. Castaño-O. 2014. Inhibitory effects of curcumin on dengue virus type 2-infected cells *in vitro*. Arch. Virol. 159: 573–579.

Padmanaban, G. and P.N. Rangarajan. 2016. Curcumin as an adjunct drug for infectious diseases. Trends Pharmacol. Sci. 37: 1–3.

Padmanaban, G. and V.A. Nagaraj. 2017. Curcumin may defy medicinal chemists. ACS Med. Chem. Lett. 8: 274⁻274.

Pan, M.H., T.M. Huang and J.K. Lin. 1999. Biotransformation of curcumin through reduction and glucuronidation in mice. Drug. Metab. Dispos. 27: 486–494.

Parimita, S.P., Y.V. Ramshankar, S. Suresh and T.N. Guru. 2007. Redetermination of curcumin: (1E,4Z,6E)-5-hydroxy-1,7-bis(4-hydroxy-3-methoxyphenyl)hepta-1,4,6-trien-3-one. Acta Cryst. E63: o860–o862.

Patel, V.R. and Y.K. Agrawal. 2011. Nanosuspension: An approach to enhance solubility of drugs. J. Adv. Pharm. Technol. Res. 2: 81–87.

Patravale, V.B., A.A. Date and R.M. Kulkarni. 2004. Nanosuspensions: a promising drug delivery strategy. J. Pharm. Pharmacol. 56: 827–840.

Payton, F., P. Sandusky and W.L. Alworth. 2007. NMR study of the solution structure of curcumin. J. Nat. Prod. 70: 143–146.

Peng, G., U. Tisch, O. Adams, M. Hakim, N. Shehada, Y.Y. Broza et al. 2009. Diagnosing lung cancer in exhaled breath using gold nanoparticles. Nat. Nanotechnol. 4: 669–673.

Pensel, P.E., M.A. Maggiore, L.B. Gende, M.J. Eguaras, M.G. Denegri and M.C. Elissondo. 2014. Efficacy of essential oils of *Thymus vulgaris* and *Origanum vulgare* on *Echinococcus granulosus*. Interdiscipl. Perspect. Infect. Dis. 2014: 1–12.

Pérez-Arriaga, L., M.L. Mendoza-Magaña, R. Cortés-Zárate, A. Corona-Rivera, L. Bobadilla-Morales, R. Troyo-Sanromán et al. 2006. Cytotoxic effect of curcumin on Giardia lamblia trophozoites. Acta Trop. 98: 152–161.

Perkins, S., R.D. Verschoyle, K. Hill, I. Parveen, M.D. Threadgill, R.A. Sharma et al. 2002. Chemopreventive efficacy and pharmacokinetics of curcumin in the min/+ mouse, a model of familial adenomatous polyposis. Cancer Epidemiol. Biomarkers Prev. 11: 535–540.

Peschel, D., R. Koerting and N. Nass. 2007. Curcumin induces changes in expression of genes involved in cholesterol homeostasis. J. Nutr. Biochem. 18: 113–119.

Peters, K., S. Leitzke, J.E. Diederichs, K. Borner, H. Hahn, R.H. Müller et al. 2000. Preparation of a clofazimine nanosuspensions for intravenous use and evaluation of its therapeutic efficacy in murine mycobacterium avium infection. J. Antimicrob. Chemother. 45: 77–83.

Pignatello, R., C. Bucolo, G. Spedalieri, A. Maltese and G. Puglisi. 2002. Flurbiprofen-loaded acrylate polymer nanosuspensions for ophthalmic application. Biomaterials. 23: 3247–3255.

Pinto, J.G., L.C. Fontana, M.A. de Oliveira, C. Kurachi, L.J. Raniero and J. Ferreira-Strixino. 2016. *In vitro* evaluation of photodynamic therapy using curcumin on Leishmania major and *Leishmania braziliensis*. Lasers Med. Sci. 31: 883–890.

Pol, A., M. Bergers and J. Schalkwijk. 2003. Comparison of antiproliferative effects of experimental and established antipsoriatic drugs on human keratinocytes, using a simple 96-well-plate assay. *In Vitro* Cell Dev. Biol. Anim. 39: 36–42.

Potroz, M.G. and N.-J. Cho. 2015. Natural products for the treatment of trachoma and chlamydia trachomatis. Molecules. 20: 4180–4203.

Priyadarsini, K. 2009. Photophysics, photochemistry and photobiology of curcumin: Studies from organic solutions, bio-mimetics and living cells. J. Photochem. Photobiol. C: Photochem. Rev. 10: 81–95.

Priyadarsini, K.I. 2014. The chemistry of curcumin: from extraction to therapeutic agent. Molecules. 19: 20091–20112.

Rabinow, B.E. 2004. Nanosuspensions in drug delivery. Nat. Rev. Drug Discov. 3: 785–796.

Rachmawati, H., L. Al Shaal, R.H. Müller and C.M. Keck. 2013. Development of curcumin nanocrystal: physical aspects. J. Pharm. Sci. 102: 204–214.

Raghav, N. 2015. Curcumin: a magnificent therapeutic molecule from traditional medicinal system. Biochem. Anal. Biochem. 4: e160.

Rajabloo, M., S.H. Hosseini and F. Jalousian. 2012. Morphological and molecular characterization of *Echinococcus granulosus* from goat isolates in Iran. Acta Trop. 123: 67–71.

Rahimi, M., P. Valeh-e-Sheyda and H. Rashidi. 2017. Statistical optimization of curcumin nanosuspension through liquid anti-solvent precipitation (LASP) process in a microfluidic platform: Box-Behnken design approach. Korean J. Chem. Eng. 34: 3017–3027.

Rao, C.V. 2007. Regulation of COX and LOX by curcumin. Adv. Exp. Med. Biol. 595: 213–26.

Rassi, A. Jr, A. Rassi and J.A. Marin-Neto. 2010. Chagas disease. Lancet. 375: 1388–1402.

Raul, S.K., G.K. Padhy, J.P. Charly and K.V. Kumar. 2012. An *in-vitro* evaluation of the anthelmintic activity of rhizome extracts of *Zingiber officinalis*, *Zingiber zerumbet* and *Curcuma longa*, a comparative study. J. Pharm. Res. 5: 3813–3814.

Raveendran, R., G. Bhuvaneshwar and C.P. Sharma. 2013. *In vitro* cytotoxicity and cellular uptake of curcumin-loaded fluronic/Polycaprolactone micelles in colorectal adenocarcinoma cells. J. Biomater. Appl. 27: 811–827.

Ravindranath, V. and N. Chandrasekhara. 1980. Absorption and tissue distribution of curcumin in rats. Toxicology. 16: 259–265.

Ravindranath, V. and N. Chandrasekhara. 1981a. *In vitro* studies on the intestinal absorption of curcumin in rats. Toxicology. 20: 251–257.

Ravindranath, V. and N. Chandrasekhara. 1981b–1982. Metabolism of curcumin-studies with [3H]curcumin. Toxicology. 22: 337–344.

Roughley, P.J. and D.A. Whiting. 1973. Experiments in the biosynthesis of curcumin. J. Chem. Soc., Perkin Trans. 1: 2379–2388.

Ruslay, S., F. Abas, K. Shaari, Z. Zainal, H. Sirat, D.A. Israf et al. 2007. Characterization of the components present in the active fractions of health gingers (*Curcuma xanthorrhiza* and *Zingiber zerumbet*) by HPLC–DAD–ESIMS. Food Chem. 104: 1183–1191.

Sahoo, S.K. and V. Labhasetwar. 2003. Nanotech approaches to drug delivery and imaging. Drug Discov. Today. 8: 1112–1120.

Saleheen, D., S.A. Ali, K. Ashfaq, A.A. Siddiqui, A. Agha and M.M. Yasinzai. 2002. Latent activity of curcumin against leishmaniasis *in vitro*. Biol. Pharm. Bull. 25: 386–9.

Saxena, S., P. Dravid, I.H. Sheikh, N.A. Kaushal and D.C. Kaushal. 2016. Antigenic characterization of embryo stage of *Setaria cervi*. Int. J. Life Sci. Biotechnol. Pharma. Res. 5: 7–13.

Schiffelers, R.M., G. Storm and I.A. Bakker-Woudenberg. 2001. Host factors influencing the preferential localization of sterically stabilized liposomes in *Klebsiella pneumoniae*-infected rat lung tissue. Pharm. Res. 18: 780–787.

Selvan, M.T., K.G. Thomas and K. Manojkumar. 2002. Ginger (*Zingiber officinale* Rosc.). pp. 110–131. *In:* H.P. Singh, K. Sivaraman and M.T. Selvan [eds.]. Indian Spices—Production and Utilization. Coconut Development Board, India.

Shang, Y.J., X.L. Jin, X.L. Shang, J.J. Tang, G.Y. Liu, F. Dai et al. 2010. Antioxidant capacity of curcumin-directed analogues: Structure–activity relationship and influence of microenvironment. J. Food Chem. 119: 1435–1442.

Sharma, R.A., H.R. McLelland, K.A. Hill, C.R. Ireson, S.A. Euden, M.M. Manson et al. 2001. Pharmacodynamic and pharmacokinetic study of oral *Curcuma* extract in patients with colorectal cancer. Clin. Cancer Res. 7: 1894–1900.

Sharma, R.A., S.A. Euden, S.L. Platton, D.N. Cooke, A. Shafayat, H.R. Hewitt et al. 2004. Phase I clinical trial of oral curcumin: biomarkers of systemic activity and compliance. Clin. Cancer Res. 10: 6847–6854.

Sharma, R.A., A.J. Gescher and W.P. Steward. 2005. Curcumin: the story so far. Eur. J. Cancer. 41: 1955–68.

Sharma, R.A., W.P. Steward and A.J. Gescher. 2007. Pharmacokinetics and pharmacodynamics of curcumin. Adv. Exp. Med. Biol. 595: 453–470.

Shishu, M.M. 2010. Comparative bioavailability of curcumin, turmeric, and Biocurcumax™ in traditional vehicles using non-everted rat intestinal sac model. J. Funct. Foods. 2: 60–65.

Shoba, G., D. Joy, T. Joseph, M. Majeed, R. Rajendran and P.S. Srinivas. 1998. Influence of piperine on the pharmacokinetics of curcumin in animals and human volunteers. Planta Med. 64: 353–356.

Siles-Lucas, M., A. Casulli, R. Cirilli and D. Carmena. 2018. Progress in the pharmacological treatment of human cystic and alveolar echinococcosis: Compounds and therapeutic targets. PLoS Negl. Trop. Dis. 12: e0006422.

Singh, R., A. Mehta, P. Mehta and K. Shukla. 2011. Anthelmintic activity of rhizome extracts of *Curcuma longa* and *Zingiber officinale* (*Zingiberaceae*). Int. J. Pharm. Pharm. Sci. 3: 236–237.

Singh, D.K., R. Jagannathan, P. Khandelwal, P.M. Abraham and P. Poddar. 2013. *In situ* synthesis and surface functionalization of gold nanoparticles with curcumin and their antioxidant properties: An experimental and density functional theory investigation. Nanoscale. 5: 1882–1893.

Snow, J.M. 1995. *Curcuma longa* L (Zingiberaceae). Protocol J. Botan. Med. 1: 43–46.

Song, M.Y., J.Y. Yim, J.M. Yim, I.J. Kang, H.W. Rho, H.S. Kim et al. 2011a. Use of curcumin to decrease nitric oxide production during the induction of antitumor responses by IL-2. J. Immunother. 34: 149–164.

Song, Z., R. Feng and M. Sun. 2011b. Curcumin-loaded PLGA-PEG-PLGA triblock copolymeric micelles: Preparation, pharmacokinetics and distribution *in vivo*. J. Colloid Interface Sci. 354: 116–123.

Stano, P., S. Bufali, C. Pisano, F. Bucci, M. Barbarino, M. Santaniello et al. 2004. Novel camptothecin analogue (gimatecan)-containing liposomes prepared by the ethanol injection method. J. Liposome Res. 14: 87–109.

Steigerwalt, R., M. Nebbioso, G. Appendino, G. Belcaro, G. Ciammaichella, U. Cornelli et al. 2012. Meriva®, a lecithinized curcumin delivery system, in diabetic microangiopathy and retinopathy. Panminerva Med. 54: 11–16.

Subudhi, B.B., C. Soma, M. Priyadarsee and K. Abhishek. 2018. Current strategies for inhibition of Chikungunya infection. Viruses. 10: 235.

Sugiyama, Y., S. Kawakishi and T. Osawa. 1996. Involvement of the β-diketone moiety in the antioxidative mechanism of tetrahydrocurcumin. Biochem. Pharmacol. 52: 519–525.

Sun, A., M. Shoji, Y.J. Lu, D.C. Liotta and J.P. Snyder. 2006. Synthesis of EF24-tripeptide chloromethyl ketone: a novel curcumin-related anticancer drug delivery system. J. Med. Chem. 49: 3153–3158.

Sundaryono, A., A. Nourmamode, C. Gardrat, S. Grelier, G. Bravic, D. Chasseau et al. 2003. Studies on the photochemistry of 1,7-diphenyl-1,6-heptadiene-3,5-dione, a non-phenolic curcuminoid model. Photochem. Photobiol. Sci. 2: 914–920.

Sweet, M.J. and I. Singleton. 2011. Silver nanoparticles: a microbial perspective. Adv. App. Microbiol. 77: 115–133.

Thakur, A., S. Manohar, C.E. Vélez Gerena, B. Zayas, V. Kumar, S.V. Malhotra et al. 2014. Novel 3,5-bis(arylidene)-4-piperidone based monocarbonyl analogs of curcumin: anticancer activity evaluation and mode of action study. Med. Chem. Commun. 5: 576–586.

Tiwari, B., R. Pahuja, P. Kumar, S.K. Rath, K.C. Gupta and N. Goyala. 2017. Nanotized curcumin and miltefosine, a potential combination for treatment of experimental visceral leishmaniasis. Antimicrob. Agents Chemother. 61: e01169–16.

Toda, S., T. Miyase, H. Arichi, H. Tanizawa and Y. Takino. 1985. Natural antioxidants. III. Antioxidative components isolated from rhizome of *Curcuma longa* L. Chem. Pharm. Bull. 33: 1725–1728.

Tønnesen, H.H., J.K. Gerard and B. van Henegouwen. 1986. Studies on curcumin and curcuminoids VIII. Photochemical stability of curcumin. Z. Lebensm. Unters. Forsch. 183: 116–122.

Tønnesen, H.H., H. de Vries, J. Karlsen and G.B. van Henegouwen. 1987. Studies on curcumin and curcuminoids. IX: Investigation of the photobiological activity of curcumin using bacterial indicator systems. J. Pharm. Sci. 76: 371–373.

Tønnesen, H.H., M. Masson and T. Loftsson. 2002. Studies of curcumin and curcuminoids. XXVII. Cyclodextrin complexation: solubility, chemical and photochemical stability. Int. J. Pharm. 244; 127–135.

Vathsala, P.G., C. Dende, V.A. Nagaraj, D. Bhattacharya, G. Das, P.N. Rangarajan et al. 2012. Curcumin-arteether combination therapy of *Plasmodium berghei*-infected mice prevents recrudescence through immunomodulation. PLoS One. 7: e29442.

Velayudhan, K.C., V.K. Muralidharan, V.A. Amalraj, P.L. Gautam, S. Mandal and D. Kumar. 1999. Curcuma genetic resources. pp. 149. *In*: Scientific Monograph No.4, National Bureau of Plant Genetic Resources, New Delhi, India.

Venkatesan, P. and M.N.A. Rao. 2000. Structure-activity relationships for the inhibition of lipid peroxidation and the scavenging of free radicals by synthetic symmetrical curcumin analogues. J. Pharm. Pharmacol. 52: 1123–1128.

Vogel, H.A. and J. Pelletier. 1815. Chemische untersuchung der gilbwurzel (kurkume). J. Pharma. 7: 20.

von Rhein, C., T. Weidner, L. Henß, J. Martin, C. Weber, K. Sliva et al. 2016. Curcumin and Boswellia serrata gum resin extract inhibit chikungunya and vesicular stomatitis virus infections *in vitro*. Antiviral Res. 125: 51–57.

Wachter, B., M. Syrowatka, A. Obwaller and J. Walochnik. 2014. *In vitro* efficacy of curcumin on *Trichomonas vaginalis*. Wien. Klin. Wochenschr. 126: S32–36.

Wahlstrom, B. and G. Blennow. 1978. A study on the fate of curcumin in the rat. Acta Pharmacol. Toxicol. 43: 86–92.

Wang, Y.-J., M.-H. Pana, A.-L. Cheng, L.-I. Lin, Y.-S. Ho, C.-Y. Hsieh et al. 1997. Stability of curcumin in buffer solutions and characterization of its degradation products. J. Pharm. Biomed. Anal. 15: 1867–1876.

Wang, Z., M.H.M. Leung, T.W. Kee and D.S. English. 2010. The role of charge in the surfactant-assisted stabilization of the natural product curcumin. Langmuir. 26: 5520–5526.

Wang, P., L. Zhang, H. Peng, Y. Li, J. Xiong and Z. Xu. 2013. The formulation and delivery of curcumin with solid lipid nanoparticles for the treatment of on non-small cell lung cancer both *in vitro* and *in vivo*. Mater. Sci. Eng. C Mater. Biol. Appl. 33: 4802–4808.

Wink, M. 2012. Medicinal plants: a source of anti-parasitic secondary metabolites. Molecules. 17: 12771-12791.

Wright, J.S. 2002. Predicting the antioxidant activity of curcumin and curcuminoids. Theochem (J. Mol. Struct.) 591: 207–217.

Wu, X., J. Xu, X. Huang and C. Wen. 2011. Self-microemulsifying drug delivery system improves curcumin dissolution and bioavailability. Drug Dev. Ind. Pharm. 37: 15–23.

Yallapu, M.M., M. Jaggi and S.C. Chauhan. 2010a. Scope of nanotechnology in ovarian cancer therapeutics. J. Ovarian Res. 3: 19.

Yallapu, M.M., B.K. Gupta, M. Jaggi and S.C. Chauhan. 2010b. Fabrication of curcumin encapsulated PLGA nanoparticles for improved therapeutic effects in metastatic cancer cells. J. Colloid Interface Sci. 351: 19–29.

Yallapu, M.M., S.F. Othman, E.T. Curtis, B.K. Gupta, M. Jaggi and S.C. Chauhan. 2011. Multi-functional magnetic nanoparticles for magnetic resonance imaging and cancer therapy. Biomaterials. 32: 1890–1905.

Yang, K.Y., L.C. Lin, T.Y. Tseng, S.C. Wang and T.H. Tsai. 2007. Oral bioavailability of curcumin in rat and the herbal analysis from *Curcuma longa* by LC-MS/MS. J. Chromatogr. B Analyt. Technol. Biomed Life Sci. 853: 183–189.

Yang, Y., J.S. Jiang, B. Du, Z.F. Gan, M. Qian and P. Zhang. 2009. Preparation and properties of a novel drug delivery system with both magnetic and biomolecular targeting. J. Mater. Sci. 20: 301–307.

Yue, G.G., B.C. Chan, P.M. Hon, M.Y. Lee, K.P. Fung, P.C. Leung et al. 2010. Evaluation of *in vitro* anti-proliferative and immunomodulatory activities of compounds isolated from *Curcuma longa*. Food Chem. Toxicol. 48: 2011–2020.

Yue, G.G., S.W. Cheng, H. Yu, Z.S. Xu, J.K. Lee, P.M. Hon et al. 2012. The role of turmerones on curcumin transportation and P-glycoprotein activities in intestinal Caco-2 cells. J. Med. Food. 15: 242–252.

Zhang, X., Y. Tian, H. Zhang, A. Kavishwar, M. Lynes, A.-L. Brownell et al. 2015. Curcumin analogues as selective fluorescence imaging probes for brown adipose tissue and monitoring browning. Sci. Rep. 5: 13116.

Chapter **15**

An Overview of Helminthiasis
Current State and Future Directions

Leyla Yurttaş,* Betül Kaya Çavuşoğlu, Derya Osmaniye and
Ulviye Acar Çevik

Introduction

Parasitic infections and infestations are widespread all over the world especially in underdeveloped and developing countries. It has been estimated that 25% of the world population is infected with helminths which cause damage in human health as well as economic losses in the endemic regions. These diseases can be controlled by vector control, improvement of nutrition, sanitation and folk health conditions. In recent years, new parasitic infections are emerging due to travel, immigration, immunosuppressive drug use and the spread of AIDS cases (Balcıoğlu et al. 2004, Akyön-Yılmaz 2012).

Helminthiasis, also known as worm infection, is a systemic or intestinal parasitic disease that is common in tropical and subtropical regions and is a major health problem especially in third world countries. Particularly, intestinal infestations caused by helminths may not be noticed and herewith severe infestations can cause serious anemia and sometimes even death (Akgün et al. 2013). Helminth parasites are complex multicellular organisms which and can be divided into the subgroups of nematodes, cestodes, trematodes and filarians according to the zoological classification. The most common helminths in humans are *Ascaris lumbricoides, Trichuris trichiura, Necator americanus Ancylostoma duodenale, Strongyloides stercoralis Brugia* sp., *Wuchereria bancrofti, Onchocerca volvulus, Taenia solium, Taenia saginata, Hymenolepis nana, Hymenolepis disminuta* and *Dypylidium caninum* (Romero-Benavides et al. 2017). Due to variations in their life cycles, structures, developments and resident differentiation on tissues, the diseases caused by helminths and the applied chemotherapy may vary. Only a limited number of drugs have been approved in the last decades and is used against helminths infections. Clinically used antihelminthic drugs are mebendazole, pyrantel, diethylcarbamazepine, ivermectin, oxamniquine, niclosamide, metrifonate and levamisole. Mostly, single or multiple dose drug administration respond to helminthiasis positively, but the currently available antihelminthic drugs are not sufficient in case of treating helminth-related systemic infections such as echinococcosis and toxocariasis (trichinosis, cysticercosis and filariasis) (Korkmaz 2012). Moreover, the development of resistance to these drugs has been reported for almost all the species of worms which infect

Anadolu University, Faculty of Pharmacy, Department of Pharmaceutical Chemistry, 26470, Eskişehir TURKEY.
* Corresponding author: lyurttas@anadolu.edu.tr

humans in cities and also for all the species that infect animals in rural farms (Ramos et al. 2016). Thereby, studies to discover new and more effective drugs to improve physicochemical properties of clinically used antihelminthics as well as to develop treatments in combination with existing chemotheurapeutic drugs, such as antiprotozoans, anticancers and antibacterials, have been carried out, in addition to surgery or other interventions (prophylaxis). Besides, targeting helminth proteins and inhibiting their enzymes are recent focused approaches for the treatment of all kinds of worm-related diseases.

Helminths

The word "*Helminth*" derives from the Greek word ἕλμινς (hélmins) which indicates an intestinal worm. The helminths are invertebrates with long, flat or round bodies and their size ranges from a few millimeters to 35 centimeters. Humans are important for helminths because they are definitive hosts in their complex life cycle (Linquist and Cross 2017, Ayi 2007).

Helminths are divided into two major phyla; (1) the platyhelminths (also recognized as flatworms) which include the trematodes (also recognized as flukes) and the cestodes (also recognized as the tapeworms) and (2) the nemathelminths or nematodes (known as roundworms) which include the major intestinal worms (also recognized as soil transmitted helminths) and the filarial worms that cause lymphatic filariasis (LF) and onchocerciasis (Rana and Misra-Bhattacharya 2013, Kim et al. 2016).

Helminth parasitism remains an underestimated problem to humans in most of the developing countries. Soil transmitted helminths like hookworm and *Ascaris* infect more than 24% of the world's population, and 200 million of people are affected with schistosomiasis according to the World Health Organization. Helminths can affect humans, animals and plants, with an estimated number of between 75,000 and 300,000 species.

In general, the most common parasitic infections in humans are helminthic infections. The highest prevalence happens in tropical and subtropical countries where there is poor sanitation, lack of formal education, contaminated food and lack of fresh water supply. However, some infections also occur in the developed world because of organic farming, the popularity of raw or uncooked foodstuff, and the import of diseases to northern/western countries where the diagnostic accuracy may be poor due to a lack of profound knowledge. Social, economic, genetic and nutritional factors play an important role in hookworm infections (Linquist and Cross 2017, Ayi 2007).

Platyhelminths and nematodes infecting humans exhibit similar anatomical features as they have common physiological needs and functions. Helminths surfaces include external and, for some helminths, internal structures. The cuticle or tegument is the outer covering of helminths. The external surfaces of parasitic helminths, called the tegument in trematodes and cestodes and the cuticle in nematodes, is highly modified in a stage- and species-dependent manner for the varied environments occupied by these organisms. The external surfaces of helminths play roles in regulation, locomotion and excretion of osmotic and electrochemical gradients. This tegument may be rough or slight and it defends the worm from digestion in the host intestinal tract and from the external environment. Other important roles of external surfaces include the regulation of the transport of water, inorganic ions, and nutrients (Thompson and Geary 2003, Gamble et al. 1995).

Nematode (roundworms)

Nematodes or roundworms constitute the phylum Nematoda (or Nemata) and belong to the superphylum Ecdysozoa (which include insects and moulting animals). Freshwater, terrestrial and marine environments are the habitats of nematodes.

Estimates of nematode variety range between 0.5 and 1 million species, with only about 26,000 species presently described. Among these species, nearly 14,000 are free-living, invertebrate and plant-associated nematodes. Nematodes are mostly small in size (plant parasites and free-living are 0.25 mm to 12 mm long, animal parasites are 5 cm to 10 meters long) and have a colourless body. These features make them extraordinary organisms.

Nematodes have a complete digestive system. They possess a pharynx, a lumen and the intestine, which is a simple tube made of single cell thickness on the peritoneal side and internally lined with microvilli. They do not have any respiratory system. Circumcentric nerve rings generally constitute the nervous system. Reproductive organs are posterior to the middle of the nematode in female. Proliferation in nematodes is asexual by paedogenesis. Examples of nematotic parasites are described in Table 1 (Khan 2015, Abate 2017, Zarowiecki and Berriman 2015, Linquist and Cross 2017).

Filariasis is a parasitic disease caused by an infection with roundworms of the Filarioidea type common in tropical regions, coastal areas and island in the Pacific, Africa, America, and Asia. The disease has been seen in people aged 10 years and older. Filarial worms cause a variety of clinical pathologies depending on the degree of host immune reaction. The subcutaneous filariasis causes skin itching, scratch marks and papules until the entire skin is dry and tempered. Filariases that affect the skin are caused by *Wuchereria bancrofti*, *Brugia malayi*, *Loa loa*, and *Onchocerca volvulus* (Kalungi et al. 2017).

Dracunculus medinensis is a nematode that causes drancunculosis, a parasitic dermatosis that has affected humans for centuries. *Dracunculus medinensis* known as "Guinea worm" has been reported in 17 African countries including Yemen, Saudi Arabia, India and Pakistan. The disease remains asymptomatic till completion of puberty and fertilisation of female larvea during incubation period. Systemic infections may cause cutaneous manifestations as well as diarrhea, nausea, dyspnea, syncope and vomiting. The diagnosis of drancunculosis can be favored by worm extrusion from a skin lesion or wet smears showing motile larvae on microscopy (Linquist and Cross 2017, Assimwe and Hengge 2017).

Ascaris is a genus of parasitic nematode worms known as the "small intestinal roundworms" and it is usually prevalent in tropical regions and expected to infect 1/4 of the world's population. Most patients who are infected with *Ascaris lumbricoides* are asymptomatic. When the number of worms increases, abdominal pain and intestinal obstruction may occur. Pulmonary symptoms, including cough, shortness of breath, and haemoptysis may occur and eosinophilic pneumonia may develop due to larval migration to lungs. These round worms live in the lumen of the small intestine for 2 years and release a large number of eggs with faeces. The eggs bear rhabditiform larvae that hatch in the intestine. The resulting larvae are released, burrow through the intestinal wall and enter the hepatic circulation via capillaries and lymphatics. The larvae migrate via the right side of the heart into the lungs and then up the bronchial tree, where they are swallowed and make their way to the duodenum where they mature into adults after several months. (Kim et al. 2010, Linquist and Cross 2017).

Trichinellosis is a parasitic disease caused by *Trichinella spiralis*, a nematode typically recognized as the "pork worm". The parasitic cycle has two stages recognized as intestinal (or enteral) phase and systemic or parenteral phase. This cycle covers a period of several days to weeks. Infections occur due to consumption of infected meat including coiled larvae 0.7–1.1 mm long. Trichinellosis may be a serious disease for elderly people, especially due to severe complications such as myocarditis or encephalitis

Table 1. Examples of nematode parasites.

Nematode	Common name	Host tissue	Symptoms
Enterobius vermicularis	Pinworm	Intestine	Rash in anal area
Ascaris lumbricoides	Giant worm	Intestine	Anaemia and intestinal blockage
Necator americanus	Hookworm	Intestine	Iron-deficiency anemia develops, accompanied by intermittent abdominal pain, loss of appetite
Ancylostoma duodenale	Hookworm	Intestine	Iron-deficiency anemia develops, accompanied by intermittent abdominal pain, loss of appetite
Wuchereria bancrofti	Filarial worm	Blood and tissues	Fever and chills, elephantiasis (swelling of the limbs), pain in the swollen areas
Dracunculus medinensis	Guinea worm	Tissue	Skin itch, scratch marks and papules
Brugia malayi	Guinea worm	Blood and tissues	Fever, inflammation and swelling of the lymph nodes, inflammation of the lymphatic vessels

that may result in death (Linquist and Cross 2017, Bruschi and Dupouy-Camet 2014, Dupouy-Camet et al. 2017).

Trematodes (flukes)

Trematodes, commonly referred to as flukes, are a class of worms within the phylum Platyhelminthes. They are internal parasites of molluscs and vertebrates. Most trematodes have a complex life cycle with at least two hosts. The primary host, where the flukes sexually reproduce, is a vertebrate. The intermediate host, in which asexual reproduction occurs, is usually a snail. Food-borne trematodes infect over 10 million people worldwide. Mature trematodes possess a gastro-vascular cavity (gastrodermis) on an internal surface with a single opening that joins both the mouth and the anus (Aeby 2016, Kim et al. 2016, Linquist and Cross 2017, de Oliveira and Neves-Filho 2014).

Liver-lung trematodes infections are frequent in older males and females with a tendency against familial accumulation. The lung flukes of the genus *Paragonimus* are involved in numerous types of human diseases. Humans can be infected with raw, partially cooked or pickled or crab crayfish containing the larval form which penetrate the duodenum and intestinal wall and finally, the peritoneal cavity. Larval forms can penetrate into the diaphragm and reach the pleural space and lung parenchyma, where they turn into adult worms that live in cystic cavities near bronchial passages and produce eggs (Kim et al. 2016).

Schistosomiasis is a disease caused by blood flukes (trematodes) belonging to the genus *Schistosoma*. First described by Theodor Bilharz in the 19th century, schistosomiasis is one of the most common parasitic infections in humans. *S. intercalatum*, *S. mansoni*, *S. japonicum*, *S. haematobium* and *S. mekongi* species are the most common etiologic agents. The World Health Organization (WHO) estimates that more than 200 million people are infected by these parasites, making schistosomiasis the second most destructive parasitic disease after malaria. Schistosomiasis affects a large proportion of children under the age of 14 years. Humans are infected when in contact with schistosoma-infested water. Infection is developed when the cercariae, the larval form of the parasite, penetrates the skin during contact with fresh water while bathing, wading or doing laundry. Eggs, larvae, or antigen-antibody immunecomplex deposits of the *Schistosoma* spp. can settle in any organ or body tissue, including the eyes. The symptoms of human schistosomiasis are mainly due to immune reaction against the invading and migrating larvae and later against the parasite eggs present in the host tissue (Leutscher and Magnussen 2017, Orefice et al. 2016, Kim et al. 2016, Linquist and Cross 2017).

The life cycle of schistosoma worms begins with the release of eggs into the aquatic environment. When the eggs come in contact with the water, the larvae come out and infect the snails (intermediate host for the parasite). In the snail, the larvae divide asexually and turns into sporocysts that form the cercariae. After a few weeks, a large number of cercariae is released from infected snails into the water with a daily circadian rhythm. They can survive 24 hours floating on the water surface after being released from snails. Cercariae can infect humans in 3–5 minutes by penetrating in the skin of people working with or washing infected water through the use of proteolytic enzymes. Parasites remain on the skin for 1–2 days, after which they lose their forked tails and become schistosomes. At the penetration site, an erythematous itchy spot known as cercarial dermatitis occurs. Schistosomes enter capillaries and lymphatic vessels. Migration continues in the venous system and the parasite reaches the lungs. This period leads to a self-limiting subacute disease known as Katayama fever. They start to feed on red blood cells and become adults within 6–8 weeks. In the portal venous system, adult parasites mate and begin to produce eggs. The ovum crosses the vessel wall and reaches the intestine and the lumen of the bladder where is thrown out with the faeces or the urine making the cycle to start again (Sen 2017, de Oliveira and Neves-Filho 2014).

The diagnosis of schistosomiasis is made by analysis of the urine or by rectal biopsy. Serological tests can identify persons who have previously been exposed to schistosomes. The test is more useful for patients in non-endemic regions (Sen 2017, Kim et al. 2016).

Although several mechanisms such as parasitic artery embolization, pulmonary arteriopathy and portopulmonary hypertension are thought to play a role in the pathogenesis, the actual pathogenesis is not yet fully understood. A large number of parasite eggs were seen in the lungs of people who died from this disease so that for a long time pulmonary hypertension (PHT) and right heart failure were thought to be due to the mechanical obstruction caused by parasite eggs. The presence of plexiform lesions and other pathological findings similar to idiopathic pulmonary arterial hypertension (IPAH) was shown in studies performed on the lungs of diseased persons. Thus, schizosoma-associated PAH (S-PAH) was classified by the WHO as group one disease such as connective tissue disease and IPAH (Orefice et al. 2016, Sen 2017).

Schistosomiasis presents separate clinical stages: cercarial dermatitis, acute schistosomiasis syndrome, chronic visceral schistosomiasis and late cutaneous schistosomiasis. Schistosomiasis infections can be prevented only by escaping contact with cercariae-infested water. If water contact is inevitable, clothes to cover skin exposed to contaminated water may provide some security. In addition, *N,N*-diethyl-m-toluamide (DEET), a well-known insect repellent, has been successfully used as topical agent for avoiding skin penetration by *S. mansoni cercariae*. However, DEET efficacy has yet to be confirmed in controlled studies. In the presence of active schistosoma infection, praziquantel, an antihelmintic drug, should be used (da Silva et al. 2017, Leutscher and Magnussen 2017, da Paixão Siqueiraa et al. 2017, Sen 2017).

Cestodes (tapeworms)

Cestodes are a complex group of organisms, usually recognised as tapeworms, having a flat, ribbon-like white to yellowish body consisting of an anterior attachment organ (scolex) and a body (strobila) consisting of a chain of segments called proglottids. Proglottids are essentially packages of eggs which are regularly shed into the environment to infect other organisms. The width and length of tapeworms are different with some worms being several meters long (i.e., *Diphyllobothrium latum* is 2–15 m long, *Taenids* are 1–4 m long), while others can be very small (i.e., *Hymenolepis nana* is 1.5–4 cm long, *H. diminuta* is 1–6 cm long) (Kotra and Dixit 2007).

Cestodes are widespread and can infect all classes of vertebrates on all continents, even if they principally affect populations in resource-poor countries (Beveridge and Jones 2002). Cestodes includes species allocated into two genera of tapeworms: *Diphyllobothriidae* and *Taeniidae*. The family *Taeniidae* consists of two types of worms: *Taenia*, which mainly causes cysticercosis in intermediate hosts, and *Echinococcus*, leading to echinococcosis at the larval stage (Hagg et al. 2008).

Tapeworms are responsible of diseases in humans in either of the two stages of their life cycle: (1) the larval stage which causes symptoms due to the growth of larval cysts in various tissues of a mammalian host, (2) the adult stage which takes place in the intestines, where it causes mild or non-existent clinical manifestations. *Taenia solium* (pork tapeworm), *T. saginata* (beef tapeworm), *Diphyllobotrium latum* (fish tapeworm), and *Hymenolepis nana* are the most commonly known human tapeworms (Machado-Pinto and Laborne 2006). *Taenia solium* (pork tapeworm) and *Taenia saginata* (beef tapeworm) are the most important human pathogens in the genus (Moore and Chiodini 2009). In their adult stage, they are morphologically homogenous. They are commonly flat and large, showing a tape-like morphology often exceeding several meters in length, with a distinctly segmented strobila and a characteristic arrangement of rostellar hooks on their scolex (Moore and Chiodini 2009). The adult form of *Taenia saginata* survives in the human small intestine and can achieve a length of 20 m. Humans are the single ultimate host for *T. saginata* and infections are well-known especially in poor countries. The cows are the intermediate hosts of oncospheres, the larval forms of tapeworms. Oncospheres migrate to the skeletal muscles of cows where they encyst to become 'bladderworms' or cysticercoids. Each of these juveniles remains calm until human eat the uncooked muscle. Once inside the human host, the bladderworm establishes itself by anchoring in the host's digestive tract where it will grow in length and will become an adult tapeworm. Eventually, the tapeworm will produce proglottids which will exit the intestinal tract with other waste material and then burst, releasing the worm's eggs and completing the cycle.

The life cycle of *T. saginata* is very similar to that of *T. solium* except that the eggs of *T. saginata* are not infective to humans. Another important difference is that the intermediate hosts include cattle, buffalo, and reindeer instead of pigs. Humans can act also as secondary hosts.

T. solium spread happens in over 75 countries affecting mostly people in the South Americas, parts of Africa, and Southeast Asia; neurocysticercosis and taeniasis are also diagnosed in Europe and North America, mostly among immigrants (Geerts 2015).

T. solium can cause two separate diseases in the human population: taeniasis, when the human is a primary host; and cysticercosis (a cyst containing an invaginated scolex) when the human is the secondary host (Berman 2012). When the intermediate host ingests a *T. solium* egg, the oncosphere is liberated after its passage through the stomach. After that it penetrates the intestinal wall and is transported through the blood or lymphatics to the muscles where it develops into a cysticercus. Cysticercoids move from the muscle to the brain and they cause cysticercosis, which can be lethal after moving to the brain. The analysis of human faeces is used in the diagnosis of taeniasis. Sedimentation, flotation, and Kato–Katz tests are concentration methods, but they have low sensitivity for Taenia eggs and cannot differentiate between *T. solium* and *T. saginata* taeniasis. In addition to this, serologic tests for a *T. solium* tapeworm stage-specific antibody have been advanced as a research technique (Geerts 2015).

Four species of *Echinococcus* are of public health concern: *E. granulosus, E. vogeli, E. oligarthus* and *E. multilocularis*. Tapeworms of this genus are small in contrast to *T. solium* and *T. saginata*. The adult *E. granulosus* can reach 3–6 mm long and resides in the small bowel of the definitive hosts like dogs and other canids as well as domestic and wild ungulates (Moro and Schantz 2009). *Echinococcus multilocularis* and *Echinococcus granulosus* cause two distinct diseases in humans and animals, namely alveolar echinococcosis (AE) and cystic echinococcosis (CE). In humans, cystic echinococcosis, known as hydatid disease, develops in the liver, followed by the kidneys, lungs, spleen, muscle, soft tissues, bone and brain (Tappe et al. 2010). Hepatic cysts are usually not palpable until 20 cm. In addition, they may cause jaundice and portal hypertension. *E. granulosus* preferentially targets the liver and the lung. Pulmonary hydatid *E. granulosus* cysts are a major public health problem in countries where dogs are used to care for large herds. Approximately 90% of the pulmonary hydatid cysts are solitary, and 10% are associated with a concomitant cyst in the liver (Tappe et al. 2010).

E. multilocularis aggressively invades host tissues via external buds that can be released and metastasise to other organs or tissues, exacerbating the disease and requiring liver transplantation in some patients. Though infection with *E. multilocularis* is less common than *E. granulosus*, it has a greater morbidity and mortality. *E. multilocularis* is a rapidly growing parasite and has invasive characteristic, resulting in rapid dissemination and high mortality (Haque 2013, Webb and Cabada).

Diphyllobothrium is a genus of tapeworms which can cause diphyllobothriasis in humans through consumption of raw or undercooked fish. The principal species causing diphyllobothriasis is *Diphyllobothrium latum*, known as the broad or fish tapeworm, or broad fish tapeworm. *Diphyllobothrium latum* uses humans as a primary host. Most infections are asymptomatic. Stool microscopy for eggs and inspection of stools for the presence of proglottids provides the mainstay of diagnosis, whilst treatment with praziquantel 25 mg/kg as a single dose or niclosamide as a single oral dose of 2 g for adults is effective (Moore and Chiodini 2009, Berman 2012).

Finally, *Hymenolepis nana* (the Greek, "nana", means dwarf) is the most common human tapeworm, particularly in young children. *Hymenolepis nana* is unique in having a direct human life-cycle. Most infections are asymptomatic but symptoms can occur with higher worm burdens. If present, symptoms are mostly nonspecific: abdominal discomfort and, occasionally, diarrhoea and malabsorption (Moore and Chiodini 2009, Thompson 2015).

Anthelminthic Drugs

A few chemotherapeutic drugs are currently used in the treatment of helminthiasis. Most of the antihelminthtic drugs were developed for veterinary use, and later have been used by physicians as effective and broad-spectrum medications for the treatment of worm infections in humans. The drugs currently available are generally effective against helminths settled in the intestines with a single dose treatment (Korkmaz 2012) and allow the removal of local, systemic or developing helminths in the human gastrointestinal system or tissues. Although natural substances isolated from leaves of sagebrush and ferns, pinene derivatives, arecoline, emetine alkaloids and various synthetic compounds such as carbohydrates, naphtaquinones, phenothiazines have been previously used to treat helminthiasis (Vardanyan and Hruby 2006), recent anthelminthic therapy consists of a few number of drugs, as shown in Table 2.

Table 2. Current drugs used in helminthiasis diseases.

Drug	Disease	Drug	Disease
Piperazine (1)	enterobiasis, ascariasis, hookworm infections	Ivermectin (9)	strongyloides, ascariasis, trichuriasis, enterobiasis, cutaneous larva migrans
Diethylcarbamazepine (2)	filariasis	Paromomycin (10)	tapeworm infections
Thiabendazole (3)	strongyloidiasis, trichinosis, visceral larva migrans, cutaneous larva migrans	Levamisole (11)	ascariasis, hookworm infections
Mebendazole (4)	enterobiasis, ascariasis, hookworm infections, ankylostomiasis, trichuriasis, strongyloidiasis, trichocephaliasis, trichostrongyliasis, mixed helminthosis	Pyrantel (12)	enterobiasis, ascariasis, ankylostomiasis, trichostrongyliasis, hookworm infections
Albendazole (5)	enterobiasis, ascariasis, hookworm infections, ankylostomiasis, strongyloidiasis, tapeworm infections, trichuriasis, trichinosis, cutaneous larva migrans	Niclosamide (13)	tapeworm infections, echinostomiasis, fasciolopsiasis, heterophyiasis
Niridazole (6)	schistosomiasis, amebiasis	Bephenium (14)	ankylostomiasis, enterobiasis, trichostrongyliasis, tricocefalosis
Praziquantel (7)	schistosomiasis, tapeworm infections	Metrifonate (15)	schistosomiasis
Oxamniquine (8)	schistosomiasis	Bithionol (16)	fascioliasis, paragonimiasis

In the 1950s, piperazine (1) was first employed as anthelminthic drug and used in the therapy of helminth infections, in particular enterobiasis and ascariasis. Piperazine acts as a weak GABA agonist and leads to a flaccid paralysis of the parasite body muscle. Paralyzed worms are eliminated from the gastrointestinal tract by intestinal peristalsis. Piperazine, synthesized via heating ethanolamine in ammonia at a pressure of 100–250 atm, is contraindicated in patients with epilepsy and patients suffer from liver or kidney deficiency (Holden-Dye and Walker 2007, Abbas and Newsholme 2011, Akgün et al. 2013, Vardanyan and Hruby 2006).

Diethylcarbamazine (2) is a piperazine derivative used in the treatment of filariasis. It is known that diethylcarbamazine interferes with arachidonic acid metabolism of parasites and activates an innate immune response in filarial parasites and host. Diethylcarbamazine is effective against filarial worms of *Brugia malayi*, *Loa loa*, *Wuchereria bancrofti*, *Onchocerca volvulus* and *Mansonella streptocerca*. Diethylcarbamazine, *N,N*-diethyl-4-methylpiperazinecarboxamide, can be easily obtained by acylating

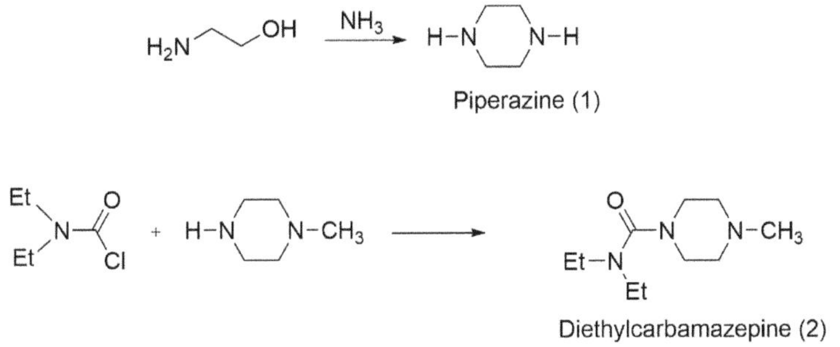

Scheme 1. Synthesis of Piperazine (1) and Diethylcarbamazepine (2).

1-methylpiperazine with diethylcarbamoyl chloride, and it is available as diethylcarbamazine citrate (Vardanyan and Hruby 2006, de Silva et al. 1997, Martin et al. 1997).

Thiabendazole (3) was the first broad spectrum benzimidazole anthelmintic drug and it was introduced in the market 1961. Thiabendazole inhibits the helminth-specific mitochondrial fumarate reductase. The other effect of thiabendazole is to bind selectively to parasite β-tubulin and prevent microtubule formation. Thiabendazole is an effective oral drug and it is generally used in the treatment of strongyloidiasis, trichinosis, visceral larva migrans and cutaneous larva migrans (Martin et al. 1997, Köhler 2001, Finch et al. 2010).

The use of thiabendazole may cause gastrointestinal and neuropsychological side effects including nausea, vomiting, diarrhea, dizziness, tinnitus, drowsiness, erythema multiforme, liver damage, and central nervous system effects. It is contraindicated during pregnancy. Thiabendazole (3) can be synthesized by the reaction between *o*-phenylenediamine and 1,3-thiazole-4-carboxylic acid as shown in Scheme 2 (Vardanyan and Hruby 2006, Shorr et al. 2007, Guerrant et al. 2011).

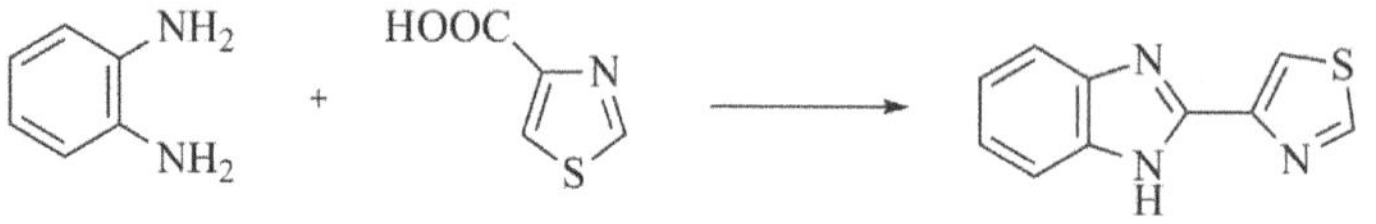

Thiabendazole (3)

Scheme 2. The synthesis of Thiabendazole (3).

Mebendazole (4), a synthetic benzimidazole, is the agent most widely used against enterobiasis, ascariasis, ankylostomiasis, strongyloidiasis, trichocephaliasis, trichostrongyliasis and mixed helminthosis. Mebendazole binds to parasite tubulin thereby inhibiting irreversibly the uptake and utilization of glucose, which causes glucose depletion in the worm. The treatment of massive worm infections with mebendazole is accompanied by abdominal pain and diarrhea. Mebendazole is contraindicated during pregnancy (Vardanyan and Hruby 2006, Kuhlmann and Fleckenstein 2017). Mebendazole can be synthesized by the reaction of 3,4-diaminobenzophenone with *N*-methoxycarbonyl-*S*-methylthiourea according to Scheme 3. The building scaffold 3,4-diaminobenzophenone is synthesized by a three-step procedure. Firstly, the nitration of 4-chlorobenzophenone with nitric acid at a temperature lower than 5°C is resulted in the formation of 4-chloro-3-nitrobenzophenone. In the second step, the obtained intermediate is heated to 125°C in a solution of ammonia in methanol to obtain 4-amino-3-nitrobenzophenone. Finally, the reduction of nitro group in this compound with hydrogen using a palladium on carbon catalyst provides 3,4-diaminobenzophenone. *N*-methoxycarbonyl-*S*-methylthiourea is synthesized by the reaction of methyl chloroformate with S-methylthiourea (Vardanyan and Hruby 2006).

Albendazole (5) is another benzimidazole derivative with a broad spectrum anthelmintic activity against *Ascaris lumbricoides*, *Enterobius vermicularis*, *Ancylostoma duodenale*, *Necator americanus*, *Strongyloides stercoralis*, *Echinococcus* spp. and *T. solium cysticerci*. The mechanism of action is similar to that of mebendazole. Albendazole acts by interfering with glucose uptake and disruption of microtubule aggregation. Abdominal discomfort, nausea, diarrhoea, headaches, dizziness, lassitude and insomnia are common short-term use side effects of albendazole (Kuhlmann and Fleckenstein 2017). In order to synthesize albendazole, the 2-nitro-5-mercaptoaniline is initially reacted with a propyl halide in alkaline medium. After the reduction of the obtained intermediate compound, the reaction with *N*-carbmethoxy-*S*-methylisothiourea gives albendazole (Vardanyan and Hruby 2006) (Scheme 3).

Niridazole (6) is a nitro-thiazole compound used to treat schistosomiasis and amebiasis. The mechanism of action is still not known. One of the hypothesised mechanisms of action of niridazole involves the inhibition of phosphorylase activation, which causes the depletion of glycogen reserves in worms. Another possible mechanism could be the inhibition of spermatogenesis of parasites (Akgün et al. 2013, Vardanyan and Hruby 2006). To synthesize niridazole, the 2-amino-5-nitrothiazole is reacted with 2-chloroethylisocyanate to obtain an intermediate disubstituted urea. This latter compound is heated to yield niridazole via an intramolecular *N*-alkylation reaction (Vardanyan and Hruby 2006) (Scheme 3).

Synthesis of mebendazole

3,4-diaminobenzophenone

N-methoxycarbonyl-*S*-methylthiourea

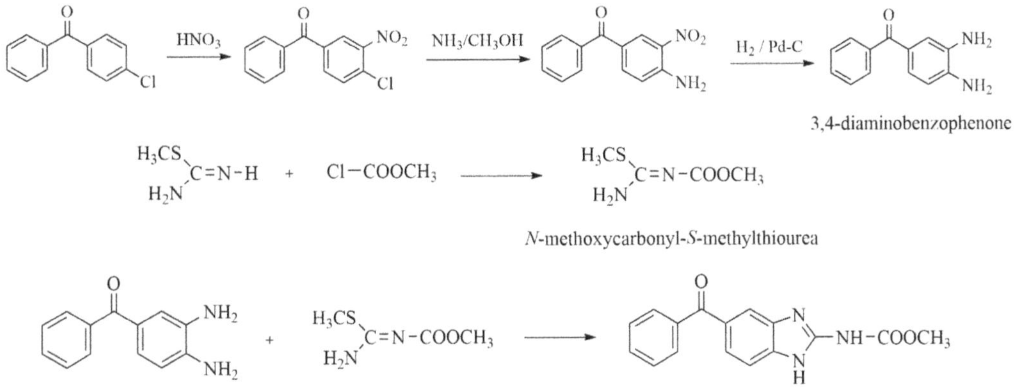

Mebendazole (4)

Synthesis of albendazole

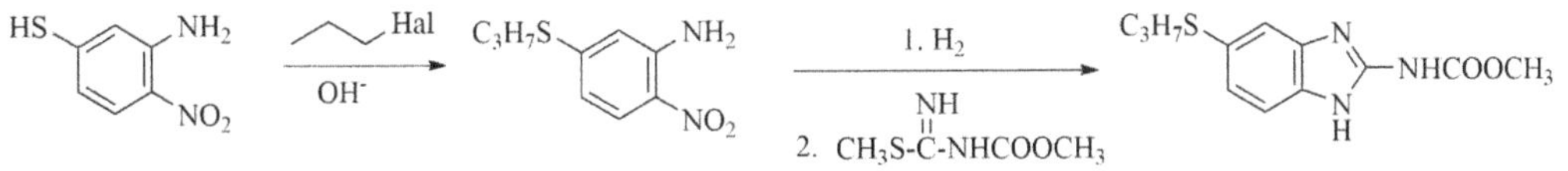

Albendazole (5)

Synthesis of niridazole

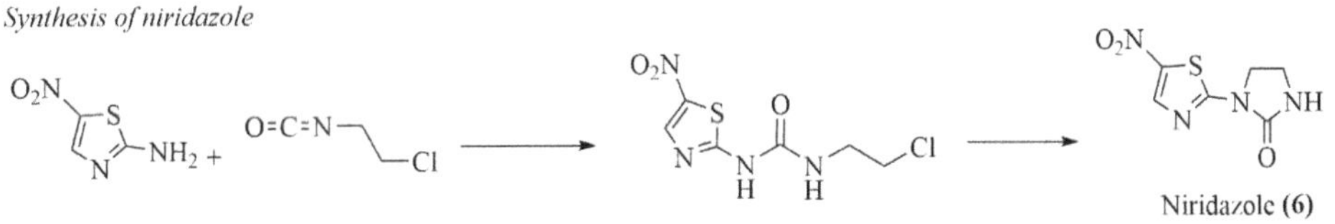

Niridazole (6)

Scheme 3. The synthesis of Mebendazole (4), Albendazole (5) and Niridazole (6).

Praziquantel (7) is a highly effective broad-spectrum agent which is used for the control of schistosomiasis and some species of cestodes and trematodes. Praziquantel is the drug of choice in the therapy of *Shistosoma mansoni, S. haematobium, S. japonicum, S. intercalatum, S. mecongi* and *Taenia solium*. The antihelminth action of praziquantel has not been fully elucidated yet, however considerable research assumes that its activity is due to the disruption of calcium homeostasis. As a result, increasing permeability of the helminth membrane to monovalent and bivalent cations, mainly Ca^{2+}, causes contractions and spastic paralysis of the worm. The side effects include abdominal pain, bloody diarrhoea, dizziness, nausea, headache, pruritus, lassitude and drowsiness. Praziquantel is a pregnancy category B drug (Vardanyan and Hruby 2006, Siqueira et al. 2017, Posey and Stauffer 2007). The synthesis of praziquantel is reported in Scheme 4. Isoquinoline is reacted with a mixture of cyclohexanecarbonyl chloride/potassium cyanide. The obtained product is reduced by hydrogen over Raney nickel. After the acylation of the reduced compound with chloroacetyl chloride, praziquantel is synthesized with the heating of chloroacetyl derivative in the presence of diethylamine via intramolecular alkylation reaction (Vardanyan and Hruby 2006).

Oxamniquine (8) is a tetrahydroquinoline derivative used in the treatment of worm infections. Oxamniquine is effective against *Schistosoma mansoni* at all stages, from acute toxaemic to chronic and complicated infections. Besides, it has no effect on *S. haematobium* and *S. japonicum*. Its mode of action is to shift worms from the mesenteric veins to the liver and thereby cause their death. The adverse effects of the oxamniquine are similar to praziquantel and commonly include headache, dizziness, drowsiness, and abdominal pain (Akgün et al. 2013). In the synthesis of oxamniquine, 2,6-dimethylquinoline is chlorinated to give 2-chloromethyl-6-methylquinoline. After replacing the chlorine with isopropylamine, the heterocyclic

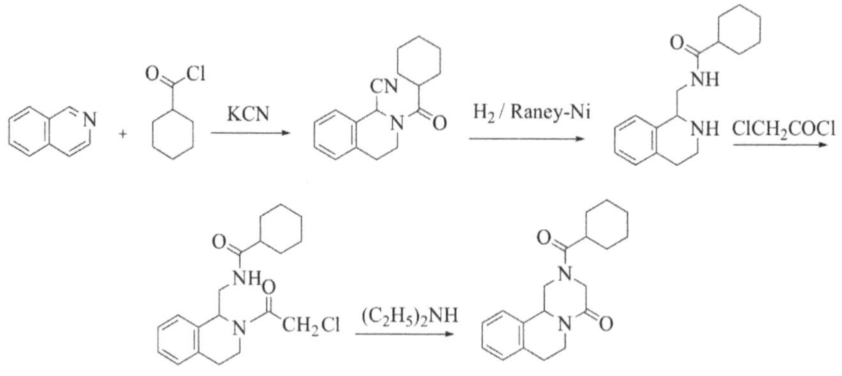

Scheme 4. The synthesis of Praziquantel (**7**).

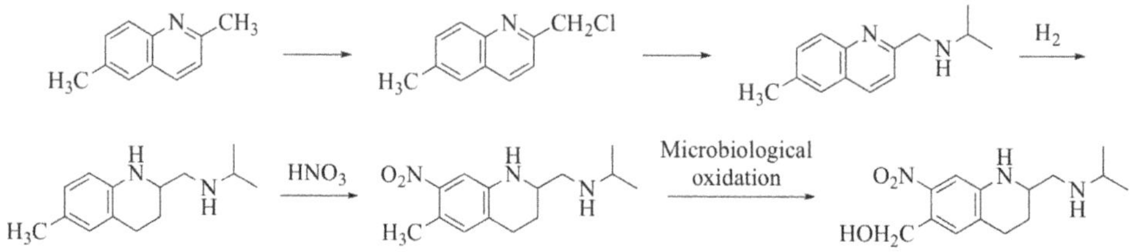

Scheme 5. The synthesis of Oxamniquine (**8**).

quinoline ring is reduced via catalytic hydrogenation. Finally, nitration and microbiologically oxidation of the methyl group with *Aspergillus sclerotium* afford oxamniquine (Vardanyan and Hruby 2006) (Scheme 5).

Ivermectin (**9**) is a mixture of two macrocyclic lactone isomers, namely 22,23-dihydroavermectin B_{1a} and 22,23-dihydroavermectin B_{1b}, derived from avermectin, a naturally occurring compound generated as fermentation product by *Streptomyces avermitilis*. Ivermectin can be obtained by catalytic reduction of avermectin. In 2015, William C. Campbell and Satoshi Ōmura were awarded the Nobel Prize in Physiology or Medicine for discovering the natural compounds avermectins, which showed to be highly effective against a broad spectrum of parasitic worm infections. The discovery of the avermectin family of compounds, from which ivermectin is chemically derived, started in Japan, where Ōmura isolated avermectins from the bacterium *Streptomyces avermitilis* and sent them to the research team led by Campbell at the Merck Therapeutic Research Institute in Rahway, New Jersey. Campbell's team purified avermectins from the bacterial cultures sent by Ōmura and later discovered the synthetic derivative ivermectin which showed greater potency and lower toxicity than avermectin. Ivermectin was finally introduced in the market in 1981 by Campbell's team (https://www.nature.com/collections/xgntcpxznb, Callaway and Cyranoski 2015). Ivermectin is the most effective drug in the treatment of onchocerciasis and lymphatic filariasis. Ivermectin is preferred to diethylcarbamazepine in the treatment of *Oncocerca volvulus* since it causes less inflammation. The drug also has activity against *Strongyloides*, *Ascaris*, *Trichuris* and *Oxyuris* infections. Ivermectin acts as antihelminthic drug by blocking the glutamate-gated chloride ion channels in the worm nervous system and therefore producing paralysis of the parasite. Side effects of ivermectin treatments include pruritus, oedema, rash, fever, headache and tender lymphadenopathy (Akgün et al. 2013, Kuhlmann and Fleckenstein 2017).

Paromomycin (**10**) is an aminoglycoside antibiotic isolated from strains of *Streptomyces*, with activity against gram-negative and various gram-positive bacteria. The taenicidal activity of paromomycin was discovered by chance during amoebiasis treatments in the 1960s. Paromomycin is the third drug of choice, after niclosamide and praziquantel, in the therapy of *Taenia saginata*, *T. solium*, *Hymenolepis nana* and

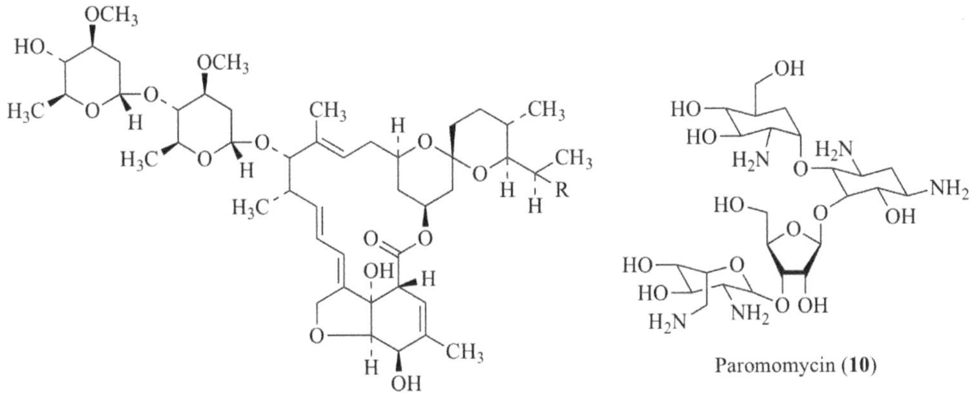

Paromomycin (**10**)

Ivermecitn (**9**)
R= CH_3 22,23-Dihydroavermectin B $_{1b}$
R= C_2H_5 22,23-Dihydroavermectin B $_{1a}$

Scheme 6. Structure of Ivermectin (**9**) and Paramomycin (**10**).

Diphyllobothrium latum infections. The most common side effect of paromomycin is diarrhoea (Akgün et al. 2013).

Levamisole (**11**) is a large-spectrum anthelmintic agent that is effective against ascardiasis and hookworm infections. It is a nicotinic receptor agonist and lead to spastic paralysis. The side effects of levamisole are mild and include nausea, headache, dizziness, skin rash and gastrointestinal disturbance. For the synthesis of levamisole, styrene oxide is initially reacted with ethanolamine followed by subsequent replacement of the hydroxyl groups using thionyl chloride to give 2-chloro-*N*-(2-chloroethyl)-2-phenylethan-1-amine. Acidic hydrolysis followed by reaction with thiourea led to a thiazolidine ring. The reaction of the latter molecule with thionyl chloride and alkaline treatment affords the racemic tetramizol, which is in turn separated into its dextro- and levo-isomers. Levamisole is the levo isomer of tetramizol (Akgün et al. 2013).

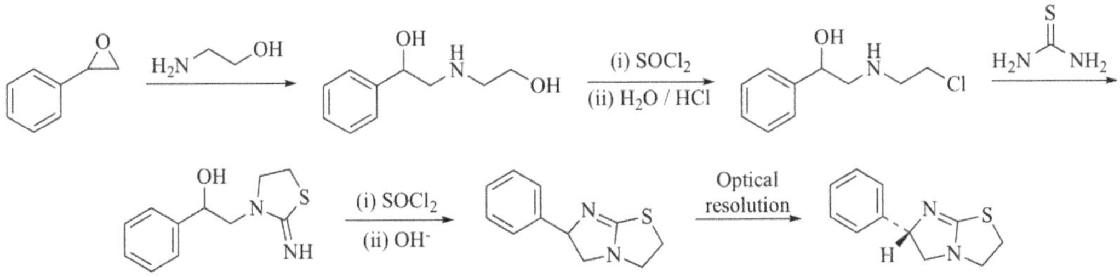

Tetramisol
(rasemic form)

Levamisole (**11**)

Scheme 7. The synthesis of Levamisole (**11**).

Pyrantel (**12**) is a broad-spectrum agent that was originally developed as a veterinary anthelmintic. It has a wide range of activity in humans for *Ascaris*, *Oxyuris*, *Ancylostoma*, *Necator* and *Trichostrongylus* infections. The drug acts by binding cholinergic receptors which leads to inhibition of neuromuscular transmission in the parasite, resulting in spastic muscle paralysis. It is used as the treatment of choice for *Enterobius vermicularis*, *Ascaris lumbricoides*, *Ancylostoma duodenale*, hookworm, *Moniliformis moniliformis*, *Necator americanus* and *Trichostrongylus* spp. Pyrantel should not be given with piperazine because piperazine antagonizes the effect of pyrantel in worm muscle cells. Pyrantel is synthesised via the Knoevangel condensation of thiophen-2-carboxaldehyde and cyanoacetic acid to give 3-(2-thienyl)-acrylonitrile which in turn undergoes acidic hydrolysis to afford 3-(2-thienyl)acrylamide.

The reaction of the latter compound with propansulfone gives an iminoester which is then reacted with *N*-methyltrimethylenediamine to afford pyrantel (Akgün et al. 2013, Vardanyan and Hruby 2006, Kuhlmann and Fleckenstein 2017).

Niclosamide (13) is a salicylamide derivative antihelmintic drug that has been used for nearly half a century as effective treatment of *Diphyllobothrium latum, D. caninum, Hymenolepis nana, Taenia saginata* and *T. solium*, as well as *Echinostoma* spp., *Fasciolopsis buski* and *Heterophyes heterophyes* infections. The antihelmintic action of niclosamide is due to the inhibition of mitochondrial oxidative phosphorylation and glucose and oxygen uptake in tapeworms. The reaction of 5-chlorosalisilic acid with 2-chloro-4-nitroaniline in the presence of phosphorus trichloride affords niclosamide, as shown in Scheme 10. The side effects of the drug are rare and include nausea, vomiting and abdominal pain (Vardanyan and Hruby 2006, Kuhlmann and Fleckenstein 2017).

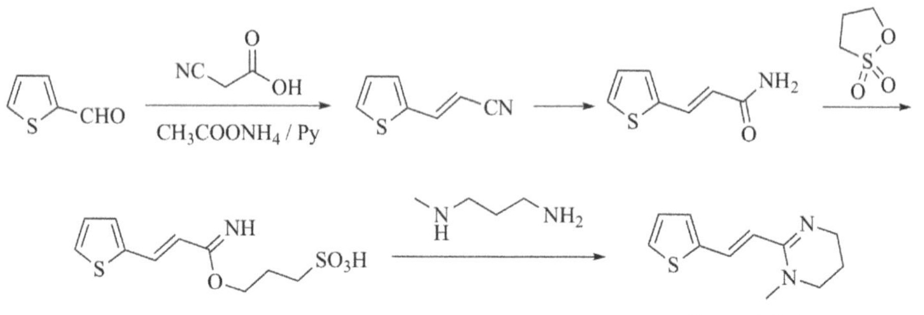

Scheme 8. Synthesis of Pyrantel (**12**).

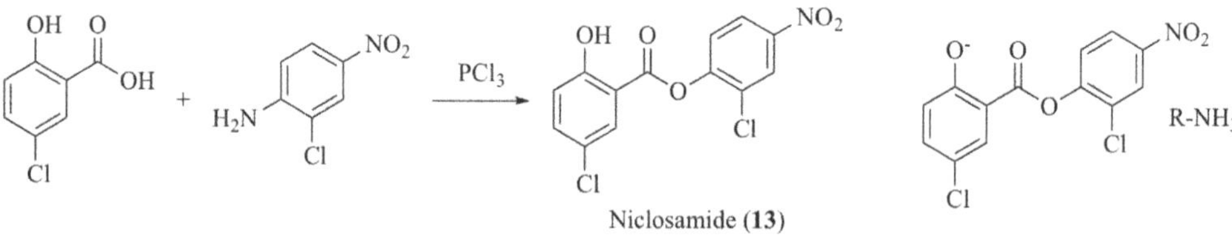

Scheme 9. Synthesis of Niclosamide (**13**).

Niclosamide is an insoluble molecule in water and this causes a decrease in its activity and efficiency and a problem in dose determination. Niclosamide has been prepared as dodecan and hexadecane ammonium salt derivatives to improve its water-solubility. The lipophilic moiety is supposed to hold on to the surface of parasites and their larvae biomembranes, thus leading to biomembrane degradation, penetration of host digestive juice into parasites and finally death of the worms (Galkinaa et al. 2014).

Bephenium (14) is a quaternary ammonium derivative effective in the treatment of ascariasis, ankylostomiasis, enterobiasis, trichostrongyliasis and tricocefalosis. It is a cholinergic agonist resulting in paralysis of the parasite musculature. For the synthesis of bephenium, sodium phenolate and 2-dimethylaminoethylchloride are first reacted to give *N*-(2-phenoxyethyl)dimethylamine which is then treated with benzyl chloride. The resulting ammonium compound is reacted with the sodium salt of 3-hydroxy-2-naphthoic acid to afford bephenium (Vardanyan and Hruby 2006).

Metrifonate (15), originally developed as an insecticide, is an alternative drug for the therapy of urinary schistosomiasis including *Schistosoma haematobium* and *S. mansoni*. It is an organophosphate inhibitor of acetylcholinesterase. Side effects include nausea, vomiting, vertigo, headache, lethargy, abdominal pain and diarrhea. It has largely been replaced by praziquantel as primary therapy. Metrifonate is made by the condensation of dimethyl phosphite with 2,2,2-trichloroacetaldehyde (Akgün et al. 2013, Kuhlmann and Fleckenstein 2017).

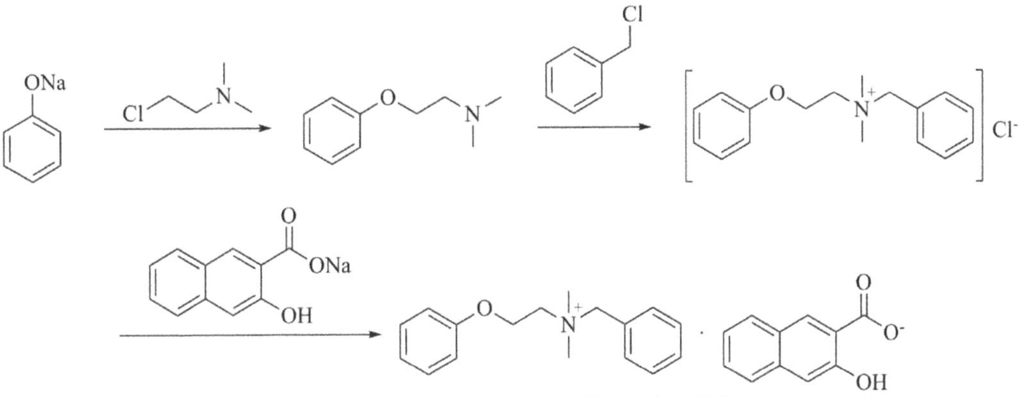

Bephenium (**14**)

Scheme 10. Synthesis of Bephenium (**14**).

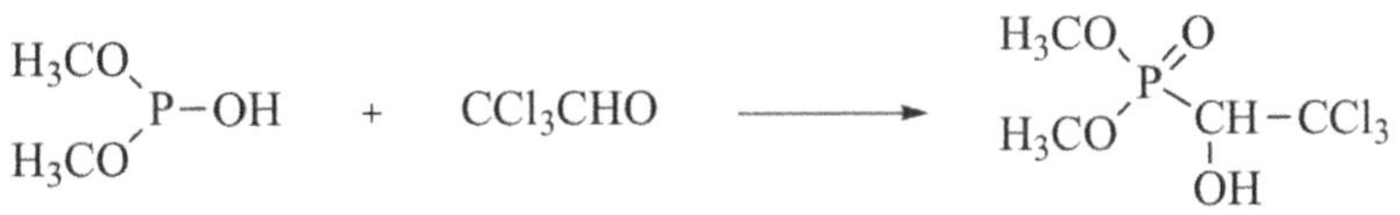

Metrifonate (**15**)

Scheme 11. Synthesis of Metrifonate (**15**).

Bithionol (**16**) is a chlorinated bisphenol and the drug of choice in the treatment of humans infected with *Fasciola hepatica*. It is an alternative drug to praziquantel in the therapy of paragonimiasis. Its mode of action is poorly understood. Side effects include anorexia, abdominal pain, nausea, vomiting, headache, dizziness, diarrhoea, urticaria and proteinuria. Bithionol is made from 2,4-dichlorophenol via reaction with sulphur chloride in the presence of aluminium chloride (Vardanyan and Hruby 2006, Kuhlmann and Fleckenstein 2017).

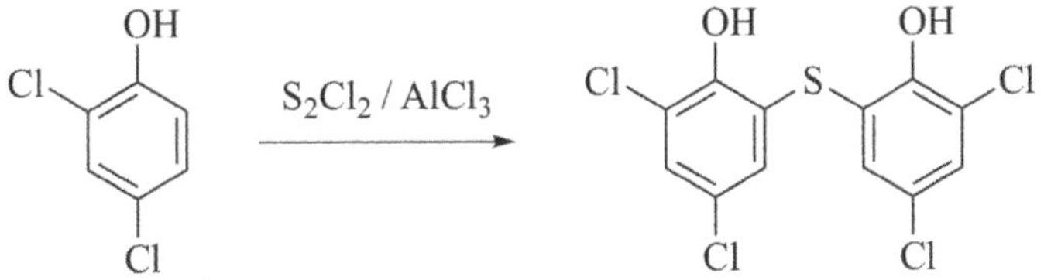

Bithionol (**16**)

Scheme 12. Synthesis of Bithionol (**16**).

The drugs mentioned above have been used in public health since 1950s. These drugs have been used on people suffering from different types of helminthiasis at various doses. Recently accepted antihelminthic drug therapy according to single dose administration is shown in Table 3.

Besides the treatment being applied at single dose, double and triple combinations of the different drugs have being implemented. Mebendazole, albendazole and pyrantel pamoate triple combination is administered against enterobiasis, ancylostomiasis, necatoriasis diseases. Niclozamide and praziquantel combination is used in the treatment of taeniazis and diphyllobothriasis whereas mebendazole and pyrantel pamoate double combination is used for the treatment of ascariasis (Akgün 2013). Co-administration of ivermectin, albendazole and praziquantel was also determined safe in areas infected with lymphatic filariasis, soil-transmitted helminthiasis and schistosomiasis (Mohammed et al. 2008).

Table 3. The single dose antihelminthic drug therapy recommended by WHO and cure percentage rates (Krolewiecki et al. 2013).

Drug	Dose	*Strongyloides stercoralis*	*Ascaris lumbricoides*	Hookworms	*Trichuris trichiura*
Albendazole	400 mg	–	88–98.4	78.4–100	10–52.7
Mebendazole	500 mg	–	95–96.5	22.9	19–36
Ivermectin	200 µg/kg	56.6–68.1	78.4–94.2	–	35.1–44.3
Pyrantel	10 mg/kg	–	88	31	28.1
Levamisole	2.5 mg/kg or 80 mg	–	91.5	10–38.2	9.6
Albendazole/Ivermectin	400 mg/ 200 µg/kg	56.6–68.1	78.4–100	78.4–100	38–79.6
Mebendazole/Ivermectin	500 mg/ 200 µg/kg	56.6–68.1	22.9	22.9	55.1–96.7

Development of Novel Antihelminthic Drugs

In addition to existing therapies, new molecular targets have been recently studied to overcome the difficulties encountered in chemotherapeutic treatments due to resistance and tolerance development. Three novel strategies for the discovery of antiparasitic drugs were developed. The first is to treat animals with parasites and then measure the changes in parasite burdens. The second is to evaluate the viability and behavior of parasites in culture or model organism. This strategy was used in discovery of benzimidazole antihelminthics. The last strategy is based on molecular biology and high throughput screening using phenotypic or whole-organisms to define new specific protein targets (Geary et al. 2015).

New antihelminthic drugs recently developed are emodepside (**17**), monepantel (**18**), derquantel (**19**), tribendimin (**20**) and nitazoxanide (**21**) (Scheme 13). Emodepside (**17**) is a semi-synthetic derivative obtained from fungus *Mycelia sterilia*. It was administered in several *in vitro* and *in vivo* studies against various nematodes (Olliaro et al. 2011). Monepantel (**18**) (*S*-enantiomer) (MOP) is an amino-acetonitrile synthetic derivative. It was discovered in 2008 and approved in the market in 2010. MOP is a broad spectrum

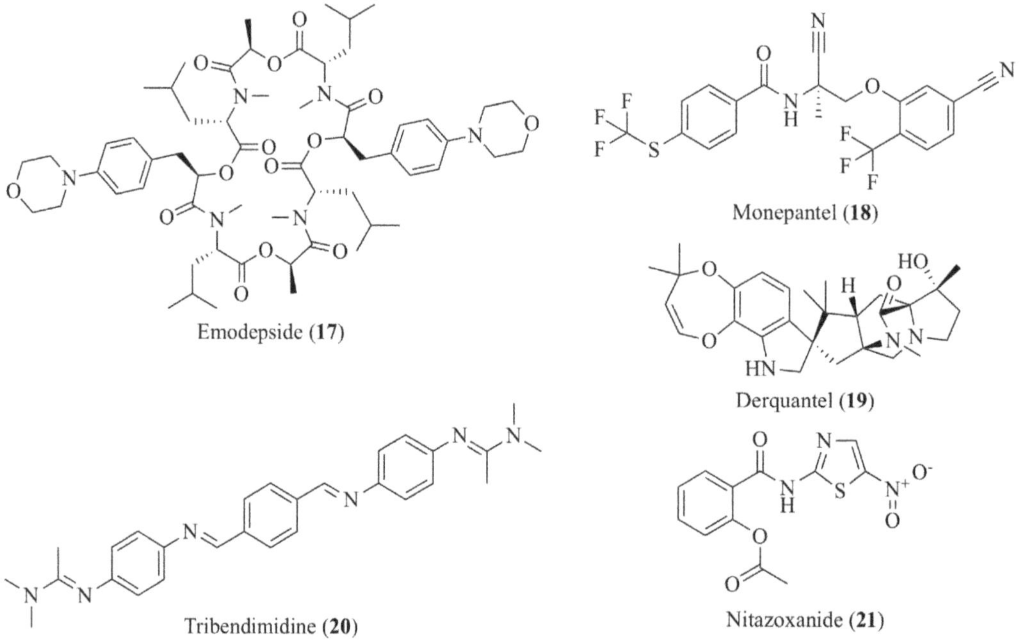

Emodepside (**17**)

Monepantel (**18**)

Derquantel (**19**)

Tribendimidine (**20**)

Nitazoxanide (**21**)

Scheme 13. New antihelminthic drugs recently developed.

antihelminthic active against gastrointestinal nematodes of sheep, including adults and larvae of the most important species. Its effectiveness is determined against nematode strains resistant to benzimidazoles, levamisole, macrocyclic lactones and closantel. MOP has a mode of action based on nematode-specific clade of nicotinic acetylcholine receptor (nAChR) that causes hypercontraction leading to the paralysis and death of adult nematodes (Lecova et al. 2014). Nitazoxanide **(21)**, a salicylic acid derivative, possesses protozoacide, anthelmintic and anti-bacterial properties. It was described previously for cryptosporidiosis and giardiasis, afterwards it was determined that this drug is effective against a number of non-protozoan parasites, including the intestinal tapeworm *Hymenolepis nana*. Nitazoxanide has variable efficacies against the soil transmitted nematodes, including *Ascaris lumbricoides* and *Trichuris trichiura* (Ashour et al. 2016). Derquantel **(19)** is also a semi-synthetic natural spyroindole derivative produced from *Penicillium paraherquei*. Because of its short plasma life and efficacy against only fourth stage larvae (L4) of *some helminths*, it is used in combination with abamectin (Bartram et al. 2012). Tribendimidine **(20)** is an old molecule which has been recently identified with antinematode activity. Tribendimidine is safe and has good clinical activity against *Ascaris* and hookworms. It is reported to act as an L-subtype nAChR agonist like levamisole and pyrantel (Hu et al 2019, Dzhafarov and Vasilevich 2014).

Recently, 1-(1*H*-benzimidazol-2-yl)-3-aryl-2-propen-1-one compounds **(22)** were investigated and found to be effective against helminth infections such as classical drugs ivermectin and febendazole. The 2-arylpropenonebenzimidazole structure was considered as a new potential pharmacophore for nematicidal activity (Quattara et al. 2011).

The combination of the antimalarial agent artemisinin **(23)** and naphthoquine phosphate **(24)** has been studied in *Schistosoma mansoni* and it gave promising results. Oral administration of this combination in single dose of 400 mg/kg resulted in the death of all female worms before depositing eggs, complete absence of eggs in hepatic and intestinal tissues and reduction of total and female worm burdens by 93.36% and 94.17% (El-Beshbishi et al. 2013, Taman and Azab 2014).

Dibenzo[b,e]oxepin-11(6*H*)-one derivatives **(25)** have been also evaluated as promising lead oxygenated tricyclic compounds in the search for novel anthelmintic drugs (Scoccia et al. 2017).

Some isoquinoline derivatives **(26)** were also found to be active antihelmintic agent (Surikova et al. 2017).

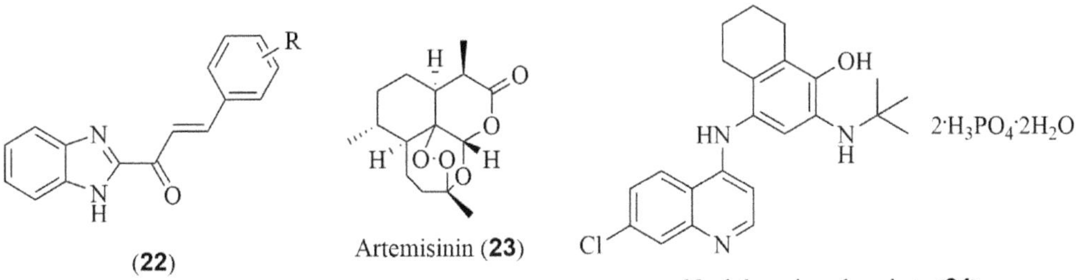

(22)   Artemisinin **(23)**   Naphthoquine phosphate **(24)**

Scheme 14. Structures of benzimidazole derivatives **(22)**, artemisinin **(23)** and naphthoquine phosphate **(24)**.

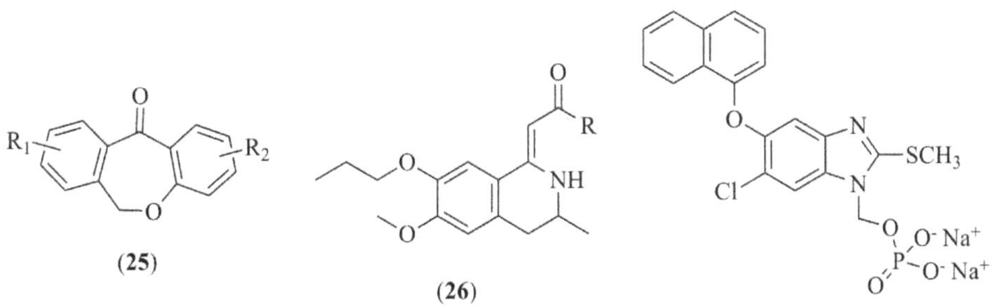

(25)   **(26)**   **(27)**

Scheme 15. Novel Antihelminthic drugs.

Finally, studies for increasing water solubility of the currently existing drugs have been recently carried out, affording successful results. The fasciolicidal agent triclabendazole has been converted into the bioisosteric phosphate salt **(27)** to increase its water-solubility (Flores-Ramos et al. 2014).

As an alternative therapy, tetracycline antibiotics such as doxycycline, are used against filariasis as second line treatment (Werren et al. 2008, Hoerauf et al. 2008). Doxycycline proved to be effective against *W. bancrofti* with a strong macrofilaricidal activity. It causes reduction in plasma levels of VEGF-C/sVEGFR-3 which provides amelioration of supratesticular dilated lymphatic vessels and this physiological condition allows the healing of the lymphatic filariasis (Debrah et al. 2006).

It has been suggested that the nicotinic acetylcholine receptor (nAChR) subunit ACR-16 from *Ascaris suum* could be an attractive new anthelmintic drug target with 'resistance-busting' properties for therapeutic drug development (Abongwa 2017).

Also, targeting excretory/secretory proteins is a remarkable way for therapeutic evaluation in helminth infections (Garg and Ranganathan 2012).

A recent approach in antihelminthic therapy is to evaluate the changes in RNA levels which could play a role in drug resistance. However, there is not enough information in cestodes to date. In a recent study, the miRNA repertoires of *T. crassiceps* and *T. solium* have been identified and the expression profile of *T. crassiceps cysticerci* with and without drug treatment has been analysed. Also, miRNA-targeted genes have been predicted (Perez et al. 2017).

Enzyme inhibition evaluation is a prominent approach for a lot of diseases as well as in helminthiasis. NADH-fumarate reductase (NFRD) has been recognized as a novel target for treating helminthiasis besides cancer chemotherapy (Liu et al. 2016).

Vaccines for helminthiasis are not currently available for human use. However, recent advances in vaccination with recombinant helminth antigens have been accomplished against nematode parasites of animals. Numerous vaccine antigens are being identified for a wide range of helminth parasite species (Hewitson and Maizels 2014).

Finally, as an alternative strategy, probiotics of the genera *Lactobacillus*, *Enterococcus*, and *Bifidobacterium* have been evaluated for the control of schistosomiasis, trichinellosis, ascariasis, and toxocariasis. Probiotics are suggested to stimulate the host immune system and to enhance the secretion of antimicrobial substances, like bacteriocins and organic acids (i.e., lactic, acetic, and butyric acid) causing larvicidal activity (Reda 2018).

References

Abate, B.A., M.J. Wingfield, B. Slippers and B.P. Harley. 2017. Commercialisation of entomopathogenic nematodes: should import regulations be revised? Biocontrol. Sci. Technol. 27: 149–168.

Abbas, A. and W. Newsholme. 2009. Diagnosis and recommended treatment of helminth infections. Drug Review Worms. 31–40.

Abbas, A. and W. Newsholme. 2011. Diagnosis and recommended treatment of helminth infections. Prescriber. 22: 56–64.

Abongwa, M. 2017. Potential New Drug Targets and Therapeutic Approaches for Parasitic Nematode Infections. Ph.D Thesis, Iowa State University, Iowa, USA.

Aeby, G.S. 2016. Porites trematodiasis. pp. 387. *In*: C.M. Woodley, C.A. Downs, A.W. Bruckner and J.W. Porter [eds.]. Diseases of Coral. John Wiley & Sons, Inc., Hoboken, New Jersey, Canada.

Akgün, H., A. Bilgin, Ü. Çalış, A. Balkan, S. Dalkara, D.D. Erol et al. 2013. *In*: A.A. Bilgin and C. Şafak [eds.]. Farmasötik Kimya. Hacettepe Üniversitesi Yayınları, Ankara, Turkey.

Akyön-Yılmaz, Y. 2012. Barsak protozoonlarina karşi kullanilan yeni ilaçlar. ANKEM Derg. 26: 116–120.

Anand, S. and S. Sharma. 1997. Approaches to Design and Synthesis of Antiparasitic Drugs. Elsevier Science, Amsterdam, The Netherlands.

Assimwe, F.T., U.R. Hengge, R. Mejia, S.K. Tyring, J. Machado-Pinto, L. Laborne et al. 2017. Other helminths. pp. 69–78. *In*: S.K. Tyring, O. Lupi and U.R. Hengge [eds.]. Tropical Dermatology. Elsevier, Beijing, China.

Ayi, B. 2007. Diseases caused by helminths (Worms). Ref. Mod. Biomed. Sci. doi.org/10.1016/B978-008055232-3.60936-5.

Balcıoğlu, İ.C., Ö. Kurt and A. Özbilgin. 2004. Antiparaziter ilaçlar. ANKEM Derg. 18(4): 237–244.

Bartram, D.J., D.M. Leathwick, M.A. Taylor, T. Geurdend and S.J. Maeder. 2012. The role of combination anthelmintic formulations in the sustainable control of sheep nematodes. Vet. Parasitol. 186: 151–158.

Berman, J.J. 2012. Taxonomic guide to infectious diseases. pp. 135–145. Elsevier, Chennai, India.

Beveridge, I. and M.K. Jones. 2002. Diversity and biogeographical relationships of the Australian cestode fauna. Int. J. Parasit. 32: 343–351.

Bruschi, F. and J. Dupouy-Camet. 2014. Trichinellosis. pp. 229–263. *In*: F. Bruschi [ed.]. Helminth Infections and their Impact on Global Public Health. Springer, New York, London.

Callaway, E. and D. Cyranoski. 2015. Anti-parasite drugs sweep Nobel prize in medicine 2015. Nature. 526: 174–175.

Campbell, W.C. and R.S. Rew. 1986. Chemotherapy of Parasitic Diseases. Plenum Press, New York, USA.

Conder, G.A. 2010. Anthelmintics. pp. 395–405. *In*: D. Greenwood, R.J. Whitley, R.G. Finch and S.R. Norrby [eds.]. Antibiotic and Chemotherapy (Ninth Edition), Elsevier Saunders, Edinburgh, Scotland.

da Paixão Siqueiraa, L., D.A.F. Fontes, C.S.B. Aguilera, T.R.R. Timoteo, M.A. Angelos, L.C.P.B.B. Silva et al. 2017. Schistosomiasis: Drugs used and treatment strategies. Acta Tropica. 176: 179–187.

da Silva, V.B.R., B.R.K.L. Campos, J.F. de Oliveira, J.L. Decout and M.C.A. de Lima. 2017. Medicinal chemistry of antischistosomal drugs: Praziquantel and oxamniquine. Bioor. Med. Chem. 25: 3259–3277.

de Oliveira, R.N. and R.A.W. Neves-Filho. 2014. Schistosomiasis. pp. 197–228. *In*: A. Beatriz and D.P. de Lima [eds.]. Recent Advances in the Synthesis of Organic Compounds to Combat Neglected Tropical Diseases. Bentham, Sharjah, U.A.E.

de Silva, N., H. Guyatt and D. Bundy. 1997. Anthelmintics. A comparative review of their clinical pharmacology. Drugs. 53: 769–88.

Debrah, A.Y., S. Mand, S. Specht, Y. Marfo-Debrekyei, L. Batsa, K. Pfarr et al. 2006. Doxycycline reduces plasma VEGF-C/sVEGFR-3 and improves pathology in lymphatic filariasis. PLoS Pathog. 2(9): e92.

Dupouy-Camet, J., P. Bouree and H. Year. 2017. Trichinella and polar bears: a limited risk for humans. J. Helmintol. 91: 440–446.

Dzhafarov, M.Kh. and F.I. Vasilevich. 2014. Ecological, physiological and biochemical adaptation in helminth: Trends in evolution of anthelminthic chemical agents. Adv. Pharmacol. and Pharm. 2: 30–45.

El-Beshbishi, S.N., A. Taman, M. El-Malky, M.S. Azab, A.K. El-Hawary and D.A. El-Tantawy. 2013. First insight into the effect of single oral dose therapy with artemisinin–naphthoquine phosphate combination in a mouse model of *Schistosoma mansoni* infection. Int. J. Parasitol. 43: 521–530.

Finch, R.G., D. Greenwood, R.J. Whitley and S. Ragnar Norrby. 2010. Antibiotic and Chemotherapy (Ninth Edition), Elsevier Saunders, Edinburgh, Scotland.

Flores-Ramos, M., F. Ibarra-Velarde, A. Hernández-Campos, Y. Vera-Montenegro, H. Jung-Cook, G.J. Cantó-Alarcón et al. 2014. A highly water soluble benzimidazole derivative useful for the treatment of fasciolosis. Bioorg. Med. Chem. Lett. 24: 5814–5817.

Frayha, G.J., J.D. Smyth, J.G. Gobert and J. Savel. 1997. The mechanisms of action of antiprotozoal and antihelminthic drugs in man. Gen. Pharmacol. 28: 273–299.

Galkinaa, I.V., D.R. Chubukaevaa, Y.V. Bakhtiyarovaa, V.I. Galkina, R.A. Cherkasova, D.R. Islamova et al. 2014. Modification of the anticestodal drug 5-chloro-N-(2-chloro-4-nitrophenyl)-2-hydroxybenzamide with a view to improve its biological effect. Russ. J. Org. Chem. 50: 800–804.

Gamble, H.R., R.H. Fetterer and J.F. Urban. 1995. Reproduction and in helminths development. pp. 289–305. *In*: J. Marr and M. Müller [eds.]. Biochemistry and Molecular Biology of Parasites. Academic Press, Beltsville, USA.

Garg, G. and S. Ranganathan. 2012. Helminth secretome database (HSD): a collection of helminth excretory/secretory proteins predicted from expressed sequence tags (ESTs). BMC Genomics. 13(Suppl 7): S8.

Geary, T.G., K. Woo, J.S. McCarthy, C.D. Mackenzie, J. Horton, R.K. Prichard et al. 2010. Unresolved issues in anthelmintic pharmacology for helminthiases of humans. Int. J. Parasitol. 40: 1–13.

Geary, T.G., J.A. Sakanari and C.R. Caffrey. 2015. Anthelmintic drug discovery: Into the future. J. Parasitol. 101(2): 125–133.

Geerts, S. 2015. Foodborne cestodes. pp. 201–216. *In*: A.A. Gajadhar [ed.]. Foodborne Parasites in the Food Supply Web. Elsevier, Cambridge, UK.

Guerrant, R.L., D.H. Walker and P.F. Weller. 2011. Tropical Infectious Diseases: Principles, Pathogens and Practice (Third Edition), Elsevier Saunders, Philadelphia, USA.

Haag, K.L., B. Gottstein and F.J. Ayala. 2008. Taeniid history, natural selection and antigenic diversity: evolutionary theory meets helminthology. Trends Parasitol. 24: 96–102.

Haque, A.K. 2013. Cestoda. pp 81–84. *In*: R. Barrios and A.K. Haque [eds.]. Parasitic Diseases of the Lungs. Springer-Verlag, Berlin, Germany.

Hewitson, J.P. and R.M. Maizels. 2014. Vaccination against helminth parasite infections. Expert. Rev. Vaccines. 13(4): 473–487.

Hoerauf, A., S. Specht, M. Büttner, K. Pfarr, S. Mand, R. Fimmers et al. 2008. Wolbachia endobacteria depletion by doxycycline as antifilarial therapy has macrofilaricidal activity in onchocerciasis: a randomized placebo-controlled study. Med. Microbiol. Immunol. 197: 295–311.

Holden-Dye, L. and R.J. Walker. 2007. Anthelmintic drugs. Wormbook. 1–13. https://www.nature.com/collections/xgntcpxznb.

Hu, Y., S.H. Xiao and R.V. Aroian. 2009. The new anthelmintic tribendimidine is an L-type (levamisole and pyrantel) nicotinic acetylcholine receptor agonist. PLoS. Negl.Trop. Dis. 3: e499.

Kalungi, S., L. Tumwine, W. Rehmus, J. Nguyen, F.T. Assımwe and U.R. Hengge. 2017. Nematodal helminths. pp. 56–68. *In*: S.K. Tyring, O. Lupi and U.R. Hengge [eds.]. Tropical Dermatology. Elsevier, Beijing, China.

Khan, M.R. 2015. Nematode diseases of crops in India. pp. 183–200. *In*: L.P. Awasthi [ed.]. Recent Advances in the Diagnosis and Management of Plant Diseases. Springer, West Bendal, India.

Kim, K., L.M. Weiss and H.B. Tanowitz. 2016. Parasitic infections. pp. 682–698. *In*: V.C. Broaddus, R.J. Mason, J.D. Ernst, T.E. King, S.C. Lazarus, J.F. Murray et al. [eds.]. Textbook of Respiratory Medicine. Murray & Nadel's. Elsevier, Philadelphia, Canada.

Korkmaz, M. 2012. Helmintlere karşi kullanilan yeni ilaçlar. ANKEM Derg. 26(Ek 2): 121–126.

Kotra, L.P. and P. Dixit. 2007. Cestode disease. pp. 1–4. Elsevier Inc. All rights reserved. University of Toronto, Toronto, Canada.

Köhler, P. 2001. The biochemical basis of anthelmintic action and resistance. Int. J. Parasitol. 31: 336–45.

Krolewiecki, A.J., P. Lammie, J. Jacobson, A.-F. Gabrielli, B. Levecke, E. Socias et al. 2013. A public health response against *Strongyloides stercoralis*: Time to look at soil-transmitted helminthiasis in full. PLoS Negl. Trop. Dis. 7: e2165.

Kuhlmann, F.M. and J.M. Fleckenstein. 2017. Antiparasitic agents. pp. 1345–1372. *In*: J. Cohen, W.G. Powderly and S.M. Opal [eds.]. Infectious Diseases (Fourth Edition), Elsevier, Amsterdam, The Netherlands.

Lecová, L., L. Stuchlíková, L. Prchal and L. Skálová. 2014. Monepantel: the most studied new anthelmintic drug of recent years. Parasitology. 141: 1686–1698.

Leutscher, P. and P. Magnussen. 2017. Trematodes. pp. 82–88. *In*: S.K. Tyring, O. Lupi and U.R. Hengge [eds.]. Tropical Dermatology. Elsevier, Beijing, China.

Lindquist, H.D.A. and J.H. Cross. 2017. Helminths. pp. 1763–1779. *In*: J. Cohen. W.G. Powderly and S.M. Opal [eds.]. Infectious Diseases. Elsevier, Amsterdam, Netherlands.

Liu, W.C., Y.Y. Wanga, J.H. Liu, A.B. Ke, Z.H. Zheng, X.H. Lu et al. 2016. Wortmannilactones I–L, new NADH-fumarate reductase inhibitors, induced by adding suberoylanilide hydroxamic acid to the culture medium of *Talaromyces wortmannii*. Bioorg. Med. Chem. Lett. 26: 5328–5333.

Machado-Pinto, J. and L. Laborne. 2006. Cestodes. pp 79–81. *In*: S.K. Tyring, O. Lupi and U.R. Hengge [eds.]. Tropical Dermatology. Elsevier, Beijing, China.

Martin, R.J., A.P. Robertson and H. Bjorn. 1997. Target sites of anthelmintics. Parasitology. 114: 111–124.

Mohammed, K.A., H.J. Haji, A.-F. Gabrielli, L. Mubila, G. Biswas, L. Chitsulo et al. 2008. Triple co-administration of ivermectin, albendazole and praziquantel in Zanzibar: a safety study. PLoS Negl. Trop. Dis. 2: e171.

Moore, L.S.P. and P.L. Chiodini. 2009. Tropical helminths. Medicine. 38: 47–51.

Moro, P. and P.M. Schantz. 2009. Echinococcosis: a review. Int. J. Infec. Dis. 13: 125–133.

Olliaro, P., J. Seiler, A. Kuesel, J. Horton, J.N. Clark, R. Don et al. 2011. Potential drug development candidates for human soil- transmitted helminthiases. PLoS Negl. Trop. Dis. 5: e1138.

Orefice, F., R.S. Fernandes and A.C. Delgado. 2016. Schistosomiasis. pp. 1367–1370. *In*: M. Zierhur, C. Pavesio, S. Ohno, F. Orefice and N.A. Rao. [eds.]. Intraocular Inflammation. Springer, Los Angeles, USA.

Ouattara, M., D. Sissouma, M.W. Kone, H.E. Menan, S.A. Toure and L. Ouattara. 2011. Synthesis and anthelmintic activity of some hybrid benzimidazolyl-chalcone derivatives. Trop. J. Pharm. Res. 6: 767–75.

Page, S.W. 2008. Antiparasitic drugs. pp. 198–260. *In*: J.E. Maddison, S.W. Page and D.B. Church [eds.]. Small Animal Clinical Pharmacology (Second Edition). Elsevier Saunders, Edinburgh, London.

Pérez, M.G., N. Macchiaroli, G. Lichtenstein, G. Conti, S. Asurmendi, D.H. Milone et al. 2017. microRNA analysis of *Taenia crassiceps cysticerci* under praziquantel treatment and genome-wide identification of *Taenia solium* miRNAs. International Journal for Parasitology. 47: 643–653.

Posey, D.L. and W. Stauffer. 2007. Schistosomiasis. pp. 499–508. Immigrant Medicine, Elsevier Inc, Philadelphia, USA.

Ramos, F., L.P. Portella, F. de, S. Rodrigues, C.Z. Reginato, L. Potter et al. 2016. Anthelmintic resistance in gastrointestinal nematodes of beef cattle in the state of Rio Grande do Sul, Brazil. Int. J. Parasitol. Drugs Drug Resist. 6: 93–101.

Rana, A.K. and S. Misra-Bhattacharya. 2013. Current drug targets for helminthic diseases. Parasitol. Res. 112: 1819–1831.

Reda, A.A. 2018. Probiotics for the control of helminth zoonosis. J. Am. Vet. Med. 2018: 1–9.

Romero-Benavides, J.C., A.L. Ruano, R. Silva-Rivas, P. Castillo-Veintimilla, S. Vivanco-Jaramillo and N. Bailon-Moscoso 2017. Medicinal plants used as anthelmintics: Ethnomedical, pharmacological, and phytochemical studies. Eur. J. Med. Chem. 129: 209–217.

Ross, A.G., P.B. Bartley, A.C. Sleigh, G.R. Olds, Y. Li, G.M. Williams et al. 2002. Schistosomiasis. N. Engl. J. Med. 346: 1212–1220.

Salem, H.H. and G. el-Allaf. 1969. Treatment of *Taenia saginata* and *Hymenolepis nana* infections with paromomycin. Trans. R. Soc. Trop. Med. Hyg. 63: 833–836.

Scoccia, J., M. Julia Castro, M.B. Faraoni, C. Bouzat, V.S. Martín and D.C. Gerbino. 2017. Iron(II) promoted direct synthesis of dibenzo[b,e]oxepin-11(6H)-one derivatives with biological activity. A short synthesis of doxepin. Tetrahedron. 73: 2913–2922.

Sen, N. 2017. Şistosomiyazis ve pulmoner hipertansiyon. Tuberk Toraks. 65: 237–244.

Shorr, R.I., A.B. Hoth and N. Rawls. 2007. Drugs for the Geriatric Patient. Saunders Elsevier, Philadelphia, USA.

Siqueira, L.D.P., D.A.F. Fontes, C.S.B. Aguilera, T.R.R. Timóteo, M.A. Ângelos, L.C.P.B.B. Silva et al. 2017. Schistosomiasis: Drugs used and treatment strategies. Acta Trop. 179–187.

Surikova, O.V., G. Mikhailovskii, B.Y. Syropyatov, A.S. Yusov and Y.D. Khudyakova. 2017. Synthesis, antihelminthic and insecticidal activity of 2-[3-methyl-6-methoxy-7-(N-propoxy)-3,4- dihydroisoquinolin-1]ethanoic acid amides. Pharmaceut. Chem. J. 51: 22–25.

Taman, A. and M. Azab. 2014. Present-day anthelmintics and perspectives on future new targets. Parasitol. Res. 113: 2425–2433.

Tappe, D., P. Kern, M. Frosch and P. Kern. 2010. A hundred years of controversy about the taxonomic status of Echinococcus species. Acta Tropica. 115: 167–174.

Thompson, D.P. and T.G. Geary. 2003. Helminth surfaces: structural, molecular and functional properties. pp. 297–338. *In*: J.J. Marr, T.W. Nilsen and R.W. Komuniecki [eds.]. Molecular Medical Parasitology. Elsevier.

Thompson, R.C.A. 2015. Neglected zoonotic helminths: Hymenolepis nana, Echinococcus canadensis and Ancylostoma ceylanicum. Clin. Microbiol. Infect. 21: 426–432.

van Genderen, P.J.J. 2005. Antihelminthic drugs. pp. 346–355. *In*: J.K. Aronson [ed.]. Side Effects of Drugs Annual Volume 28. Elsevier Science, Amsterdam, The Netherlands.

Vardanyan, R.S. and V.J. Hruby. 2006. Antihelmintic drugs. pp. 583–593. *In:* V.J. Hruby [ed.]. Synthesis of Essential Drugs. Elsevier, Amsterdam, The Netherlands.

Werren J.H., L. Baldo and M.E. Clark. 2008. Wolbachia: master manipulators of invertebrate biology. Nature rev./ Microbiol. 6: 741–751.

Wilson, C.M. 2012. Antiparasitic agents. pp. 1518–1545. *In*: S.S. Long, L.K. Pickering and C.G. Prober [eds.]. Principles and Practice of Pediatric Infectious Diseases (Fourth Edition). Elsevier Saunders, Edinburgh, Scotland.

Zarowiecki, M. and M. Berriman. 2015. What helminth genomes have taught us about parasite evolution. Parasitology. 142: 85–97.

Index

Color Plate Section

Chapter 2

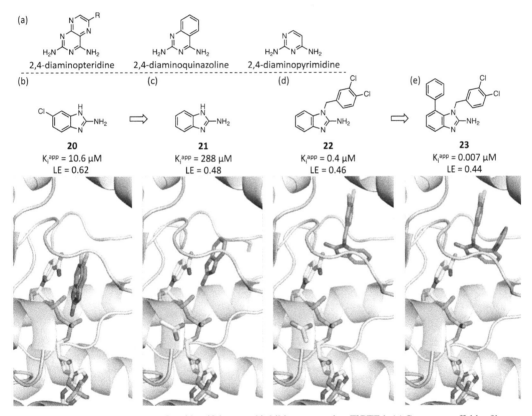

Figure 4. Fragment-based approach to identifying novel inhibitors targeting *Tb*PTR1. **(a)** Common scaffolds of known PTR1 and DHFR inhibitors. **(b)** Crystal structure showing binding of an aminobenzimidazole fragment hit (carbons in magenta) identified in a virtual fragment screen, to *Tb*PTR1 (with bound NADP⁺ cofactor, carbons in yellow) [PDB ID: 2WD7]. The fragment was observed to bind in two overlapping poses. **(c–e)** Crystal structures of analogues of fragment **20** in complex with *Tb*PTR1-NADP⁺ [PDB IDs: 3GN1, 3GN2, 2WD8]. An acetate molecule (carbons in grey) can be seen in the crystal structures shown in (c) and (d). LE = $(-RT\ln(K_i^{app}))/NHA$, in kcal.mol⁻¹.NHA⁻¹.

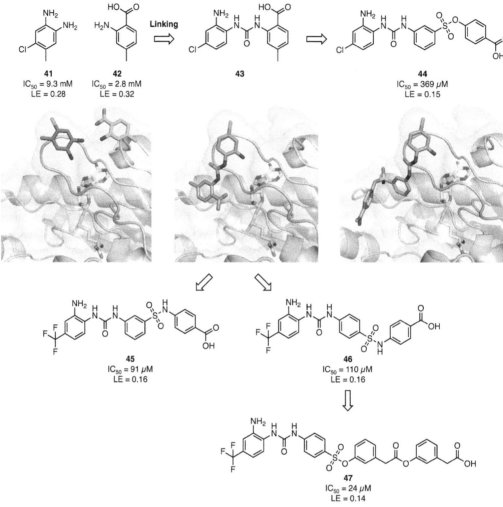

Figure 7. Fragment-based approach to targeting DENV MTase. Crystal structures showing binding of fragment hits **41** and **42** (carbons in magenta or cyan, respectively) and elaborated compounds **43** and **44** (carbons in orange) to DENV-3 MTase (with bound SAM, carbons in yellow) [PDB IDs: 5EKX, 5EIF, 5EC8 and 5EHG]. IC_{50} values measured in a 2'-*O*-MTase activity assay, and the corresponding LE values in kcal.mol^{-1}.NHA, are shown.

Chapter 3

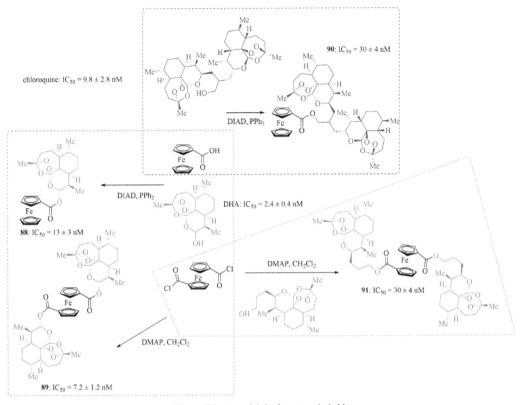

Figure 24. Artemisinin-ferrocene hybrids.

Chapter 4

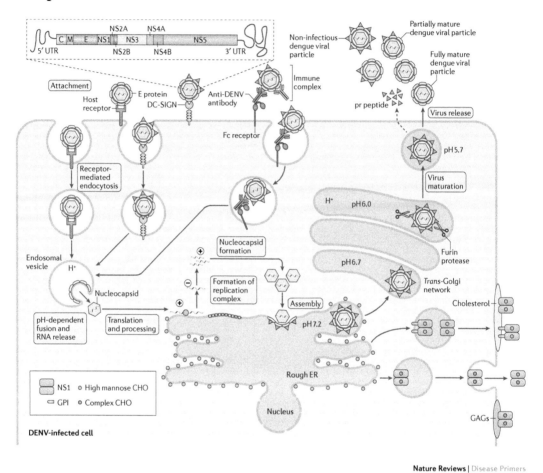

Figure 1. DENV lifecycle (printed with permission from Nature publishers, Guzman et al. 2016).

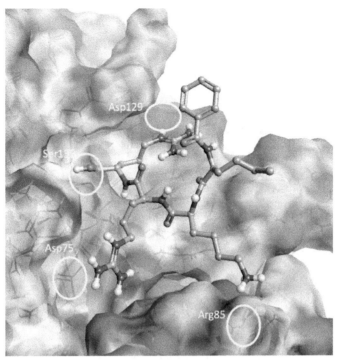

Figure 4. Tetrapeptide inhibitor shown as a ball and stick figure (Bz-*N*-Leu-Lys-Arg-Arg-H) covalently bound to the shallow and open binding pocket of DENV3 protease (3U1I). Key interactions are shown in yellow including the covalent link via the side chain of serine₁₃₅. The molecular surface is coloured by atom type; nitrogen in blue, oxygen in red and carbon in grey (Nitsche et al. 2014 and references therein).

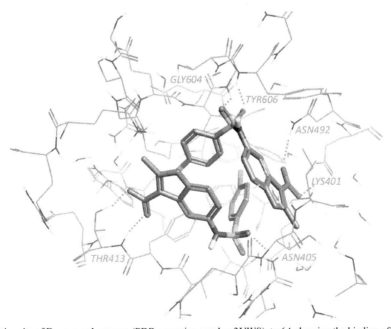

Figure 6a. Active site of Dengue polymerase (PDB accession number 3VWS) to 6A showing the binding of two molecules of Benzofuran **6-4**. Key hydrogen bond interactions are shown in green dotted lines and the relevant amino acids are labelled in green. The figure was generated using Flare™, Cressett Group UK.

Table 1. DENV Genome (Adapted from Guzman et al. 2016 and Dung et al. 2014).

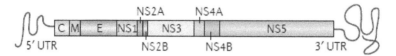

Name	Size (kDa)	Length (aa)	Key features	Functions
C		114	Highly basic. Contains bipartite nuclear location sequence that targets the protein to the nucleus. Binds RNA genome.	Nucleocapsid protein
M		166	Cleaved by furin in the Golgi to form mature membrane protein prior to virus release. Membrane remains associated with viron until virus leaves the cell by exocytosis.	Glycoprotein which protects envelope glycoprotein from low pH induced rearrangement and premature fusion during intracellular life cycle of the virus.
E		495	Dimerises with membrane protein in the immature virus or with second envelope molecule in the mature virus.	Envelope glycoprotein required for receptor-mediated endocytosis, antibody function and membrane fusion.
NS1	46	352	Can be endoplasmic reticulum-anchored, membrane associated or secreted (sNS1). Multiple oligomeric states, glycosylated secreted as hexamer.	Intracellular NS1 is involved in early viral RNA replication. sNS1 activates the innate immune system and is implicated in vascular cleavage.
NS2A	22	218	Hydrophobic integral membrane protein which forms part of the replication complex.	Involved in RNA replication and possible regulator of NS1 function.
NS2B	14	130	Small hydrophobic protein which forms part of the active site binding pocket of NS3.	Co-factor for NS3 protease. Mediates membrane association.
NS3	69	618	Multifunctional protein with several catalytic domains. Highly conserved and interacts with NS5. Involved in virus assembly and also interacts with NS4B.	Involved in nucleoside triphosphatase and helicase functions during RNA synthesis.
NS4A	16	150	Hydrophobic integral membrane protein binding to non-structural proteins in replication process.	Required for the formation of replication vesicles and postulated to play a role in protein targeting and anchoring.
NS4B	30	248	Small hydrophobic membrane protein like NS4A.	Supresses Interferon β and γ cytokine signalling
NS5	105	900	Largest and most highly conserved DENV protein which contains nuclear location sequence as both nuclear and cytoplasmic forms.	Involved in RNA synthesis and blockade of the Interferon system. The C-terminal RNA-dependent RNA polymerase is the viral replicase.

Chapter 5

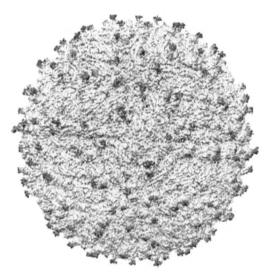

Figure 1. Overall structure of ZIKV (Sirohi et al. 2016).

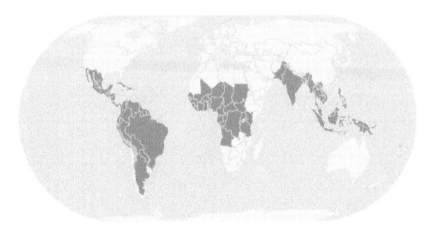

Area with risk of ZIKV infection
Area with low likelihood of ZIKV infection
Area with no known risk of ZIKV infection

Figure 2. World map of area with risk of ZIKV, according to the Centers for Disease Control and Prevention Centers for Disease Control and Prevention (CDC), 2018.

Chapter 6

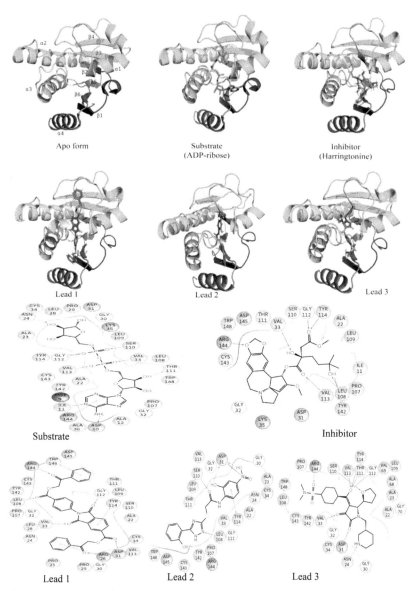

Figure 6. Binding mode and binding interactions of substrate (ADP ribose), inhibitor (harringtonine) and top identified lead compounds.

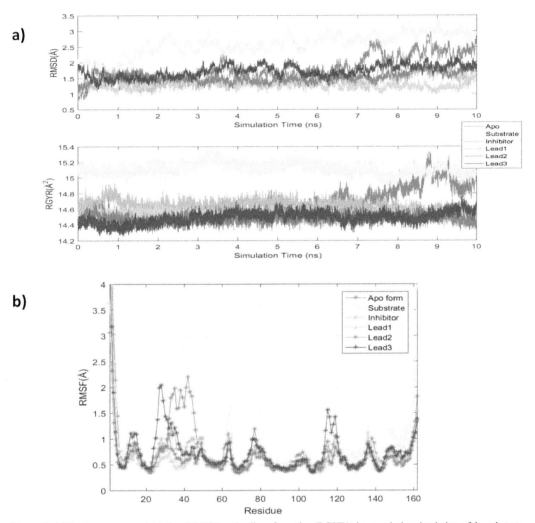

Figure 7. (a) Root mean square deviation (RMSD) and radius of gyration (RGYR) changes during simulation of the substrate (ADP ribose), inhibitor (harringtonine) and top identified lead compounds. (b) Root mean square fluctuation (RMSF) in residues wise of the substrate (ADP ribose), inhibitor (harringtonine) and top identified lead compounds.

Chapter 9

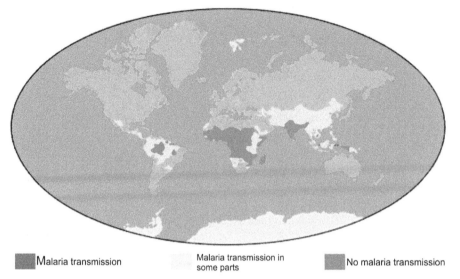

Malaria transmission   Malaria transmission in
                                some parts   No malaria transmission

Figure 1. Populations at risk of malaria. Source: Centers for Disease Control and prevention (CDC)—https://www.cdc.gov/malaria/about/distribution.html. Used with permission.

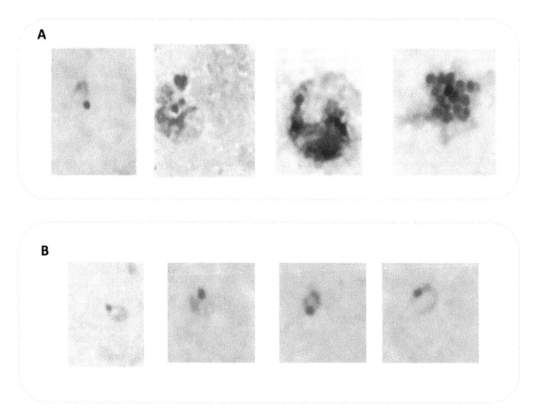

Figure 2. *P. vivax* (A) and *P. falciparum* (B) forms found on thick slides.

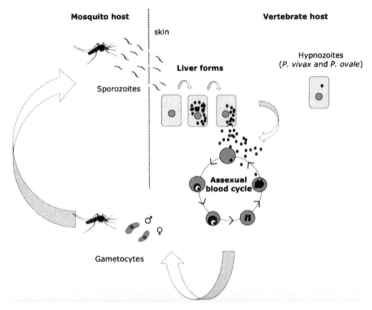

Figure 3. *Plasmodium* spp. life cycle.

Chapter 10

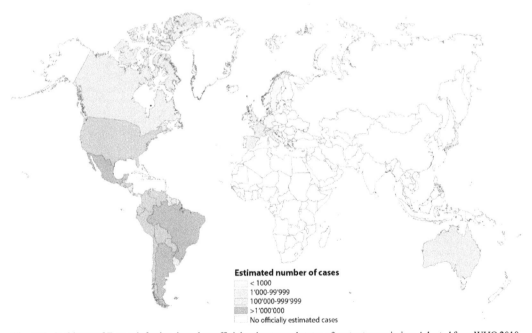

Figure 1. Incidence of *T. cruzi* infection, based on official estimates and status of vector transmission. Adapted from WHO 2010.

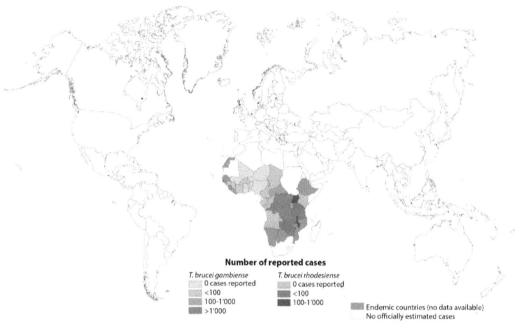

Figure 3. Distribution of Human African Trypanosomiasis (*T. b. gambiense* in green and *T. b. rhodesiense* in blue) worldwide. Adapted from WHO 2017.

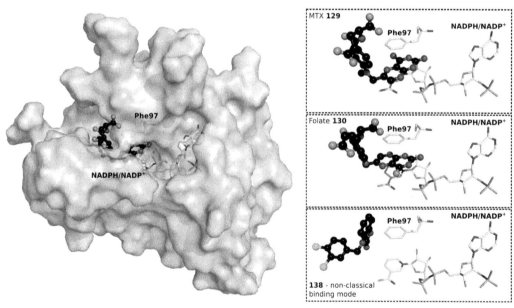

Figure 46. Illustration of compounds binding in the π-sandwich between Phe97 and the nicotinamide of the NADPH/NADP⁺ cofactor of TbPTR1 or in alternative modes adjacent to the active site. On the left, a monomer of the homotetrameric enzyme is shown as a semi-transparent surface representation with bound MTX **129** in dark ball-and-stick representation, and the cofactor and Phe97 in white sticks. In the right-hand panel, the same representation is used, omitting the protein apart from Phe 97. The complex with MTX **129** is based on PDB-ID 2c7v (Dawson et al. 2006), with folate **130**—on PDB-ID 3bmc (Tulloch et al. 2010) and with **138**, illustrating the non-classical binding mode outside the π-sandwich—on PDB-ID 3gn2 (Mpamhanga et al. 2009).

Chapter 11

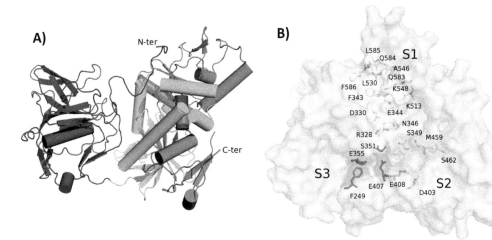

Figure 2. (A). TSA (TryS) overall fold. The amidase domain is colored blue (residues 1-215; 634-652). The synthetase domain is composed by three subdomains: A, residues 216-393 and 595-633, colored in green; B, residues 394-511, colored in magenta; C, residues 512-595, colored in red. (**B). The synthetase active site.** The protein surface is depicted as a *gray* semi-transparent van der Waals surface, except for ATP binding site (*yellow*) (S1), GSH binding site (*cyan*) (S2), spermidine binding site (magenta) (S3). The residues lining the three binding sites are indicated and depicted as sticks.

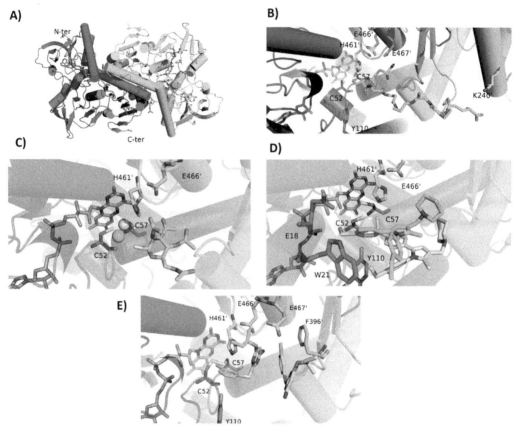

Figure 4. (A). TR overall fold (PDB code 4ADW). The two TR monomers are colored cyan and violet. The NADPH, FAD and trypanothione molecules are depicted as sticks. **(B).** Blow-up of TR-trypanothione complex catalytic cavity. The trypanothione molecule is depicted as sticks and colored green. The residues interacting with trypanothione are depicted as sticks. **(C).** Blow-up of the Auranofin-TR complex catalytic cavity (PDB code 2YAU). The 3,4,5-triacetyloxy-6-(acetyloxymethyl)oxane-2-thiol moiety is depicted as sticks and colored green, the gold ion is depicted as sphere and colored yellow, the chloride ion is depicted as sphere and colored green. The residues interacting with trypanothione are depicted as sticks. **(D).** Blow-up of the compound1-TR complex catalytic cavity (PDB code 4APN). The two compound 1 molecules present in the cavity are colored in green and lime green. All the residues interacting with the compound 1 molecules as well as the residues important for catalysis are indicated and depicted as sticks. **(E)** Blow-up of the RDS 777-TR complex catalytic cavity (PDB code 5EBK). The two RDS 777 molecules present in the cavity of TR monomer 1 are colored in green and lime green. All the residues interacting with the RDS 777 molecules as well as the residues important for catalysis are indicated and depicted as sticks.

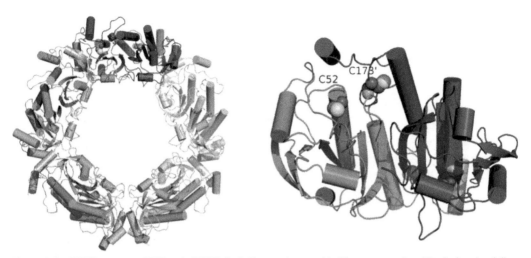

Figure 6. LmTXNPx structure (PDB code 3TUE). **Left:** Decameric assembly. The monomer A and B of a functional dimer are colored clear gray and dark gray, respectively. The two catalytic cysteines are represented as spheres. **Right:** Functional dimer. The two monomers A and B are colored clear grey and dark grey, respectively. The two catalytic cysteines are represented as spheres.

Chapter 14

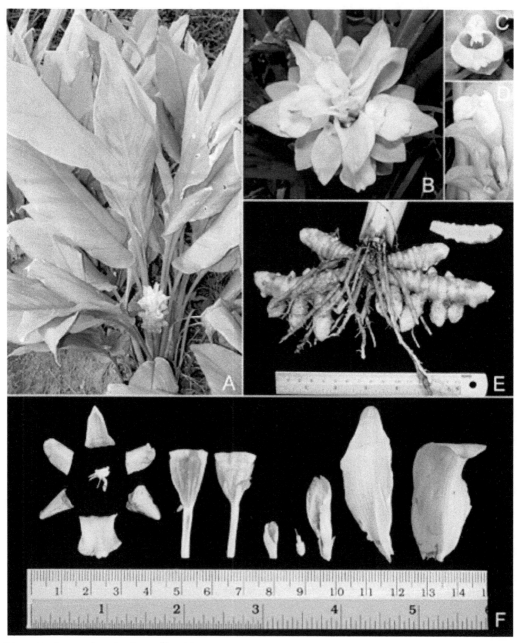

Figure 1. *Curcuma longa* L. (Leong-Škorničková et al. 2008): (A) plant habit; (B) inflorescence; (C) flower in fertile bract (front view); (D) flower in fertile bract (side view); (E) rhizome; (F) flower dissection.

Milton Keynes UK
Ingram Content Group UK Ltd.
UKHW032233151223
434481UK00022B/555